The Causes and Treatment of Arthritis

The Causes and Treatment of Arthritis

Editor: Sharlton Pierce

AMERICAN
MEDICAL PUBLISHERS
www.americanmedicalpublishers.com

AMERICAN
MEDICAL PUBLISHERS
www.americanmedicalpublishers.com

Cataloging-in-Publication Data

The causes and treatment of arthritis / edited by Sharlton Pierce.
p. cm.
Includes bibliographical references and index.
ISBN 978-1-63927-403-1
1. Arthritis. 2. Arthritis--Treatment. 3. Arthritis--Diagnosis. I. Pierce, Sharlton.
RC933 .A683 2022
616.72--dc23

American Medical Publishers,
41 Flatbush Avenue,
1st Floor, New York,
NY 11217, USA

ISBN 978-1-63927-403-1 (Hardback)

Contents

Preface

I am honored to present to you this unique book which encompasses the most up-to-date data in the field. I was extremely pleased to get this opportunity of editing the work of experts from across the globe. I have also written papers in this field and researched the various aspects revolving around the progress of the discipline. I have tried to unify my knowledge along with that of stalwarts from every corner of the world, to produce a text which not only benefits the readers but also facilitates the growth of the field.

Any disorder that affects the joints can be termed as arthritis. Joint pain and stiffness are its key characteristics. Some other symptoms may also occur, such as warmth, swelling, redness and decreased range of motion around the affected joints. The onset of arthritis can be sudden or gradual. Osteoarthritis, ankylosing spondylitis, rheumatoid arthritis, juvenile idiopathic arthritis, septic arthritis, gout and pseudo-gout are some of the different forms of the disease. The diagnosis of arthritis is based on a physical examination, blood tests and radiology. There is no cure for rheumatoid arthritis or osteoarthritis. The mode of treatment recommended varies according to the form of arthritis and may include orthopedic bracing, physical therapy, lifestyle changes and in certain cases, joint replacement surgery. Research in arthritis seeks alternative approaches to the management of the condition, such as transcutaneous electrical nerve stimulation, low level laser therapy and pulsed electromagnetic field therapy. The topics included in this book on arthritis are of utmost significance and bound to provide incredible insights to readers. It presents researches and studies performed by experts across the globe on the pathophysiology and management of arthritis. This book will prove to be immensely beneficial to students and researchers involved in the study of arthritis.

Finally, I would like to thank all the contributing authors for their valuable time and contributions. This book would not have been possible without their efforts. I would also like to thank my friends and family for their constant support.

Editor

1

Prevalence of methotrexate intolerance in rheumatoid arthritis and psoriatic arthritis

Maja Bulatović Ćalasan[1*], Oscar FC van den Bosch[1], Marjonne CW Creemers[2], Martijn Custers[3], Antonius HM Heurkens[4], Jan Maarten van Woerkom[5] and Nico M Wulffraat[1]

Abstract

Introduction: The aim of this study was to determine the prevalence of gastrointestinal and behavioural symptoms occurring before (anticipatory/associative) and after methotrexate (MTX) administration, termed MTX intolerance, in rheumatoid (RA) and psoriatic arthritis (PsA).

Methods: Methotrexate Intolerance Severity Score (MISS), previously validated in juvenile idiopathic arthritis patients, was used to determine MTX intolerance prevalence in 291 RA/PsA patients. The MISS consisted of four domains: abdominal pain, nausea, vomiting and behavioural symptoms, occurring upon, prior to (anticipatory) and when thinking of MTX (associative). MTX intolerance was defined as ≥6 on the MISS with ≥1 point on anticipatory and/or associative and/or behavioural items.

Results: A total of 123 patients (42.3%) experienced at least one gastrointestinal adverse effect. The prevalence of MTX intolerance was 11%. MTX intolerance prevalence was higher in patients on parenteral (20.6%) than on oral MTX (6.2%) ($p < 0.001$).

Conclusion: Besides well-known gastrointestinal symptoms after MTX, RA and PsA patients experienced these symptoms also before MTX intake. RA and PsA patients on MTX should be closely monitored with the MISS for early detection of MTX intolerance, in order to intervene timely and avoid discontinuation of an effective treatment.

Introduction

Rheumatoid arthritis (RA) and psoriatic arthritis (PsA) are inflammatory disorders characterized by chronic arthritis [1,2]. In RA and PsA treatment, methotrexate (MTX) is the first-choice disease-modifying anti-rheumatic drug (DMARD) due to low costs, efficacy and an acceptable safety profile [3,4]. Serious adverse effects such as pulmonary toxicity, hepatotoxicity and bone marrow suppression are rare or transient if MTX is stopped [5]. In contrast, gastrointestinal adverse effects are common, affecting as many as 66% of patients [2,6-11]. Due to these adverse effects, up to 12% of RA and PsA patients discontinue MTX after 6 months to 2 years of treatment [6-8,12].

Previously, we showed in juvenile idiopathic arthritis (JIA) that 50.5% of patients suffered not only from a myriad of gastrointestinal adverse effects after MTX intake, but also from adverse effects before MTX intake (anticipatory) and when thinking of MTX (associative) [13]. The latter symptoms arise as a classical conditioning response to gastrointestinal symptoms after MTX administration. Therefore, the nature of MTX-induced gastrointestinal adverse effects, which we termed MTX intolerance, is complex, and could even further impede the use of an otherwise effective drug. Although MTX-induced gastrointestinal adverse effects occur frequently in RA and PsA, severity and the type - in particular the occurrence of anticipatory and associative symptoms - have not been assessed.

The aim of this study was to determine the type and prevalence of MTX-induced gastrointestinal adverse effects, with a standardized questionnaire, in a large cohort of RA and PsA patients.

Methods

Study design and patients

A cross-sectional descriptive study (ISRCTN13524271) included RA and PsA patients attending the outpatient wards of four general hospitals between May 2011 and

* Correspondence: m.bulatovic@umcutrecht.nl
[1]Department of Pediatric Immunology, Room KC 03.063.0, University Medical Center, Wilhelmina Children's Hospital, Utrecht 3508 AB, The Netherlands
Full list of author information is available at the end of the article

June 2012. All patients were treated with MTX for at least 3 months and received weekly folic acid (5 to 15 mg) [5]. Patients' data on disease activity, MTX dose and route of administration, co-medication, history of peptic ulcers and smoking was collected. The study was approved by the medical ethics committees of the University Medical Center Utrecht and the four general hospitals in 's-Hertogenbosch, Woerden, Amersfoort and Apeldoorn where the patients were included. As the study burden for patients was low and required no treatment changes, the ethics committees waived the need for informed consent.

MTX intolerance severity score

To determine the prevalence of MTX-induced gastrointestinal adverse effects, patients completed the methotrexate intolerance severity score (MISS), previously developed and validated in JIA [13]. The MISS consists of four domains: abdominal pain, nausea, vomiting and behavioural symptoms, assessing symptoms after MTX administration, anticipatory (before MTX) and associative symptoms (when thinking of MTX). The behavioural symptoms domain includes restlessness, irritability and refusal of MTX, which develop in response to MTX-induced gastrointestinal symptoms and anticipation thereof. A patient could score 0 (no symptoms), 1 (mild symptoms), 2 (moderate symptoms) or 3 (severe symptoms) points on each item. MTX intolerance was defined as ≥6 points, including at least one anticipatory, associative or behavioural symptom [13].

MTX intolerance prevalence

The prevalence was determined of: a) individual symptoms in all patients; b) MTX intolerance, defined as above; c) individual symptoms in MTX intolerant versus tolerant patients. MTX intolerance prevalence was compared between patients on oral and parenteral MTX (chi-square test). MTX intolerance severity, age, MTX dose, disease activity parameters and medication use were compared in tolerant versus intolerant patients, and in intolerant patients on oral versus parenteral MTX (*t*-test, Mann–Whitney *U*-test). To evaluate associations of MTX intolerance with clinically relevant covariates - disease activity score (DAS)-28, physician global assessment (PGA), age, MTX dose, MTX route and non-steroidal anti-inflammatory drug (NSAID) use - multivariate logistic regression was performed. Statistical analyses were carried out with IBM SPSS Statistics, version 20.

Results

Baseline characteristics

Of 296 patients, 5 were excluded due to diagnosis other than RA or PsA (n = 3 with ankylosing spondylitis; n = 1 with peripheral spondyloarthritis; and n = 1 with scleroderma). Table 1 shows the baseline characteristics of 291 patients; the majority was female (62.2%), 249 (85.6%) had RA and 42 (14.4%) had PsA with low to moderate DAS-28.

Table 1 Baseline characteristics of 291 patients at the time of completing the MISS

Characteristic	Value in patient sample
Sex, female	181 (62.2)
Age, mean +/− SD years	59.4 +/− 12.4
Diagnosis	
Rheumatoid arthritis	249 (85.6)
Psoriatic arthritis	42 (14.4)
Disease activity	
Disease activity score 28, median (IQR)[a]	2.5 (1.7 to 3.2)
Physician's global assessment, median (IQR), (0 to 10 scale)[b]	2.0 (1.0 to 3.0)
Erythrocyte sedimentation rate (mm/hour)	11.0 (5.0 to 22.0)
MTX use	
Route of administration, oral	194 (66.7)
Dose, mg/week, median (IQR)	20.0 (12.5 to 25.0)
Other medication	
NSAIDs	145 (49.9)
Proton-pump inhibitors	127 (43.6)
Anti-emetics	5 (1.7)
Oral steroids	31 (10.7)
Other DMARDs[c]	72 (24.7)

Characteristics are as calculated at the time of completing the MISS except where indicated otherwise. Values are number (%), except where indicated otherwise. [a]Disease activity score 28 was determined in 266 patients (274 rheumatoid arthritis and 19 psoriatic arthritis patients); [b]physician's global assessment was determined in 268 patients; [c]of 72 patients on other DMARDs, 26 were on DMARDs (plaquenil, n = 24; leflunomide, n = 2) and 46 were on biologic agents (infliximab, n = 24; adalimumab, n = 10; etanercept, n = 9; abatecept, n = 2; golimumab, n = 1). MISS, methotrexate intolerance severity score; MTX, methotrexate; NSAIDs, nonsteroidal anti-inflammatory drugs; DMARDs, disease-modifying anti-rheumatic drugs.

MTX intolerance prevalence in RA and PsA

One hundred and twenty-three (42.3%) RA and PsA patients experienced at least one gastrointestinal symptom during MTX treatment. The most prevalent gastrointestinal symptom after MTX administration was nausea, affecting 93 (32.0%) patients, whereas abdominal pain occurred in 11.3% and vomiting in 6.5% (Table 2). Pre-treatment nausea was the most prevalent; 8.6% had anticipatory and 11.0% associative nausea. Anticipatory vomiting was the least prevalent, affecting 1.7% (Table 2). Behavioural symptoms, overall, affected 16.5% of patients, with restlessness being the most prominent symptom in 13.1% of patients (Table 2).

Table 2 Prevalence of MTX-related gastrointestinal symptoms in all patients and in intolerant patients by route of MTX administration

	All patients	Tolerant to MTX	Intolerant to MTX	Oral MTX	Parenteral MTX
Total	291 (100)	259 (89.0)	32 (11.0)	194 (66.7)	97 (33.3)
Cutoff score ≥6	32 (11.0)	0 (0)	32 (100)	12 (6.2)	20 (20.6)[a]
Abdominal pain	44 (15.1)	24 (9.3)	20 (62.5)	7 (58.3)	13 (65.0)
After MTX	33 (11.3)	18 (6.9)	15 (46.9)	5 (41.7)	10 (50.0)
Anticipatory	17 (5.8)	5 (1.9)	12 (37.5)	5 (41.7)	7 (35.0)
Associative	17 (5.8)	6 (2.3)	11 (34.4)	4 (33.3)	7 (35.0)
Nausea	100 (34.4)	68 (26.3)	32 (100)	12 (100)	20 (100)
After MTX	93 (32.0)	61 (23.6)	32 (100)	12 (100)	20 (100)
Anticipatory	25 (8.6)	7 (2.7)	18 (56.3)	6 (50.0)	12 (60.0)
Associative	32 (11.0)	15 (5.8)	17 (53.1)	5 (41.7)	12 (60.0)
Vomiting	22 (7.6)	11 (4.2)	11 (34.4)	5 (41.7)	6 (30.0)
After MTX	19 (6.5)	9 (3.5)	10 (31.3)	5 (41.7)	5 (25.0)
Anticipatory	5 (1.7)	0 (0)	5 (15.6)	2 (16.7)	3 (15.0)
Behavioural symptoms	48 (16.5)	22 (8.5)	26 (81.3)	7 (58.3)	19 (95.0)[b]
Restlessness	38 (13.1)	16 (6.2)	22 (68.8)	6 (50.0)	16 (80)
Irritability	29 (10.0)	7 (2.7)	22 (68.8)	5 (41.7)	17 (85.0)[c]
Refusal of MTX	13 (4.5)	1 (0.4)	12 (37.5)	2 (16.7)	10 (50.0)

Values are number (%) of patients. All domains and individual items differentiate between tolerant and intolerant patients ($P < 0.001$). [a]$P < 0.001$ versus oral MTX, by chi-square test; [b]$P = 0.02$ versus oral MTX, by chi-square test, [c]$P = 0.02$ versus oral MTX, by chi-square test. MTX, methotrexate.

MTX intolerance was found in 32 (11.0%) patients having a median score of 9 (IQR: 6.25 to 12.00). The prevalence and severity of MTX intolerance was similar in RA (n = 26 (10.4%), score 9 (6.8 to 12.3)) and PsA (n = 6 (14.3%), score 7 (6.0 to 13.0)). All intolerant patients (100%) experienced post-treatment nausea, whereas 46.9% had post-treatment abdominal pain and 31.3% had post-treatment vomiting (Table 2). The most prevalent pre-treatment gastrointestinal symptoms were anticipatory and associative nausea, affecting 56.3% and 53.1% of intolerant patients respectively, followed by anticipatory abdominal pain in 37.5% and associative abdominal pain in 34.4%. Anticipatory vomiting occurred in 15.6% of intolerant patients, whereas this symptom did not occur in tolerant patients. Overall, behavioural symptoms occurred in 81.3% of intolerant patients, of whom 37.5% refused MTX.

MTX-intolerant patients were younger than the MTX-tolerant (mean age 51.6 +/− 12.2 versus 60.4 +/− 12.1 years, $P < 0.001$). MTX dose, DAS-28, PGA, erythrocyte sedimentation rate (ESR), co-medication use, history of peptic ulcers (3.8% of all patients) and smoking (25.8% of all patients) did not differ between the two groups. Gender distribution did not differ between MTX-intolerant and MTX-tolerant patients (female, 75.0% versus 60.6%; male, 25.0% versus 39.4%), but more female (75%) than male patients (25%) were intolerant, although this was not statistically significant.

MTX intolerance prevalence in patients on oral and parenteral MTX

MTX intolerance prevalence was significantly higher in patients on parenteral (20 of 97, 20.6%) than on oral MTX (12 of 194 m 6.2%, $P < 0.001$) (Table 2). Significantly more patients on parenteral than on oral MTX exhibited behavioural symptoms ($P = 0.02$), whereas other symptoms were comparable between the two groups. The median MTX intolerance score was higher in intolerant patients on parenteral than on oral MTX, although not significantly (9.5, IQR 7.0 to 15.5) versus 7.5, IQR 6.0 to 9.0), $P = 0.08$). Patients on parenteral MTX received the same MTX dose (20.0 mg/week, IQR 15.0 to 25.0) as patients on oral MTX (20.0 mg/week, IQR 15.0 to 20.0).

In the multivariate analysis, older patients were less likely to have MTX intolerance (odds ratio (OR) 0.93, 95% m, CI 0.89, 0.97; $P = 0.001$). If age was stratified into two groups, namely ≥65 and <65 years, older patients were again less likely to have MTX intolerance (OR 0.21, 95% CI 0.06, 0.85; $P = 0.03$) whereas patients with higher PGA (OR 1.26, 95% CI 1.05, 1.51; $P = 0.01$) and those receiving parenteral MTX (OR 3.88, 95% CI 1.41, 10.62; $P = 0.01$) were more likely to have MTX intolerance.

Discussion

We showed that besides the well-known MTX-induced gastrointestinal symptoms upon MTX administration, RA and PsA patients also had anticipatory and associative gastrointestinal and behavioural symptoms before MTX administration, collectively termed MTX intolerance. MTX intolerance prevalence in RA and PsA patients was 11%.

Studies in RA have found similar occurrence rates compared to our study [7,11]; nausea was the most prevalent symptom, occurring in 14.4 to 28.0% compared to 32.0% in our cohort, followed by abdominal pain in 9.7 to 10.6% compared to 11.3% in our cohort and vomiting in 3.4% compared to 6.5% in our cohort. Of note is that comparisons were made between symptoms occurring only after MTX, as it is likely that previous studies took solely these symptoms into account (not the pre-treatment symptoms).

In contrast to JIA in which the prevalence of MTX intolerance reached 50.5%, the prevalence in RA/PsA was considerably lower at 11%. MTX intolerance severity was lower in adults (score 9) than in children (score 12) (P = 0.003). Substantially lower MTX intolerance prevalence in RA/PsA was due to: a) lower percentage of adults with score ≥6, and b) lower percentage of adults (24.4% versus 67% in JIA) with at least one anticipatory, associative and/or behavioural symptoms. As anticipatory and associative symptoms arise as classic conditioning responses to physical symptoms upon MTX use, the lower percentage of RA/PsA patients with pre-treatment symptoms suggests a weaker, classic, conditioning response in adults than in children taking MTX. This is supported by the fact that, whereas 82% of 204 JIA patients with symptoms after MTX also had symptoms before MTX intake, only 51% of 106 RA/PsA patients with symptoms after MTX had symptoms before MTX intake.

MTX intolerance prevalence was higher in patients on parenteral (20.8%) than on oral MTX (6.2%), which we also demonstrated for JIA [13,14]. This difference was caused by more behavioural symptoms in the parenteral group. Aversion towards needles, besides aversion towards MTX, could have contributed to a higher prevalence of these symptoms. It is common to switch patients from oral to parenteral MTX due to gastrointestinal symptoms [5]. Indeed, 13 of 20 intolerant patients on parental MTX had been switched to this route from oral MTX due to gastrointestinal symptoms. Considering their past symptoms on oral MTX, the patients who switched may have been more prone to develop gastrointestinal and behavioural symptoms on parenteral MTX, resulting in higher MTX intolerance prevalence in the parenteral group.

Besides the observed association between parenteral MTX and MTX intolerance, age was also associated with MTX intolerance, namely older patients (>65 years) were less likely to have MTX intolerance than younger patients (≤65 years). In previous studies, neither younger nor older age (>65 years) was associated with occurrence of MTX-related gastrointestinal and other side effects [15,16]. Validation studies are required to determine whether younger age is a risk factor for MTX intolerance.

Anticipatory and associative gastrointestinal symptoms could have a negative impact on patients' quality of life [14] and impede the use of MTX. Nevertheless, these symptoms are clinically not very evident [13]. Consequently, they cannot be easily detected by physician assessment only, but can be detected using the MISS [13]. Therefore, using the MISS is advantageous as it allows early detection of symptoms. This could create a window of opportunity for timely treatment of MTX intolerance, as well as for early treatment of emerging physical symptoms, which could prevent the development of conditioned responses and therefore MTX intolerance. Similar to JIA, treatment of (physical) symptoms could include lowering the MTX dose [17], switching to parenteral MTX [14,18,19] or starting behavioural therapy [20] or anti-emetics [19].

Although the MISS was validated and employed to measure MTX intolerance prevalence in JIA, it provided a structured platform to assess the type of MTX-induced gastrointestinal symptoms in RA/PsA. Nevertheless, the MISS should be validated in adults with rheumatic diseases. Furthermore, this study does not reveal variables associated with MTX intolerance development, nor does it demonstrate the frequency of MTX discontinuation or of switching to other medication due to MTX intolerance. Prospective trials are required to address these issues.

This is the first study to demonstrate using a standardized questionnaire, that MTX intolerance occurs in 11%, more frequently in patients on parenteral than on oral MTX, and possibly persists after a switch from oral to parenteral MTX. Since persistent gastrointestinal symptoms are the major reason to discontinue MTX, intolerant patients could be more prone to stop MTX or switch to (less effective) DMARDs or expensive biological agents [12]. Upon validation in adults, the MISS may be used in daily clinical practice to closely monitor patients and to intervene timely using the abovementioned approaches in order to prevent or reduce the negative impact of MTX intolerance on patients' daily lives, compliance and continuation of an effective treatment.

Conclusions

Using a standardized MISS questionnaire, we showed that besides the well-known MTX-induced gastrointestinal symptoms upon MTX administration, RA and PsA patients also experienced anticipatory and associative gastrointestinal and behavioural symptoms before MTX administration, which develop as a classical conditioning response to physical symptoms after MTX. The prevalence of MTX intolerance was 11%. MTX intolerance occurred more often in patients on parenteral (20.6%) than in those on oral MTX (6.2%) and persisted after a switch from oral to parenteral MTX. As persisting MTX intolerance could have a negative impact on patients' quality of life and hamper the use of MTX, RA and PsA patients on MTX should be monitored with the MISS for early detection of MTX intolerance. This would create a window of opportunity to intervene timely and avoid incompliance and discontinuation of an otherwise efficacious treatment.

Abbreviations
DAS: Disease activity score; DMARD: Disease-modifying anti-rheumatic drug; ESR: Erythrocyte sedimentation rate; JIA: Juvenile idiopathic arthritis; MISS: Methotrexate intolerance severity score; MTX: Methotrexate; NSAID: Non-steroidal anti-inflammatory drug; OR: Odds ratio; PGA: Physician global assessment; PsA: Psoriatic arthritis; RA: Rheumatoid arthritis.

Competing interests
The authors declare that they have no competing interests.

Authors' contributions
MBĆ: substantial contribution to conception and design, acquisition of data, analysis and interpretation of data; involved in drafting the manuscript and revising it critically for important intellectual content; final approval of the version to be published. OvdB: substantial contribution to acquisition of data, analysis and interpretation of data; involved in drafting the manuscript; final approval of the version to be published. MCr: substantial contribution to acquisition of data; involved in revising the manuscript critically for important intellectual content; final approval of the version to be published. MCu: substantial contribution to acquisition of data; involved in revising the manuscript critically for important intellectual content; final approval of the version to be published. AH: substantial contribution to acquisition of data; involved in revising the manuscript critically for important intellectual content; final approval of the version to be published. JMvW: substantial contribution to acquisition of data; involved in revising the manuscript critically for important intellectual content; final approval of the version to be published. NW: substantial contribution to conception and design and interpretation of data; involved in revising the manuscript critically for important intellectual content; final approval of the version to be published. All authors read and approved the final manuscript.

Author details
[1]Department of Pediatric Immunology, Room KC 03.063.0, University Medical Center, Wilhelmina Children's Hospital, Utrecht 3508 AB, The Netherlands. [2]Department of Rheumatology, Jeroen Bosch Hospital, 's-Hertogenbosch, The Netherlands. [3]Department of Rheumatology, Woerden, Maartenskliniek, The Netherlands. [4]Department of Rheumatology, Meander Medical Center, Amersfoort, The Netherlands. [5]Department of Rheumatology, Gelre Hospitals, Apeldoorn and Zutphen, The Netherlands.

References
1. Scott DL, Wolfe F, Huizinga TW: **Rheumatoid arthritis.** *Lancet* 2010, **376**:1094–1108.
2. Ceponis A, Kavanaugh A: **Use of methotrexate in patients with psoriatic arthritis.** *Clin Exp Rheumatol* 2010, **28**:S132–S137.
3. Smolen JS, Landewe R, Breedveld FC, Dougados M, Emery P, Gaujoux-Viala C, Gorter S, Knevel R, Nam J, Schoels M, Aletaha D, Buch M, Gossec L, Huizinga T, Bijlsma JW, Burmester G, Combe B, Cutolo M, Gabay C, Gomez-Reino J, Kouloumas M, Kvien TK, Martin-Mola E, McInnes I, Pavelka K, van Riel P, Scholte M, Scott DL, Sokka T, Valesini G, *et al*: **EULAR recommendations for the management of rheumatoid arthritis with synthetic and biological disease-modifying antirheumatic drugs.** *Ann Rheum Dis* 2010, **69**:964–975.
4. Gossec L, Smolen JS, Gaujoux-Viala C, Ash Z, Marzo-Ortega H, van der Heijde D, FitzGerald O, Aletaha D, Balint P, Boumpas D, Braun J, Breedveld FC, Burmester G, Cañete JD, de Wit M, Dagfinrud H, de Vlam K, Dougados M, Helliwell P, Kavanaugh A, Kvien TK, Landewé R, Luger T, Maccarone M, McGonagle D, McHugh N, McInnes IB, Ritchlin C, Sieper J, Tak PP, *et al*: **European league against rheumatism recommendations for the management of psoriatic arthritis with pharmacological therapies.** *Ann Rheum Dis* 2012, **71**:4–12.
5. Visser K, Katchamart W, Loza E, Martinez-Lopez JA, Salliot C, Trudeau J, Bombardier C, Carmona L, van der Heijde D, Bijlsma JW, Boumpas DT, Canhao H, Edwards CJ, Hamuryudan V, Kvien TK, Leeb BF, Martín-Mola EM, Mielants H, Müller-Ladner U, Murphy G, Østergaard M, Pereira IA, Ramos-Remus C, Valentini G, Zochling J, Dougados M: **Multinational evidence-based recommendations for the use of methotrexate in rheumatic disorders with a focus on rheumatoid arthritis: integrating systematic literature research and expert opinion of a broad international panel of rheumatologists in the 3E Initiative.** *Ann Rheum Dis* 2009, **68**:1086–1093.
6. Verstappen SM, Bakker MF, Heurkens AH, van der Veen MJ, Kruize AA, Geurts MA, Bijlsma JW, Jacobs JW, Utrecht Rheumatoid Arthritis Cohort Study Group: **Adverse events and factors associated with toxicity in patients with early rheumatoid arthritis treated with methotrexate tight control therapy: the CAMERA study.** *Ann Rheum Dis* 2010, **69**:1044–1048.
7. Jacobs JW, Bakker MF, Bijlsma JW: **Low-dose prednisone inclusion in a methotrexate-based, tight control strategy for early rheumatoid arthritis.** *Ann Intern Med* 2012, **157**:300.
8. Schnabel A, Herlyn K, Burchardi C, Reinhold-Keller E, Gross WL: **Long-term tolerability of methotrexate at doses exceeding 15 mg per week in rheumatoid arthritis.** *Rheumatol Int* 1996, **15**:195–200.
9. McKendry RJ, Dale P: **Adverse effects of low dose methotrexate therapy in rheumatoid arthritis.** *J Rheumatol* 1993, **20**:1850–1856.
10. Braun J, Kastner P, Flaxenberg P, Wahrisch J, Hanke P, Demary W, von Hinüber U, Rockwitz K, Heitz W, Pichlmeier U, Guimbal-Schmolck C, Brandt A, MC-MTX.6/RH Study Group: **Comparison of the clinical efficacy and safety of subcutaneous versus oral administration of methotrexate in patients with active rheumatoid arthritis: results of a six-month, multicenter, randomized, double-blind, controlled, phase IV trial.** *Arthritis Rheum* 2008, **58**:73–81.
11. Kremer JM, Phelps CT: **Long-term prospective study of the use of methotrexate in the treatment of rheumatoid arthritis. Update after a mean of 90 months.** *Arthritis Rheum* 1992, **35**:138–145.
12. Lie E, van der Heijde D, Uhlig T, Heiberg MS, Koldingsnes W, Rodevand E, Kaufmann C, Mikkelsen K, Kvien TK: **Effectiveness and retention rates of methotrexate in psoriatic arthritis in comparison with methotrexate-treated patients with rheumatoid arthritis.** *Ann Rheum Dis* 2010, **69**:671–676.
13. Bulatovic M, Heijstek MW, Verkaaik M, van Dijkhuizen EH, Armbrust W, Hoppenreijs EP, Kamphuis S, Kuis W, Egberts TC, Sinnema G, Rademaker CM: **High prevalence of methotrexate intolerance in juvenile idiopathic arthritis: development and validation of a methotrexate intolerance severity score.** *Arthritis Rheum* 2011, **63**:2007–2013.
14. Brunner HI, Johnson AL, Barron AC, Passo MH, Griffin TA, Graham TB, Lovell TJ: **Gastrointestinal symptoms and their association with health-related quality of life of children with juvenile rheumatoid arthritis: validation of a gastrointestinal symptom questionnaire.** *J Clin Rheumatol* 2005, **11**:194–204.
15. Rheumatoid Arthritis Clinical Trial Archive Group: **The effect of age and renal function on the efficacy and toxicity of methotrexate in rheumatoid arthritis.** *J Rheumatol* 1995, **22**:218–223.
16. Bologna C, Viu P, Jorgensen C, Sany J: **Effect of age on the efficacy and tolerance of methotrexate in rheumatoid arthritis.** *Br J Rheumatol* 1996, **35**:453–457.
17. Murray KJ, Lovell DJ: **Advanced therapy for juvenile arthritis.** *Best Pract Res Clin Rheumatol* 2002, **16**:361–378.
18. Alsufyani K, Ortiz-Alvarez O, Cabral DA, Tucker LB, Petty RE, Malleson PN: **The role of subcutaneous administration of methotrexate in children with juvenile idiopathic arthritis who have failed oral methotrexate.** *J Rheumatol* 2004, **31**:179–182.
19. Ravelli A, Martini A: **Methotrexate in juvenile idiopathic arthritis: answers and questions.** *J Rheumatol* 2000, **27**:1830–1833.
20. van der Meer A, Wulffraat NM, Prakken BJ, Gijsbers B, Rademaker CM, Sinnema G: **Psychological side effects of MTX treatment in juvenile idiopathic arthritis: a pilot study.** *Clin Exp Rheumatol* 2007, **25**:480–485.

2

Kinetics of gene expression and bone remodelling in the clinical phase of collagen-induced arthritis

Katja CM Denninger[1,2*], Thomas Litman[2], Troels Marstrand[2], Kristian Moller[2], Lars Svensson[2], Tord Labuda[2] and Åsa Andersson[1]

Abstract

Introduction: Pathological bone changes differ considerably between inflammatory arthritic diseases and most studies have focused on bone erosion. Collagen-induced arthritis (CIA) is a model for rheumatoid arthritis, which, in addition to bone erosion, demonstrates bone formation at the time of clinical manifestations. The objective of this study was to use this model to characterise the histological and molecular changes in bone remodelling, and relate these to the clinical disease development.

Methods: A histological and gene expression profiling time-course study on bone remodelling in CIA was linked to onset of clinical symptoms. Global gene expression was studied with a gene chip array system.

Results: The main histopathological changes in bone structure and inflammation occurred during the first two weeks following the onset of clinical symptoms in the joint. Hereafter, the inflammation declined and remodelling of formed bone dominated.

Global gene expression profiling showed simultaneous upregulation of genes related to bone changes and inflammation in week 0 to 2 after onset of clinical disease. Furthermore, we observed time-dependent expression of genes involved in early and late osteoblast differentiation and function, which mirrored the histopathological bone changes. The differentially expressed genes belong to the bone morphogenetic pathway (BMP) and, in addition, include the osteoblast markers integrin-binding sialoprotein (*Ibsp*), bone gamma-carboxyglutamate protein (*Bglap1*), and secreted phosphoprotein 1 (*Spp1*). Pregnancy-associated protein A (*Pappa*) and periostin (*Postn*), differentially expressed in the early disease phase, are proposed to participate in bone formation, and we suggest that they play a role in early bone formation in the CIA model. Comparison to human genome-wide association studies (GWAS) revealed differential expression of several genes associated with human arthritis.

Conclusions: In the CIA model, bone formation in the joint starts shortly after onset of clinical symptoms, which results in bony fusion within one to two weeks. This makes it a candidate model for investigating the relationship between inflammation and bone formation in inflammatory arthritis.

Introduction

Inflammatory arthritis is characterised by joint destruction, often resulting in severe distortion of the joint architecture, and leading to impaired function of the joints. The balance between anabolic and catabolic bone remodelling, however, differs between the inflammatory arthritic diseases rheumatoid arthritis (RA), psoriatic arthritis (PsA), and ankylosing spondylitis (AS). While RA primarily is an erosive disease, bone erosion and bone formation co-exist in patients with PsA and AS [1]. Why the bone responds differently to an inflammatory insult is not clarified, but may be important in directing future treatment strategies.

Collagen-induced arthritis (CIA) is a model for RA both due to its construct validity, including autoimmune reaction to collagen type II and MHC class II dependency, and due to its face validity, that is severe bone destruction. Moreover, disease development ends in bony fusion (ankylosis) of the destroyed joints, which could

* Correspondence: katjadenninger@gmail.com
[1]Department of Drug Design and Pharmacology, Faculty of Health and Medical Sciences, University of Copenhagen, Universitetsparken 2, Copenhagen Ø DK-2100, Denmark
[2]Disease Pharmacology/Molecular Biomedicine, LEO Pharma A/S, Industriparken 55, Ballerup DK-2750, Denmark

make it a relevant model for bone-forming inflammatory arthritic diseases.

Bone formation in CIA has been described as starting two to four weeks after onset of arthritis, but mainly playing a role in the healing state two to three months after onset [2]. However, in a kinetic study of new bone formation in CIA and adjuvant-induced arthritis (AIA) in rat, periosteal proliferation was reported as early as day 3 (CIA) and day 5 (AIA) after onset of arthritis, and new bone formation peaked at day 27 in both models [3].

Bone formation may occur directly within the mesenchyme (intramembranous) or via a cartilage scaffold (endochondral ossification). In both processes, the extracellular matrix (ECM) is mineralised. In particular two pathways have been implicated in osteoblast differentiation and bone formation: the bone morphogenetic protein (BMP) signalling pathway, of which several proteins induce ectopic bone formation [4], and the wingless-type (WNT) signalling pathway [5].

With the aim to understand the molecular mechanisms linking inflammation with new bone formation, the present study was initiated to histologically characterise bone remodelling in the CIA model throughout the disease course, and to relate this to gene expression. To minimise variation between the data and enable correlation to clinical duration of arthritis, we used tarsal joints with a clinical score of 3. By grouping the tarsal joints according to onset and duration of symptoms, we show that the process of bone formation runs in parallel with the local inflammatory process in the joint, with a concomitant differential expression of genes involved in bone remodelling.

Methods

Animal model

Arthritis was induced in male DBA/1JBom mice by intradermal injection of 100 µl chicken collagen type II (CII) (2 mg/ml) (Sigma-Aldrich, St Louis, MO, USA) in complete Freund's adjuvant (CFA) (0.5 mg/ml) (Sigma-Aldrich) on day 1 and boosted on day 21 with CII in incomplete Freund's adjuvant (IFA) (Sigma-Aldrich). The control group received CFA and IFA without collagen, respectively. The mice were scored for onset, severity and duration of arthritis in the tarsal joints. Severity in this joint was scored from 0 (no erythema or swelling) to 3 (severe erythema and swelling). Tarsal joints were collected for histology and gene expression analysis. The mice were, in addition, assigned a total score for all four paws (with a theoretical maximum of 24 points for all paws). This additional scoring system was used to judge when the animals should be euthanized as required by Danish legislation (score exceeding 10 points). The mice were housed under standard conditions, and provided pellets and water *ad libitum*. The Danish Ethics Authorities 'The Animal Experiments Inspectorate' approved the studies (permit number: 2008/561 – 1532).

Histology

Fifty-two tarsal joints were collected for histology. The tarsal joints were divided into groups according to duration of arthritis in the joint: day 0 to 3, day 4 to 7, week 1 to 2, > 2 weeks, and > 2 weeks with declining inflammation ('declined'). In the group 'declined' the joints previously had a clinical score of 3 for minimum two weeks, after which the clinical score had declined > 1 score at the time the joint was sampled. For all other joints, the clinical score was 3 at the sampling time. For number of joints per time-point, see Table S2A in Additional file 1. The joints were fixed in formalin and decalcified in 10% Na-EDTA for two to three weeks.

Haematoxylin and eosin-stained sections were assigned a score for bone erosion, bone formation, synovitis, tendinitis, and peritendinitis. Bone remodelling was judged by the degree of modulation of joint structure, presence of osteoclasts (OCs) and osteoblasts (OBs), and formation of cartilage and woven bone (Figure S1 in Additional file 2). Synovitis, tendinitis and peritendinitis were scored by the degree of infiltrating cells and fibrosis. All features were scored from 0 (no pathologic changes) to 4 (severe pathologic changes).

RNA extraction and microarray analysis

Three tarsal joints were sampled per group (twelve joints in total). For the group 'More than two weeks, with declined inflammation' the joints had had a clinical score of 3 for minimum two weeks, after which the clinical score had declined > 1 score at the time for sampling. For all other joints, the clinical score was 3 when sampled (Table S2B in Additional file 1). The twelve joints were compared to three joints from non-immunised control animals. The joints were processed and analysed separately (unpooled). Skin, visible muscle tissue and fur were removed and tarsal joints collected by transverse sectioning of the metatarsus bones and the tibia/fibula under the fur border. This procedure ensured that all joints in the tarsus were included in each sample. Except for the skin and visible muscle, all other soft tissues were included in the sample. The joints were subsequently snap-frozen in liquid N_2 and stored at −80°C. RNA was extracted using the *mir*Vana™ miRNA isolation kit (Ambion, Exiqon A/S, Vedbæk Denmark), amplified and labelled using the Pico amplification kit (Nugen Technologies, San Carlos, CA, USA), according to the manufacturers' instructions, followed by hybridisation to Mouse Gene 1.0ST microarrays (Affymetrix, Santa Clara, CA, USA).

The quality of the RNA was evaluated using the RNA integrity number (RIN), and only samples with RIN >8.3 were included for further analysis.

Arrays were normalized using RMA background correction and quantile normalisation in R v.2.15 (Additional file 3). Significance of differentially expressed genes was assessed by analysis of variance (ANOVA), and adjusted for multiple testing by estimating false discovery rates (FDR). Data visualisation was performed in Qlucore Omics Explorer v.2.2 (Qlucore AB, Lund, Sweden). The expression data are deposited in Gene Expression Omnibus [6]; accession number: Series record GSE61140).

Functional analysis and network representation of differentially expressed genes was performed in Ingenuity Pathway Analysis (IPA, Ingenuity™ Systems). Gene expression levels are indicated in the IPA networks as red (upregulated) or green (downregulated) in comparison to non-induced controls.

The differentially regulated genes assigned to Bio Functions of bone and skeleton, were used to compile a comprehensive list of genes potentially involved in bone remodelling in the CIA model.

Quantitative PCR

For qPCR analysis of *Bmp1*, RNA (90 ng per reaction) was reverse transcribed to cDNA using the High Capacity cDNA Reverse Transcription kit (Applied Biosystems, Carlsbad, CA, USA). qPCR was performed with TaqMan Universal PCR Mastermix (Applied Biosystems, USA) and primer-assays Bmp1 Mm00802225_m1 and Gapdh Mm99999915_g1 (Applied Biosystems, USA). PCR was initiated at 50°C for 2 minutes and 95°C for 10 minutes, and the cycling conditions were 95°C for 15 seconds and 60°C for 1 minute (40 cycles). For the remaining 14 genes (Table S4 in Additional file 4), qPCR analysis was performed by AROS Applied Biotechnology A/S (Aarhus, Denmark). cDNA was prepared from 100 ng RNA/sample using the High Capacity cRNA Reverse Transcription kit (Applied Biosystems, USA) and the qPCR reaction was performed with TaqMan™ Universal PCR Master Mix (Applied Biosystems, USA). Assay IDs for the specific primer/probe sets (Life Technologies, Carlsbad, CA, USA) are listed in Table S4 in Additional file 4. Samples were analysed as triplicates and normalized by subtraction of the sample mean Ct value from that of the mean Ct value of the housekeeping gene Gapdh.

Statistics

Histological scoring results were assessed using Kruskall-Wallis test followed by a Dunn's multiple comparisons test. qPCR results were analysed by ANOVA, followed by Bonferroni's multiple comparison test, and compared by linear regression to array results. The significance of the correlation coefficients was tested using Student's *t*-distribution. All statistical analyses were performed in GraphPad Prism v.5 (GraphPad Software, San Diego, CA, USA), with the statistical unit being one joint from each animal included.

Results

Development of arthritis and histopathology of CIA from onset to decline of clinical symptoms

After immunization with chicken CII, mean onset of arthritis was observed on day 31 ± 8.8. Mean score of arthritis peaked six weeks after boost with a mean score of 4.6 ± 1.8. In order to study local arthritis development, onset and severity of arthritis in the tarsal joint was recorded in detail.

For the histological study, a total of 52 tarsal joints were used. Fourteen were sampled between day 0 and 4, ten between day 4 and 7, eleven between week 1 and 2, and seventeen after week 2 of clinical inflammation onset. After week 2, twelve samples showed declining clinical symptoms. Little variation in the appearance of synovitis, peritendinitis, and bone remodelling was noted within the groups. The data are in accordance with a previously published study showing occurrence of bony spur formation early after disease onset [3].

Day 0 to 4 after clinical disease onset: The infiltration of inflammatory cells was equally pronounced when comparing the synovium (mean score 3.8 +/−0.4) and the peritendon (mean score 3.9+/−0.3) (Figure 1A). In 10/14 joints, fibroblast activity and fibrosis indicated chronic inflammation, while 4/14 joints had no signs of chronicity. Bone pathology was dominated by erosion (11/14 joints), initiated where the peritendon and synovium are attached to, or in close proximity to the bone, while the articular cartilage remained intact. Bone erosion was severe as judged by the presence of multinucleated osteoclasts (OC) and the extent of structural damage of the cartilage and bone tissue (Figure 1B). However, both OB proliferation, and collagen deposition, was observed in the periosteum and seemed, from visible staining ability, to have progressed into secretion of osteoid-like matrix in 3/14 joints (Figure 1C).

Day 4 to 7 after clinical disease onset: Severe fibrosis and synovitis approaching the articular cartilage, and resulting in erosion of the articular cartilage, was observed (Figure 1D). In areas of less severe inflammation, pronounced OB activity and onset of endochondral ossification was noted as judged from the appearance of hypertrophic cartilage. Bone erosion (mean score of 3.1+/−1.3) and bone formation (2.2+/−1.1), was observed in 9/10 joints.

Week 1 to 2 after clinical disease onset: Bone erosion (score 2.6+/−1.4) and bone formation (score 2.9+/−1.1) was pronounced and observed in 10/11 joints. Endochondral ossification was dominating (Figure 2A). Ankylosis was noted from day 8 and consisted of an inner layer of remodelled bone, followed by a cartilage layer.

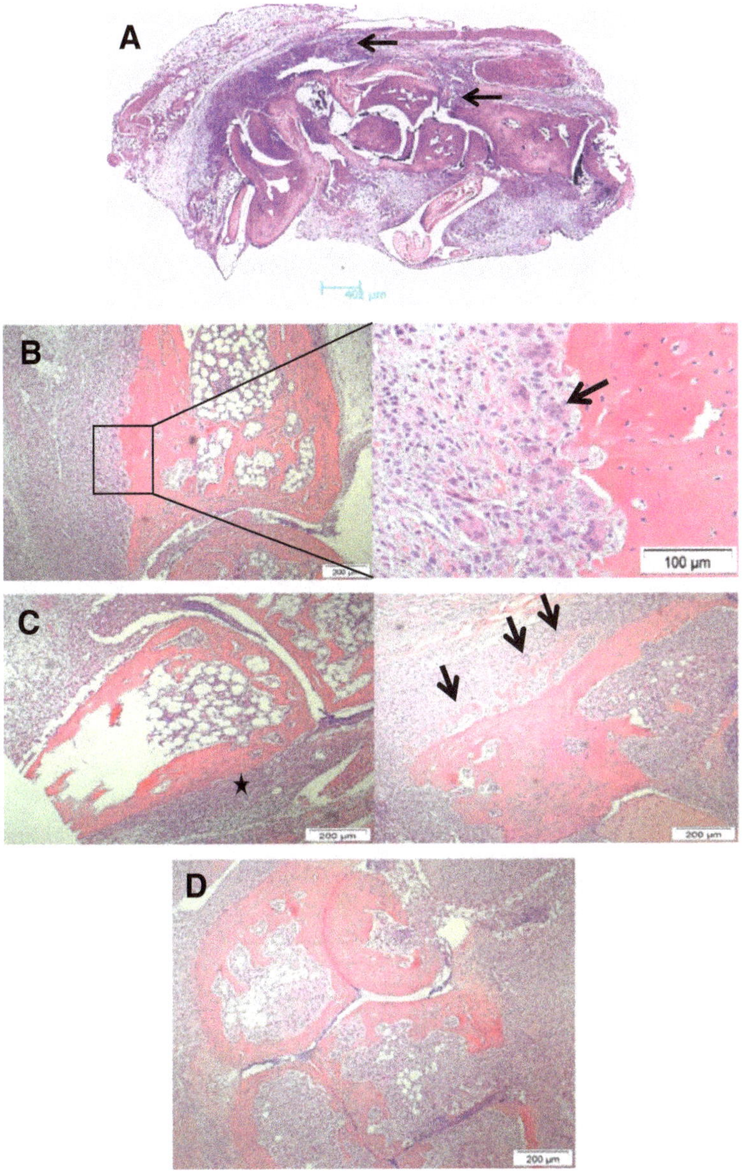

Figure 1 Histopathology of tarsal joints day 0 to 7. A) Day 0 to 4: overview of inflammation in the tarsal joint showing equal severity of inflammation in peripheral tissues and synovium (arrows). **(B-C)** Day 0 to 4: bone erosion and OC activity (arrow in B, day 3) dominates. Proliferation and collagen deposition takes place (star in C, day 0) in the periosteum and results in osteoid deposition (arrows in C, day 3). **(D)** Day 4 to 7: the joint architecture is severely distorted (day 7). OC, osteoclast.

The outer lining layer of the bone-forming lesion consisted of mesenchymal cells (Figure 2B). In most joints, inflammation was severe, but gradually disappearing and replaced by severe fibrosis with yet active fibroblast proliferation.

Two weeks after clinical disease onset: The clinical severity of inflammation was declining in most joints, although 5/17 joints still showed severe clinical signs. In the joints with severe clinical arthritis, accumulation of cartilage was still apparent, while in joints with declining clinical symptoms, an increase in what was observed as mineralisation of cartilage and newly formed bone took place, in addition to modification of the newly formed bone by OCs (Figure 2C).

By comparing the development in scores for bone erosion and bone formation, respectively, a significant difference over time was observed with the greatest development in scores of bone formation ($P = 0.0186$ vs. $P < 0.0001$) (Figure 2D).

Gene expression in joints from mice with CIA normalises after two weeks of inflammation

Having examined the bone remodelling after clinical onset of arthritis histologically, we aimed at describing the

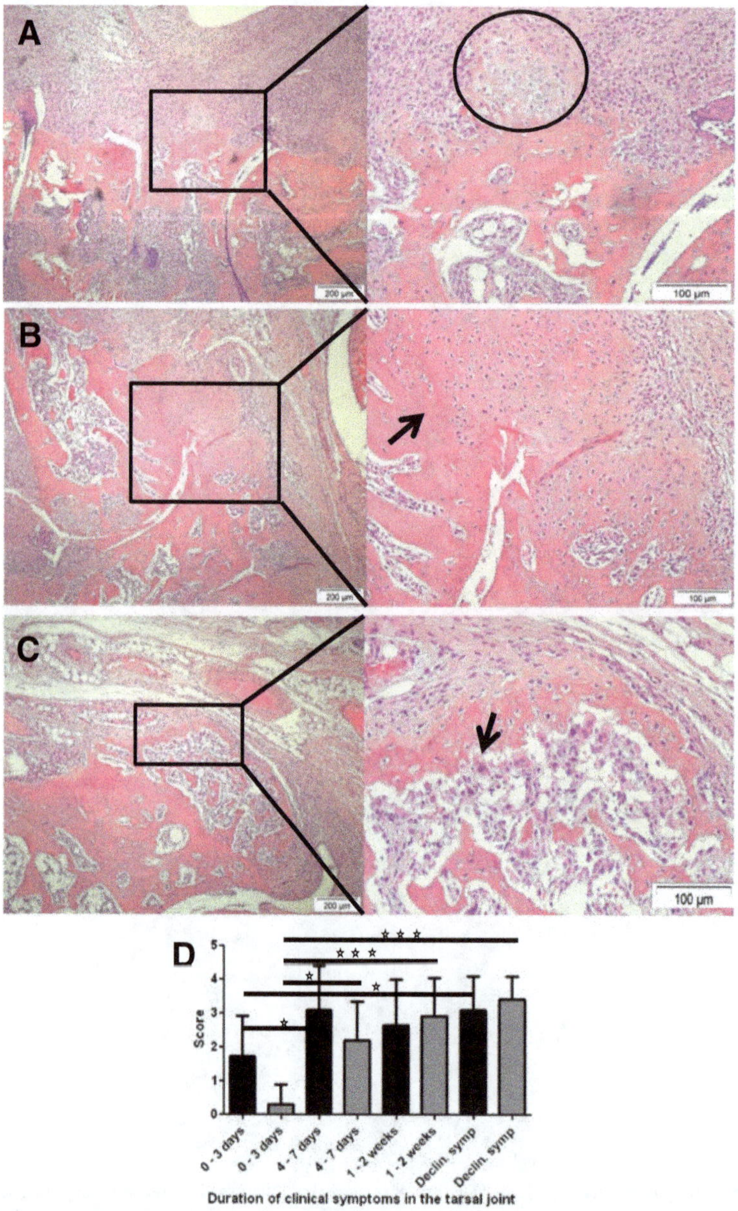

Figure 2 Histopathology of tarsal joints from day 8 and until decline of symptoms. (A) Appearance of cartilage (encircled) marks the onset of endochondral ossification (day 8). **(B)** Ankylosis has progressed from being fibrous to consist of cartilage and osteoid (day 10), with osteoid closest to the original bone (arrow). **(C)** Declining disease phase: bone formation is remodelled with OC activity observed in some animals (arrow). **(D)** Histological scores of bone erosion (black bars) and bone formation (grey bars) over time (mean +/− standard deviation (SD)). Statistics from the comparisons of individual groups is indicated by lines above the bars (Dunn's multiple comparison test, *P <0.05, **P <0.01, ***P <0.001). OC, osteoclast.

time course of bone remodelling by global gene expression profiling (Figure 3A and B).

Unsupervised hierarchical clustering grouped the samples into a phase of high transcriptional activity between week 0 and 2, and, subsequently, a period of declining transcriptional activity. One sample from the declining disease phase (decline 10) clustered together with the controls, showing that the gene expression pattern normalised in the late disease phase (Figure 3A). In the first three days, 908 genes displayed a +2-fold change in the transcriptional level, while 749 genes were differentially expressed in week 1 to 2 (>2 fold change, P <0.05). The IPA showed that the top biological functions, canonical pathways, and upregulated genes were dominated by genes involved in arthritis and the immune system in general, in connective and skeletal tissue disorders and remodelling, as well as tissue development and function (Table S5A and B in Additional file 5).

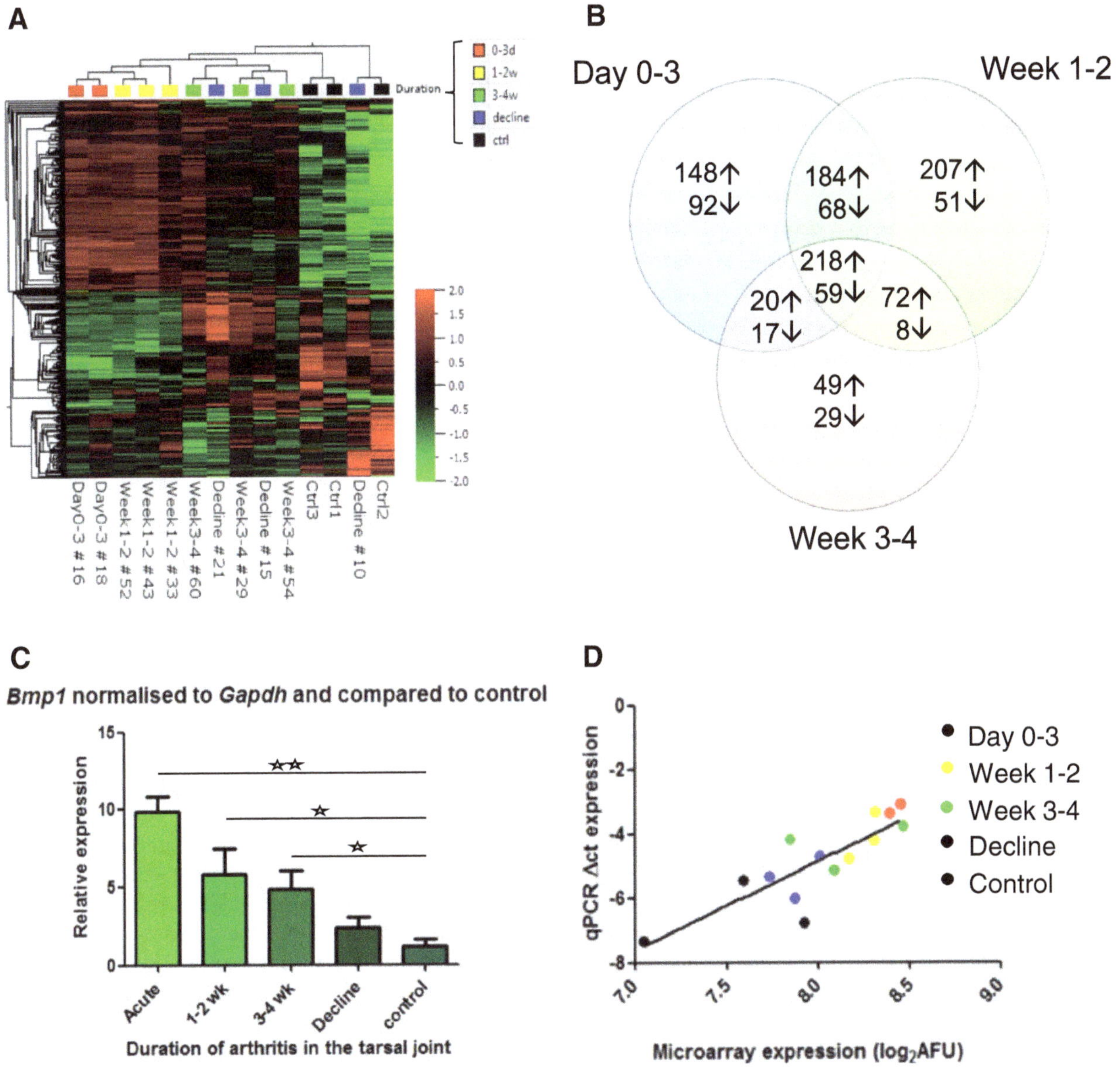

Figure 3 Cluster analysis and validation of gene expression profile. (A) Separation of samples by unsupervised hierarchical clustering. The groups are: day 0 to 3, week 1 to 2 and week 3 to 4 after onset of arthritis, and joints with declining clinical disease activity. Colours and colour intensity indicate upregulation (red) or downregulation (green) regulation of genes. **(B)** Venn diagram of the gene expression study showing the number of genes differentially expressed at the time points: day 0 to 3, week 1 to 2, week 3 to 4, and in the declining disease phase in comparison to control. **(C)** The results from the microarray study were validated with qPCR. *Bmp1* was normalised to *Gapdh* expression and compared to a control sample from non-immunised mice. Statistically significant differences between group means (δ-ct-values) are indicated with lines above the bars (Bonferroni's multiple comparison test, $^*P < 0.05$, $^{**}P < 0.01$). **(D)** The gene expression level of *Bmp1* assessed by qPCR correlated significantly ($r^2 = 0.7$, $P < 0.0002$) with the corresponding microarray data (linear regression test).

Several potentially disease-relevant genes (*Saa3*, *Timp1*, *Postn*, *Ctsk*, *Mmp3* and *Mmp13*) demonstrated very high fold changes (between 10.6 and 45.3) (Table 1). Moreover, pregnancy–associated plasma protein A (*Pappa*) was strongly upregulated when comparing day 0 to 3 with week 1 to 2 (fold change +2.3) (Table 2). A muscle- and epidermis-specific gene expression signature was found among the most downregulated genes when comparing day 0 to 3 and control samples (Table 1).

In week 3 to 4 after onset of disease, the number of two-fold differentially expressed genes had decreased to 353 (Figure 3B). The pathway profile changed accordingly, and was dominated by tissue remodelling and developmental pathways, although an inflammatory gene

Table 1 Highly differentially expressed genes grouped according to function

Gene symbol	Ctrl (Log_2AFU)[a]	Day 0 to 3[b]	week 1 to 2[c]	Week 3 to 4[d]	Decline[e]	Localisation	Ar vs. N[f]	Ar vs. N[g]
Saa3	6.8	44.1	26.2	7.8	2.7	Plasma	18.0	2.0
Mmp3	7.2	23.1	11.9	5.2	2.9	Synovium	10.1	5.3
Mmp13	7.6	13.2	17.3	8.9	4.5	Synovium	3.5	2.3
Timp1	7.5	19.4	9.3	5.3	3.4	Synovium	1.9	3.5
Ctsk	7.8	11.0	11.7	7.6	4.8	Osteoclasts	2.8	1.7
Atp6v0d2	6.97	9.03	7.18	5.94	3.67	Endosome	1.5	1.0
Postn	8.5	10.3	9.8	5.0	2.5	Osteoblasts	4.5	1.0
Krtdap	7.6	0.1	0.2	4.5	14.1	Skin*	0.4	1.1
Lce1a1/1a2	8.2	0.1	0.1	2.8	7.9	Skin	NA	1.0
Lor	8.4	0.1	0.2	3.7	5.4	Skin*	0.6	1.1
Krt1/2/5/14	7.8	0.1	0.2	3.4	10.3	Skin*	0.8	1.0
Mt4	7.40	0.32	0.36	4.63	19.15	Epithelia*	0.8	1.0
Myl2	10.5	0.1	0.8	1.0	1.0	Muscle	0.2	0.6
Pygm	10.8	0.1	0.4	0.4	0.6	Muscle	0.5	0.7
Casq1	10.78	0.12	0.85	0.57	0.72	Muscle	0.5	0.7
Myh4	11.96	0.13	0.45	0.31	0.43	Muscle	0.3	0.9
Ckm	10.78	0.14	0.44	0.46	0.76	Muscle	0.6	0.7

[a]Mean log2 expression in non-induced control mice. Mean fold change in comparison to control: [b]on day 0 to 3, [c]in week 1 to 2, [d]in week 3 to 4, [e]in the declining disease phase. Fold change of gene expression in arthritic joints from the [f]TNFα overexpressing model versus control [7], and the [g]PGIA arthritis model versus control [8], *Differentially expressed epidermal specific genes in arthritic joints from the present study and the TNFα overexpressing model [7]. Ctrl, control; PGIA, proteoglycan-induced arthritis; TNFα, tumour necrosis factor alpha.

expression signature was still present (Table S5C and D in Additional file 5).

A comparison of gene expression between week 0 to 2 and week 3 to 4 revealed considerable up-regulation of several epidermal genes (fold changes between 3.8 and 13.9) in the samples collected three to four weeks after onset of arthritis (Table 1).

The expression pattern of 15 differentially expressed genes was verified by qPCR. Of these, 12 genes correlated significantly with the gene expression pattern obtained from the microarray profile, while three genes showed the same expression pattern, but the correlation was not significant. The expression of *Bmp1* is shown in Figure 3C and D ($r^2 = 0.7$, $p < 0.0002$), and the remaining validation data are shown in Figure S6 in Additional file 6 and Figure S7 in Additional file 7 and with the corresponding r^2 and *P*-values in Table S8 in Additional file 8.

To identify genes associated with the observed bone pathology, we focused on genes, differentially expressed at the different time-points, which were related to bone and skeleton in the IPA Bio Functions. The genes and associated Bio Functions reflected the bone remodelling process (Table S9 in Additional file 9), and their number and effect size declined over time. The genes and their expression profiles are shown individually in Table S10 in Additional file 10.

Distinctive expression profiles of genes involved in osteoblast and osteoclast functions

The differentially expressed genes, related to bone, from Table S10 in Additional file 10, were divided into profiles and are shown separately in Table 2. Profile one encompassed genes with the highest expression on day 0 to 3 with a subsequently declining profile. These were in particular genes encoding proteins involved in OC differentiation and function (*Ccl9, Tyrobp, Atp6v0d2, Lif*; fold changes between 2.0 and 9.2), in addition to ECM formation and collagen type 1 assembly (*Bmp1, Crtap, Tnc, Lox*; fold changes between 1.9 and 10.6) [9-14] (Table 2, Figure 4A, and Table S10 in Additional file 10). In profile two, genes with the highest expression in week 1 to 2, followed by a declining expression pattern, were included. These were in particular genes encoding proteins involved in mineralisation and osteoblast function (*Sp7, Spp1, Mgp, Sparc, Enpp1, Bglap1, Ifitm5*; fold changes between 1.5 and 4.5) [15-21] (Table 2, Figure 4B and Table S10 in Additional file 10). Integrin-binding sialoprotein (*Ibsp*; fold change +3.0) also belongs to this group [20], but showed the highest expression in week 3 to 4. Moreover, a large group of genes showed a sustained differential expression pattern at day 0 to 3 and week 1 to 2. These included genes involved in osteoblast functions and ECM formation (*Col1a1, Col1a2, Ogn, Bgn, Col12a1, Ppib, Lum, Hapln1, Cthrc1, Postn*; fold

Table 2 Groups of genes showing a time-dependent expression pattern

Gene symbol	Ctrl[a]	Day 0 to 3[b]	Week 1 to 2[c]	Week 3 to 4[d]	Decline[e]	
	Log_2	Fold change (*P*-value)				**Protein function in relation to bone**
Osteoclast function: highest differential expression day 0 to 3						
Ccl9	6.42	***2.05 (0.01)***	1.78 (0.01)	1.61 (0.10)	1.44 (0.10)	Stimulates OC motility and polarisation through CCR1.
Tyrobp	10.21	***4.09 (0.03)***	3.31 (0.02)	2.47 (0.06)	1.56 (0.33)	Kinase involved in the generation of the actin cytoskeleton in OC, which is critical for bone resorption.
Atp6v0d2	6.97	***9.03 (0.01)***	7.18 (0.003)	5.94 (0.005)	3.67 (0.02)	ATPase proton pump involved in acidification of the extracellular resorption lacuna created by OC and early OC differentiation.
Lif	5.74	***2.20 (0.01)***	1.12 (0.22)	0.85 (0.39)	0.73 (0.10)	Expressed in OC and modulates the recruitment of OB to resorption surfaces in a TGFβ dependent manner.
Early osteoblast function: highest differentially expression day 0 to 3						
Bmp1	7.52	***1.86 (0.07)***	1.67 (0.10)	1.52 (0.13)	1.28 (0.30)	Metalloproteinase that may play a role on several levels of bone formation. It processes the c-terminal end of pro-collagen type I, activates other BMPs and processes BGN and DMP1. Expressed in patients with arthritis and acute fractures.
Crtap	6.84	***2.69 (0.02)***	2.43 (0.01)	1.66 (0.12)	1.12 (0.77)	Scaffolding protein that associates with others to hydroxylate collagen type I chains. Associated with osteogenesis imperfecta.
Tnc	9.19	***3.01 (0.03)***	2.67 (0.03)	2.09 (0.05)	1.72 (0.11)	Pro-inflammatory extracellular matrix protein, expressed in synovium and blood in RA patients. Involved in extracellular matrix remodelling, where it is bound by periostin.
Lox	7.13	***4.51 (0.11)***	3.52 (0.14)	2.49 (0.23)	1.57 (0.49)	Catalyses cross-linking of collagen type I. Is activated by BMP1.
Late osteoblast function: highest differentially expression week 1 to 2 or week 3 to 4						
Sp7	6.43	1.02 (0.90)	***1.67 (0.04)***	1.19 (0.25)	1.01 (0.95)	Transcription factor with a critical role in osteoblast differentiation.
Spp1	8.37	2.90 (0.05)	***4.46 (0.00003)***	3.49 (0.003)	1.98 (0.14)	OB marker, expressed in OB, OC, and osteocytes. Inhibits formation and growth of hydroxyapatite by binding the crystals. Promotes attachment of OC to bone under control of Acp5 phosphatase.
Mgp	10.45	2.61 (0.06)	***3.33 (0.04)***	2.45 (0.07)	1.65 (0.21)	Inhibitor of bone mineralisation.
Sparc	11.77	2.17 (0.04)	***2.48 (0.03)***	2.13 (0.04)	1.68 (0.07)	The protein binds hydroxyapatite when bound to collagen type I *in vitro*. *Sparc* null mice have normal collagen content in bone, but reduced bone formation and numbers of OC and OB.
Enpp1	9.08	2.72 (0.01)	***3.19 (0.0003)***	2.52 (0.01)	1.60 (0.15)	Expression is induced in OB by MDK. Essential for converting extracellular ATP to inorganic pyrophosphate, thus controlling the levels and functions in bone mineralization and soft tissue calcification. Essential for normal bone development.
Bglap1	9.05	0.75 (0.62)	***2.63 (0.0004)***	1.82 (0.04)	1.37 (0.13)	OB marker and serum marker of bone formation. Expressed in the late mineralisation phase. The exact role of the protein in bone is, however, debated as data is controversial.
Ifitm5	6.67	1.25 (0.11)	***1.47 (0.03)***	1.35 (0.05)	1.14 (0.27)	Expressed in OB and involved in mineralisation.
Ibsp	10.67	2.22 (0.02)	2.59 (0.01)	***2.99 (0.01)***	2.19 (0.02)	Marker of late OB differentiation. Expressed in OB, OC, hypertrophic chondrocytes and osteocytes. Binds to the AvB3 integrin and hydroxyapatite, probably mediating cell attachment to matrix. Nucleates hydroxyapatite.
Sustained high expression week 0 to 2						
Col1a2	9.94	***1.88 (0.08)***	***2.25 (0.05)***	2.03 (0.06)	1.69 (0.10)	This gene encodes the alpha2 chain of collagen type I. Collagen type I is the most abundant protein in bone and a marker of OB activity.

Table 2 Groups of genes showing a time-dependent expression pattern *(Continued)*

Col1a1	9.84	***1.80 (0.11)***	***2.25 (0.05)***	1.92 (0.09)	1.69 (0.14)	This gene encodes the alpha1 chain of collagen type I. Collagen type I is the most abundant protein in bone and a marker of OB activity.
Ogn	7.83	***2.28 (0.07)***	***3.88 (0.02)***	2.16 (0.09)	1.43 (0.34)	Proteoglycan belonging to the SLRP family. The protein is processed by BMP1 and regulates collagen type I fibrillogenesis.
Bgn	10.63	***2.18 (0.04)***	***2.21 (0.03)***	1.63 (0.09)	1.08 (0.72)	Proteoglycan belonging to the SLRP family. KO mice have reduced collagen synthesis, reduced bone mass and production of bone precursor cells. The protein is processed by BMP1.
Col12a1	8.24	***4.59 (0.04)***	***4.81 (0.04)***	2.98 (0.08)	1.75 (0.25)	Expressed by OB in areas of bone formation. COL12A1 KO mice have skeletal abnormalities with less mechanical strength and reduced matrix deposition.
Ppib	7.45	***2.17 (0.04)***	***2.27 (0.07)***	1.49 (0.14)	1.16 (0.64)	Associates with other proteins to hydroxylate collagen type I chains. Associated with osteogenesis imperfecta.
Lum	10.18	***3.37 (0.04)***	***3.97 (0.03)***	2.78 (0.05)	1.69 (0.18)	Proteoglycan belonging to the SLRP family (same as BGN).
Hapln1	6.72	***1.69 (0.15)***	***3.10 (0.01)***	2.88 (0.005)	2.08 (0.01)	Involved in cartilage biosynthesis by linking aggrecans and hyalyron acid. Polymorphism in this gene is associated with osteophyte formation in osteoarthritis and it is located in a susceptibility locus of AS.
Postn	8.52	***10.33 (0.07)***	***9.76 (0.07)***	4.97 (0.12)	2.53 (0.29)	Promotes cell survival of preosteoblasts and OB. Increases activation of pro-lysyl oxidase, which cross-links collagen type I.
Cthrc1	8.46	***4.78 (0.06)***	***6.79 (0.05)***	3.50 (0.10)	1.65 (0.43)	Molecule that stimulates bone formation, secreted by OC.
Others						
Igf1	9.68	1.94 (0.04)	***2.61 (0.03)***	1.82 (0.05)	1.18 (0.59)	Growth factor positively regulating bone formation. Regulates bone mineral density.
Pappa	5.99	***2.24 (0.0002)***	1.20 (0.06)	1.08 (0.11)	0.96 (0.68)	IGF-dependent proteinase that regulates the bioavailability of IGF. Expressed in fibroblasts, chondrocytes and OB. *Pappa* KO mice have reduced bone formation and delayed fracture-healing.
Dmp1	8.30	0.74 (0.42)	1.2 (0.59)	***1.81 (0.17)***	1.47 (0.30)	Extracellular matrix protein that is processed by BMP1 and involved in mineralisation of extracellular matrix. Expressed by hypertrophic chondrocytes, osteocytes, and OB.
Tissue degradation						
Mmp13	7.57	13.15 (0.02)	***17.33 (0.02)***	8.93 (0.02)	4.53 (0.05)	Bone resorption, OC- and osteoprogenitor differentiation.
Ctsk	7.82	11.02 (0.04)	***11.75 (0.04)***	7.58 (0.04)	4.80 (0.08)	Bone resorption. Principle enzyme degrading osteoid.
Mmp3	7.24	***23.11 (0.02)***	11.87 (0.01)	5.24 (0.04)	2.94 (0.11)	Metalloproteinase associated with arthritis.
Timp1	7.53	***19.45 (0.002)***	9.33 (0.001)	5.30 (0.03)	3.44 (0.02)	Inhibitor of metalloproteinases.
Mmp9	7.15	***4.24 (0.02)***	3.79 (0.02)	2.95 (0.04)	2.20 (0.08)	Resorption, OC- and osteoprogenitor differentiation.
Ctss	8.32	***3.62 (0.04)***	2.99 (0.05)	2.29 (0.08)	1.68 (0.20)	Expressed in hypertrophic chondrocytes and OC.
Mmp19	5.99	***2.18 (0.02)***	2.05 (0.01)	1.45 (0.16)	1.26 (0.09)	Degradation of extracellular tissue.
Mmp14	7.92	2.63 (0.02)	***2.82 (0.02)***	2.11 (0.02)	1.77 (0.05)	Involved in tissue destruction in RA.
Acp5	7.30	***3.68 (0.02)***	3.46 (0.03)	3.59 (0.03)	2.50 (0.03)	The encoded protein is a phosphatase, also called Trap. It is a marker of OC function and is extensively expressed in OC. It is activated by Cathepsin K and dephosphorylates SPP1 and IBSP. Plays an inhibitory role in collagen type I synthesis, degradation, and mineralisation.
Genes of the BMP pathway						
Bmp2	7.16	1.67 (0.30)	**1.68 (0.29)**	1.24 (0.63)	1.26 (0.59)	Ligand of the BMP pathway.
Bmpr1a	6.88	1.84 (0.13)	**2.01 (0.10)**	1.91 (0.11)	1.15 (0.72)	Type I receptor of the BMP pathway.

Table 2 Groups of genes showing a time-dependent expression pattern *(Continued)*

Bmpr2	8.36	**2.05 (0.04)**	1.65 (0.08)	1.40 (0.15)	1.30 (0.28)	Receptor type II in the BMP pathway.
Smad2	7.23	2.05 (0.14)	**2.14 (0.12)**	1.70 (0.22)	1.44 (0.37)	Regulatory Smad involved in BMP signalling.
Smad6	7.27	**0.55 (0.08)**	0.58 (0.0045)	0.72 (0.04)	0.76 (0.12)	Inhibitory Smad antagonising BMP signalling.
Smad4	8.16	**1.28 (0.18)**	1.27 (0.19)	1.18 (0.32)	1.04 (0.84)	Co-Smad associating with regulatory Smads.
Smad5	7.07	**1.40 (0.04)**	1.28 (0.06)	1.20 (0.17)	0.99 (0.92)	Regulatory Smad involved in BMP signalling.
Bmp4	7.68	**0.59 (0.04)**	0.68 (0.04)	0.99 (0.95)	0.95 (0.61)	Ligand of the BMP pathway.
Bmp6	8.44	**0.62 (0.07)**	0.75 (0.15)	0.88 (0.67)	0.93 (0.63)	Ligand of the BMP pathway.
Bmp7	5.82	**0.78 (0.19)**	0.86 (0.31)	0.94 (0.67)	1.26 (0.17)	Ligand of the BMP pathway.
Inhba	7.20	**5.65 (0.01)**	3.94 (0.01)	2.09 (0.07)	1.17 (0.77)	Non-steroidal hormone reported to increase bone formation in transgenic mice overexpressing human inhibin A. Associated with human arthritis.
Acvr2a	7.23	1.27 (0.33)	***1.29 (0.03)***	1.18 (0.04)	0.91 (0.34)	Type II receptor of the TGFβ pathway.
Acvr2b	6.21	***0.80 (0.01)***	0.73 (0.0034)	0.76 (0.03)	0.85 (0.29)	Type II receptor of the TGFβ pathway.
Genes of the WNT pathway						
Fzd1	6.91	***1.70 (0.05)***	1.57 (0.05)	1.39 (0.08)	1.18 (0.37)	Receptor of the WNT pathway.
Hif1a	8.35	***4.23 (0.02)***	3.56 (0.02)	2.49 (0.03)	1.43 (0.34)	Regulates the cellular response to hypoxia during endochondral bone formation and inhibits WNT signalling in OB in cooperation with Sp7.
Sost	7.28	***0.48 (0.03)***	0.61 (0.02)	0.62 (0.03)	0.73 (0.15)	WNT antagonist and marker of mature osteocytes.
Ndrg2	10.56	***0.18 (0.01)***	0.31 (0.0014)	0.37 (0.01)	0.52 (0.01)	Down-regulates WNT-signalling mediated TCF-promotor activity and GSK3β phosphorylation synergistically with PRA1.
Dkk1	7.19	***0.67 (0.18)***	0.85 (0.25)	1.15 (0.32)	1.09 (0.43)	Antagonist of the WNT pathway.
Tcf4	7.96	1.46 (0.09)	***1.73 (0.03)***	1.30 (0.28)	0.99 (0.94)	Transcription factor of the WNT pathway.

[a]Mean log2 expression in non-induced control mice. Mean fold change and p-value in comparison to control: [b]on day 0 to 3, [c]in week 1 to 2, [d]in week 3 to 4, [e]in the declining disease phase. The highest differential expression value and corresponding p-value of each gene are shown in bold italics. AS, ankylosing spondylitis; BMP, bone morphogenetic protein; BGN, biglycan; CCR1, C-C chemokine receptor type 1; Ctrl, control; DMP1, dentin matrix acidic phosphoprotein1; IGF, insulin-like growth factor; KO, knockout; MDK, midkine; OB, osteoblast; OC, osteoclast; RA, rheumatoid arthritis; SLRP, leucine rich repeat containing 6; TCF, T-cell-specific transcription factor; TGFβ, transforming growth factor beta.

changes between 2.2 and 10.3) [13,14,22-27] (Table 2). Finally, tissue destruction was reflected by up-regulation of the genes for four metalloproteinases (MMPs): the MMP inhibitor *Timp1;* acid phosphatase 5 (*Acp5*); cathepsin K [28]; cathepsin S [29], and additional cathepsins. These genes were among the most highly expressed, throughout disease development (Table 1, Table 2 and Table S10 in Additional file 10).

Differential expression of genes belonging to the BMP pathway

Differentially expressed genes related to the BMP pathway included the genes encoding the BMP type I and type II receptors (*Bmpr1a* and *Bmpr2,* fold change +2 at week 1 to 2 and day 0 to 3, respectively), and proteins downstream of the BMP signalling pathway (*Smad2* and *Smad6,* fold change +2.1 at week 1 to 2 and −1.8 at day 0 to 3, respectively) (Table 2, Figure 5 and Table S10 in Additional file 10). The BMP ligand *Bmp2* (fold change +1.7 at day 0 to 3) together with *Smad4* (fold change +1.3 at day 0 to 3) and *Smad5* (fold change +1.4 at day 0 to 3) showed the same marginal change in expression pattern. The BMP ligands *Bmp4, Bmp6,* and *Bmp7* were slightly downregulated (fold change between −1.7 to −1.3 at day 0 to 3).

High upregulation of the gene for Inhibin beta A (*Inhba;* fold change +5.6 at day 0 to 3) was found, in addition to minor expression changes in the genes of some of the transforming growth factor beta (TGFβ) receptors (*Acvr2a* and *Acvr2b)* bound by this protein (Table 2 and Figure 5A).

Differential expression of genes belonging to the WNT pathway

Within the group of genes related to the WNT pathway, the genes for the receptor FZD1 (fold change +1.7 at day 0 to 3) and transcription factor TCF4 (fold change +1.7 at week 1 to 2) were differentially expressed, in addition to a number of WNT inhibitors. These included the hypoxia-induced *Hif1a,* which showed more than 4-fold up-regulation and *Sost* and *Ndrg2,* which were between 2 and 5.6-fold downregulated. The well-described WNT inhibitor *Dkk1* was slightly downregulated (Table 2 and Table S10 in Additional file 10).

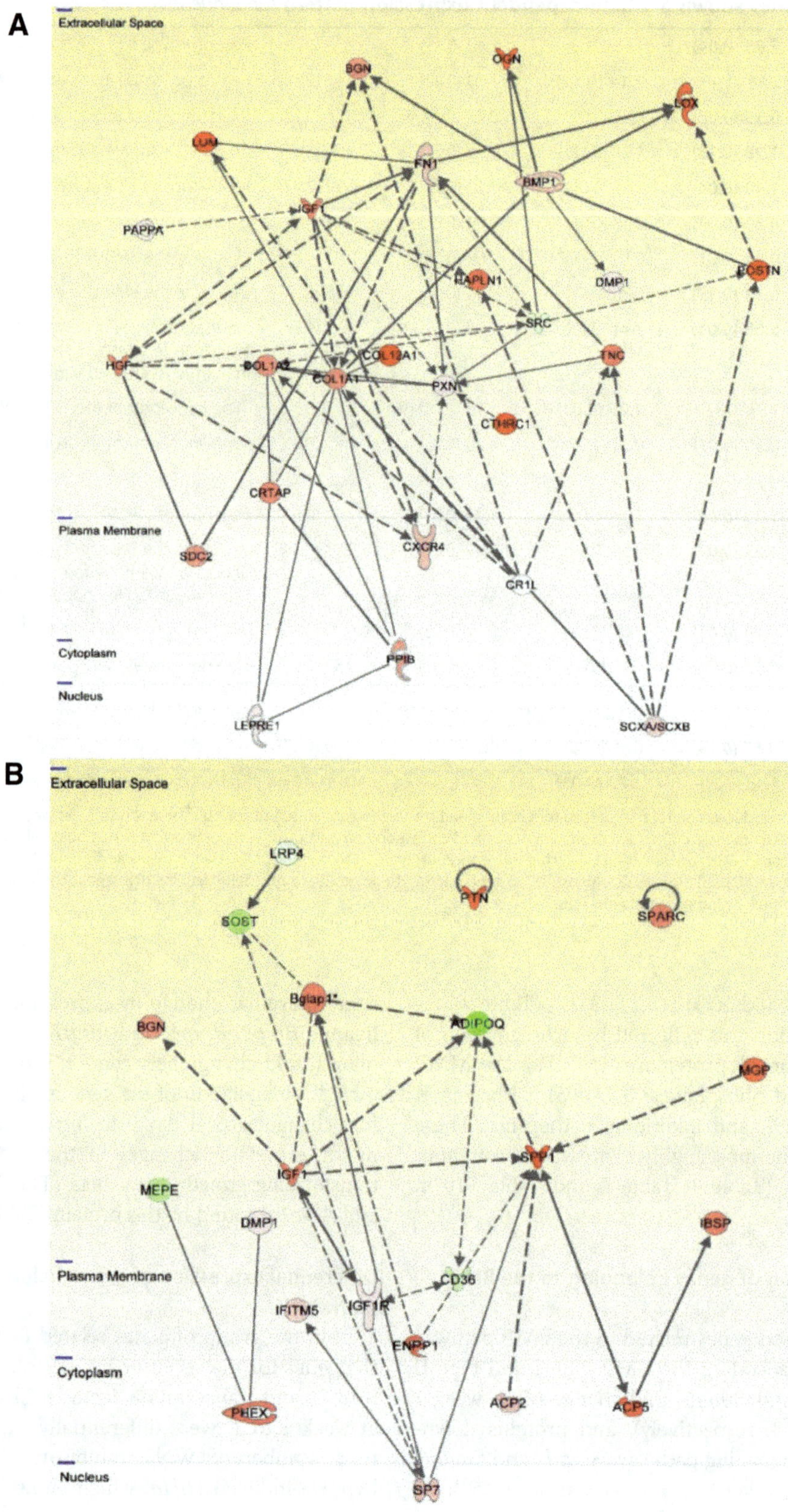

Figure 4 (See legend on next page.)

(See figure on previous page.)

Figure 4 Gene expression networks during osteoblast activity in early and late phases of joint inflammation. A) A network of genes related to osteoblast activity, in particular collagen type I assembly and cross-linking, during the early phase of clinical disease. Colours and colour intensity indicate upregulation (red) or downregulation (green) regulation of genes at day 0 to 3, where most of the genes showed the greatest fold change in comparison to non-induced controls. One exception is *Dmp1*, which became upregulated at week 3 to 4. **B)** A network of genes related to osteoblast activity, in particular mineralisation, during the late phase of clinical disease. Colours and colour intensity indicate upregulation (red) or downregulation (green) regulation of genes at week 1 to 2, where most of the genes showed the greatest fold change in comparison to non-induced controls. One exception is *Ibsp*, which was most highly upregulated in week 3 to 4.

Comparison to genome-wide association studies in human arthritis

Some of the genes differentially expressed in the herein presented study have been linked to human arthritis in genome-wide association studies (GWAS) (Table 2). Of those genes, several are involved in cartilage- and bone remodelling (underlined in Table 3).

Discussion

In this study, we have shown that in CIA, major histopathological changes, comprising inflammation as well as bone formation and ankylosis, occur within the first two weeks after the inflammatory symptoms become clinically apparent in a joint. Moreover, we have shown that the histopathology is reflected at the gene expression level, where a number of genes, coding for proteins important in inflammation and bone remodelling, are differentially expressed within the same time period after disease onset. This suggests that the CIA model is relevant for the osteoproliferative inflammatory arthritis in PsA and AS.

Bone formation in the murine CIA model has been described as starting in the subacute inflammatory disease phase, two to four weeks after onset of arthritis, but mainly playing a role in the healing state two to three months after onset [2]. However, no studies disclose any molecular details regarding bone formation throughout the arthritis disease course. Recently, Schett *et al.* [3] performed a histological study of new bone formation in the rat CIA and AIA models. In their study, periosteal proliferation was noted on day 3 (CIA) and day 5 (AIA) after onset of arthritis and new bone formation peaked at day 27 after onset of arthritis in both models.

The link between joint inflammation and bone remodelling is not clear. In human arthritis, areas with inflammation were shown to be predictive of bone formation [42], but bone formation does not seem to be blocked by anti-tumor necrosis factor alpha (TNFα) treatment [43]. In the present study, we have shown that in the murine CIA model, bone formation is (1) initiated during active inflammation, (2) develops in parallel with the inflammation, and (3) that the bone mineralises and remodels when clinical inflammatory signs are declining.

The molecular events underlying inflammation and bone remodelling were investigated using gene expression profiling. The results are based on a first kinetic mapping of global gene expression in the joint during clinical onset and development of arthritis. Expression of specific genes might differ depending on the microanatomical site within the joint and future studies of proteins important in the interplay between inflammation and bone formation should address this. We found that the bone pathology observed histologically was reflected in the Bio Functions, significantly associated with differentially expressed genes, from onset to decline of clinical arthritis in the joint. Moreover, genes involved in inflammation and bone remodelling were co-expressed during the first two weeks after onset of clinical arthritis and, hereafter, the gene expression gradually normalized to control levels, while the clinical inflammation was declining. A muscle-specific signature was observed among the most downregulated genes during the first two weeks after onset of arthritis. This may reflect muscle inactivity and atrophy observed in the model [44] and may translate to the impaired muscle function observed in arthritis patients. However, since animals in the acute disease phase also lose weight, this may partly explain some of the gene expression changes observed in muscle-specific genes.

Several metalloproteinases and cathepsins associated with human arthritis showed sustained, high expression during the entire disease course (Table 1, and Table S10 in Additional file 10). These reflect tissue destruction, in addition to being a link between bone erosion and bone formation. MMP9 and MMP13 have been shown to play a crucial role in endochondral bone formation, as well as in matrix degradation and in OC and osteoprogenitor differentiation [45,46].

Genes with the highest fold change at day 0 to 3 after onset of clinical arthritis reflected osteoclast function and differentiation, in addition to ECM formation and collagen type 1 assembly, while genes showing the highest fold change at week 1 to 2 or week 3 to 4 encompassed a well-known group of OB markers and genes involved in mineralisation (Table 2, Figure 4A and B). These variations in gene expression pattern mirror the development in OB differentiation and function, as gene expression is specific for the differential stages of the OB [47]. The gene expression profiles followed the histological observations: bone erosion, periosteal proliferation and osteoid secretion, was observed in the initial phase followed by onset of

A

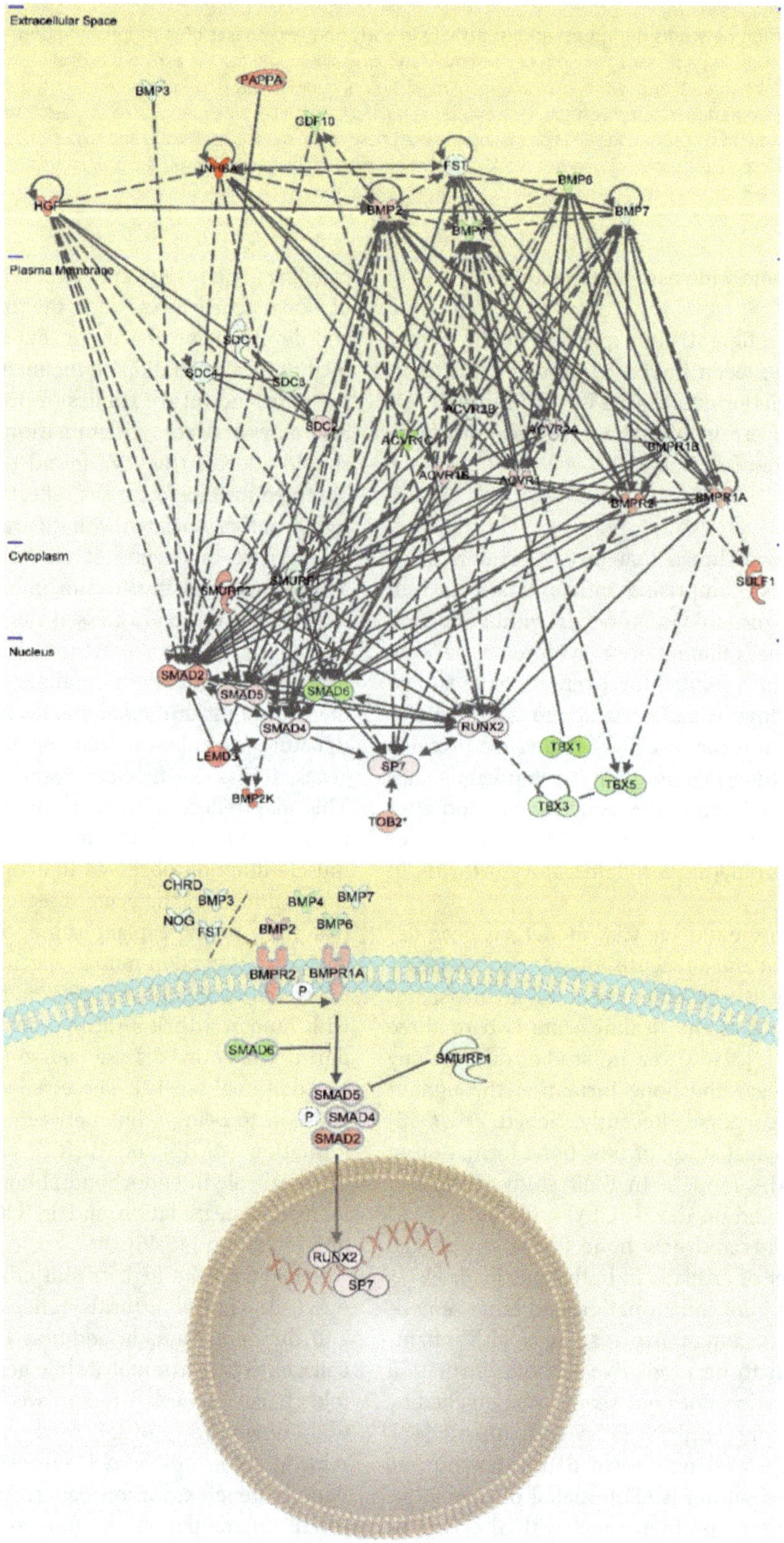

B

Figure 5 Differentially expressed genes related to BMP signalling at day 0 to 3 of arthritis in comparison to non-induced controls. Regulation of genes is indicated by colour and colour intensity (red = upregulated, green = downregulated). **(A)** Network of BMP related genes in general. **(B)** Functional pathway of BMP signalling. BMP, bone morphogenetic protein.

Table 3 Differential expression of genes associated with human arthritis in GWAS studies

Gene symbol	Ctrl[a]	0 to 3d vs. Ctrl[b]	1 to 2w vs. Ctrl[c]	3 to 4w vs. Ctrl[d]	Decline vs. Ctrl[e]	Protein function
	log2	Fold change (*P*-value)				
Ankylosing spondylitis						
Hapln1	**6.72**	**1.69 (0.15)**	**3.10 (0.01)**	**2.89 (0.005)**	**2.08 (0.01)**	**Involved in cartilage development and bone formation. Associated with osteophyte formation in OA [30].**
Edil3	**5.58**	**1.53 (0.14)**	**2.95 (0.003)**	**3.07 (0.005)**	**2.33 (0.11)**	**Integrin ligand with a proposed role in cartilage development and angiogenesis. Inhibitor of the WNT pathway [30].**
Ano6	**7.22**	**2.25 (0.05)**	**1.88 (0.04)**	**1.61 (0.14)**	**1.19 (0.60)**	**Regulates phosphatidylserine exposure on the cell surface, which is essential for mineralisation of bone and involved in osteoclast formation [30,31].**
Psmg1	6.95	2.04 (0.002)	1.91 (0.002)	1.37 (0.03)	1.03 (0.78)	Proteasome Assembly Chaperone 1. The gene is, in addition, associated with inflammatory bowel disease [32].
Rheumatoid arthritis						
Anapc4	6.85	1.77 (0.0008)	1.91 (0.0003)	1.45 (0.02)	1.18 (0.45)	An SNP close to this gene was associated with RA susceptibility [33]. The encoded protein is an E3 ubiquitin ligase involved in control of the cell cycle, muscle cell function, and function of neurons [34].
Cd84	5.61	3.07 (0.01)	3.01 (0.004)	2.17 (0.02)	1.51 (0.12)	Membrane protein involved in immune function. High expression of the gene was associated with a positive response to Etanercept treatment [35].
Il6st	**9.44**	**2.41 (0.03)**	**1.79 (0.06)**	**1.52 (0.10)**	**1.09 (0.76)**	**Signal transducing subunit for cytokines belonging to the IL-6 family. Activates Stat-3, which plays a role in OC and OB differentiation and their interaction [36].**
Ptpn2	6.68	1.74 (0.06)	1.78 (0.02)	1.32 (0.30)	1.46 (0.16)	Protein phosphatase involved in T-cell activation by regulation of the JAK/STAT signalling pathway [33,37,38].
Cdk6	5.88	2.51 (0.10)	2.35 (0.08)	2.11 (0.08)	1.64 (0.21)	Cyclin-dependent kinase involved in proliferation of lymphocytes [39].
Prkcq	7.42	0.48 (0.17)	0.65 (0.26)	0.55 (0.16)	0.61 (0.32)	Kinase involved in activation of NFκB and AP-1 transcription factors [39].
Prkch	7.20	1.36 (0.04)	1.43 (0.07)	1.58 (0.06)	0.99 (0.95)	Serine/threonine kinase. The association with RA is suggestive [38].
Osteoarthritis						
Gnl3	7.81	2.41 (0.11)	2.10 (0.08)	2.17 (0.07)	1.47 (0.34)	Nucleostemin. Increased in *in vitro* cultures of chondrocytes from patients with OA [40].
Glt8d	7.18	1.97 (0.03)	1.99 (0.02)	1.43 (0.05)	1.13 (0.71)	Involved in glycosylation of cartilage proteins [40].
Pla2g	5.96	1.47 (0.16)	1.67 (0.04)	2.06 (0.03)	1.71 (0.04)	Cytosolic phospholipase A2 enzyme. mRNA transcript was abundantly expressed in chondrocytes from OA patients [41].
Ptgs2	6.91	2.66 (0.01)	1.72 (0.07)	1.15 (0.41)	1.56 (0.03)	Cyclooxygenase 2 (COX-2). mRNA transcript was abundantly expressed in chondrocytes from OA patients [41].
Col12a1	**8.24**	**4.56 (0.04)**	**4.82 (0.01)**	**2.97 (0.04)**	**1.74 (0.22)**	**A SNP close to this gene has been associated with OA susceptibility [40]. The encoded protein is expressed by OB in areas of bone formation. KO mice have skeletal abnormalities with less mechanical strength and reduced matrix deposition [24].**

[a]Mean log2 expression in non-induced control mice. Mean fold change and *P*-value in comparison to control: [b]on day 0 to 3, [c]in week 1 to 2, [d]in week 3 to 4, [e]in the declining disease phase. Genes shown in bold are encoding proteins with a known function in cartilage- or bone remodelling. Ctrl, control; GWAS, genome-wide association studies; IL-6, interleukin 6; KO, knockout; NFκB, nuclear factor kappa B; OA, osteoarthritis; OB, osteoblast; OC, osteoclast; RA, rheumatoid arthritis; WNT, wingless-type.

endochondral bone formation and mineralisation in weeks 1 to 2. The data support a model for bone remodelling during arthritis, where bone erosion is mainly taking place during the very early phase of clinical arthritis, with the onset of tissue remodelling and bone formation following shortly after, developing in parallel with the inflammation. When the inflammatory response ceases, the addition of new bone decreases, and the hitherto created bone is remodelled and mineralised. As suggested by the histological results, the newly formed bone may be created in different processes depending on the microanatomical site. Thus, addition of bone in the periosteum takes place first, without preceding cartilage formation, while osteophytes at the joint margin are created in a process resembling endochondral ossification (Figure 6). A comparison of the present data to the proteoglycan-induced arthritis (PGIA) model reveals a high degree of similarity concerning the mixed anabolic and catabolic bone remodelling profile [8]. In contrast, the TNFα-transgenic arthritis mouse model showed a primarily catabolic bone remodelling profile, while genes representing the osteoproliferative response showed no or marginally differential expression [7]. This is in line with a general comprehension of the TNFα-transgenic mouse as a mainly erosive model, while the PGIA and CIA models demonstrate osteoproliferative arthritis. All three models showed a strong up-regulation of *Mmps* and *Timp1*. Data are compared in Table S10 Additional file 10.

Highly differentially expressed genes encoding proteins involved in bone formation between day 0 to 3 of clinical arthritis are potential links between inflammation and bone formation. Two of these genes are the insulin-like growth factor (IGF)-dependent proteinase pregnancy-associated plasma protein A gene (*Pappa*) and periostin (*Postn*). In addition, genes particularly involved in early ECM formation, preceding bone formation, are potential candidates. The PAPP-A protein is an anabolic growth factor in bone *in vivo* and *in vitro* [48,49] and regulates bioavailability of Insulin-like growth factor (IGF) involved in bone formation [50], and also differentially expressed. Expression of *Pappa* is stimulated by inflammatory cytokines in several cell types, including OBs, and macrophages isolated from artherosclerotic lesions [51,52]. It has recently been identified as a marker of inflammation in acute coronary syndrome [53]. Furthermore, *Pappa* knockout mice display disturbed bone formation [54,55], while mice overexpressing *Pappa* have increased bone formation [48,49]. Thus, *Pappa* expression might be induced in the early inflammatory environment and the protein could be involved in initiating bone formation in the CIA model.

The *Postn* gene is one of the highly differentially expressed genes with a proposed role in bone remodelling.

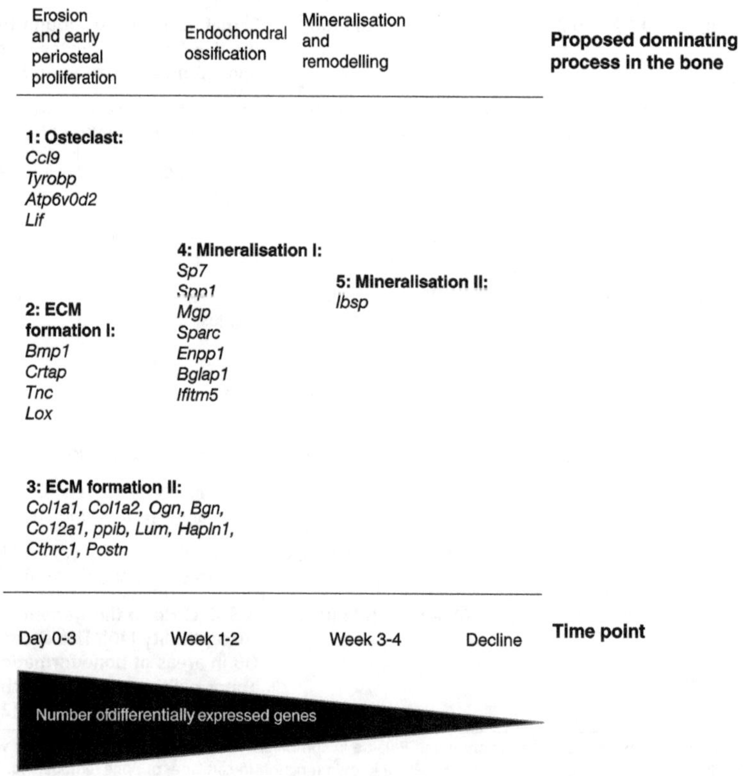

Figure 6 Bone remodelling in the CIA model. Model of bone remodelling during the course of clinical arthritis. The proposed dominating process in the bone is shown in the top part of the figure. Differentially expressed genes, encoding proteins with a function in bone remodelling, are divided into groups according to function and time point of highest differential expression in comparison to the control. All genes are upregulated in comparison to the control at the indicated time-point. Group 1: genes encoding proteins involved in osteoclast function and differentiation; Group 2: genes encoding proteins with a function in extracellular matrix formation and collagen type I assembly (highest differential expression at day 0 to 4); Group 3: genes encoding proteins with a function in extracellular matrix formation and collagen type I assembly (sustained high differential expression on day 0 to 4 and week 1 to 2); Group 4: genes with a function in mineralisation of bone (highest differential expression in week 1 to 2); Group 5: genes with a function in mineralisation of bone (highest differential expression during week 3 to 4). CIA, collagen-induced arthritis; ECM, extracellular matrix.

It is preferentially located in the periostium and is re-expressed during fracture repair, mechanical stress, and in RA [14]. The expression is regulated by BMP2 and TGFβ. Overexpression of periostin increases bone formation possibly by promoting cell survival of preosteoblasts and OBs [56]. By binding fibronectin, tenascin and BMP1, it increases the activation of pro-lysyl oxidase, which in turn cross-links collagen [14]. Moreover, BMP1 has been linked to arthritis and bone formation [57,58] and may increase bone formation in several ways.

In weeks 1 to 2 after clinical onset, many genes reflecting the mineralisation of osteoid showed the highest differential expression over time in comparison to control (Table 2 and Figure 4B). Integrin-binding sialoprotein (*Ibsp*) is involved in the formation of crystals, as well as cell attachment to hydroxyapatite [20]. Osteonectin (*Sparc*) binds and connects hydroxyapatite to collagen type I [21], while osteonectin (*Spp1*) binds hydroxyapatite crystals, inhibiting their formation [21]. Moreover, these genes also reflect the complexity of interactions between ECM, OCs and OBs, as many of them have dual functions in bone remodelling.

In summary, the network of regulated genes involved in collagen type I assembly represented in Figure 4A, might play an important role in arthritis-associated ECM formation, leading to fibrosis and osteophyte formation.

Of particular interest in arthritis-associated bone remodelling are molecules belonging to the BMP and WNT signalling pathways. In human arthritis, the BMP ligands 2 and 6 [59] and their receptors BMPR1a and BMPR2 [60] were upregulated, while BMP ligands 4 and 5 were downregulated in RA and osteoarthritis (OA) synovium in comparison to normal control samples. Our results showed a similar up-regulation of the genes for the receptors BMPR1a and BMPR2, but down-regulation of *Bmp4*, *Bmp6* and *Bmp7* (Figure 5).

One of the strongly upregulated genes in this study is *Inhba* (Inhibin beta A), which may stimulate the TGFβ signalling pathway through binding to receptors Acv1b, Avr2a and Avr2b. This non-steroidal hormone regulating follicle-stimulating hormone (FSH) secretion is reported to increase bone formation in a knock-in transgenic mouse [61], and has been associated with human arthritis [62].

A profile of WNT signalling is not distinct in our gene expression data, since most of the genes belonging to this pathway were marginally differentially expressed compared to the control samples. However, a number of WNT inhibitors were differentially expressed. These included the upregulated *Hif1a*. The encoded protein is a hypoxia inducible factor that plays a role in angiogenesis during endochondral bone formation. Together with Sp7, it inhibits the WNT signalling pathway [63]. Moreover, WNT inhibitors *Sost* and *Ndgr2* were both downregulated and *Dkk1*, the master regulator of WNT signalling, was slightly downregulated. This could be expected during anabolic bone conditions. *Sost* and *Dkk1* downregulation has been associated with proteoglycan-induced arthritis in mice, and DKK1 with human AS [8].

In Table 3, several genes identified in GWAS of human arthritis are listed together with the expression data from the CIA model found in the present study. The five underlined genes encode proteins with a function in cartilage or bone remodelling, and are potential therapeutic candidate genes. The expression of those genes highlights the importance of the CIA model for studies of osteoproliferative inflammatory arthritic diseases.

Conclusions

Bone remodelling in the CIA model results in ankylosis within one to two weeks after clinical disease onset and occurs simultaneously with the local inflammatory process in the joint. Furthermore, in this study, we have identified networks of genes involved in early and late bone formation, as well as genes associated with human arthritis, which may provide potential targets for modulating bone formation in arthritis.

Taken together, this suggests that the CIA model is an important tool in investigations of the relationship between inflammation and bone formation in the search for therapeutic targets to prevent ankylosis in inflammatory arthritis.

Additional files

Additional file 1: Table S2. A and B: Overview of samples used for histology and global gene expression study.

Additional file 2: Figure S1. Illustration of histological bone scores. **(A)** Bone erosion and formation score 0: no pathological changes. **(B)** Bone erosion score 2. **(C)** Bone formation score 2. **(D)** Bone erosion score 4. **(E)** Bone formation score 4.

Additional file 3: RMA gene default summary of array data for review.

Additional file 4: Table S4. Table of assay IDs for specific primer/probe sets (Life Techologies) used for validation of gene expression at AROS Applied Biotechnology A/S.

Additional file 5: Table S5. (A) Comparison of samples from day 0 to 3 versus control. **(B)** Comparison of samples from week 1 to 2 versus control. **C)** Comparison of samples from week 3 to 4 versus control. **(D)** Comparison of samples from the declining disease phase versus control.

Additional file 6: Figure S6. Validation of selected genes by qPCR showing correlation between the microarray data (X-axis, log2-transformed values) and the qPCR data (Y-axis, δCt values). $\delta C_{t,gene}$ is calculated as $C_{t,Gapdh}$-$C_{t,gene}$. Color coding, Red: day 0 to 3; Yellow: week 1 to 2; Green: week 3 to 4; Blue: declining disease phase; Black: control.

Additional file 7: Figure S7. Validation of selected genes by qPCR showing a non-significant correlation between the microarray data (X-axis, log2 transformed values) and the qPCR data (Y-axis, δCt values). $\delta C_{t,gene}$ is calculated as $C_{t,Gapdh}$-$C_{t,gene}$. Color coding, Red: day 0 to 3; Yellow: week 1 to 2; Green: week 3 to 4; Blue: declining disease phase; Black: control.

Additional file 8: Table S8. Correlation data and *P*-values for correlation between microarray and qPCR data.

Additional file 9: Table S9. Selected Bio Functions related to bone. The Bio Functions that form the basis of the list of genes encoding proteins with a function in bone remodelling.

Additional file 10: Table S10. List of genes encoding proteins with a suggested function in bone remodelling. The list was created from data in the selected Bio Functions and supplemented with genes based on literature search. The data are also compared to data from other gene expression studies. A list of references is available (please contact the corresponding author).

Abbreviations

AIA: antibody-induced arthritis; AS: ankylosing spondylitis; BMP: bone morphogenetic protein; CFA: complete Freund's adjuvant; CIA: collagen-induced arthritis; CII: collagen type II; ECM: extracellular matrix; ERK: extracellular signal-regulated kinases; FSH: follicle-stimulating hormone; GWAS: genome-wide association studies; IFA: incomplete Freund's adjuvant; IGF: insulin-like growth factor; IPA: Ingenuity Pathway Analysis; MMP: matrix metallopeptidase; OA: osteoarthritis; OB: osteoblast; OC: osteoclast; PGIA: proteoglycan-induced arthritis; PsA: psoriatic arthritis; RA: rheumatoid arthritis; TGFβ: transforming growth factor beta; TNFα: tumor necrosis factor alpha; WNT: wingless-type.

Competing interests

The authors declare that they have no competing interests.

Authors' contributions

KD conceived, designed and conducted the study, carried out the microscopic analysis with KM and further analysis of the array data with TLi, and drafted the manuscript. TLi analysed and interpreted the microarray data, the IPA, and assisted in drafting the manuscript. TM carried out the first-line analysis and interpretation of the microarray data, and revised the manuscript critically. KM analysed and interpreted the microscopic data, and revised the manuscript critically. LS conceived and participated in design of the study, and revised the manuscript critically. TLa conceived and participated in design of the study, and revised the manuscript critically. ÅA conceived and participated in design of the study, and assisted substantially in drafting the manuscript. All authors read and approved the final manuscript, and agree to be accountable for all aspects of the work.

Acknowledgements

We wish to thank Rikke Bøgebo and Mikala Skydsgaard for assistance with data analysis, Marianne Løvendorf for technical assistance, John Zibert and Gunnar Olsen for contributing to the design of the study.

The study was supported by: The Danish Association for Rheumatism, The Graduate Program for In vivo Pharmacology, University of Copenhagen and LEO Pharma.

References

1. Finzel S, Englbrecht M, Engelke K, Stach C, Schett G. A comparative study of periarticular bone lesions in rheumatoid arthritis and psoriatic arthritis. Ann Rheum Dis. 2011;70:122–7.
2. Holmdahl R, Andersson EC, Andersen CB, Svejgaard A, Fugger L. Transgenic mouse models of rheumatoid arthritis. Immunol Rev. 1999;169:161–73.
3. Schett G, Stolina M, Dwyer D, Zack D, Uderhardt S, Kronke G, et al. Tumor necrosis factor alpha and RANKL blockade cannot halt bony spur formation in experimental inflammatory arthritis. Arthritis Rheum. 2009;60:2644–54.
4. Wozney JM, Rosen V. Bone morphogenetic protein and bone morphogenetic protein gene family in bone formation and repair. Clin Orthop Relat Res. 1998;346:26–37.
5. Schett G, Zwerina J, David JP. The role of Wnt proteins in arthritis. Nat Clin Pract Rheumatol. 2008;4:473–80.
6. Edgar R, Domrachev M, Lash AE. Gene Expression Omnibus: NCBI gene expression and hybridization array data repository. Nucleic Acids Res. 2002;30:207–10.
7. Aidinis V, Carninci P, Armaka M, Witke W, Harokopos V, Pavelka N, et al. Cytoskeletal rearrangements in synovial fibroblasts as a novel pathophysiological determinant of modeled rheumatoid arthritis. PLoS Genet. 2005;1:e48.
8. Haynes KR, Pettit AR, Duan R, Tseng HW, Glant TT, Brown MA, et al. Excessive bone formation in a mouse model of ankylosing spondylitis is associated with decreases in Wnt pathway inhibitors. Arthritis Res Ther. 2012;14:R253.
9. Lean JM, Murphy C, Fuller K, Chambers TJ. CCL9/MIP-1gamma and its receptor CCR1 are the major chemokine ligand/receptor species expressed by osteoclasts. J Cell Biochem. 2002;87:386–93.
10. Ota K, Quint P, Weivoda MM, Ruan M, Pederson L, Westendorf JJ, et al. Transforming growth factor beta 1 induces CXCL16 and leukemia inhibitory factor expression in osteoclasts to modulate migration of osteoblast progenitors. Bone. 2013;57:68–75.
11. Wu H, Xu G, Li YP. Atp6v0d2 is an essential component of the osteoclast-specific proton pump that mediates extracellular acidification in bone resorption. J Bone Miner Res. 2009;24:871–85.
12. Zou W, Reeve JL, Liu Y, Teitelbaum SL, Ross FP. DAP12 couples c-Fms activation to the osteoclast cytoskeleton by recruitment of Syk. Mol Cell. 2008;31:422–31.
13. Eyre DR, Weis MA. Bone collagen: new clues to its mineralization mechanism from recessive osteogenesis imperfecta. Calcif Tissue Int. 2013;93:338–47.
14. Merle B, Garnero P. The multiple facets of periostin in bone metabolism. Osteoporos Int. 2012;23:1199–212.
15. Boskey AL, Christensen B, Taleb H, Sorensen ES. Post-translational modification of osteopontin: effects on in vitro hydroxyapatite formation and growth. Biochem Biophys Res Commun. 2012;419:333–8.
16. Gopalakrishnan R, Ouyang H, Somerman MJ, McCauley LK, Franceschi RT. Matrix gamma-carboxyglutamic acid protein is a key regulator of PTH-mediated inhibition of mineralization in MC3T3-E1 osteoblast-like cells. Endocrinology. 2001;142:4379–88.
17. Kaback LA, Soung DY, Naik A, Smith N, Schwarz EM, O'Keefe RJ, et al. Osterix/Sp7 regulates mesenchymal stem cell mediated endochondral ossification. J Cell Physiol. 2008;214:173–82.
18. Mackenzie NC, Zhu D, Milne EM, Van 't Hof R, Martin A, Darryl QL, et al. Altered bone development and an increase in FGF-23 expression in Enpp1(−/−) mice. PLoS One. 2012;7:e32177.
19. Moffatt P, Gaumond MH, Salois P, Sellin K, Bessette MC, Godin E, et al. Bril: a novel bone-specific modulator of mineralization. J Bone Miner Res. 2008;23:1497–508.
20. Nahar NN, Missana LR, Garimella R, Tague SE, Anderson HC. Matrix vesicles are carriers of bone morphogenetic proteins (BMPs), vascular endothelial growth factor (VEGF), and noncollagenous matrix proteins. J Bone Miner Metab. 2008;26:514–9.
21. Delany AM, Hankenson KD. Thrombospondin-2 and SPARC/osteonectin are critical regulators of bone remodeling. J Cell Commun Signal. 2009;3:227–38.
22. Chen XD, Shi S, Xu T, Robey PG, Young MF. Age-related osteoporosis in biglycan-deficient mice is related to defects in bone marrow stromal cells. J Bone Miner Res. 2002;17:331–40.
23. Ge G, Seo NS, Liang X, Hopkins DR, Hook M, Greenspan DS. Bone morphogenetic protein-1/tolloid-related metalloproteinases process osteoglycin and enhance its ability to regulate collagen fibrillogenesis. J Biol Chem. 2004;279:41626–33.
24. Izu Y, Sun M, Zwolanek D, Veit G, Williams V, Cha B, et al. Type XII collagen regulates osteoblast polarity and communication during bone formation. J Cell Biol. 2011;193:1115–30.
25. Kimura H, Kwan KM, Zhang Z, Deng JM, Darnay BG, Behringer RR, et al. Cthrc1 is a positive regulator of osteoblastic bone formation. PLoS One. 2008;3:e3174.
26. Raouf A, Ganss B, McMahon C, Vary C, Roughley PJ, Seth A. Lumican is a major proteoglycan component of the bone matrix. Matrix Biol. 2002;21:361–7.
27. Urano T, Narusawa K, Shiraki M, Sasaki N, Hosoi T, Ouchi Y, et al. Single-nucleotide polymorphism in the hyaluronan and proteoglycan link protein 1 (HAPLN1) gene is associated with spinal osteophyte formation and disc degeneration in Japanese women. Eur Spine J. 2011;20:572–7.
28. Gowen M, Lazner F, Dodds R, Kapadia R, Feild J, Tavaria M, et al. Cathepsin K knockout mice develop osteopetrosis due to a deficit in matrix degradation but not demineralization. J Bone Miner Res. 1999;14:1654–63.

29. Baumgrass R, Williamson MK, Price PA. Identification of peptide fragments generated by digestion of bovine and human osteocalcin with the lysosomal proteinases cathepsin B, D, L, H, and S. J Bone Miner Res. 1997;12:447–55.
30. Lin Z, Bei JX, Shen M, Li Q, Liao Z, Zhang Y, et al. A genome-wide association study in Han Chinese identifies new susceptibility loci for ankylosing spondylitis. Nat Genet. 2012;44:73–7.
31. Ehlen HW, Chinenkova M, Moser M, Munter HM, Krause Y, Gross S, et al. Inactivation of anoctamin-6/Tmem16f, a regulator of phosphatidylserine scrambling in osteoblasts, leads to decreased mineral deposition in skeletal tissues. J Bone Miner Res. 2013;28:246–59.
32. Reveille JD, Sims AM, Danoy P, Evans DM, Leo P, Pointon JJ, et al. Genome-wide association study of ankylosing spondylitis identifies non-MHC susceptibility loci. Nat Genet. 2010;42:123–7.
33. The Wellcome Trust Case Control Consortium. Genome-wide association study of 14,000 cases of seven common diseases and 3,000 shared controls. Nature. 2007;447:661–78.
34. Manchado E, Eguren M, Malumbres M. The anaphase-promoting complex/cyclosome (APC/C): cell-cycle-dependent and -independent functions. Biochem Soc Trans. 2010;38:65–71.
35. Cui J, Stahl EA, Saevarsdottir S, Miceli C, Diogo D, Trynka G, et al. Genome-wide association study and gene expression analysis identifies CD84 as a predictor of response to etanercept therapy in rheumatoid arthritis. PLoS Genet. 2013;9:e1003394.
36. Itoh S, Udagawa N, Takahashi N, Yoshitake F, Narita H, Ebisu S, et al. A critical role for interleukin-6 family-mediated Stat3 activation in osteoblast differentiation and bone formation. Bone. 2006;39:505–12.
37. Cobb JE, Plant D, Flynn E, Tadjeddine M, Dieude P, Cornelis F, et al. Identification of the tyrosine-protein phosphatase non-receptor type 2 as a rheumatoid arthritis susceptibility locus in Europeans. PLoS One. 2013;8:e66456.
38. Okada Y, Terao C, Ikari K, Kochi Y, Ohmura K, Suzuki A, et al. Meta-analysis identifies nine new loci associated with rheumatoid arthritis in the Japanese population. Nat Genet. 2012;44:511–6.
39. Raychaudhuri S, Remmers EF, Lee AT, Hackett R, Guiducci C, Burtt NP, et al. Common variants at CD40 and other loci confer risk of rheumatoid arthritis. Nat Genet. 2008;40:1216–23.
40. Zeggini E, Panoutsopoulou K, Southam L, Rayner NW, Day-Williams AG, Lopes MC, et al. Identification of new susceptibility loci for osteoarthritis (arcOGEN): a genome-wide association study. Lancet. 2012;380:815–23.
41. Valdes AM, Loughlin J, Timms KM, van Meurs JJ, Southam L, Wilson SG, et al. Genome-wide association scan identifies a prostaglandin-endoperoxide synthase 2 variant involved in risk of knee osteoarthritis. Am J Hum Genet. 2008;82:1231–40.
42. Baraliakos X, Listing J, Rudwaleit M, Sieper J, Braun J. The relationship between inflammation and new bone formation in patients with ankylosing spondylitis 2. Arthritis Res Ther. 2008;10:R104.
43. van der Heijde D, Landewe R, Einstein S, Ory P, Vosse D, Ni L, et al. Radiographic progression of ankylosing spondylitis after up to two years of treatment with etanercept. Arthritis Rheum. 2008;58:1324–31.
44. Filippin LI, Teixeira VN, Viacava PR, Lora PS, Xavier LL, Xavier RM. Temporal development of muscle atrophy in murine model of arthritis is related to disease severity. J Cachexia Sarcopenia Muscle. 2013;4:231–8.
45. Ortega N, Behonick D, Stickens D, Werb Z. How proteases regulate bone morphogenesis. Ann N Y Acad Sci. 2003;995:109–16.
46. Stickens D, Behonick DJ, Ortega N, Heyer B, Hartenstein B, Yu Y, et al. Altered endochondral bone development in matrix metalloproteinase 13-deficient mice. Development. 2004;131:5883–95.
47. Neve A, Corrado A, Cantatore FP. Osteoblast physiology in normal and pathological conditions. Cell Tissue Res. 2011;343:289–302.
48. Phang D, Rehage M, Bonafede B, Hou D, Xing W, Mohan S, et al. Inactivation of insulin-like-growth factors diminished the anabolic effects of pregnancy-associated plasma protein-A (PAPP-A) on bone in mice. Growth Horm IGF Res. 2010;20:192–200.
49. Qin X, Wergedal JE, Rehage M, Tran K, Newton J, Lam P, et al. Pregnancy-associated plasma protein-A increases osteoblast proliferation in vitro and bone formation in vivo. Endocrinology. 2006;147:5653–61.
50. Boldt HB, Conover CA. Pregnancy-associated plasma protein-A (PAPP-A): a local regulator of IGF bioavailability through cleavage of IGFBPs. Growth Horm IGF Res. 2007;17:10–8.
51. Conover CA, Chen BK, Resch ZT. Regulation of pregnancy-associated plasma protein-A expression in cultured human osteoblasts. Bone. 2004;34:297–302.
52. Sangiorgi G, Mauriello A, Bonanno E, Oxvig C, Conover CA, Christiansen M, et al. Pregnancy-associated plasma protein-a is markedly expressed by monocyte-macrophage cells in vulnerable and ruptured carotid atherosclerotic plaques: a link between inflammation and cerebrovascular events. J Am Coll Cardiol. 2006;47:2201–11.
53. Li W, Li H, Gu F. CRP and TNF-alpha induce PAPP-A expression in human peripheral blood mononuclear cells. Mediators Inflamm. 2012;2012:697832.
54. Miller BS, Bronk JT, Nishiyama T, Yamagiwa H, Srivastava A, Bolander ME, et al. Pregnancy associated plasma protein-A is necessary for expeditious fracture healing in mice. J Endocrinol. 2007;192:505–13.
55. Tanner SJ, Hefferan TE, Rosen CJ, Conover CA. Impact of pregnancy-associated plasma protein-a deletion on the adult murine skeleton. J Bone Miner Res. 2008;23:655–62.
56. Zhu S, Barbe MF, Liu C, Hadjiargyrou M, Popoff SN, Rani S, et al. Periostin-like-factor in osteogenesis. J Cell Physiol. 2009;218:584–92.
57. Sanchez-Sabate E, Alvarez L, Gil-Garay E, Munuera L, Vilaboa N. Identification of differentially expressed genes in trabecular bone from the iliac crest of osteoarthritic patients. Osteoarthritis Cartilage. 2009;17:1106–14.
58. Grgurevic L, Macek B, Mercep M, Jelic M, Smoljanovic T, Erjavec I, et al. Bone morphogenetic protein (BMP)1-3 enhances bone repair. Biochem Biophys Res Commun. 2011;408:25–31.
59. Lories RJ, Derese I, Ceuppens JL, Luyten FP. Bone morphogenetic proteins 2 and 6, expressed in arthritic synovium, are regulated by proinflammatory cytokines and differentially modulate fibroblast-like synoviocyte apoptosis. Arthritis Rheum. 2003;48:2807–18.
60. Marinova-Mutafchieva L, Taylor P, Funa K, Maini RN, Zvaifler NJ. Mesenchymal cells expressing bone morphogenetic protein receptors are present in the rheumatoid arthritis joint. Arthritis Rheum. 2000;43:2046–55.
61. Perrien DS, Nicks KM, Liu L, Akel NS, Bacon AW, Skinner RA, et al. Inhibin A enhances bone formation during distraction osteogenesis. J Orthop Res. 2012;30:288–95.
62. El-Gendi SS, Moniem AE, Tawfik NM, Ashmawy MM, Mohammed OA, Mostafa AK, et al. Value of serum and synovial fluid activin A and inhibin A in some rheumatic diseases. Int J Rheum Dis. 2010;13:273–9.
63. Chen D, Li Y, Zhou Z, Xing Y, Zhong Y, Zou X, et al. Synergistic inhibition of Wnt pathway by HIF-1alpha and osteoblast-specific transcription factor osterix (Osx) in osteoblasts. PLoS One. 2012;7:e52948.

3

Heterogeneous expression pattern of interleukin 17A (IL-17A), IL-17F and their receptors in synovium of rheumatoid arthritis, psoriatic arthritis and osteoarthritis: possible explanation for nonresponse to anti-IL-17 therapy?

Lisa GM van Baarsen[1,2*†], Maria C Lebre[1,2†], Dennis van der Coelen[1,2], Saïda Aarrass[1,2], Man W Tang[1], Tamara H Ramwadhdoebe[1,2], Daniëlle M Gerlag[1,3] and Paul P Tak[1,3]

Abstract

Introduction: Accumulating evidence suggests an important role for interleukin 17 (IL-17) in the pathogenesis of several inflammatory diseases, including rheumatoid arthritis (RA) and psoriatic arthritis (PsA). Accordingly, clinical trials aimed at blocking IL-17 have been initiated, but clinical results between patients and across different diseases have been highly variable. The objective was to determine the variability in expression of IL-17A, IL-17F and their receptors IL-17RA and IL-17RC in the synovia of patients with arthritis.

Methods: Synovial biopsies were obtained from patients with RA ($n = 11$), PsA ($n = 15$) and inflammatory osteoarthritis (OA, $n = 14$). For comparison, synovia from noninflamed knee joints ($n = 7$) obtained from controls were included. Frozen sections were stained for IL-17A, IL-17F, IL-17RA and IL-17RC and evaluated by digital image analysis. We used confocal microscopy to determine which cells in the synovium express IL-17A and IL-17F, double-staining with CD4, CD8, CD15, CD68, CD163, CD31, von Willebrand factor, peripheral lymph node address in, lymphatic vessel endothelial hyaluronan receptor 1, mast cell tryptase and retinoic acid receptor–related orphan receptor γt (RORγt).

Results: IL-17A, IL-17F, IL-17RA and IL-17RC were abundantly expressed in synovial tissues of all patient groups. Whereas IL-17RA was present mostly in the synovial sublining, IL-17RC was abundantly expressed in the intimal lining layer. Digital image analysis showed a significant ($P < 0.05$) increase of only IL-17A in arthritis patients compared to noninflamed control tissues. The expression of IL-17A, IL-17F and their receptors was similar in the different patient groups, but highly variable between individual patients. CD4+ and CD8+ cells coexpressed IL-17A, and few cells coexpressed IL-17F. IL-17A and IL-17F were not expressed by CD15+ neutrophils. Mast cells were only occasionally positive for IL-17A or IL-17F. Interestingly, IL-17A and IL-17F staining was also observed in macrophages, as well as in blood vessels and lymphatics. This staining probably reflects receptor-bound cytokine staining. Many infiltrated cells were positive for the transcription factor RORγt. Colocalisation between RORγt and IL-17A and IL-17F indicates local IL-17 production.
(Continued on next page)

* Correspondence: e.g.vanbaarsen@amc.uva.nl
†Equal contributors
[1]Division of Clinical Immunology and Rheumatology, Academic Medical Centre, University of Amsterdam, Meibergdreef 9, 1105, AZ, Amsterdam, the Netherlands
[2]Department of Experimental Immunology, Academic Medical Centre, University of Amsterdam, Meibergdreef 9, 1105 AZ, Amsterdam, The Netherlands
Full list of author information is available at the end of the article

(Continued from previous page)

Conclusions: Increased expression of IL-17A is not restricted to synovial tissues of RA and PsA patients; it is also observed in inflammatory OA. The heterogeneous expression levels may explain nonresponse to anti-IL-17 therapy in subsets of patients.

Introduction

Whereas initial studies focused mainly on type 1 helper T (Th1) cells as having a prominent role in rheumatoid arthritis (RA), subsequent studies suggested that Th17 cells also have an important role in this disease. The functional role of this new type of effector helper T cell has been studied extensively in recent years and shows that it has important functions in the response to microbial infection and in promoting and maintaining chronic inflammation and autoimmunity [1]. Interestingly, recent studies have demonstrated the plasticity of Th17 cells and have indicated their pathogenic role, especially when shifted towards Th1 cells [2-4].

Th17 cells were originally identified by their expression of the proinflammatory cytokine interleukin 17 (IL-17) and represent a distinct subset of CD4+ cells characterised by the expression of Retinoic acid receptor–related orphan receptor γt (RORγt) [5]. The production of IL-17 is specifically regulated by this transcription factor. The cytokine IL-17 is formally referred to as IL-17A and is part of a larger IL-17 cytokine family consisting of six members ranging from IL-17A to IL-17F. The most studied family members are IL-17A and IL-17F, which are mainly produced by Th17 cells to protect against extracellular pathogens and fungi but also have proinflammatory properties. IL-17 promotes the transcriptional activation of proinflammatory cytokines, hematopoietic cytokines, acute-phase response genes and antimicrobial mediators [6], especially in synergy with other proinflammatory cytokines such as tumour necrosis factor and IL-1β [7,8]. The common receptor for the IL-17 Family members is IL-17RA [9]. In addition to IL-17RA, IL-17RC is required for signalling in response to IL-17A or IL-17F [10,11].

Levels of IL-17 have been found to be increased in the synovial fluid and tissues of RA patients [12-14]. Furthermore, studies in several experimental animal models demonstrated a detrimental role of IL-17 in arthritis [15-17]. IL-17$^{-/-}$ mice are resistant to collagen-induced arthritis [18]. Therefore, it has been suggested that IL-17 may play a crucial role in the pathogenesis of different forms of arthritis by inducing synovial inflammation and promoting bone destruction [19,20]. Accordingly, several clinical trials targeting the IL-17 pathway in RA [21], psoriasis [22,23], psoriatic arthritis (PsA) [24] and ankylosing spondylitis [25] have been initiated (reviewed in [26]). Although psoriasis patients show marked clinical benefit of targeting IL-17A, the clinical response in RA and PsA has been limited and variable between patients [27]. Conceivably, inhibiting IL-17 is only beneficial for those arthritis patients with increased cytokine levels in the target tissue. To provide more insight into the heterogeneity of the expression of IL-17 and IL-17 receptors at the site of inflammation, we investigated the expression of IL-17A, IL-17F and their receptors at the protein level in synovial tissues from inflammatory arthritis patients.

Methods

Patients and synovial tissue collection

We included biological naïve patients with RA (according to the American College of Rheumatology (ACR) 1987 criteria [28], $n = 11$), PsA (Caspar criteria [29], $n = 15$) and inflammatory osteoarthritis (OA; according to the 1986 ACR criteria for OA [30], $n = 14$). For research purposes all patients underwent miniarthroscopic synovial biopsy sampling of an actively inflamed ankle or knee joint [31]. Six to eight samples were collected for immunohistochemistry (IHC) to correct for sampling error, as described previously [32]. For comparison non-inflammatory controls (n = 7) were included, patients who underwent orthopaedic arthroscopy for non-inflammatory joint pain. Table 1 shows the demographic and clinical features. The study was approved by the Institutional Review Board of the Academic Medical Centre and performed according to the Declaration of Helsinki. All study patients provided written informed consent.

To ensure preservation of antigenic content [31,32], synovial biopsy samples were snap-frozen *en bloc* in Tissue-Tek O.C.T. compound (Sakura Finetek Europe, Zoeterwoude, the Netherlands) immediately after collection and stored in liquid nitrogen. Synovial tissue biopsies were cut into 5-μm sections and mounted on StarFrost adhesive glass slides (Knittelgläser, Braunschweig, Germany), after which slides were sealed in parafilm (Bemis, Neenah, WI, USA) and stored at −80°C until further use.

Antibodies

To investigate the detailed expression pattern of IL-17 in synovium, tissue sections were stained using mouse monoclonal antibodies against IL-17A (immunoglobulin G1 (IgG1), clone 41802), IL-17F (IgG2a, clone 197315) and their receptors IL-17RA (IgG1, clone 133617) and IL-17RC (IgG2b, clone 309882), all from R&D Systems (Minneapolis, MN, USA). For colocalisation studies, we used antibodies against the transcription factor RORγt

Table 1 Demographic and clinical features[a]

	Controls (*n* = 7)	RA (*n* = 11)	PsA (*n* = 15)	OA (*n* = 14)
Age, yr	47 (40 to 60)	49 (45 to 62)	48 (34 to 56)	68 (54 to 77)
Females, *n* (%)	2 (29)	7 (64)	7 (47)	10 (71)
Disease duration, mo	NA	18 (8 to 88)	41 (23 to 84)[b]	42 (13 to 72)[c]
Erosive disease, *n* (%)	NA	3/8 (38)	ND	ND
RF-positive, *n*/total (%)	NA	3/11 (27)	ND	ND
ACPA-positive, *n* (%)	NA	4/7 (57)	ND	ND
VAS GDA	NA	57 (55 to 85)	67 (54 to 75)	ND
TJC28, *n*	NA	9 (7 to 13)	2 (1 to 12)	ND
SJC28	NA	11 (6 to 14)	2 (1 to 12)	ND
ESR, mm/h	NA	23 (16 to 47)	34 (8 to 56)	ND
CRP, mg/L	NA	24.3 (12.0 to 37.0)	11.0 (4.7 to 18.0)	ND
DAS28	NA	5.46 (5.33 to 6.62)	4.67 (2.83 to 5.99)	ND
NSAID use, *n* (%)	NA	7 (64)	6 (40)	6 (67)[d]
MTX use, *n* (%)	NA	6 (55)	10 (67)	0 (0)

[a]ACPA, Anticitrullinated protein antibodies; CRP, C-reactive protein; DAS28, Disease Activity Score in 28 joints; ESR, Erythrocyte sedimentation rate; MTX, Methotrexate; NA, Not applicable; ND, Not determined; NSAID, Nonsteroidal anti-inflammatory drug; OA, Osteoarthritis; PsA, Psoriatic arthritis; RA, Rheumatoid arthritis; RF, Rheumatoid factor; SJC28, Swollen joint count of 28 joints; TJC28, Tender joint count of 28 joints; VAS GDA, Visual analogue scale (range from 0 to 100 mm) global disease activity. [b]*n* = 1, [c]*n* = 6, [d]*n* = 5 with no data available. Data are presented as median (interquartile range).

(RORc, mouse IgG2a; RayBiotech, Norcross, GA, USA), T cells (biotin-conjugated mouse anti-CD4: IgG1, clone RPA-T4; Biolegend, San Diego, CA, USA; and biotin-conjugated mouse anti-CD8: IgG1, clone RFT8; SouthernBiotech, Birmingham, AL), B cells (biotin-conjugated mouse anti-CD19; IgG1, clone HIB19; Biolegend), macrophages (biotin-conjugated mouse anti-CD68; IgG2b clone Y1/82A; Biolegend; and biotin-conjugated mouse anti-CD163; IgG1 clone GHI/61; Biolegend), neutrophils (biotin-conjugated mouse anti-CD15; IgM clone HI98; eBioscience, San Diego, CA, USA), mast cells (mouse anti–mast cell tryptase (MCT); IgG1 clone AA1; Dako, Glostrup, Denmark), lymphatic vessels (goat polyclonal anti-lymphatic vessel endothelial hyaluronan receptor 1 (Lyve-1); R&D Systems), blood vessels (mouse anti–von Willebrand factor (vWF); IgG1 clone F8/86; Dako) and high endothelial venules (mouse anti–peripheral lymph node addressin (PNAd); IgM clone MECA-79; Biolegend). Because some cell-specific antibodies were of the same isotype as the IL-17A antibody, we used a rabbit polyclonal IL-17A antibody (Insight Biotechnology, Wembley, UK) to investigate colocalisation with MCT, CD31 and vWF. During this project, the anti-IL-17F antibody was removed from the market and replaced with another mouse monoclonal anti-IL-17F antibody (IgG2b clone 197301; R&D Systems). Colocalisation studies using both anti-IL-17F antibodies showed that the antibodies almost completely overlap.

Immunohistochemistry

IHC was performed using a two-step immunoperoxidase method followed by a biotin tyramide (PerkinElmer, Waltham, MA, USA) enhancement step to detect IL-17A, IL-17F and IL-17RA or followed by BrightVision (Immunologic, Duiven, the Netherlands) to detect IL-17RC. Sealed slides containing frozen sections were thawed at room temperature for 30 minutes, unpacked, and air-dried for another 20 minutes. Subsequently, sections were fixed in acetone, and endogenous peroxidase activity was blocked with 0.3% H_2O_2 in 0.1% sodium azide in phosphate-buffered saline (PBS) for 20 minutes. After washing in PBS, primary antibodies were incubated overnight at 4°C. As negative controls, irrelevant isotype-matched immunoglobulins instead of the primary antibody were applied to the sections. The next day, staining was developed using a goat anti-mouse horseradish peroxidase (HRP)–conjugated antibody (Dako), after which the intensity was enhanced using biotinylated tyramide (PerkinElmer) and streptavidin-HRP (Dako). Enhancement of the IL-17RC staining was performed using BrightVision. 3-Amino-9-ethylcarbazole; Vector Laboratories, Burlingame, CA, USA) was used as chromogen. Slides were counterstained with Gill's haematoxylin (Klinipath, Duiven, the Netherlands) and mounted in Kaiser's glycerol gelatin (Merck, Darmstadt, Germany).

The intensity of staining was analysed by digital image analysis in a blinded fashion using a Syndia algorithm on a Qwin-based analysis system (Leica, Cambridge, UK) as described previously [33]. The expression of stained

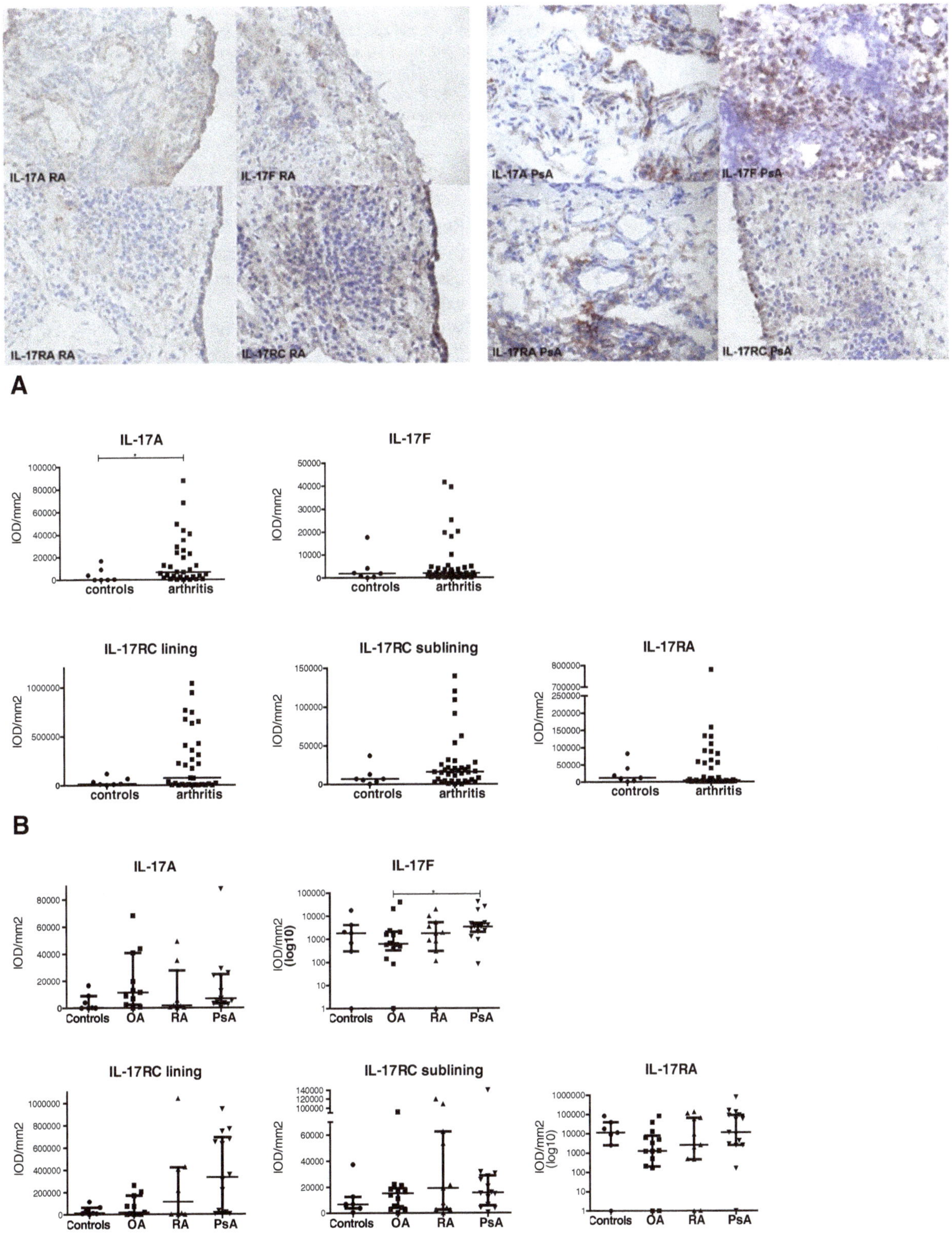

Figure 1 (See legend on next page.)

(See figure on previous page.)
Figure 1 Expression of interleukins 17A and 17F and their receptors in synovial tissue. The expression of interleukin 17A (IL-17A), IL-17F, IL-17RA and IL-17RC in rheumatoid arthritis (RA), osteoarthritis (OA), psoriatic arthritis (PsA) and noninflamed synovial tissue was determined by immunohistochemistry using monoclonal antibodies. For each marker, a representative microscopic picture is given in synovial tissue of a RA patient (left) and a PsA patient (right) **(A)**. The intensity of staining was analysed using digital image analysis, and levels were compared between the noninflammatory and arthritis groups using a Mann-Whitney *U* test **(B)** and between OA, PsA and RA patients using a Kruskal-Wallis test with *post hoc* Dunn's multiple-comparisons tests **(C)**. *$P < 0.05$. IOD, Integrated optical density.

proteins was calculated for each section as the median integrated optical density per square millimetre of tissue [34].

Colocalisation using immunofluorescence

Colocalisation studies between IL-17 and cell-specific markers were performed using a sequential double-immunofluorescence staining method. Frozen tissue sections were thawed and air-dried at room temperature and subsequently fixed in acetone. After washing in PBS, primary antibody (anti-IL17A or anti-IL-17F) was applied and incubated overnight at 4°C. As a negative control, sections were incubated with isotype-matched immunoglobulins. After incubation, bound primary antibodies were detected using isotype-specific Alexa Fluor 594–conjugated or Alexa Fluor 488–conjugated antibodies (Molecular Probes Europe, Leiden, the Netherlands). Subsequently, sections were blocked with 10% normal mouse serum to prevent nonspecific binding. Cell-specific antibodies were applied and incubated for 1 hour at room temperature, after which the staining was developed using streptavidin-Alexa Fluor 594–, streptavidin-Alexa Fluor 633– or isotype-specific Alexa Fluor 594– or Alexa Fluor 488–conjugated antibodies (Molecular Probes Europe). After staining, the slides were mounted with VECTASHIELD HardSet containing 4′,6-diamidino-2-phenylindole dihydrochloride (Vector Laboratories) for nuclear counterstaining. Colocalisation was visualised using a TCS SP2 spectral confocal and multiphoton system (Leica Microsystems, Wetzlar, Germany).

Statistical analysis

GraphPad Prism software (V.5; GraphPad Software, La Jolla, CA, USA) and SPSS version 18.0.2 software (SPSS, Chicago, IL, USA) were used for statistical analysis. Nonnormally distributed data are presented as median (interquartile range). Differences between study groups were analysed using the Kruskal-Wallis test with *post hoc* Dunn's multiple comparisons test or the Mann Whitney *U* test where appropriate. Correlations were assessed with the Spearman's rank-order correlation coefficients. *P*-values below 0.05 were considered statistically significant.

Results

Levels of IL-17A were significantly increased in synovial tissues of patients with inflammatory arthritis, but highly variable between patients

We used monoclonal antibodies against IL-17A, IL-17F, IL-17RA and IL-17RC to determine their protein expression in synovial tissue biopsies using IHC (Figure 1A). A diffuse cytoplasmic staining pattern was observed for IL-17A in the sublining as well as in the intimal lining layer of the synovium. IL-17F showed a more cellular staining pattern, mainly in the synovial sublining. In line with their ubiquitous expression, both IL-17RA and IL-17RC were abundantly present at high IL-17RC levels in the intimal lining layer. Whereas the levels of IL-17F, IL-17RA and IL-17RC were on average comparable between noninflamed synovial tissues ($n = 7$) and the levels observed in patients with inflammatory arthritis ($n = 40$), the levels of IL-17A were significantly increased in patients with inflammatory arthritis (Figure 1B).

The expression levels of IL-17A and their receptors were not different between RA, OA and PsA patients (Figure 1C). This is in line with the results of the study by Benham and colleagues, which showed no difference in synovial IL-17 expression between RA, PsA and OA patients, although those investigators did not (further) stain for the different members of the IL-17 Family and their receptors [35]. The levels of IL-17F were significantly increased in PsA compared to OA patients.

Interestingly, the overall levels of IL-17RA were positively correlated with IL-17F ($r = 0.45$, $P = 0.001$), but not with IL-17A ($r = 0.15$, $P = 0.36$). In addition, the overall IL-17RC level was positively correlated with both IL-17A and IL-17F ($r = 0.48$, $P = 0.005$; and $r = 0.39$, $P = 0.012$, respectively). In a subanalysis, similar correlations were observed for individual patients within a group of the same diagnosis (data not shown). This may suggest that targeting IL-17RC might be a more effective treatment strategy through inhibition of both the IL-17A and IL-17F pathways.

The baseline characteristics between the different groups of patients were comparable, except for age and swollen joint count 28 (SJC28). OA patients were significantly older than the other groups. The RA patients had more swollen joints compared to the PsA patients. The expression levels of IL-17A, IL-17F, IL-17RA and IL-17RC were not correlated with clinical parameters.

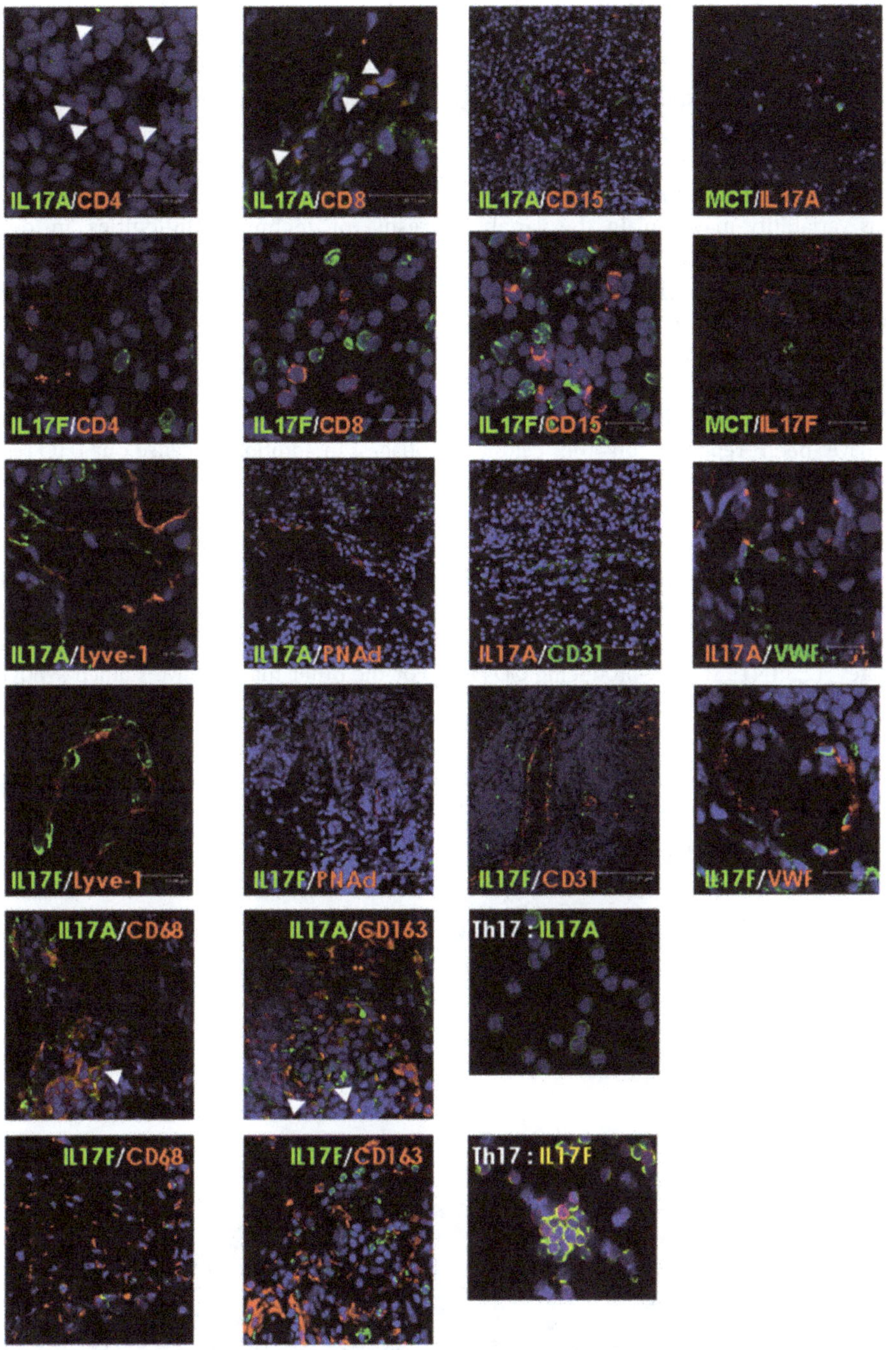

Figure 2 Colocalisation between interleukins 17A, 17F and cell-specific markers. The colocalisation between interleukin 17A (IL-17A) or IL-17F and markers for T cells, neutrophils, mast cells, macrophages, blood vessels and lymphatics was examined using double-immunofluorescence labelling and visualised by confocal microscopy. White arrowheads indicate colocalisation. Representative pictures are presented. Type 17 helper T (Th17) cells were used to show that the IL-17A and IL-17F antibodies used can detect Th17-produced IL-17. Lyve-1, Lymphatic vessel endothelial hyaluronan receptor 1; MCT, Mast cell tryptase; PNAd, Peripheral lymph node addressin; vWF, von Willebrand factor. Pictures illustrating the separate channels for CD4, CD8, CD68 and CD163 staining with IL-17 are shown in Additional file 1: Figure S1 and Additional file 2: Figure S2.

However, IL-17RA was positively correlated with the erythrocyte sedimentation rate (ESR) and C-reactive protein ($r = 0.41$ and $P = 0.040$, $r = 0.41$ and $P = 0.045$, respectively). The correlation with ESR was strongest in the PsA patients ($r = 0.50$ and $P = 0.028$). Only the levels of IL-17F showed a weak but statistically significant negative correlation with age ($r = -0.41$, $P < 0.005$). We cannot exclude the possibility that this may be explained by chance in light of multiple comparisons, although the *P*-value was quite low.

Altogether, these immunohistochemical analyses revealed a striking heterogeneous expression pattern for IL-17A, IL-17F and their receptors in inflamed synovium. Although some synovial tissues showed high expression levels, in other patients almost no expression was observed. This variability may explain the variable clinical responses observed in clinical trials in which IL-17 was targeted (reviewed in [27,36]). In addition, low levels of IL-17 may reflect the possible shift from Th17 to Th1 cells at sites of local inflammation [4,37].

Cellular sources of IL-17A and IL-17F in inflamed synovium

Conflicting data have been reported on the cellular sources of IL-17A and IL-17F in inflamed synovia of patients with different forms of arthritis. In the first studies showing IL-17 production and protein expression in RA synovial tissue biopsies using IHC, researchers reported lymphocytic morphology of IL-17-positive cells [12], and IL-17A and IL-17F staining was especially prominent in lymphocyte aggregates [12,38-41]. IL-17A-producing CD4+ T cells have also been observed in the synovial fluid of RA patients [42,43] and PsA patients [35,41,44]. Later reports suggested colocalisation of IL-17 with markers for mast cells [45,46] and neutrophils [47] in RA synovial tissue. Also, in ankylosing spondylitis, cells of the innate immune system appeared to be a major source of IL-17 [48,49]. The conflicting observations may be the result of technical difficulties in detecting IL-17 in paraffin-embedded synovial tissue, the use of polyclonal antibodies to detect IL-17, and clinical differences between patients studied.

We performed detailed double-immunofluorescence studies to investigate colocalisation of IL-17A or IL-17F and markers for T cells, neutrophils, mast cells and macrophages. In addition, because our IHC results indicated the presence of IL-17A and IL-17F in vessel-like structures, we included markers for blood vessels and lymphatics. To investigate whether the origin of IL-17A or IL-17F was different between RA, PsA and OA patients, synovial tissue was stained from at least five different patients per diagnosis for the analysis of T cells, mast cells and macrophages. For the other markers, we stained synovial tissues from at

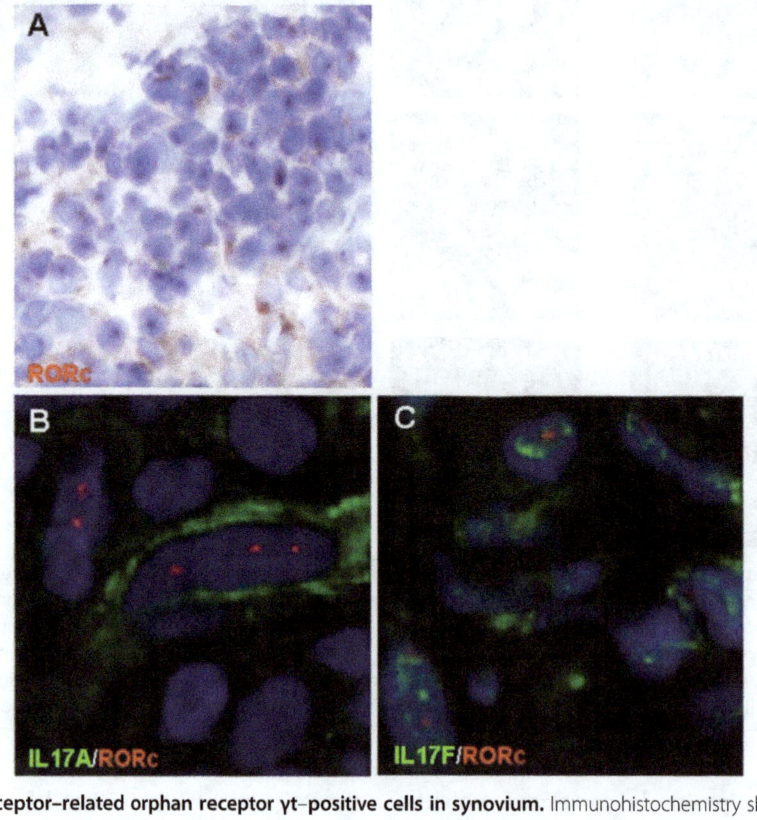

Figure 3 Retinoic acid receptor-related orphan receptor γt-positive cells in synovium. Immunohistochemistry showed an abundant nuclear expression of the IL-17-specific transcription factor retinoic acid receptor-related orphan receptor γt (RORγt) (shown in red) in synovial tissue biopsies **(A)**. Immunofluorescence showed that RORγt-positive cells (red nuclei) in synovial tissue were indeed positive for interleukin 17A (IL-17A) **(B)** or IL-17F **(C)**.

least two different patients per diagnosis. Representative confocal pictures are shown in Figure 2, Additional file 1: Figure S1 and Additional file 2: Figure S2.

The frequency of CD15+ neutrophils in the synovium was very low, and no colocalisation with IL-17A or IL-17F was observed, suggesting that, in inflamed synovium, these cells do not contribute to IL-17 production. CD4+ and CD8+ T cells stained positive for IL-17A, and few cells were positive for IL-17F. CD68+ and CD163+ macrophages showed colocalisation with IL-17A and, to a lesser extent, with IL-17F. We only occasionally observed colocalisation between MCT + mast cells and IL-17A or IL-17F, mainly in PsA patients. Interestingly, we observed IL-17A- and IL-17F-positive cells in vWF+, CD31+ and PNad + blood vessels, as well as in Lyve-1 positive lymphatics. Overall, no clear differences were observed between RA, PsA and OA patients.

Colocalisation between IL-17 and specific cell markers does not necessarily mean that IL-17 is produced by this specific cell. Because the used IL-17 antibodies are non-neutralising, we may detect IL-17 bound to its receptor, which probably is the case in the IL-17-positive blood vessels and lymphatics. To investigate whether IL-17 can be produced by infiltrated cells in the synovium, we stained for the transcription factor RORγt, which is essential for IL-17 production. RORγt-positive cells were abundantly present throughout the synovial tissues (Figure 3A). As expected, most RORγt-positive cells were CD3+ T cells (data not shown). More importantly, RORγt nuclear staining colocalised with IL-17A and IL-17F around the same cell, indicating local cytokine production (Figures 3B and C).

Discussion

We observed increased IL-17A expression in synovial tissues from inflammatory arthritis patients compared with noninflamed control synovium, supporting the concept that IL-17 is a key cytokine in chronic inflammatory arthritis. The levels of IL-17A, IL-17F and their receptors are comparable, on average, between RA, PsA and OA. Using double-immunofluorescence we show that T cells and macrophages can contribute to the production of IL-17A and IL-17F. Colocalisation between the transcription factor RORγt and IL-17 indicate local cytokine production. The heterogeneous expression patterns of IL-17A, IL-17F and their receptors could perhaps explain the limited clinical response observed in clinical trials in which IL-17A in arthritis is targeted, as many patients exhibit very low IL-17 levels at the site of inflammation. These results suggest that patient stratification based on IL-17 expression may be required to demonstrate the beneficial effect of anti-IL-17 therapy in subsets of patients.

Abbreviations

ACPA: Anticitrullinated protein antibody; CD: Cluster of differentiation; CRP: C-reactive protein; ESR: Erythrocyte sedimentation rate; HRP: Horseradish peroxidase; IHC: Immunohistochemistry; IL: Interleukin; Lyve-1: Lymphatic vessel endothelial hyaluronan receptor 1; MCT: Mast cell tryptase; MTX: Methotrexate; OA: Osteoarthritis; PBS: Phosphate-buffered saline; PNAd: Peripheral lymph node addressin; PsA: Psoriatic arthritis; RA: Rheumatoid arthritis; RF: Rheumatoid factor; RORc: Retinoic acid receptor-related orphan receptor C; RORγ: Retinoic acid receptor related orphan receptor γ; SJC28: Swollen joint count of 28 joints; TJC28: Tender joint count of 28 joints; VAS GDA: Visual analogue scale (range 0 to 100 mm) of global disease activity; VWF: von Willebrand factor.

Competing interests

DMG and PPT are currently employees of GlaxoSmithKline, Stevenage, UK. GlaxoSmithKline had no involvement in this project.

Authors' contributions

LGMvB, MCL and PPT were responsible for study conception and experiment design. DMG, PPT and MWT were responsible for recruitment of patients, acquisition of clinical data and collection of synovial tissue. LGMvB, DC, SA and THR were responsible for acquisition of experimental data. LGMvB, MCL, DC, THR, MWT and PPT were responsible for analysis and interpretation of data. LGMvB and MCL drafted the manuscript under the close supervision of PPT. All authors read and revised the manuscript critically for important intellectual content and approved the final version.

Acknowledgements

We thank our study subjects for participating in the study, the arthroscopy team for obtaining synovial tissue biopsies and the AMC KIR laboratory for sample processing. In addition, we thank Barbara Snoek and Geurt Schilders for setting up several immunohistochemistry stainings and the van Leeuwenhoek Centre for Advanced Microscopy at the AMC for confocal microscopy. We also thank Dr Y Souwer for providing Th17 cells. This study was sponsored by the European Union–funded Innovative Medicines Initiative BeTheCure project (115142).

Author details

[1]Division of Clinical Immunology and Rheumatology, Academic Medical Centre, University of Amsterdam, Meibergdreef 9, 1105, AZ, Amsterdam, the Netherlands. [2]Department of Experimental Immunology, Academic Medical Centre, University of Amsterdam, Meibergdreef 9, 1105 AZ, Amsterdam, The Netherlands. [3]Current address: University of Cambridge, U.K. Trinity Lane, Cambridge CB2 1TN, UK, and GlaxoSmithKline, Stevenage UK Gunnels Wood Road, Stevenage Herts SG1 2NY, UK.

References

1. Miossec P, Korn T, Kuchroo VK: **Interleukin-17 and type 17 helper T cells.** *N Engl J Med* 2009, **361**:888–898.
2. Annunziato F, Romagnani S: **The transient nature of the Th17 phenotype.** *Eur J Immunol* 2010, **40**:3312–3316.
3. Muranski P, Restifo NP: **Essentials of Th17 cell commitment and plasticity.** *Blood* 2013, **121**:2402–2414.
4. Nistala K, Adams S, Cambrook H, Ursu S, Olivito B, de Jager W, Evans JG, Cimaz R, Bajaj-Elliott M, Wedderburn LR: **Th17 plasticity in human**

autoimmune arthritis is driven by the inflammatory environment. *Proc Natl Acad Sci U S A* 2010, **107**:14751–14756.

5. Harrington LE, Hatton RD, Mangan PR, Turner H, Murphy TL, Murphy KM, Weaver CT: **Interleukin 17-producing CD4+ effector T cells develop via a lineage distinct from the T helper type 1 and 2 lineages.** *Nat Immunol* 2005, **6**:1123–1132.
6. Shen F, Gaffen SL: **Structure-function relationships in the IL-17 receptor: implications for signal transduction and therapy.** *Cytokine* 2008, **41**:92–104.
7. Chabaud M, Fossiez F, Taupin JL, Miossec P: **Enhancing effect of IL-17 on IL-1-induced IL-6 and leukemia inhibitory factor production by rheumatoid arthritis synoviocytes and its regulation by Th2 cytokines.** *J Immunol* 1998, **161**:409–414.
8. Katz Y, Nadiv O, Beer Y: **Interleukin-17 enhances tumor necrosis factor α-induced synthesis of interleukins 1, 6, and 8 in skin and synovial fibroblasts: a possible role as a "fine-tuning cytokine" in inflammation processes.** *Arthritis Rheum* 2001, **44**:2176–2184.
9. Yao Z, Fanslow WC, Seldin MF, Rousseau AM, Painter SL, Comeau MR, Cohen JI, Spriggs MK: ***Herpesvirus saimiri*** **encodes a new cytokine, IL-17, which binds to a novel cytokine receptor.** *Immunity* 1995, **3**:811–821.
10. Toy D, Kugler D, Wolfson M, Vanden Bos T, Gurgel J, Derry J, Tocker J, Peschon J: **Cutting edge: interleukin 17 signals through a heteromeric receptor complex.** *J Immunol* 2006, **177**:36–39.
11. Gaffen SL: **Structure and signalling in the IL-17 receptor family.** *Nat Rev Immunol* 2009, **9**:556–567.
12. Chabaud M, Durand JM, Buchs N, Fossiez F, Page G, Frappart L, Miossec P: **Human interleukin-17: A T cell-derived proinflammatory cytokine produced by the rheumatoid synovium.** *Arthritis Rheum* 1999, **42**:963–970.
13. Kotake S, Udagawa N, Takahashi N, Matsuzaki K, Itoh K, Ishiyama S, Saito S, Inoue K, Kamatani N, Gillespie MT, Martin TJ, Suda T: **IL-17 in synovial fluids from patients with rheumatoid arthritis is a potent stimulator of osteoclastogenesis.** *J Clin Invest* 1999, **103**:1345–1352.
14. Ziolkowska M, Koc A, Luszczykiewicz G, Ksiezopolska-Pietrzak K, Klimczak E, Chwalinska-Sadowska H, Maslinski W: **High levels of IL-17 in rheumatoid arthritis patients: IL-15 triggers in vitro IL-17 production via cyclosporin A-sensitive mechanism.** *J Immunol* 2000, **164**:2832–2838.
15. Koenders MI, Kolls JK, Oppers-Walgreen B, van den Bersselaar LV, Joosten LA, Schurr JR, Schwarzenberger P, van den Berg WB, Lubberts E: **Interleukin-17 receptor deficiency results in impaired synovial expression of interleukin-1 and matrix metalloproteinases 3, 9, and 13 and prevents cartilage destruction during chronic reactivated streptococcal cell wall–induced arthritis.** *Arthritis Rheum* 2005, **52**:3239–3247.
16. Lubberts E, Koenders MI, Oppers-Walgreen B, van den Bersselaar L, Coenen-de Roo CJ, Joosten LA, van den Berg WB: **Treatment with a neutralizing anti-murine interleukin-17 antibody after the onset of collagen-induced arthritis reduces joint inflammation, cartilage destruction, and bone erosion.** *Arthritis Rheum* 2004, **50**:650–659.
17. Plater-Zyberk C, Joosten LA, Helsen MM, Koenders MI, Baeuerle PA, van den Berg WB: **Combined blockade of granulocyte-macrophage colony stimulating factor and interleukin 17 pathways potently suppresses chronic destructive arthritis in a tumour necrosis factor α-independent mouse model.** *Ann Rheum Dis* 2009, **68**:721–728.
18. Nakae S, Nambu A, Sudo K, Iwakura Y: **Suppression of immune induction of collagen-induced arthritis in IL-17-deficient mice.** *J Immunol* 2003, **171**:6173–6177.
19. Kirkham BW, Lassere MN, Edmonds JP, Juhasz KM, Bird PA, Lee CS, Shnier R, Portek IJ: **Synovial membrane cytokine expression is predictive of joint damage progression in rheumatoid arthritis: a two-year prospective study (the DAMAGE study cohort).** *Arthritis Rheum* 2006, **54**:1122–1131.
20. Peck A, Mellins ED: **Breaking old paradigms: Th17 cells in autoimmune arthritis.** *Clin Immunol* 2009, **132**:295–304.
21. Genovese MC, Van den Bosch F, Roberson SA, Bojin S, Biagini IM, Ryan P, Sloan-Lancaster J: **LY2439821, a humanized anti-interleukin-17 monoclonal antibody, in the treatment of patients with rheumatoid arthritis: A phase I randomized, double-blind, placebo-controlled, proof-of-concept study.** *Arthritis Rheum* 2010, **62**:929–939.
22. Hueber W, Patel DD, Dryja T, Wright AM, Koroleva I, Bruin G, Antoni C, Draelos Z, Gold MH, the Psoriasis Study Group, Durez P, Tak PP, Gomez-Reino JJ, the Rheumatoid Arthritis Study Group, Foster CS, Kim RY, Samson CM, Falk NS, Chu DS, Callanan D, Nguyen QD, the Uveitis Study Group, Rose K, Haider A, Di Padova F: **Effects of AIN457, a fully human antibody to interleukin-17A, on psoriasis, rheumatoid arthritis, and uveitis.** *Sci Transl Med* 2010, **2**:52ra72.
23. Papp KA, Leonardi C, Menter A, Ortonne JP, Krueger JG, Kricorian G, Aras G, Li J, Russell CB, Thompson EH, Baumgartner S: **Brodalumab, an anti-interleukin-17-receptor antibody for psoriasis.** *N Engl J Med* 2012, **366**:1181–1189.
24. McInnes IB, Sieper J, Braun J, Emery P, van der Heijde D, Isaacs JD, Dahmen G, Wollenhaupt J, Schulze-Koops H, Kogan J, Ma S, Schumacher MM, Bertolino AP, Hueber W, Tak PP: **Efficacy and safety of secukinumab, a fully human anti-interleukin-17A monoclonal antibody, in patients with moderate-to-severe psoriatic arthritis: a 24-week, randomised, double-blind, placebo-controlled, phase II proof-of-concept trial.** *Ann Rheum Dis* 2014, **73**:349–356.
25. Baeten D, Baraliakos X, Braun J, Sieper J, Emery P, van der Heijde D, McInnes I, van Laar JM, Landewé R, Wordsworth P, Wollenhaupt J, Kellner H, Paramarta J, Wei J, Brachat A, Bek S, Laurent D, Li Y, Wang YA, Bertolino AP, Gsteiger S, Wright AM, Hueber W: **Anti-interleukin-17A monoclonal antibody secukinumab in treatment of ankylosing spondylitis: a randomised, double-blind, placebo-controlled trial.** *Lancet* 2013, **382**:1705–1713.
26. Miossec P, Kolls JK: **Targeting IL-17 and TH17 cells in chronic inflammation.** *Nat Rev Drug Discov* 2012, **11**:763–776.
27. Patel DD, Lee DM, Kolbinger F, Antoni C: **Effect of IL-17A blockade with secukinumab in autoimmune diseases.** *Ann Rheum Dis* 2013, **72**:ii116–ii123.
28. Arnett FC, Edworthy SM, Bloch DA, McShane DJ, Fries JF, Cooper NS, Healey LA, Kaplan SR, Liang MH, Luthra HS, Medsger TA Jr, Mitchell DM, Neustadt DH, Pinals RS, Schaller JG, Sharp JT, Wilder RL, Hunder GG: **The American Rheumatism Association 1987 revised criteria for the classification of rheumatoid arthritis.** *Arthritis Rheum* 1988, **31**:315–324.
29. Taylor W, Gladman D, Helliwell P, Marchesoni A, Mease P, Mielants H: **Classification criteria for psoriatic arthritis: development of new criteria from a large international study.** *Arthritis Rheum* 2006, **54**:2665–2673.
30. Altman R, Asch E, Bloch D, Bole G, Borenstein D, Brandt K, Christy W, Cooke TD, Greenwald R, Hochberg M, Diagnostic and Therapeutic Criteria Committee of the American Rheumatism Association: **Development of criteria for the classification and reporting of osteoarthritis: classification of osteoarthritis of the knee.** *Arthritis Rheum* 1986, **29**:1039–1049.
31. Gerlag DM, Tak PP: **How to perform and analyse synovial biopsies.** *Best Pract Res Clin Rheumatol* 2009, **23**:221–232.
32. van de Sande MG, Gerlag DM, Lodde BM, van Baarsen LG, Alivernini S, Codullo V, Felea I, Vieira-Sousa E, Fearon U, Reece R, Montecucco C, Veale DJ, Pitzalis C, Emery P, Klareskog L, McInnes IB, Tak PP: **Evaluating antirheumatic treatments using synovial biopsy: a recommendation for standardisation to be used in clinical trials.** *Ann Rheum Dis* 2011, **70**:423–427.
33. Haringman JJ, Vinkenoog M, Gerlag DM, Smeets TJ, Zwinderman AH, Tak PP: **Reliability of computerized image analysis for the evaluation of serial synovial biopsies in randomized controlled trials in rheumatoid arthritis.** *Arthritis Res Ther* 2005, **7**:R862–R867.
34. Smeets TJ, Kraan MC, Galjaard S, Youssef PP, Smith MD, Tak PP: **Analysis of the cell infiltrate and expression of matrix metalloproteinases and granzyme B in paired synovial biopsy specimens from the cartilage-pannus junction in patients with RA.** *Ann Rheum Dis* 2001, **60**:561–565.
35. Benham H, Norris P, Goodall J, Wechalekar MD, FitzGerald O, Szentpetery A, Smith M, Thomas R, Gaston H: **Th17 and Th22 cells in psoriatic arthritis and psoriasis.** *Arthritis Res Ther* 2013, **15**:R136.
36. Kellner H: **Targeting interleukin-17 in patients with active rheumatoid arthritis: rationale and clinical potential.** *Ther Adv Musculoskelet Dis* 2013, **5**:141–152.
37. Cosmi L, Cimaz R, Maggi L, Santarlasci V, Capone M, Borriello F, Frosali F, Querci V, Simonini G, Barra G, Piccinni MP, Liotta F, De Palma R, Maggi E, Romagnani S, Annunziato F: **Evidence of the transient nature of the Th17 phenotype of CD4 + CD161+ T cells in the synovial fluid of patients with juvenile idiopathic arthritis.** *Arthritis Rheum* 2011, **63**:2504–2515.
38. Zrioual S, Ecochard R, Tournadre A, Lenief V, Cazalis MA, Miossec P: **Genome-wide comparison between IL-17A- and IL-17F-induced effects in human rheumatoid arthritis synoviocytes.** *J Immunol* 2009, **182**:3112–3120.
39. Evans HG, Gullick NJ, Kelly S, Pitzalis C, Lord GM, Kirkham BW, Taams LS: **In vivo activated monocytes from the site of inflammation in humans**

specifically promote Th17 responses. *Proc Natl Acad Sci U S A* 2009, **106**:6232–6237.

40. Stamp LK, Easson A, Pettersson L, Highton J, Hessian PA: **Monocyte derived interleukin (IL)-23 is an important determinant of synovial IL-17A expression in rheumatoid arthritis.** *J Rheumatol* 2009, **36**:2403–2408.
41. Raychaudhuri SP, Raychaudhuri SK, Genovese MC: **IL-17 receptor and its functional significance in psoriatic arthritis.** *Mol Cell Biochem* 2012, **359**:419–429.
42. Gullick NJ, Evans HG, Church LD, Jayaraj DM, Filer A, Kirkham BW, Taams LS: **Linking power Doppler ultrasound to the presence of th17 cells in the rheumatoid arthritis joint.** *PLoS One* 2010, **5**:e12516.
43. Arroyo-Villa I, Bautista-Caro MB, Balsa A, Aguado-Acín P, Nuño L, Bonilla-Hernán MG, Puig-Kröger A, Martín-Mola E, Miranda-Carús ME: **Frequency of Th17 CD4+ T cells in early rheumatoid arthritis: a marker of anti-CCP seropositivity.** *PLoS One* 2012, **7**:e42189.
44. Fiocco U, Accordi B, Martini V, Oliviero F, Facco M, Cabrelle A, Piva L, Molena B, Caso F, Costa L, Scanu A, Pagnin E, Atteno M, Scarpa R, Basso G, Semenzato G, Punzi L, Doria A, Dayer JM: **JAK/STAT/PKCδ molecular pathways in synovial fluid T lymphocytes reflect the in vivo T helper-17 expansion in psoriatic arthritis.** *Immunol Res* 2014, **58**:61–69.
45. Hueber AJ, Asquith DL, Miller AM, Reilly J, Kerr S, Leipe J, Melendez AJ, McInnes IB: **Mast cells express IL-17A in rheumatoid arthritis synovium.** *J Immunol* 2010, **184**:3336–3340.
46. Suurmond J, Dorée AL, Boon MR, Knol EF, Huizinga TW, Toes RE, Schuerwegh AJ: **Mast cells are the main interleukin 17-positive cells in anticitrullinated protein antibody-positive and -negative rheumatoid arthritis and osteoarthritis synovium.** *Arthritis Res Ther* 2011, **13**:R150.
47. Moran EM, Heydrich R, Ng CT, Saber TP, McCormick J, Sieper J, Appel H, Fearon U, Veale DJ: **IL-17A expression is localised to both mononuclear and polymorphonuclear synovial cell infiltrates.** *PLoS One* 2011, **6**:e24048.
48. Appel H, Maier R, Wu P, Scheer R, Hempfing A, Kayser R, Thiel A, Radbruch A, Loddenkemper C, Sieper J: **Analysis of IL-17^{+} cells in facet joints of patients with spondyloarthritis suggests that the innate immune pathway might be of greater relevance than the Th17-mediated adaptive immune response.** *Arthritis Res Ther* 2011, **13**:R95.
49. Noordenbos T, Yeremenko N, Gofita I, van de Sande M, Tak PP, Cañete JD, Baeten D: **Interleukin-17-positive mast cells contribute to synovial inflammation in spondylarthritis.** *Arthritis Rheum* 2012, **64**:99–109.

4

Interleukin-37 is increased in adult-onset Still's disease and associated with disease activity

Huihui Chi[1†], Dongzhou Liu[2†], Yue Sun[1], Qiongyi Hu[1], Honglei Liu[1], Xiaobing Cheng[1], Junna Ye[1], Hui Shi[1], Yufeng Yin[1], Mengru Liu[1], Xinyao Wu[1], Zhuochao Zhou[1], Jialin Teng[1], Chengde Yang[1*] and Yutong Su[1*]

Abstract

Background: Interleukin (IL)-37 has been known to play an immunosuppressive role in various inflammatory disorders, but whether it participates in the regulation of pathogenesis of adult-onset Still's disease (AOSD) has not been investigated. In this study, we examined serum IL-37 levels and their clinical association with AOSD, and we explored the anti-inflammatory effects of IL-37 on peripheral blood mononuclear cells (PBMCs) from patients with AOSD.

Methods: Blood samples were collected from 62 patients with AOSD and 50 healthy control subjects (HC). The serum IL-37 levels were determined using an enzyme-linked immunosorbent assay (ELISA). The correlations of serum IL-37 levels with disease activity, laboratory values, and inflammatory cytokines in AOSD were analyzed by Spearman's correlation test. The correlations between serum IL-37 levels and clinical manifestations were analyzed by Mann-Whitney *U* test. PBMCs from ten patients with AOSD were stimulated with recombinant human IL-37 protein, and expression levels of tumor necrosis factor (TNF)-α, IL-6, IL-10, IL-1β, and IL-18 were determined by qRT-PCR and ELISA.

Results: A significantly higher IL-37 protein level was observed in patients with AOSD than in HC. Serum IL-37 levels correlated with systemic score, laboratory values, IL-1β, IL-18, and IL-10 in patients with AOSD. The expression levels of IL-37 were closely related to the patients with AOSD who also had fever, skin rash, lymphadenopathy, splenomegaly, myalgia, and arthralgia. Moreover, the production of proinflammatory cytokines such as IL-6, IL-1β, TNF-α, and IL-18 in PBMCs from patients with AOSD was obviously attenuated after recombinant human IL-37 stimulation.

Conclusions: Increased expression of IL-37 and its positive correlation with disease activity suggest its involvement in AOSD pathogenesis. More importantly, IL-37 inhibits the expression of proinflammatory cytokines in PBMCs from patients with AOSD, indicating the potential anti-inflammatory role of IL-37 in AOSD. Thus, IL-37 may be a novel disease activity biomarker and research target in AOSD.

Keywords: Adult-onset Still's disease, IL-37, Cytokines, Peripheral blood mononuclear cells

* Correspondence: yangchengde@sina.com; allenylcheng@yahoo.com
†Equal contributors
[1]Department of Rheumatology and Immunology, Ruijin Hospital, Shanghai Jiao Tong University School of Medicine, No. 197 Ruijin Second Road, Shanghai 200025, China
Full list of author information is available at the end of the article

Background

Adult-onset Still's disease (AOSD) is a rare systemic inflammatory disorder characterized by spiking fever, evanescent rash, arthralgia or arthritis, sore throat, lymphadenopathy, hepatosplenomegaly, and myalgia [1–4]. Although the pathogenic mechanism of AOSD is still largely unknown, multiple factors, including a predisposing genetic background, viral infections, and aberrant immune response, have been suggested to be involved in the development of this disease [4–7].

Proinflammatory cytokines, such as interleukin (IL)-1β, IL-6, IL-18, tumor necrosis factor-α (TNF-α), and interferon-γ (IFN-γ), have been found to be elevated during AOSD and are thought to be involved in the pathogenesis of AOSD [8–13]. IL-18 and IL-1β, two proinflammatory cytokines processed through the inflammasome machinery, are key factors in the pathogenesis of AOSD; they cause IL-6 and Th1 cytokine secretion as well as natural killer cell dysregulation leading to macrophage activation [3]. A growing body of clinical trials support the hypothesis that blocking these cytokines could partly relieve inflammatory symptoms of AOSD and reduce disease severity, such as TNF-α blockers and IL-1β and IL-6 antagonists [8, 14, 15]. Increasing evidence regarding the efficacy of IL-1 inhibitors such as anakinra (IL-1 receptor antagonist) and canakinumab (monoclonal anti-IL-1β antibody) has been collected from patients with refractory AOSD [16, 17]. Indeed, there is accumulating evidence that the clinical course of AOSD can be divided into systemic monophasic, polycyclic, and chronic articular patterns or a systemic pattern and an articular pattern, based on cytokine profile, clinical presentation, and outcome [3, 8, 18–20]. Anakinra may prove to be more effective in patients with the systemic disease pattern than in the chronic articular one, especially in those patients experiencing severe complications such as macrophage activation syndrome [21, 22]. In the event of an insufficient response to anakinra, canakinumab can be considered because of its longer half-life. Both agents have been reported to be effective in AOSD [23]. On the basis of these studies, IL-1 inhibitors seem to represent the best biologic disease-modifying antirheumatic drugs available and should be considered the first-line biologic treatment for patients not responding to conventional treatment. Recent studies have indicated that IL-37 downregulated the expression of proinflammatory cytokines in chronic inflammatory diseases such as systemic lupus erythematosus (SLE) [24], rheumatoid arthritis (RA) [25–27], and ankylosing spondylitis (AS) [28], suggesting that IL-37 might abrogate proinflammatory cytokine production to reduce inflammatory responses in AOSD.

IL-37, a newly discovered member of the IL-1 family, has been identified as a natural inhibitor of immune responses [29]. The IL-37 expression level was markedly upregulated in peripheral blood monocular cells (PBMCs), epithelial cells, macrophages, dendritic cells (DCs), and T cells following the stimulation of proinflammatory cytokines, including IL-1β, IL-18, TNF-α, and IFN-γ, and the Toll-like receptor (TLR) ligand lipopolysaccharide (LPS) [30–32]. The anti-inflammatory properties of IL-37 were first revealed by transfection of human IL-37 into mouse macrophages, resulting in suppression of TLR-induced proinflammatory cytokines [31]. Unlike other IL-1 family members, a homolog gene for IL-37 has not been identified in the mouse. Nevertheless, transgenic mice expressing the human IL-37 gene were generated (IL-37-transgenic [IL37-tg]) and have extensively revealed IL-37 anti-inflammatory properties [29]. IL37-tg mice exhibited a remarkable protection of spinal cord contusion injury [33]. Similarly, recombinant IL-37 treatment in wild-type mice was effective in inflammatory arthritis [27] and revealed a property of IL-37 that induced metabolic reprogramming and limited metabolic costs of inflammation, thus ameliorating inflammation-induced fatigue [34]. Another study demonstrated that IL-37 inhibited nuclear factor-κB (NF-κB) activation induced by oxidized low-density lipoprotein in human aortic valve cells [35]. In recent years, the inhibitory activity of IL-37 has also been investigated in autoimmune diseases. Upregulated expression of IL-37 in serum has been reported in many inflammation-related disorders, such as SLE, RA, AS, and Graves' disease [24–28, 30, 36]. Concomitantly, upregulated IL-37 significantly suppresses the production of proinflammatory cytokines in PBMCs from subjects with SLE, RA, and AS in vitro [24–26, 28]. However, whether immunosuppressive features of IL-37 contribute to the pathogenesis of autoinflammatory diseases such as AOSD is still unclear.

In the present study, we investigated the expression of IL-37 in the serum of patients with AOSD. In addition, we determined the correlation of serum IL-37 levels with disease activity, laboratory parameters, inflammatory cytokines, and disease manifestations in patients with AOSD. We further studied the effect of IL-37 on cytokine production in PBMCs from patients with AOSD.

Methods

Patients and healthy control subjects

A total of 62 patients with AOSD were enrolled in this study. Patients with AOSD were diagnosed according to Yamaguchi et al.'s criteria [37] after infections, malignancy, and other autoimmune diseases were excluded. Fifty age- and sex-matched volunteers with no history of autoimmune, rheumatic, or other diseases were recruited as healthy control subjects (HC). The study was performed in accordance with the Declaration of

Helsinki and the principles of good clinical practice. Biological samples were obtained under a protocol approved by the Institutional Research Ethics Committee of Ruijin Hospital (identifier 2016-62), Shanghai, China. Informed consent was obtained from recruited subjects.

The medical histories and clinical characteristics, including those identified during a physical examination, of all subjects were collected. Serum samples of the patients with active AOSD were collected before steroid or synthetic disease-modifying antirheumatic drug treatment. Follow-up samples were collected from ten patients with active AOSD after resolution of disease activity. Laboratory findings, including a complete blood count, erythrocyte sedimentation rate (ESR), C-reactive protein (CRP), rheumatoid factor, antinuclear antibody, ferritin, and liver function tests were reviewed. AOSD disease activity was assessed according to the systemic disease score method widely accepted and used [38, 39], which scores disease activity from 0 to 12 and adds 1 point for each of the following manifestations: fever, evanescent rashes, sore throat, arthritis, myalgia, pleuritis, pericarditis, pneumonitis, lymphadenopathy, hepatomegaly or abnormal liver function tests, elevated leukocyte count > 15,000/μl, and serum ferritin > 3000 μg/L. Patients with AOSD were considered to have clinically active disease if they had fever and/or inflammatory arthralgia/arthritis and/or any suggestive cutaneous lesions and/or sore throat. Their disease was otherwise considered inactive [40].

Blood collection and PBMC isolation

Venous blood samples were obtained. PBMCs were isolated from patients with AOSD and HC using Lymphoprep™ (STEMCELL Technologies, Vancouver, BC, Canada) under sterile conditions following the manufacturer's instructions [41]. The collected cells were used for cell cultures or frozen at – 80 °C until RNA extraction. Serum samples were stored at – 80 °C until cytokines were determined.

Cell culture

Whole-blood PBMCs were cultured in RPMI 1640 medium (Thermo Fisher Scientific, Waltham, MA, USA) with 100 μg/ml streptomycin (Thermo Fisher Scientific), 100 IU/ml penicillin, and 10% FBS (Thermo Fisher Scientific) as culture medium in a humidified atmosphere of 5% CO_2 at 37 °C. PBMCs were stimulated with or without recombinant human IL-37 (rhIL-37, catalogue number 1975-IL-025; R&D Systems, Minneapolis, MN, USA) at various concentrations for 24 h, then incubated further with 1 μg/ml LPS (Sigma-Aldrich, St. Louis, MO, USA) for 4 h. Total RNA was extracted [42], and cytokine transcription was analyzed by qRT-PCR. To determine cytokine protein expression in PBMCs, cells were stimulated with or without rhIL-37 at 100 ng/ml for 24 h, then incubated further with LPS (1 μg/ml) for 8 h, and culture supernatants were harvested and frozen at – 80 °C for later cytokine analysis by enzyme-linked immunosorbent assay (ELISA).

RNA extraction and qRT-PCR

Total RNA was extracted with TRIzol reagent (Thermo Fisher Scientific) according to the manufacturer's instructions. For messenger RNA (mRNA) reverse transcription, 1 μg of the total RNA was converted into complementary DNA in a 20-μl reaction volume using a reverse transcription kit (Promega, Madison, WI, USA) following the manufacturer's instructions. PCR primers used for qRT-PCR were as follows: human IL-37: forward 5′-AGTGAGGT CAGCGATTAGGA-3′ and reverse 5′-TTTTAGTGAG CAGGTTTGGT-3′; human glyceraldehyde 3-phosphate dehydrogenase (GAPDH): forward 5′- CTGGGCTACACT GAGCACC-3′ and reverse 5′-AAGTGGTCGTTGAGGG-CAATG-3′; human IL-6: forward 5′-ACTCACCTCTTCA-GAACGAATTG-3′ and reverse 5′- CCATCTTTGGAA GGTTCAGGTTG-3′; human IL-18: forward 5′- TCTTC ATTGACCAAGGAAATCGG-3′ and reverse 5′- TCCGG GGTGCATTATCTCTAC-3′; human TNF-α: forward 5′-GAGGCCAAGCCCTGGTATG-3′ and reverse 5′-CGG GCCGATTGATCTCAGC-3′; human IL-10: forward 5′-GACTTTAAGGGTTACCTGGGTTG-3′ and reverse 5′-TCACATGCGCCTTGATGTCTG-3′; human IL-1β: forward 5′- ATGATGGCTTATTACAGTGGCAA-3′ and reverse 5′-GTCGGAGATTCGTAGCTGGA-3′. qPCR was performed using a LightCycler 480 real-time PCR system (Roche Applied Science, Indianapolis, IN, USA). RNA samples were normalized to control housekeeping genes (human GAPDH), and relative mRNA levels of target genes were calculated using the $2^{-\Delta\Delta Ct}$ comparative cycle threshold method.

Cytokine assessment

Serum IL-37 levels and cell culture supernatant TNF-α, IL-1β, IL-18, IL-6, and IL-10 levels were determined by ELISA following the manufacturer's instructions. Serum IL-37 levels were quantified using commercial ELISA reagent kits purchased from AdipoGen Life Sciences (San Diego, CA, USA). Detection of the TNF-α, IL-1β, IL-18, IL-6, and IL-10 in the cell culture supernatant was accomplished using an ELISA kit (R&D Systems). Serum TNF-α, IL-1β, IL-18, IL-6, and IL-10 levels were measured using the Meso Scale Discovery electrochemiluminescence assay (MSD, Rockville, MD, USA).

Statistical analysis

Data were expressed as mean ± SD and analyzed by Prism version 5.00 software (GraphPad Software, La Jolla, CA, USA). Spearman's correlation test was used to assess the association between serum IL-37 levels and different variables. Comparisons between groups were made using the nonparametric Mann-Whitney *U* test. The Wilcoxon signed-rank test was used to compare IL-37 levels in patients who underwent follow-up serum sampling. The differences were considered significant at $P < 0.05$.

Results

Serum IL-37 levels were higher in patients with AOSD compared with healthy control subjects

The serum IL-37 levels of 62 patients with AOSD and 50 age- and sex-matched HC were measured by ELISA. Patients with AOSD and HC did not have significant differences in terms of mean age or sex distribution

Table 1 Clinical characteristics of patients at enrollment

	AOSD (*n* = 62)		
	Active (*n* = 41)	Inactive (*n* = 21)	HC (*n* = 50)
Age, years	43.4 ± 14.1	37.5 ± 14.2	38.6 ± 11.7
Sex, F/M	31/10	15/6	37/13
Duration, months	2.4 ± 2.7	13.7 ± 13.0	
Clinical features			
Fever	38 (92.7)	0	
Sore throat	30 (73.2)	0	
Skin rash	32 (78.0)	2 (9.5)	
Lymphadenopathy	30 (73.2)	2 (9.5)	
Splenomegaly	15 (36.6)	0	
Hepatomegaly	1 (2.4)	0	
Pericarditis	8 (19.5)	0	
Pleuritis	10 (24.4)	0	
Myalgia	14 (34.1)	0	
Arthralgia	37 (90.2)	0	
Arthritis	17 (41.5)	1 (4.8)	
Systemic score	6.9 ± 2.0	0.2 ± 0.5	
Laboratory markers			
Hemoglobin, g/L	110.2 ± 25.8	130.0 ± 16.5	
Leukocytes, 10^9/L	17.0 ± 5.5	8.1 ± 2.5	
Platelets, 10^9/L	285.7 ± 119.6	248.9 ± 74.9	
ESR, mm/h	73.2 ± 27.1	17.0 ± 27.9	
CRP, mg/L	91.5 ± 54.8	13.5 ± 16.6	
ALT, U/L	63.1 ± 58.9	27.1 ± 12.0	
AST, U/L	49.1 ± 20.1	31.1 ± 10.3	
Ferritin, ng/ml	9665.2 ± 4692.7	181.8 ± 162.6	
ANA positivity	6 (14.6)	1 (4.8)	
RF positivity	2 (4.9)	0	
Treatments			
Steroid- and sDMARD-naïve	41 (100)	2[a] (9.5)	
Low-dose steroid monotherapy	0	0	
High-dose steroid monotherapy	0	0	
sDMARD(s)	0	6 (28.6)	
Combination therapy, steroids + sDMARD(s)	0	13 (61.9)	

Abbreviations: AOSD Adult-onset Still's disease, *HC* Healthy control, *ESR* Erythrocyte sedimentation rate, *CRP* C-reactive protein, *AST* Aspartate transaminase, *ALT* Alanine transaminase, *ANA* Antinuclear antibody, *RF* Rheumatoid factor, *sDMARD* Synthetic disease-modifying antirheumatic drug

Low dose of steroids was defined as ≤ 0.5 mg/kg/day of prednisone; high dose of steroids was defined as > 0.5 mg/kg/day of prednisone

All values are presented as number (percent) or mean ± SD

[a]Drug withdrawal

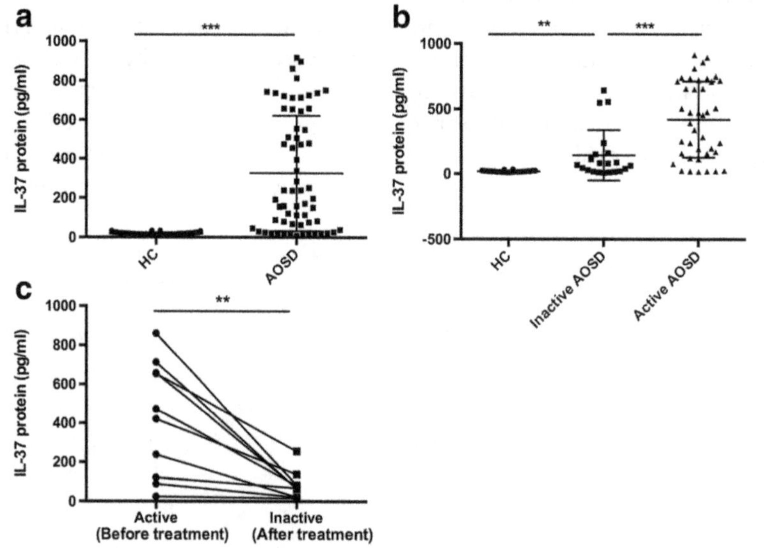

Fig. 1 The expression of interleukin (IL)-37 protein levels in patients with adult-onset Still's disease (AOSD). **a** Comparison of IL-37 protein levels between patients with AOSD (n = 62) and healthy control subjects (HC) (n = 50). **b** Comparison of IL-37 protein levels among patients with AOSD with active and inactive disease activity (active [n = 41] versus inactive [n = 21]) as well as in HC (n = 50). **c** Change in IL-37 protein levels in ten patients with active AOSD according to disease activity. Serum IL-37 protein levels were determined by enzyme-linked immunosorbent assay. Each symbol represents an individual patient with AOSD and an HC. *Horizontal lines* indicate median values. The data represent the mean ± SD. ** $P < 0.01$, *** $P < 0.001$ by Student's t test in (**a**) and (**b**). The Wilcoxon signed-rank test was used to perform statistical analysis in (**c**)

(Table 1). As shown in Fig. 1a, patients with AOSD had significantly higher serum IL-37 protein levels than HC, indicating that IL-37 probably participated in the pathogenesis of AOSD. We next investigated whether IL-37 was related to disease activity in patients with AOSD. We divided patients with AOSD into active and inactive groups according clinical manifestations mentioned above (Table 1). As seen in Fig. 1b, significant differences in IL-37 protein levels were found between patients with active versus inactive disease activity. Moreover, patients with inactive disease displayed higher serum IL-37 protein levels than HC. During serial follow-up, IL-37 showed a significant decrease in the inactive phase (Fig. 1c). Thus, we speculated that IL-37 was probably associated with AOSD disease activity.

Table 2 Correlation of serum IL-37 levels with disease activity score and laboratory values

Disease activity markers	Correlation coefficient r (P value)
Leukocytes	0.3019 (0.018)
ESR	0.3071 (0.0161)
CRP	0.3573 (0.0047)
AST	0.1366 (0.3883)
ALT	− 0.0424 (0.7562)
Ferritin	0.5303 (0.0001)
Systemic score	0.4152 (0.0008)

Abbreviations: ESR Erythrocyte sedimentation rate, *CRP* C-reactive protein, *AST* Aspartate transaminase, *ALT* Alanine transaminase
These data were analyzed using Spearman's correlation coefficient
The systemic score described by Rau et al. [39] assigns a score from 0 to 12 and adds 1 point for each of the following manifestations: fever, evanescent rashes, sore throat, arthritis, myalgia, pleuritis, pericarditis, pneumonitis, lymphadenopathy, hepatomegaly or abnormal liver function tests, elevated leukocyte count > 15,000/μl, and serum ferritin > 3000 μg/L

Correlation between IL-37 levels and AOSD disease activity score as well as laboratory values

To further survey the relationship between serum IL-37 protein levels and disease activity, we next detected the correlations between IL-37 and AOSD disease activity score as well as laboratory values such as leukocytes, ESR, ferritin, CRP, alanine transaminase, and aspartate transaminase. A significantly positive correlation was observed between serum IL-37 levels and systemic score (r = 0.4152, P = 0.0008), as well as leukocytes (r = 0.3019, P = 0.018), ESR (r = 0.3071, P = 0.0161), ferritin (r = 0.5303, P = 0.0001), and CRP (r = 0.3573, P = 0.0047) (Table 2). No significant correlations were found between serum IL-37 levels and liver function.

Associations of serum IL-37 levels with inflammatory cytokines levels

Published studies have demonstrated that proinflammatory cytokines IL-1β, TNF-α, IL-6, IL-18, and IL-17 play an important role in promoting AOSD disease development [14, 19, 40, 43, 44]. Consistent with these findings, we also demonstrated that the levels of serum IL-1β, IL-1Rα, TNF-α, soluble tumor necrosis factor receptor, IL-6, IL-18, and IL-17 were significantly higher in patients

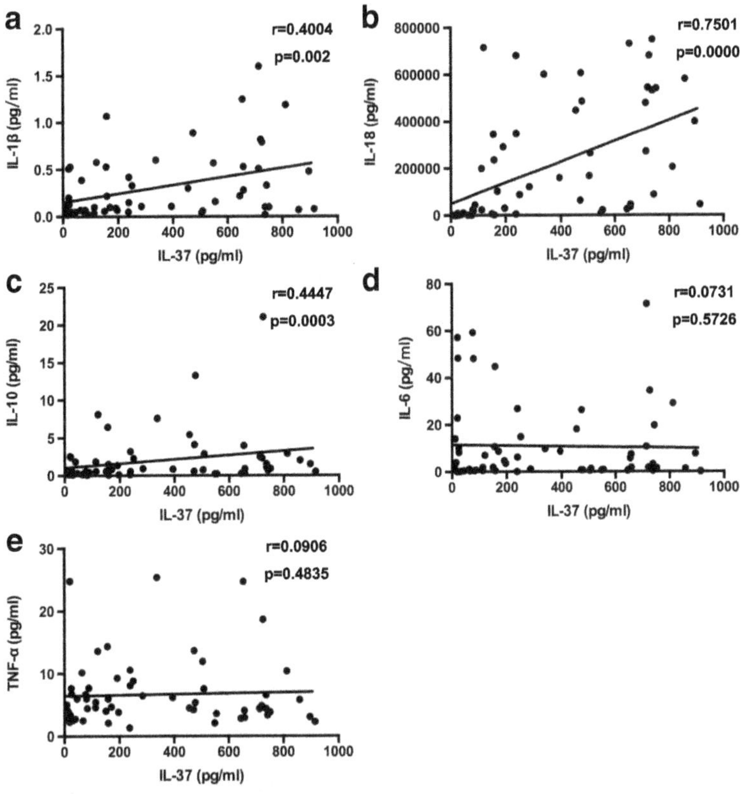

Fig. 2 Associations between serum interleukin (IL)-37 levels and inflammatory cytokines in patients with adult-onset Still's disease. Serum IL-37 levels were positively correlated with IL-1β (**a**), IL-18 (**b**), and IL-10 (**c**) respectively except for IL-6 (**d**) and TNF-α (**e**). Each symbol represents an individual patient. The correlations were evaluated with Spearman's nonparametric test. $P < 0.05$ represents a significant difference. *TNF-α* Tumor necrosis factor-α

with active AOSD than in those with inactive AOSD and in HC. Moreover, serum TNF-α, IL-1Rα, and IL-18 were still higher in the inactive group than in HC (*see* Additional file 1: Figure S1). To assess the potential relationships of serum IL-37 levels with the levels of the proinflammatory cytokines mentioned above in patients with AOSD, the correlations between IL-37 and IL-1β, TNF-α, IL-6, and IL-18 were analyzed by Spearman's correlation test. The results indicated that the concentrations of serum IL-37 were positively correlated with the concentrations of serum IL-1β (r = 0.4004, P = 0.002) (Fig. 2a) and IL-18 (r = 0.7501, P = 0.0000) (Fig. 2b). IL-10, an anti-inflammatory cytokine, showed higher expression levels in patients with active AOSD than in those with inactive AOSD and in HC (*see* Additional file 1: Figure S1). Interestingly, the levels of the anti-inflammatory cytokine IL-37 were positively correlated with IL-10 (r = 0.4447, P = 0.0003) (Fig. 2c).

Association of serum IL-37 protein levels with clinical features in patients with AOSD

To assess associations between serum IL-37 protein levels and clinical manifestations in patients with AOSD, serum IL-37 protein levels were compared among patients with and those without certain clinical features. When the serum IL-37 levels were analyzed with regard to the manifestations of AOSD, the patients who had fever had a higher serum IL-37 level (428.42 ± 291.4 pg/ml) than the patients who did not have fever (165.33 ± 221.06 pg/ml) (P = 0.0003) (Table 3), and the patients who had a skin rash had a higher level (416.33 ± 308.19 pg/ml) than those who did not have a rash (217.60 ± 239.06 pg/ml) (P = 0.0041) (Table 3). Moreover, the patients who had sore throat, lymphadenopathy, splenomegaly, myalgia, and arthralgia had a higher level of IL-37 than those who did not have these symptoms (Table 3). Together, these data demonstrate that serum IL-37 protein levels correlated significantly with clinical features in patients with AOSD. On the basis of the proposed classification of disease courses of AOSD [45], we had follow-up of the patients with AOSD for at least 1 year, and we classified them into three kinds of courses: monophasic (n = 39), polycyclic (n = 20), and chronic articular patterns (n = 3). The serum IL-37 levels were comparable between these three groups (Additional file 1: Figure S2b). We also divided our patients with AOSD into those with a systemic pattern (n = 59) and those with a chronic articular pattern (n = 3). Again, the serum IL-37 levels were

Table 3 Comparison of the serum IL-37 levels according to disease manifestations in 62 patients with adult-onset Still's disease

Manifestations	Serum IL-37 levels		*P* value
Fever	(+), *n* = 38	428.42 ± 291.40	0.0003
	(−), *n* = 24	165.33 ± 221.06	
Sore throat	(+), *n* = 30	419.32 ± 294.61	0.0127
	(−), *n* = 32	239.64 ± 270.42	
Skin rash	(+), *n* = 34	416.33 ± 308.19	0.0041
	(−), *n* = 28	217.60 ± 239.06	
Lymphadenopathy	(+), *n* = 32	436.64 ± 288.01	0.0005
	(−), *n* = 30	209.18 ± 256.72	
Hepatomegaly	(+), *n* = 1	156.63	0.7586
	(−), *n* = 61	329.37 ± 295.93	
Splenomegaly	(+), *n* = 15	477.52 ± 311.97	0.015
	(−), *n* = 47	278.41 ± 274.67	
Pericarditis	(+), *n* = 8	432.69 ± 301.64	0.1824
	(−), *n* = 54	310.86 ± 292.79	
Pneumonia	(+), *n* = 20	379.57 ± 310.59	0.3544
	(−), *n* = 42	301.34 ± 286.62	
Pleuritis	(+), *n* = 10	479.63 ± 336.37	0.0978
	(−), *n* = 52	297.15 ± 279.57	
Myalgia	(+), *n* = 14	449.08 ± 222.11	0.0211
	(−), *n* = 48	290.85 ± 304.96	
Arthritis	(+), *n* = 18	427.91 ± 324.91	0.1068
	(−), *n* = 44	285.13 ± 274.02	
Arthralgia	(+), *n* = 38	405.41 ± 297.41	0.0026
	(−), *n* = 24	201.77 ± 246.81	

IL Interleukin
Serum IL-37 levels are shown as mean ± SD, and differences between two groups were analyzed using the Mann-Whitney *U* test for nonparametric data

comparable between these two groups (Additional file 1: Figure S2a).

IL-37 inhibits the productions of inflammatory cytokines in PBMCs of patients with AOSD

IL-37 has been reported to be an inhibitor of innate immunity [31]. To assess whether IL-37 has a similar capacity to regulate the expression of inflammatory cytokines involved in the pathogenesis of AOSD, we evaluated the effects of IL-37 on LPS-induced cytokine expression in PBMCs of patients with AOSD. The PBMCs isolated from patients with AOSD were cultured in the presence or absence of rhIL-37 and further with LPS stimulation. The cell pellets and cultural supernatants were harvested for later qRT-PCR and ELISA analysis, respectively. We found that IL-37 significantly reduced spontaneous and LPS-induced IL-1β, IL-6, and TNF-α mRNA (Fig. 3a–c) and protein (Fig. 3f–h) expression, but the expression of IL-10 and IL-18 mRNA (Fig. 3d, e) and protein (Fig. 3i, j) was not clearly inhibited. However, we further incubated the PBMCs with 5 mM adenosine triphosphate (ATP) after IL-37 and LPS treatment, and we observed that IL-37 significantly reduced IL-18 mRNA (Fig. 3e) and protein (Fig. 3j) expression induced by ATP and LPS in patients with AOSD.

Discussion

Previous studies have demonstrated that IL-37 acts as an immune mediator to restrain the inflammatory response of many inflammatory and autoimmune diseases. Yet, it is still not clear whether IL-37 is involved in the pathogenesis of AOSD. Our present results show that serum IL-37 levels were dramatically higher in patients with AOSD than in HC, and the levels of IL-37 were positively correlated with systemic score and laboratory features that represented AOSD disease activity. Serum IL-37 levels fell when disease activity was reduced upon follow-up of patients with AOSD. We confirmed the presence of high serum IL-37 levels in AOSD and demonstrated a possible role of IL-37 as a disease biomarker. In addition, we found that serum IL-37 protein levels were correlated with expression of proinflammatory cytokines IL-1β and IL-18 as well as anti-inflammatory cytokine IL-10. Moreover, serum IL-37 levels correlated significantly with clinical features of fever, skin rash, lymphadenopathy, splenomegaly, myalgia, and arthralgia in patients with AOSD. Consequently, it is likely that IL-37, as an important anti-inflammatory cytokine, may play a specific role in the systemic inflammation of AOSD. The disease course and prognosis for patients with AOSD may vary considerably [46]. Several studies demonstrate that IL-18, IFN-γ, IL-10, and IL-4 are associated with systemic AOSD, whereas IL-6, IL-17, and IL-23 are associated with arthritic AOSD [20, 47, 48]. Our studies showed that serum levels of IL-37 were comparable between patients who had a chronic articular pattern and those who had a systemic pattern (Additional file 1: Figure S2a) or between monophasic, polycyclic, and articular patterns (Additional file 1: Figure S2b). Because in our study patients with limited chronic articular AOSD were enrolled, further studies are needed to explore the role of IL-37 in different AOSD disease patterns.

Although the pathogenesis of AOSD is poorly understood, the published data have indicated that proinflammatory cytokines play an important role in the development of inflammation in AOSD. Previous studies demonstrated that serum levels of TNF-α, IL-6, IL-1β, and IL-18 are significantly elevated in patients with AOSD and that blocking these proinflammatory cytokines with antibodies or recombinant soluble receptor dramatically alleviated the disease severity in patients with AOSD [11, 12, 14, 18, 40, 43, 49, 50]. In this study, we observed higher serum levels of these cytokines in patients with AOSD (*see* Additional file 1: Figure S1).

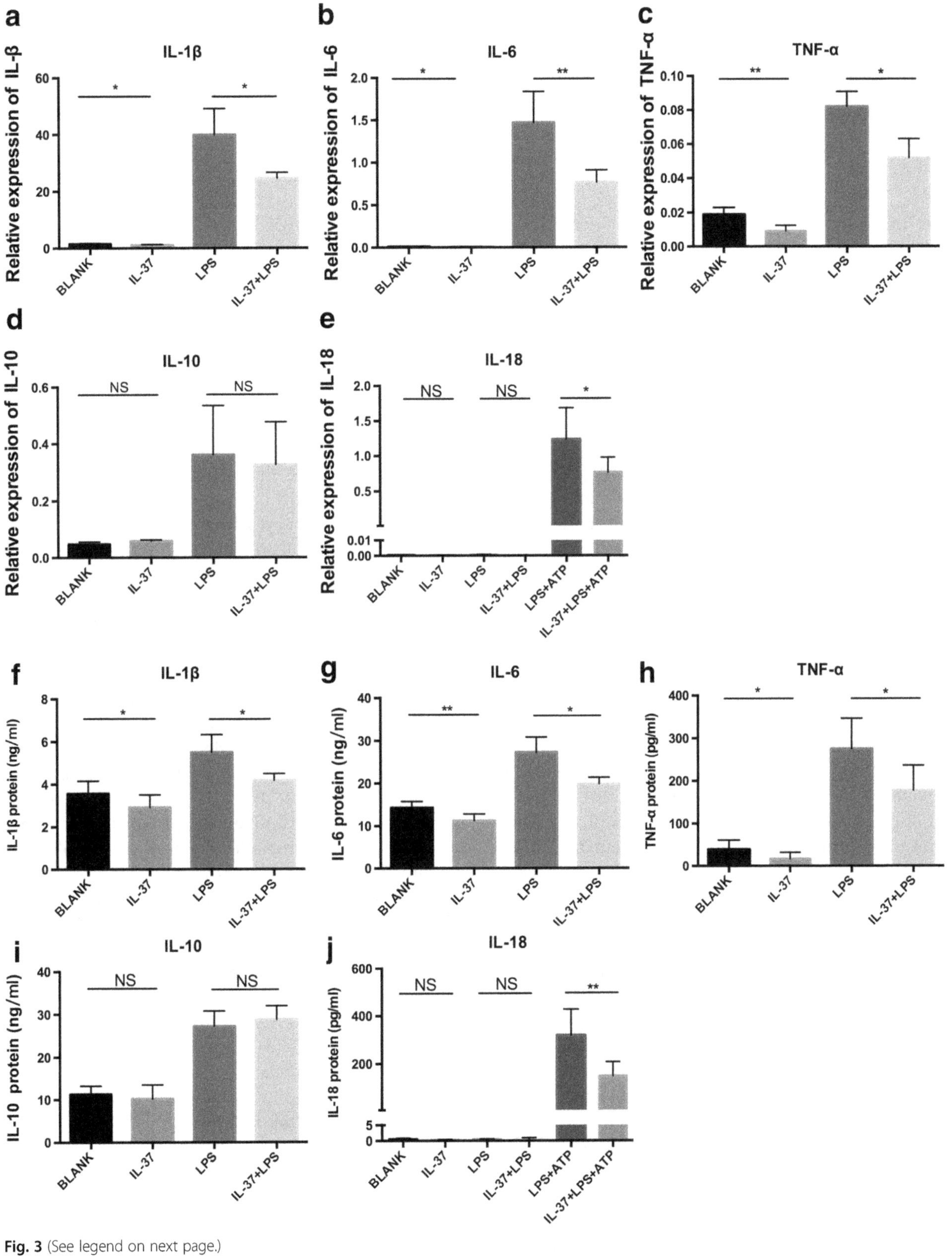

Fig. 3 (See legend on next page.)

(See figure on previous page.)

Fig. 3 Interleukin (IL)-37 inhibits the expression of proinflammatory cytokines in peripheral blood mononuclear cells (PBMCs) of patients with adult-onset Still's disease (AOSD). PBMCs of patients with AOSD (n = 10) were stimulated with human recombinant IL-37 (100 ng/ml) for 24 h, then incubated further with lipopolysaccharide (LPS) (1 μg/ml) for 4 h. **a–e** The total RNA was harvested for qRT-PCR analysis or incubated further with LPS (1 μg/ml) for 8 h. **f–j** The total protein was harvested for enzyme-linked immunosorbent assay analysis. The cells were further stimulated with 5 mM adenosine triphosphate (ATP) for 20 minutes for IL-18 messenger RNA (**e**) and protein (**j**) analysis. The data represent the mean ± SD. * $P < 0.05$, ** $P < 0.01$ by Student's t test. *TNF-α* Tumor necrosis factor-α

More importantly, we also found elevated serum IL-37 levels in patients with AOSD. Spearman's correlation analysis showed that serum IL-37 levels were positively correlated with major proinflammatory cytokines such as IL-1β and IL-18 in patients with AOSD. IL-37 is expressed at low levels in PBMCs and DCs and is upregulated in an inducible manner. IL-37 is induced mainly in an inflammatory context. IL-1β, IL-18, TNF-α, IFN-γ, and transforming growth factor-β increase IL-37 synthesis, whereas IL-4 plus granulocyte-macrophage colony-stimulating factor inhibits IL-37 expression [31]. It has been demonstrated that the IL-37 mRNA and protein expression can be induced by TNF-α via activation of NF-κB and activator protein 1 signaling pathways in intestinal epithelial cells [51]. These results indicate that these proinflammatory cytokines act as positive feedback loops for upregulation of IL-37 production. Therefore, it is reasonable to explain the correlation between higher disease activity and higher IL-37 expression levels in AOSD, and an increase in IL-37 levels may result from an excessive inflammatory response in AOSD.

Moreover, our results show that serum IL-37 levels were positively correlated with the anti-inflammatory cytokine IL-10. Previous studies showed that upregulation of genes encoding negative regulators of innate immunity, such as IL-10 [39], IL-1 receptor antagonist, and SOCS3 [52], were elevated in patients with active AOSD, and IL-10 showed a trend similar to that of the AOSD disease activity [53]. These anti-inflammatory responses were presumably an attempt to quell aberrant inflammation in active AOSD [54]. The activation of anti-inflammatory mechanisms was also supported by the M2 polarization of macrophages of patients with systemic juvenile idiopathic arthritis, who shared clinical similarities with patients with AOSD. Contrary to classically activated macrophages (M1) that were highly pro-inflammatory, M2 macrophages were intended to resolve inflammation, perform scavenger functions, and promote tissue repair. The M2 polarization could result from stimulation by anti-inflammatory cytokines such as IL-4, IL-37, or IL-10 [55]. In our study, serum IL-37 levels in patients with AOSD were positively correlated with IL-10; thus, we speculate that M2 macrophages may have a role in the pathogenesis of AOSD. Several other studies showed that the expression level of IL-10 in PBMCs was increased after rhIL-37 treatment, which is different from our results [56–58]. In IL37-tg mice subjected to a model of inflammatory colitis, there was also an increase in IL-10 production by colon tissue; however, the protective effects of IL-37 were shown to be IL-10-independent because antibody blockade of the IL-10 receptor did not abrogate the effects. In mice subjected to inflammatory arthritis, the efficacy of treatment with recombinant IL-37 was also unrelated to induction of IL-10 [27]. We speculate that inflammation signaling not only exacerbated the inflammatory response in the pathogenesis of AOSD but also promoted the expression of anti-inflammatory cytokines such as IL-37 and IL-10 to limit excessive inflammation in AOSD through specific and distinct anti-inflammatory properties [29].

In recent reports, IL-37 was shown to be a negative mediator reducing proinflammatory cytokine production in inflammatory diseases. Nold et al. found that inhibition of endogenous IL-37 with small interfering RNAs in human PBMCs increased the production of IL-1β, IL-6, and TNF-α [31], suggesting that IL-37 is crucial for inflammation control. In addition, IL-37 significantly suppresses the production of proinflammatory cytokines and the activation of DCs [31, 32, 59]. To further explore the effects of IL-37 on the proinflammatory cytokines that are responsible for the pathogenesis of AOSD, the rhIL-37 protein was used to stimulate PBMCs from patients with AOSD. In our study, we showed that rhIL-37 remarkably attenuated spontaneous and LPS-induced TNF-α, IL-6, and IL-1β expression in PBMCs from patients with AOSD. Although the inhibition of proinflammatory cytokine signaling pathways by IL-37 remains elusive, Nold et al. revealed that IL-37 can reduce the expression of STAT3 [31], whereas STAT3 has been reported to be closely related to AOSD pathogenesis [60]. We suspect that IL-37 may attenuate the production of proinflammatory cytokines through regulating several critical signal transducers, such as STAT3, to smother the excessive inflammation in patients with AOSD.

Conclusions

In the present study, we showed that the upregulation of IL-37 was positively correlated with AOSD disease activity, indicating its involvement in AOSD pathogenesis, and it may become a novel disease activity biomarker.

Our results derived from the cell-based functional assay suggest that IL-37 may participate in the course of AOSD through the reduction of proinflammatory cytokines. Further studies are required to confirm the regulatory mechanism of IL-37 in the pathogenesis of AOSD and extend the present findings.

Additional file

Additional file 1: Figure S1. Comparison of serum cytokines between AOSD and HC. Serum IL-1β (**a**), IL-1Rα (**b**), TNF-α (**c**), soluble tumor necrosis factor receptor (**d**), IL-6 (**e**), IL-18 (**f**), IL-17 (**g**), and IL-10 (**h**) protein levels among patients with AOSD with active and inactive disease activity (active [$n = 41$] versus inactive [$n = 21$]) as well as HC ($n = 50$) were determined by ELISA. Each symbol represents an individual patient with AOSD and an HC. *Horizontal lines* indicate median values. The data represent the mean ± SD. *** $P < 0.001$ by Student's t test. **Figure S2.** Comparison of serum IL-37 levels between patients with AOSD with different disease patterns. (**a**) The serum IL-37 levels in 59 patients with AOSD with a systemic course and 3 with an articular course. (**b**) The serum IL-37 levels in 39 patients with AOSD with a monophasic course, 20 with a polycyclic course and 3 with an articular course. Data are expressed as the mean ± SD. The Mann-Whitney U test was used to perform the statistical analysis. (ZIP 2677 kb)

Abbreviations

ALT: Alanine transaminase; ANA: Antinuclear antibody; AOSD: Adult-onset Still's disease; AS: Ankylosing spondylitis; AST: Aspartate transaminase; ATP: Adenosine triphosphate; CRP: C-reactive protein; DC: Dendritic cell; ELISA: Enzyme-linked immunosorbent assay; ESR: Erythrocyte sedimentation rate; GAPDH: Glyceraldehyde 3-phosphate dehydrogenase; HC: Healthy control subject; rhIL-37: Recombinant human interleukin-37; IFN-γ: Interferon-γ; IL: Interleukin; IL37-tg: Interleukin-37-transgenic; LPS: Lipopolysaccharide; mRNA: Messenger RNA; NF-κB: Nuclear factor-κB; PBMC: Peripheral blood mononuclear cell; RA: Rheumatoid arthritis; RF: Rheumatoid factor; sDMARD: Synthetic disease-modifying antirheumatic drug; SLE: Systemic lupus erythematosus; TLR: Toll-like receptor; TNF-α: Tumor necrosis factor-α

Acknowledgements

Not applicable.

Funding

This work was supported by the Shanghai Jiao Tong University Medicine-Engineering Cross-Disciplinary Research Foundation (YG2016QN62), the Guangxi Excellent Youth Program (GCQN-2017-B04), the National Natural Science Foundation of China (81671589, 81601400), the Shanghai Sailing Program (16YF1407000), and the Science and Technology Commission of Shanghai Municipality (17411965100).

Authors' contributions

HC participated in experiments, provided the figures, and performed statistical analysis. DL conceived of and designed the experiments. YS and QH carried out RNA extraction and qRT-PCR assays. HL helped to revise the manuscript. XC participated in study design and coordination. JY and HS carried out PBMC isolation and cell culture. YY and ML carried out ELISAs. XW, ZZ, and JT collected samples and clinical information. CY contributed to the discussion, edited the manuscript, and helped with coordination. YS conceived of the study, designed and participated in experiments, analyzed data, and wrote the manuscript. All authors read and approved the final manuscript.

Authors' information

Not applicable.

Competing interests

The authors declare that they have no competing interests.

Author details

[1]Department of Rheumatology and Immunology, Ruijin Hospital, Shanghai Jiao Tong University School of Medicine, No. 197 Ruijin Second Road, Shanghai 200025, China. [2]Department of Rheumatology and Immunology, Shenzhen People's Hospital, the Second Clinical Medical College of Jinan University, Shenzhen, China.

References

1. Castañeda S, Blanco R, González-Gay MA. Adult-onset Still's disease: advances in the treatment. Best Pract Res Clin Rheumatol. 2016;30(2):222–38.
2. Kadavath S, Efthimiou P. Adult-onset Still's disease-pathogenesis, clinical manifestations, and new treatment options. Ann Med 2015;47(1):6–14.
3. Gerfaud-Valentin M, Jamilloux Y, Iwaz J, Sève P. Adult-onset Still's disease. Autoimmun Rev. 2014;13(7):708–22.
4. Fautrel B. Adult-onset Still disease. Best Pract Res Clin Rheumatol. 2008; 22(5):773–92.
5. Efthimiou P, Moorthy LN, Mavragani CP, Skokos D, Fautrel B. Adult onset Still's disease and autoinflammation. Int J Inflamm. 2012;2012:964751.
6. Wouters JM, van der Veen J, van de Putte LB, de Rooij DJ. Adult onset Still's disease and viral infections. Ann Rheum Dis. 1988;47(9):764–7.
7. Pouchot J, Ouakil H, Debin ML, Vinceneux P. Adult Still's disease associated with acute human parvovirus B19 infection. Lancet. 1993;341(8855):1280–1.
8. Maria AT, Le Quellec A, Jorgensen C, Touitou I, Rivière S, Guilpain P. Adult onset Still's disease (AOSD) in the era of biologic therapies: dichotomous view for cytokine and clinical expressions. Autoimmun Rev. 2014;13(11): 1149–59.
9. Sugiura T, Kawaguchi Y, Harigai M, Terajima-Ichida H, Kitamura Y, Furuya T, Ichikawa N, Kotake S, Tanaka M, Hara M, et al. Association between adult-onset Still's disease and interleukin-18 gene polymorphisms. Genes Immun. 2002;3(7):394–9.
10. Kawashima M, Yamamura M, Taniai M, Yamauchi H, Tanimoto T, Kurimoto M, Miyawaki S, Amano T, Takeuchi T, Makino H. Levels of interleukin-18 and its binding inhibitors in the blood circulation of patients with adult-onset Still's disease. Arthritis Rheum. 2001;44(3):550–60.
11. Kawaguchi Y, Terajima H, Harigai M, Hara M, Kamatani N. Interleukin-18 as a novel diagnostic marker and indicator of disease severity in adult-onset Still's disease. Arthritis Rheum. 2001;44(7):1716–7.
12. Hoshino T, Ohta A, Yang D, Kawamoto M, Kikuchi M, Inoue Y, Kamizono S, Ota T, Itoh K, Oizumi K. Elevated serum interleukin 6, interferon-γ, and tumor necrosis factor-α levels in patients with adult Still's disease. J Rheumatol. 1998;25(2):396–8.
13. Colafrancesco S, Priori R, Alessandri C, Perricone C, Pendolino M, Picarelli G, Valesini G. IL-18 serum level in adult onset Still's disease: a marker of disease activity. Int J Inflamm. 2012;2012:156890.
14. Giampietro C, Fautrel B. Anti-interleukin-1 agents in adult onset Still's disease. Int J Inflamm. 2012;2012:317820.
15. Cipriani P, Ruscitti P, Carubbi F, Pantano I, Liakouli V, Berardicurti O, Giacomelli R. Tocilizumab for the treatment of adult-onset Still's disease: results from a case series. Clin Rheumatol. 2014;33(1):49–55.
16. Kontzias A, Efthimiou P. The use of canakinumab, a novel IL-1β long-acting inhibitor, in refractory adult-onset Still's disease. Semin Arthritis Rheum. 2012;42(2):201–5.
17. Ortiz-Sanjuán F, Blanco R, Riancho-Zarrabeitia L, Castañeda S, Olivé A, Riveros A, Velloso-Feijoo ML, Narváez J, Jiménez-Moleón I, Maiz-Alonso O, et al. Efficacy of anakinra in refractory adult-onset Still's disease: multicenter study of 41 patients and literature review. Medicine (Baltimore). 2015;94(39):e1554.
18. Chen DY, Lan JL, Lin FJ, Hsieh TY. Proinflammatory cytokine profiles in sera and pathological tissues of patients with active untreated adult onset Still's disease. J Rheumatol. 2004;31(11):2189–98.
19. Fujii T, Nojima T, Yasuoka H, Satoh S, Nakamura K, Kuwana M, Suwa A, Hirakata M, Mimori T. Cytokine and immunogenetic profiles in Japanese patients with adult Still's disease: association with chronic articular disease. Rheumatology (Oxford). 2001;40(12):1398–404.

20. Ichida H, Kawaguchi Y, Sugiura T, Takagi K, Katsumata Y, Gono T, Ota Y, Kataoka S, Kawasumi H, Yamanaka H. Clinical manifestations of Adult-onset Still's disease presenting with erosive arthritis: association with low levels of ferritin and interleukin-18. Arthritis Care Res. 2014;66(4):642–6.
21. Govoni M, Bortoluzzi A, Rossi D, Modena V. How I treat patients with adult onset Still's disease in clinical practice. Autoimmun Rev. 2017; 16(10):1016–23.
22. Cavalli G, Franchini S, Aiello P, Guglielmi B, Berti A, Campochiaro C, Sabbadini MG, Baldissera E, Dagna L. Efficacy and safety of biological agents in adult-onset Still's disease. Scand J Rheumatol. 2015;44(4):309–14.
23. Colafrancesco S, Priori R, Valesini G, Argolini L, Baldissera E, Bartoloni E, Cammelli D, Canestrari G, Cantarini L, Cavallaro E, et al. Response to interleukin-1 inhibitors in 140 Italian patients with adult-onset Still's disease: a multicentre retrospective observational study. Front Pharmacol. 2017;8:369.
24. Ye L, Ji L, Wen Z, Zhou Y, Hu D, Li Y, Yu T, Chen B, Zhang J, Ding L, et al. IL-37 inhibits the production of inflammatory cytokines in peripheral blood mononuclear cells of patients with systemic lupus erythematosus: its correlation with disease activity. J Transl Med. 2014;12:69.
25. Xia L, Shen H, Lu J. Elevated serum and synovial fluid levels of interleukin-37 in patients with rheumatoid arthritis: attenuated the production of inflammatory cytokines. Cytokine. 2015;76(2):553–7.
26. Ye L, Jiang B, Deng J, Du J, Xiong W, Guan Y, Wen Z, Huang K, Huang Z. IL-37 alleviates rheumatoid arthritis by suppressing IL-17 and IL-17-triggering cytokine production and limiting Th17 cell proliferation. J Immunol. 2015; 194(11):5110–9.
27. Cavalli G, Koenders M, Kalabokis V, Kim J, Tan AC, Garlanda C, Mantovani A, Dagna L, Joosten LA, Dinarello CA. Treating experimental arthritis with the innate immune inhibitor interleukin-37 reduces joint and systemic inflammation. Rheumatology (Oxford). 2016;55(12):2220–9.
28. Chen B, Huang K, Ye L, Li Y, Zhang J, Zhang J, Fan X, Liu X, Li L, Sun J, et al. Interleukin-37 is increased in ankylosing spondylitis patients and associated with disease activity. J Transl Med. 2015;13:36.
29. Cavalli G, Dinarello CA. Suppression of inflammation and acquired immunity by IL-37. Immunol Rev. 2018;281(1):179–90.
30. Zhao PW, Jiang WG, Wang L, Jiang ZY, Shan YX, Jiang YF. Plasma levels of IL-37 and correlation with TNF-α, IL-17A, and disease activity during DMARD treatment of rheumatoid arthritis. PLoS One. 2014;9(5):e95346.
31. Nold MF, Nold-Petry CA, Zepp JA, Palmer BE, Bufler P, Dinarello CA. IL-37 is a fundamental inhibitor of innate immunity. Nat Immunol. 2010;11(11): 1014–22.
32. Boraschi D, Lucchesi D, Hainzl S, Leitner M, Maier E, Mangelberger D, Oostingh GJ, Pfaller T, Pixner C, Posselt G, et al. IL-37: a new anti-inflammatory cytokine of the IL-1 family. Eur Cytokine Netw. 2011; 22(3):127–47.
33. Coll-Miró M, Francos-Quijorna I, Santos-Nogueira E, Torres-Espin A, Bufler P, Dinarello CA, López-Vales R. Beneficial effects of IL-37 after spinal cord injury in mice. Proc Natl Acad Sci U S A. 2016;113(5):1411–6.
34. Cavalli G, Justice JN, Boyle KE, D'Alessandro A, Eisenmesser EZ, Herrera JJ, Hansen KC, Nemkov T, Stienstra R, Garlanda C, et al. Interleukin 37 reverses the metabolic cost of inflammation, increases oxidative respiration, and improves exercise tolerance. Proc Natl Acad Sci U S A. 2017;114(9):2313–8.
35. Zeng Q, Song R, Fullerton DA, Ao L, Zhai Y, Li S, Ballak DB, Cleveland JC Jr, Reece TB, McKinsey TA, et al. Interleukin-37 suppresses the osteogenic responses of human aortic valve interstitial cells in vitro and alleviates valve lesions in mice. Proc Natl Acad Sci U S A. 2017;114(7):1631–6.
36. Li Y, Wang Z, Yu T, Chen B, Zhang J, Huang K, Huang Z. Increased expression of IL-37 in patients with Graves' disease and its contribution to suppression of proinflammatory cytokines production in peripheral blood mononuclear cells. PLoS One. 2014;9(9):e107183.
37. Yamaguchi M, Ohta A, Tsunematsu T, Kasukawa R, Mizushima Y, Kashiwagi H, Kashiwazaki S, Tanimoto K, Matsumoto Y, Ota T, et al. Preliminary criteria for classification of adult Still's disease. J Rheumatol. 1992;19(3):424–30.
38. Pouchot J, Sampalis JS, Beaudet F, Carette S, Decary F, Salusinsky-Sternbach M, Hill RO, Gutkowski A, Harth M, Myhal D, et al. Adult Still's disease: manifestations, disease course, and outcome in 62 patients. Medicine (Baltimore). 1991;70(2):118–36.
39. Rau M, Schiller M, Krienke S, Heyder P, Lorenz H, Blank N. Clinical manifestations but not cytokine profiles differentiate adult-onset Still's disease and sepsis. J Rheumatol. 2010;37(11):2369–76.
40. Girard C, Rech J, Brown M, Allali D, Roux-Lombard P, Spertini F, Schiffrin EJ, Schett G, Manger B, Bas S, et al. Elevated serum levels of free interleukin-18 in adult-onset Still's disease. Rheumatology (Oxford). 2016;55(12):2237–47.
41. Grievink HW, Luisman T, Kluft C, Moerland M, Malone KE. Comparison of three isolation techniques for human peripheral blood mononuclear cells: cell recovery and viability, population composition, and cell functionality. Biopreserv Biobank. 2016;14(5):410–5.
42. Su Y, Jiang X, Li Y, Li F, Cheng Y, Peng Y, Song D, Hong J, Ning G, Cao Y, et al. Maternal low protein isocaloric diet suppresses pancreatic β-cell proliferation in mouse offspring via miR-15b. Endocrinology. 2016;157(12):4782–93.
43. Al-Homood IA. Biologic treatments for adult-onset Still's disease. Rheumatology (Oxford). 2014;53(1):32–8.
44. Chen DY, Chen YM, Lan JL, Lin CC, Chen HH, Hsieh CW. Potential role of Th17 cells in the pathogenesis of adult-onset Still's disease. Rheumatology (Oxford). 2010;49(12):2305–12.
45. Mavragani CP, Spyridakis EG, Koutsilieris M. Adult-onset Still's disease: from pathophysiology to targeted therapies. Int J Inflamm. 2012;2012:879020.
46. Cush JJ, Medsger TA Jr, Christy WC, Herbert DC, Cooperstein LA. Adult-onset Still's disease: clinical course and outcome. Arthritis Rheum. 1987; 30(2):186–94.
47. Shimizu M, Yokoyama T, Yamada K, Kaneda H, Wada H, Wada T, Toma T, Ohta K, Kasahara Y, Yachie A. Distinct cytokine profiles of systemic-onset juvenile idiopathic arthritis-associated macrophage activation syndrome with particular emphasis on the role of interleukin-18 in its pathogenesis. Rheumatology (Oxford). 2010;49(9):1645–53.
48. Shimizu M, Nakagishi Y, Yachie A. Distinct subsets of patients with systemic juvenile idiopathic arthritis based on their cytokine profiles. Cytokine. 2013; 61(2):345–8.
49. Chen DY, Lan JL, Lin FJ, Hsieh TY, Wen MC. Predominance of Th1 cytokine in peripheral blood and pathological tissues of patients with active untreated adult onset Still's disease. Ann Rheum Dis. 2004;63(10):1300–6.
50. Choi JH, Suh CH, Lee YM, Suh YJ, Lee SK, Kim SS, Nahm DH, Park HS. Serum cytokine profiles in patients with adult onset Still's disease. J Rheumatol. 2003;30(11):2422–7.
51. Imaeda H, Takahashi K, Fujimoto T, Kasumi E, Ban H, Bamba S, Sonoda H, Shimizu T, Fujiyama Y, Andoh A. Epithelial expression of interleukin-37b in inflammatory bowel disease. Clin Exp Immunol. 2013;172(3):410–6.
52. Fall N, Barnes M, Thornton S, Luyrink L, Olson J, Ilowite NT, Gottlieb BS, Griffin T, Sherry DD, Thompson S, et al. Gene expression profiling of peripheral blood from patients with untreated new-onset systemic juvenile idiopathic arthritis reveals molecular heterogeneity that may predict macrophage activation syndrome. Arthritis Rheum. 2007;56(11):3793–804.
53. Ito T, Ozaki Y, Shimamoto K, Amuro H, Tanijiri T, Yokoi T, Son Y, Tajima K, Fukuhara S. Successful treatment with plasma exchange in adult-onset Still's disease with hyper-IL-18-naemia and hyperallergic state. Mod Rheumatol. 2008;18(4):407–10.
54. Mellins ED, Macaubas C, Grom AA. Pathogenesis of systemic juvenile idiopathic arthritis: some answers, more questions. Nat Rev Rheumatol. 2011;7(7):416–26.
55. Huang J, Hou FL, Zhang AY, Li ZL. Protective effect of the polarity of macrophages regulated by IL-37 on atherosclerosis. Genet Mol Res. 2016; 15(2):gmr.15027616.
56. Lunding L, Schroder A, Wegmann M. Allergic airway inflammation: unravelling the relationship between IL-37, IL-18Rα and Tir8/SIGIRR. Expert Rev Respir Med. 2015;9(6):739–50.
57. Luo Y, Cai X, Liu S, Wang S, Nold-Petry CA, Nold MF, Bufler P, Norris D, Dinarello CA, Fujita M. Suppression of antigen-specific adaptive immunity by IL-37 via induction of tolerogenic dendritic cells. Proc Natl Acad Sci U S A. 2014;111(42):15178–83.
58. Moretti S, Bozza S, Oikonomou V, Renga G, Casagrande A, Iannitti RG, Puccetti M, Garlanda C, Kim S, Li S, et al. IL-37 inhibits inflammasome activation and disease severity in murine aspergillosis. PLoS Pathog. 2014; 10(11):e1004462.
59. Chen HM, Fujita M. IL-37: a new player in immune tolerance. Cytokine. 2015; 72(1):113–4.
60. Takeichi T, Watanabe N, Muro Y, Teshigawara S, Sato M, Ban N, Akiyama M. Phosphorylated signal transducer and activator of transcription 3 in the epidermis in adult-onset Still's disease. J Dermatol. 2017;44(10):1172–5.

5

Comorbidities in polymyalgia rheumatica

Richard Partington*, Toby Helliwell, Sara Muller, Alyshah Abdul Sultan and Christian Mallen

Abstract

Background and aim: Comorbidities are known to exist in many rheumatological conditions. Polymyalgia rheumatica (PMR) is a common inflammatory rheumatological condition affecting older people which, prior to effective treatment, causes severe disability. Our understanding of associated comorbidities in PMR is based only on case reports or series and small cohort studies. The objective of this study is to review systematically the existing literature on the comorbidities associated with PMR.

Methods: MEDLINE, EMBASE, PsycINFO and CINAHL databases were searched for original observational research from inception to November 2016. Papers containing the words 'Polymyalgia Rheumatica' OR 'Giant Cell Arteritis' OR the terms 'PMR' OR 'GCA' were included. Article titles were reviewed based on pre-defined criteria by two reviewers. Following selection for inclusion, studies were quality assessed using the Newcastle–Ottawa tool and data were extracted.

Results: A total of 17,329 papers were reviewed and 41 were incorporated in this review, including three published after the search took place. Wide variations were found in study design, comorbidities reported and populations studied. Positive associations were found between PMR diagnosis and stroke, cardiovascular disease, peripheral arterial disease, diverticular disease and hypothyroidism. Two studies reported a positive association between PMR and overall malignancy rate. Seven studies reported an association between PMR and specific types of cancer, such as leukaemia, lymphoma, myeloproliferative disease and specified solid tumours, although nine studies found either no or negative association between cancer and PMR.

Conclusion: Quantification of the prevalence of comorbidities in PMR is important to accurately plan service provision and enable identification of cases of PMR which may be more difficult to treat. This review highlights that research into comorbidities in PMR is, overall, methodologically inadequate and does not comprehensively cover all comorbidities. Future studies should consider a range of comorbidities in patients with a validated diagnosis of PMR in representative populations.

Keywords: Polymyalgia rheumatica, Giant cell arteritis, Systematic review, Comorbidities, Multimorbidity, Epidemiology

Introduction

Polymyalgia rheumatica (PMR) is the most common inflammatory rheumatological condition affecting people over the age of 50 years [1]. Symptoms include muscle stiffness and pain, predominantly around the neck or shoulder and pelvic girdles [2], as well as a low-grade fever, depression, fatigue, anorexia and weight loss [3, 4]. Raised inflammatory markers (erythrocyte sedimentation rate (ESR) or C-reactive protein (CRP)) are a hallmark of this condition. PMR is usually treated with medium/low dose oral glucocorticoids (GCs) which are gradually reduced and stopped over several years [5].

Patients with common inflammatory rheumatological conditions, for example gout [6] and rheumatoid arthritis (RA) [7], are predisposed to developing cardiovascular disease (CVD). In patients with RA, this risk has been attributed to an increased prevalence of arterial atherosclerotic plaques [8, 9], the quantity of which are correlated with levels of systemic inflammation [10] and duration of

* Correspondence: r.partington@keele.ac.uk
Arthritis Research UK Primary Care Centre, Primary Care Sciences, Keele University, Keele ST5 5BG, UK

rheumatological disease [11]. Patients with RA are also known to have a higher risk of lung diseases [12] and certain types of cancers, particularly haematological cancers [13]. PMR, like RA, is a rheumatological condition characterised by increased levels of inflammation, and therefore patients with PMR may have a similar predisposition to increased risks of certain conditions.

In order to diagnose PMR, guidelines endorsed by the American College of Rheumatology and the European League Against Rheumatism advise the exclusion of conditions which may cause similar symptoms [14]. These include core exclusion conditions (GCA, cancer and infections) as well as RA, fibromyalgia, hypothyroidism and drug-induced myalgia. The guidelines also suggest an evaluation of whether patients have comorbidities that put them at greater risk of side effects from GC treatment [14]. Quantifying the burden of comorbidities in this group of patients is therefore important.

The age group (typically over 50 years) most commonly affected by PMR frequently has more than one comorbidity. Aging is an important predictor of multimorbidity; a recent Scottish study found the number of adults with two or more chronic conditions increased from 30.4% between age 45 and 64 years, to 64.9% in those aged 65–84 years, to greater than 80% in those aged over 85 years [15]. This systematic review aims to summarise the available evidence of the comorbidity profile of people with PMR, and will be the first review to assess comprehensively the evidence for all comorbidities and whether there is evidence for multiple comorbidities existing together. If the evidence shows that patients with PMR commonly have multiple comorbidities then these may no longer be viewed as exclusion criteria precluding a diagnosis of PMR, potentially revealing the true burden of PMR to be higher than currently recognised.

Methods

We conducted a systematic review and narrative synthesis of research literature. We searched medical bibliographic databases to identify articles containing data on any comorbidity either preceding or following a diagnosis of PMR.

Data sources, searches and study selection

The search was conducted in MEDLINE, EMBASE, PsyciINFO and CINAHL from their inception until the date of search in November 2016. Additional articles were found by examining reference lists of included studies and an updated search was run in June 2018 which led to the inclusion of a further study. The exploded MeSH terms 'polymyalgia rheumatica' and 'giant cell arteritis' were used in combination with text word searches for the same as well as for 'PMR' and 'Giant Cell Arteritis' (GCA). GCA is a vasculitis which very commonly co-occurs with PMR; around 10–30% of patients with PMR develop GCA during the course of their illness [16, 17]. Given this overlap in conditions, GCA was included to increase the likelihood of ensuring that all studies in which PMR comorbidities were considered were included in the review. PRISMA guidelines were followed throughout the review process [18].

All article titles identified were screened by a single reviewer (RP) against the inclusion and exclusion criteria. A random sample of 100 of these titles was reviewed by a second reviewer (TH) and agreement between decisions was assessed using adjusted κ calculation [19]. All selected abstracts were then assessed by two reviewers (RP and TH). Any citation thought to be eligible by either reviewer was carried forward to full text review. Reasons for exclusion were recorded. Finally, the remaining full texts were reviewed by the same two authors and a list of papers to be included in the narrative synthesis was created.

Inclusion and exclusion criteria

The inclusion criteria for this review included: a sample of patients with PMR and at least one comorbidity; and the study design must be either cross-sectional, case–control or a prospective or retrospective cohort study. Exclusion criteria were: patients under the age of 40 years; randomised control trials (RCTs); and review articles or conference abstracts. PMR is a disease of older adults. In order to make a diagnosis of PMR, clinical guidelines suggest patients must be aged over 50 years [20], therefore patients under 40 years old are likely to represent misdiagnosis. RCTs were excluded as we wished to look at representative samples of patients with PMR drawn from real-world, observational data. Review articles and conference abstracts were not included to ensure all articles were peer reviewed and fully referenced. In order to ensure that all conditions represented true comorbidities, rather than secondary complications of GC treatment in PMR, we excluded trials which reported only complications of GC therapy [3, 21–27].

There were no date or language restrictions although all included studies were in English. Potentially relevant studies that contained data on GCA were included until full text review due to the overlap between PMR and GCA. If, at that point, the paper only contained data about GCA, it was excluded. The reference lists of other systematic reviews that had assessed individual comorbidities related to PMR were also reviewed to reduce the chance of missing relevant studies.

Quality assessment

Both reviewers, using the Newcastle–Ottawa Scale for case–control and/or cohort studies [28], evaluated the quality of studies. This scale was chosen as it is endorsed for use in systematic reviews of non-randomised trials by the Cochrane Collaboration [29].

Data extraction

A standardised form was developed and used by both reviewers independently to ensure the accuracy of data extraction (Additional file 1). The primary outcome of interest was the total number of patients with PMR who developed a comorbidity of interest compared to controls (without PMR). Other data extracted included clinical criteria used to diagnose PMR, study design, comorbidity under investigation and its temporal relationship to PMR. Meta-data from each study, such as lead author name, publication year, sex, age, country and healthcare setting, were also extracted. Comorbidities were categorised into four groups: malignant disease, particularly haematological malignancies; vascular disease, including coronary, cerebroarterial and peripheral arterial disease; mortality; and other comorbidities (e.g. endocrine, psychiatric and neurological diseases).

Data analysis

Using the total number of patients with PMR and, if present, their controls we attempted to aggregate data to obtain pooled estimates of prevalence of comorbidities and odds ratios to quantify the strength of any apparent association.

Results

Search results

A total of 27,698 articles were identified in this search with a further seven identified following review of references of other articles. Of this total, 10,376 were removed due to duplications, leaving 17,329 unique articles. Following application of inclusion and exclusion criteria during screening of titles, 17,042 further citations were excluded. Of the random selection of 100 of these articles which were reviewed by a second author, agreement between authors was excellent (κ = 0.86).

The abstracts of 287 studies were assessed for eligibility, and 131 were excluded at this stage. The full texts of articles were reviewed and 41 were retained for data extraction [30–70]. This process, which followed PRISMA guidelines, including reasons for exclusion of studies [18], is illustrated in Fig. 1.

Articles included in the review

Of the 41 included studies, 32 were cohort studies [30–61] and nine were case–control studies [62–70]. Eighteen of the cohort studies did not use a formal comparator group. Of the 14 cohort studies with controls, six were based on national datasets, whereas eight were based either on local datasets or on patients presenting to clinics at the same hospital. PMR cases were defined from medical records in 16 studies, national registries in 19 studies and national databases in the remaining six studies. Co-existent GCA cases were formally excluded in six studies and included, or not explicitly excluded, in 35 studies. All but one study was from Europe (predominantly Scandinavia) or the United States. Included studies are tabulated in Additional file 2.

PMR and cancer

Seven studies, reporting 12 outcome measures, have assessed the risk of cancer diagnosis prior to PMR onset (Table 1). All of these studies excluded PMR diagnoses made in the year prior to diagnosis of cancer, to reduce the risk of reverse causality (i.e. cancer causing PMR or PMR symptoms). Of these, the rate of haematogenous cancers was significantly higher among patients with PMR in five cases, while the other seven were non-significantly different.

Six studies reported prospective rates of any cancer diagnosis after diagnosis with PMR (Table 2); two showed an increase in the proportion of people with PMR who developed cancer compared to controls, two were equivocal and the remaining two found the opposite.

In six prospective cohort studies the risk of 17 types of cancer following diagnosis with PMR was considered. Two studies showed an increase in the risk of Hodgkin's lymphoma [55] and non-Hodgkin's lymphoma [56]. Of the remaining four studies, three reported no difference in the rates of female cancers [51], upper gastrointestinal cancers [47] or myeloma [54]. The final study reported no difference in mortality following diagnosis with gastrointestinal cancers [50] among people with or without PMR.

PMR and vascular disease

A number of studies (n = 8) have assessed a variety of different vascular diseases in patients with PMR (Table 3). Fifteen outcome measures were reported, although only seven gave comparable figures for patients without PMR. In each study with a comparator group the proportion of people with PMR who developed vascular disease was higher compared to controls.

PMR and mortality

Few studies have assessed the association between PMR and mortality (n = 4). Three studies reported reduced mortality among patients diagnosed with PMR [35, 38, 39] while one study found an increase, but this study did not differentiate between patients with PMR and GCA [36].

PMR and other comorbidities

An association between thyroid disease and PMR is unproven. Bowness et al. [31] found an increase in the risk of hypothyroid disease (RR 3.2 (95% confidence interval 1.71, 5.91)), but Juchet et al. [33] did not. One recent case–control study found a significantly increased rate of diverticular disease prior to a diagnosis with PMR (OR 4.06 (95% CI 1.76–9.35)) [70].

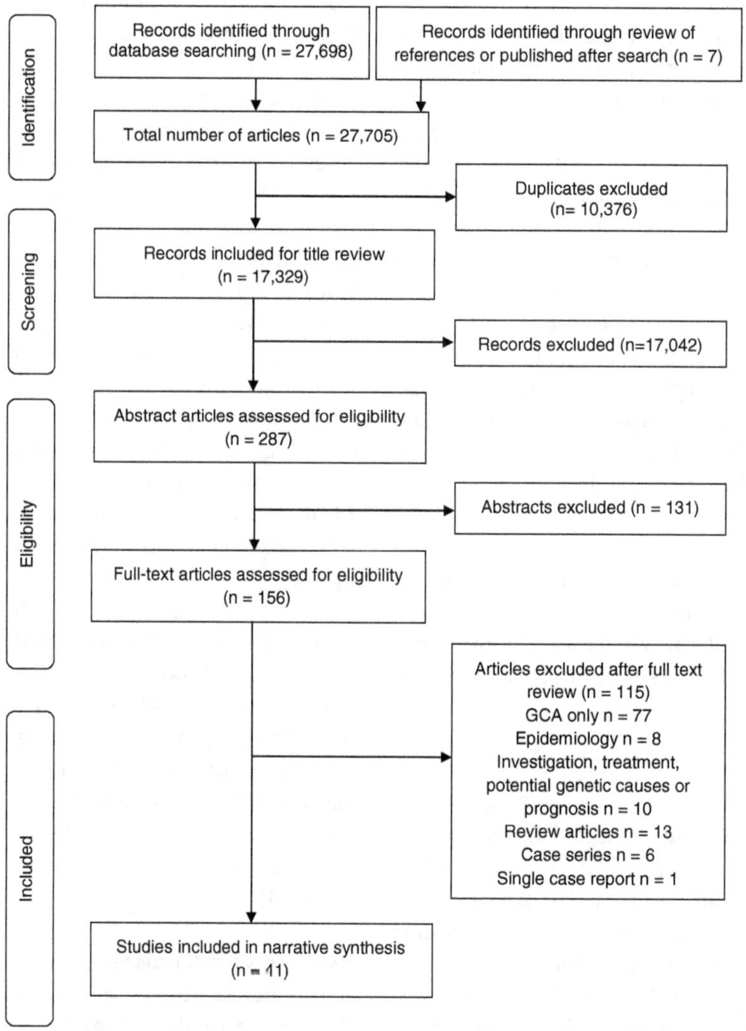

Fig. 1 Flowchart of study inclusion, adopted from Preferred Reporting Items for Systematic Reviews and Meta-Analyses (PRISMA) guidelines [18]. GCA giant cell arteritis

No evidence has been found to associate PMR with psychiatric comorbidities, including schizophrenia [44, 69] and bipolar disease [44]. Li et al. [49] found a potential association between PMR and Parkinson's disease (SIR 1.25 (95% CI 1.01, 1.53)). Hemminki et al. [53] also reported an association between PMR and hospitalisation due to obesity (SIR 1.65 (95% CI 1.22, 2.19)).

A small number of studies from the United States (n = 2) [40, 59] looked at wide ranges of different comorbidities but their sample size was insufficient to find significant associations for the majority of the comorbidities.

Quality assessment

All of the articles in this study used medical records or nationwide registries (based on medical records) to corroborate diagnosis of PMR and the comorbidity; therefore, they were awarded three or four stars for cohort or case selection using the Newcastle–Ottawa criteria. All studies also achieved at least two stars for outcome measurement. However, many of the studies failed to recruit a comparator group, instead using the population as a reference, and therefore comparability scores were low (Additional file 2).

Many of the cohort studies identified failed to include comparison groups (n = 18), instead using indirect standardisation to calculate incidence or mortality ratios. The lack of comparison groups limits the generalisability of many of the studies. Further to this, almost half of the studies (n = 19) sourced their sample of patients with PMR based on hospital discharge data. This may be an appropriate approach for some autoimmune conditions, but the majority of patients with PMR are managed in primary care settings [71, 72].

Aggregation of data to calculate pooled odds and hazard ratios was attempted for vascular disease and cancer diagnoses; however, high levels of heterogeneity were

Table 1 Cancer prior to diagnosis with PMR

Retrospective case–control study								
Study	Diagnosis	Cases (*n*)	PMR cases (*n*)	Controls (*n*)	PMR controls (*n*)	Odds ratio (95% CI)	Case rate (%)	Control rate (%)
Anderson et al. [64]	Lymphoid malignancies	33,721	344	122,531	1244	0.9 (0.8–1.0)	1.02	1.02
Anderson et al. [63]	Myeloid malignancy	9998	125	160,086	1288	1.7 (1.4–2.1)	1.25	0.80
	Myelodysplastic malignancy	3758	55	42,886	518	1.5 (1.1–2)	1.46	1.21
Anderson et al. [67]	HCL	418	9	160,086	2721	1.5 (0.5–3.9)	2.15	1.70
Askling et al. [62]	All lymphoma	42,676	114	78,487	250	0.8 (0.7–1.0)	0.27	0.32
	NHL	28,355	88	52,164	187	0.9 (0.7–1.1)	0.31	0.36
	HL	4037	3	7394	15	0.4 (0.1–1.3)	0.07	0.2
	CLL	10,555	24	19,391	52	0.8 (0.5–1.4)	0.23	0.27
Kristinsson et al. [66]	Any MPN	11,039	46	43,550	104	1.7 (1.2–2.5)	0.42	0.24
Lanoy and Engels [65]	Cutaneous NHL	2652	19	178,452	1731	0.7 (0.5–1.1)	0.72	0.97
Lindqvist et al. [68]	MM	19,112	56	75,408	116	1.9 (1.4–2.6)	0.29	0.15
	MGUS	5403	58	21,209	79	2.9 (2.1–4.1)	1.07	0.37

PMR polymyalgia rheumatica, *HCL* hairy cell leukaemia, *NHL* non-Hodgkin's lymphoma, *HL* Hodgkin's lymphoma, *CLL* chronic lymphocytic leukaemia, *MM* multiple myeloma, *MPN* myeloproliferative neoplasm, *MGUS* monoclonal gammopathy of undetermined significance

found between the studies (88–100%) and therefore this was not reported.

Many of the studies limited themselves to a small number of comorbid conditions, thus not allowing a picture of the overall health of patients with PMR to develop. Two studies [34, 40] did attempt to look at a range of comorbidities but they were underpowered.

Discussion

Statement of principle findings

This review found some evidence of an association between PMR and vascular disease, and possibly cancer, particularly in the first 6 months following diagnosis. However, the evidence for this is not robust.

Table 2 Cancer following diagnosis with PMR

Prospective cohort with combined cancer cases						
	PMR patients			Control patients		
Study	PMR cases (*n*)	Cancer cases (*n*)	Proportion (%)	Controls (*n*)	Cancer cases (*n*)	Proportion (%)
Muller et al. [57]	2877	667	23.18	9942	1938	19.49
Bellan et al. [61]	100	24	24.00	702	41	5.84
Ji et al. [45]	35,918	3941	10.97	–	–	–
Myklebust et al. [37]	366	34	9.29	1324	143	10.80
Haga et al. [32]	91	10	10.99	794	131	16.50
Pfeifer et al. [59]	359	66	18.38	357	62	17.37
Total[a]	39,711	4742	21.12	13,119	2315	17.65

PMR polymyalgia rheumatica
[a]Ji et al. [45] not included in calculation as no control group

The concentration of the apparent association between PMR and cancer in the first 6 months following diagnosis suggests the possibility of an element of misdiagnosis. This could occur as some of the features of PMR (myalgia, fatigue, weight loss, raised inflammatory markers) are also non-specific early features of some cancers. Furthermore, as time passed, the rate of diagnosis of cancer was found to drop down to the background population rate.

Regarding specific types of cancer, some studies have proposed there could be associations between PMR and haematological cancers. This includes Hodgkin's and non-Hodgkin's lymphoma [56], myeloma [68] and other myeloid malignancies [63, 66]. An increase in the risk of lymphoma has been observed with RA, which has been postulated to be due to higher accumulated inflammatory activity in RA [73]; a similar mechanism may lie behind the apparent increase in patients with PMR.

The overall trend of results suggests that PMR may be associated with an increased risk of the development of vascular disease. Knowing that both PMR and RA are inflammatory conditions, there is biological plausibility that PMR and vascular disease could be associated. However, the two largest studies, both based on population data from the UK, reported conflicting results: Hancock et al. [58] stated that PMR was significantly associated with vascular disease, while Pujades-Rodriguez et al. [60] reported a reduction in the risk (incidence rate ratio 0.88 (95% CI 0.83–, 0.94)). However, in the latter study when only patients with PMR were included, there was a slight increase in the proportion of patients with the condition who went on to have a vascular event compared to controls (23.24% compared to 20.43%).

These two studies employed similar approaches selecting with PMR from linked UK databases. However, a number of differences existed between the studies, including the age of participants (> 50 years only for Hancock et al. [58] and > 18 years for Pujades-Rodriguez et al. [60]), average years of follow up (7.8 and 3.13 years respectively) as well as the total number of patients found with PMR (3249 compared to 11,320 patients). Potentially, the variation in risk of vascular events between these studies could be explained by the differences in follow up or the age distribution of the study population.

Another reason for inconsistent evidence of an increase in vascular risk for patients with PMR may be the modulating effect that GCs have upon levels on inflammation. If the risk of vascular disease correlates with the presence of inflammation in the body, GC therapy would reduce this, which may then also reduce vascular risk. The study by Kremers et al. [42] appears to bear this out. In this study, the risk of vascular events was lower in patients with PMR who were treated with GCs compared to those who were not. Further to this, Hancock et al. [58] reported that the excess vascular risk in PMR reduced over time; this could reflect declining levels of inflammation.

Overall, although some studies dissent from this view, it appears that a diagnosis of PMR increases an individual's risk of vascular disease. However, further research in this area is needed to add clarity.

Conversely, it appears that a diagnosis with PMR is associated with a reduction in mortality. This was demonstrated in three out of the four studies that reported it as an independent outcome. A possible explanation for this could again be surveillance bias. Patients with chronic illness (and especially PMR where regular assessment, follow up and monitoring are advised) are more likely to be under active follow up for their condition and any developing morbidity, particularly if related to well-recognised adverse effects of treatment, is likely to be identified and managed earlier.

There is a small amount of evidence that patients with PMR may be more likely to develop hypothyroidism [31] and Parkinson's disease [49]. PMR and hypothyroidism both preferentially affect females, and therefore a similar autoimmune pathway may be present in both conditions. However, as has been pointed out, PMR does not share all of the characteristics of traditional autoimmune conditions, for example it lacks specific autoantibodies [74].

Table 3 Vascular disease and PMR

Study	PMR patients			Control patients		
	PMR cases (*n*)	Comorbid condition (*n*)	Proportion (%)	Controls (*n*)	Comorbid condition (*n*)	Proportion (%)
Stroke						
Kang et al. [46]	781	113	14.47	3905	273	6.99
Zoller et al. [48]	16,496	1981	12.01			
Kremers et al. [42]	276	58	21.01			
Hancock et al. [58]	3249	397	12.22	12,735	556	4.37
Myocardial infarction						
Kremers et al. [42]	276	47	17.03			
Hancock et al. [58]	3249	460	14.16	12,735	575	4.52
Zoller et al. [48]	21,351	5669	26.55			
Heart failure						
Kremers et al. [42]	276	68	24.64			
Peripheral vascular disease						
Kremers et al. [42]	276	35	12.68			
Hancock et al. [58]	3249	140	4.31	12,735	151	1.19
Warrington et al. [43]	353	38	10.76	705	28	3.97
Combined						
Kremers et al. [42]	276	208	75.36			
Hancock et al. [58]	3249	918	28.25	12,735	1150	9.03
Pujades-Rodriguez et al. [60]	9776	2272	23.24	105,504	21,559	20.43
Bengtsson and Malmvall [30]	73	16	21.92			

PMR polymyalgia rheumatica

Furthermore, it seems that PMR is not associated as strongly with other autoimmune conditions as would be expected if it was a pure autoimmune disease. Parkinson's disease is a condition which predominantly affects older people, as does PMR, and therefore this association may just be a result of clustering of diagnoses in an older population.

Strengths and weaknesses

The main strength of the study was its deliberately broad scope and aim to include any study in which the risk of any comorbidity either before or after diagnosis with PMR was to be reviewed. Following the initial broad search, articles from the 'grey literature' were excluded and only articles fully published in peer-reviewed journals were included.

The potential limitations in this study arose not due to the protocol but rather because the majority of studies were of relatively poor quality. These risks included selection bias, surveillance bias and a lack of adequate control groups.

Selection bias within the included studies is a possibility in this review, as the majority of studies drew PMR cases from secondary care, either from hospital discharge data or from rheumatology outpatient clinics. Current UK guidelines suggest only referring atypical cases, cases of diagnostic uncertainty or treatment predicaments [5, 14], meaning that in the UK 71–84% of patients with PMR are treated in the community by primary care physicians [71, 72]. Therefore, the patient population in these studies may not accurately reflect the majority of those who are diagnosed with PMR. This may have artificially inflated the apparent differences in development of comorbidities between patients with and without PMR.

Another limitation is the risk of surveillance bias as discussed earlier around the apparent reduction in mortality [75]. Some case–control studies attempted to deal with this by excluding comorbid disease found in the year prior to diagnosis [63, 64, 67, 68], while in two observational cohort studies [58, 60], controls were selected that had contacted a primary care service in the year the index cases were diagnosed. Finally, many of these studies assessed multiple variables, often > 30 different autoimmune conditions, increasing the likelihood of a chance finding (type II error).

Furthermore, we also noted that the range of comorbidities reported in the literature was more limited than we expected; for example, there were no studies which explicitly examined the risks of important and common conditions such as diabetes mellitus and asthma or other chronic respiratory conditions.

A further potential bias is the effect of GC therapy and the impact of this on the risks of comorbidities. As GC is the only widely accepted treatment for PMR, we could not exclude studies where patients were treated with GC. To reduce the impact of potential bias from GC treatment, we excluded studies in which direct complications of GC therapy were assessed. However, as discussed previously in relation to vascular risk, GC therapy is inevitable in PMR and therefore we could not completely mitigate this effect.

Conclusion

This review has found the overall standard of evidence regarding the association of comorbidities with PMR to be weak. There may be an increased risk of vascular disease and possibly cancer in patients with PMR. Weaker quality evidence also suggests that patients with PMR have a reduced mortality rate. Currently, there is little evidence around the wider health of patients with PMR either at the time of diagnosis or in the period following.

This lack of firm evidence around which comorbidities exist alongside or are potentially associated with PMR presents a problem for the pragmatic clinician. Current clinical guidelines suggest that in order to diagnose PMR, a large number of other conditions which may mimic the symptoms of PMR should be excluded. This list includes, but is not limited to, rheumatoid arthritis and endocrine, infective and neoplastic conditions [14]. However, comorbidities are very common in the age group affected by PMR [76], and therefore the coexistence of one of these comorbidities with PMR should not necessarily prevent or invalidate the diagnosis of PMR.

The uncertainty around the general health of patients with PMR and comorbidities that may coexist with it presents a challenge for healthcare practitioners who deal most with this condition, be they from primary or secondary care. A rigorous diagnostic and follow-up process is crucial to ensure this uncertainty does not translate into misdiagnosis. In the future, it is important to confirm whether, and if so to what extent, a diagnosis of PMR imparts an excess risk of vascular disease or cancer.

Further research in the form of large observational studies, based in primary care, of the health of patients with PMR, including the prevalence of comorbidities before and after diagnosis, would allow clinicians to better monitor for these outcomes.

Abbreviations

CRP: C-reactive protein; CVD: Cardiovascular disease; ESR: Erythrocyte sedimentation rate; GC: Glucocorticoid; GCA: Giant cell arteritis; PMR: Polymyalgia rheumatica; RA: Rheumatoid arthritis; RCT: Randomised control trial

Acknowledgements
Thanks to Opeyemi Babatunde (Research Associate: Systematic Reviews, Keele University) and Jo Jordan (Research Information Manager, Keele University) for assistance with the protocol and search strategy.

Funding
RP is funded by NHS Research and Infrastructure funds. CM is funded by the NIHR Collaborations for Leadership in Applied Health Research and Care West Midlands, the NIHR School for Primary Care Research and an NIHR Research Professorship in General Practice, which also supports AAS (NIHR-RP-2014-04-026). TH is funded by an NIHR Clinical Lectureship in General Practice. The views expressed are those of the authors and not necessarily those of the NHS, the NIHR or the Department of Health and Social Care. The funder was not involved in the study design; in the collection, analysis and interpretation of data; in the writing of the report; or in the decision to submit the article for publication.

Authors' contributions
RP, TH, SM, CM and AAS contributed to study design. RP performed the literature search, RP and TH the title, abstract and full text review. RP produced the first draft of the manuscript and the tables. SM, TH, CM and AS performed critical revision of the manuscript drafts. All authors read and approved the final manuscript.

Competing interests
The authors declare that they have no competing interests.

References

1. Michet CJ, Matteson EL. Polymyalgia rheumatica. Br Med J. 2008;336:765–9. https://doi.org/10.1016/S0140-6736(97)05001-0.
2. Salvarani C, Cantini F, Hunder GG. Polymyalgia rheumatica and giant-cell arteritis. Lancet. 2008;372(9634):234–45. https://doi.org/10.1016/S0140-6736(08)61077-6.
3. Chuang TY, Hunder GG, Ilstrup DM, Kurland LT. Polymyalgia rheumatica: a 10-year epidemiologic and clinical study. Ann Intern Med. 1982;97(5):672–80.
4. Salvarani C, Macchioni PL, Tartoni PL, et al. Polymyalgia rheumatica and giant cell arteritis: a 5-year epidemiologic and clinical study in Reggio Emilia, Italy. Clin Exp Rheumatol. 1987;5(3):205–15.
5. Dasgupta B, Borg FA, Hassan N, et al. BSR and BHPR guidelines for the management of polymyalgia rheumatica. Rheumatology. 2010;49(1):186–90. https://doi.org/10.1093/rheumatology/kep303a.
6. Clarson L, Chandratre P, Hider S, et al. Increased cardiovascular mortality associated with gout: a systematic review and meta-analysis. Eur J Prev Cardiol. 2013;22(3):335–43. https://doi.org/10.1177/2047487313514895.
7. Avina-Zubieta JA, Thomas J, Sadatsafavi M, Lehman AJ, Lacaille D. Risk of incident cardiovascular events in patients with rheumatoid arthritis: a meta-analysis of observational studies. Ann Rheum Dis. 2012;71(9):1524–9. https://doi.org/10.1136/annrheumdis-2011-200726.
8. Pamuk ÖN, Ünlü E, Çakir N. Role of insulin resistance in increased frequency of atherosclerosis detected by carotid ultrasonography in rheumatoid arthritis. J Rheumatol. 2006;33(12):2447–52.
9. Jonsson SW, Backman C, Johnson O, et al. Increased prevalence of atherosclerosis in patients with medium term rheumatoid arthritis. J Rheumatol. 2001;28(12):2597–602 pmid: 11764203.
10. Kumeda Y, Inaba M, Goto H, et al. Increased thickness of the arterial intima-media detected by ultrasonography in patients with rheumatoid arthritis. Arthritis Rheum. 2002;46(6):1489–97. https://doi.org/10.1002/art.10269.
11. Dessein PH, Norton GR, Woodiwiss AJ, Joffe BI, Wolfe F. Influence of nonclassical cardiovascular-risk factors on the accuracy of predicting subclinical atherosclerosis in rheumatoid arthritis. J Rheumatol. 2007;34(5):943–51.
12. Brown K. Rheumatoid lung disease. Proc Am Thorac Soc. 2007;4:443–8. https://doi.org/10.1513/pats.200703-045MS.
13. Chen Y-J, Chang Y-T, Wang C-B, Wu C-Y. The risk of cancer in patients with rheumatoid arthritis: A nationwide cohort study in Taiwan. Arthritis Rheum. 2011;63(2):352–8. https://doi.org/10.1002/art.30134.
14. Dejaco C, Singh YP, Perel P, et al. 2015 Recommendations for the management of polymyalgia rheumatica: a European League Against Rheumatism/American College of Rheumatology collaborative initiative. Ann Rheum Dis. 2015;74:1799–807. https://doi.org/10.1136/annrheumdis-2015-207492.
15. Barnett K, Mercer SW, Norbury M, Watt G, Wyke S, Guthrie B. Epidemiology of multimorbidity and implications for health care, research, and medical education: a cross-sectional study. Lancet. 2012;380(9836):37–43. https://doi.org/10.1016/S0140-6736(12)60240-2.
16. Salvarani C, Cantini F, Boiardi L, Hunder GG. Polymyalgia rheumatica and giant-cell arteritis. N Engl J Med. 2002;347(4):261–71.
17. Weyand CM, Goronzy J. Giant-cell arteritis and polymyalgia rheumatica. Ann Intern Med. 2003;139:505–16.
18. Moher D, Liberati A, Tetzlaff J, Altman DG, Grp P. Preferred Reporting Items for Systematic Reviews and Meta-Analyses: the PRISMA statement (reprinted from Annals of Internal Medicine). PLoS ONE. 2009;6(7):1-6. https://doi.org/10.1371/journal.pmed.1000097.
19. Byrt T, Bishop J, Carlin JB. Bias, prevalence and kappa. J Clin Epidemiol. 1993; 46(5):423–9. https://doi.org/10.1016/0895-4356(93)90018-V.
20. Dasgupta B, Cimmino MA, Kremers HM, et al. 2012 Provisional classification criteria for polymyalgia rheumatica: a European League Against Rheumatism/American College of Rheumatology collaborative initiative. Arthritis Rheum. 2012;64(4):943–54. https://doi.org/10.1002/art.34356.
21. Behn AR, Perera T, Myles AB. Polymyalgia rheumatica and corticosteroids: how much for how long? Ann Rheum Dis. 1983;42(4):374–8. https://doi.org/10.1136/ard.42.4.374.
22. Gabriel SE, Sunku J, Salvarani C, O'Fallon WM, Hunder GG. Adverse outcomes of antiinflammatory therapy among patients with polymyalgia rheumatica. Arthritis Rheum. 1997;40(10):1873–8. https://doi.org/10.1002/art.1780401022.
23. Mazzantini M, Torre C, Miccoli M, et al. Adverse events during longterm low-dose glucocorticoid treatment of polymyalgia rheumatica: a retrospective study. J Rheumatol. 2012;39(3):552–7. https://doi.org/10.3899/jrheum.110851.
24. Proven A, Gabriel SE, Orces C, O'Fallon WM, Hunder GG. Glucocorticoid therapy in giant cell arteritis: duration and adverse outcomes. Arthritis Rheum. 2003;49(5):703–8. https://doi.org/10.1002/art.11388.
25. Paskins Z, Whittle R, Sultan AA, et al. Risk of fracture among patients with polymyalgia rheumatica and giant cell arteritis: a population-based study. BMC Med. 2018;16(4):1–9. https://doi.org/10.1186/s12916-017-0987-1.
26. Shbeeb I, Challah D, Raheel S, Crowson CS, Matteson EL. Comparable rates of glucocorticoid associated adverse events in patients with polymyalgia rheumatica and comorbidities in the general population. Arthritis Care Res. 2018;70(4):643–7. https://doi.org/10.1002/acr.23320.
27. Albrecht K, Huscher D, Buttgereit F, et al. Long-term glucocorticoid treatment in patients with polymyalgia rheumatica, giant cell arteritis, or both diseases: results from a national rheumatology database. Rheumatol Int. 2018;38(4):569–77. https://doi.org/10.1007/s00296-017-3874-3.
28. Wells G, Shea B, O'Connell D, Peterson J, Welch V, Losos M. The Newcastle-Ottawa Scale (NOS) for assessing the quality if nonrandomized studies in meta-analyses. Available from: http://www.ohri.ca/programs/clinical_epidemiology/oxford.htm. Accessed 1 Nov 2016.
29. Higgins JPT, Green S. Cochrane Handbook for Systematic Reviews of Interventions. Version 5.1.0 [updated March 2011]. The Cochrane Collaboration; 2011. Available from http://handbook.cochrane.org.
30. Bengtsson BA, Malmvall BE. The epidemiology of giant cell arteritis including temporal arteritis and polymyalgia rheumatica. Incidences of different clinical presentations and eye complications. Arthritis Rheum. 1981; 24(7):899–904.
31. Bowness P, Shotliff K, Middlemiss A, Myles AB. Prevalence of hypothyroidism in patients with polymyalgia rheumatica and giant cell arteritis. Br J Rheumatol. 1991;30(5):349–51.
32. Haga H, Eide G, Brun J, Johansen A, Langmark F. Cancer in association with polymyalgia rheumatica and temporal arteritis. J Rheumatol. 1993;20(8): 1335–9.
33. Juchet H, Labarthe M, Ollier S, Vilain C, Arlet P. Prevalence of hypothyroidism and hyperthyroidism in patients with giant cell arteritis or polymyalgia rheumatica: a controlled study in one hundred and four cases. Rev du Rhum English Ed. 1993;60(7–8):406–11.

34. Schaufelberger C, Bengtsson BA, Andersson R. Epidemiology and mortality in 220 patients with polymyalgia rheumatica. Br J Rheumatol. 1995;34(3): 261–4. https://doi.org/10.1093/rheumatology/34.3.261.
35. Gran JT, Myklebust G, Wilsgaard T, Jacobsen BK. Survival in polymyalgia rheumatica and temporal arteritis: a study of 398 cases and matched population controls. Rheumatology. 2001;40(11):1238–42 http://www.ncbi.nlm.nih.gov/pubmed/11709607.
36. Uddhammar A, Eriksson A-L, Nyström L, et al. Increased mortality due to cardiovascular disease in patients with giant cell arteritis in northern Sweden. J Rheumatol. 2002;29(4):737–42.
37. Myklebust G, Wilsgaard T, Jacobsen BK, Gran TJ. No increased frequency of malignant neoplasms in polymyalgia rheumatica and temporal arteritis. A prospective longitudinal study of 398 cases and matched population controls. J Rheumatol. 2002;29(10):2143–7.
38. Doran MF, Crowson CS, O'Fallon WM, Hunder GG, Gabriel SE. Trends in the incidence of polymyalgia rheumatica over a 30 year period in Olmsted County, Minnesota, USA. J Rheumatol. 2002;29(8):1694–7.
39. Myklebust G, Wilsgaard T, Jacobsen BK, Gran JT. Causes of death in polymyalgia rheumatica. A prospective longitudinal study of 315 cases and matched population controls. Scand J Rheumatol. 2003;32(1):38–41. https://doi.org/10.1080/03009740310000382.
40. Kremers HM, Reinalda MS, Crowson CS, Zinsmeister AR, Hunder GG, Gabriel SE. Direct medical costs of polymyalgia rheumatica. Arthritis Rheum. 2005; 53(4):578–84. https://doi.org/10.1002/art.21311.
41. Eaton WW, Rose NR, Kalaydjian A, Pedersen MG, Mortensen PB. Epidemiology of autoimmune diseases in Denmark. J Autoimmun. 2007; 29(1):1–9.
42. Kremers HMH, Reinalda MMS, Crowson CCS, Davis JMJ, Hunder GGG, Gabriel SES. Glucocorticoids and cardiovascular and cerebrovascular events in polymyalgia rheumatica. Arthritis Care Res. 2007;57(2):279–86. https://doi.org/10.1002/art.22548.
43. Warrington KJ, Jarpa EP, Crowson CS, et al. Increased risk of peripheral arterial disease in polymyalgia rheumatica: a population-based cohort study. Arthritis Res Ther. 2009;11(2):R50. https://doi.org/10.1186/ar2664.
44. Eaton WW, Byrne M, Ewald H, et al. Association of schizophrenia and autoimmune diseases: linkage of Danish national registers. Am J Psychiatry. 2006;163(3):521–8. https://doi.org/10.1176/appi.ajp.163.3.521.
45. Ji J, Liu X, Sundquist K, Sundquist J, Hemminki K. Cancer risk in patients hospitalized with polymyalgia rheumatica and giant cell arteritis: a follow-up study in Sweden. Rheumatology. 2010;49(6):1158–63.
46. Kang J-H, Sheu J-J, Lin H-C. Polymyalgia rheumatica and the risk of stroke: a three-year follow-up study. Cerebrovasc Dis. 2011;32(5):497–503. https://doi.org/10.1159/000332031.
47. Hemminki K, Liu X, Ji J, Sundquist J, Sundquist K. Autoimmune disease and subsequent digestive tract cancer by histology. Ann Oncol. 2012;23(4):927–33. https://doi.org/10.1093/annonc/mdr333.
48. Zoller B, Li X, Sundquist J, Sundquist K. Risk of subsequent ischemic and hemorrhagic stroke in patients hospitalized for immune-mediated diseases: a nationwide follow-up study from Sweden. BMC Neurol. 2012;12:41. https://doi.org/10.1186/1471-2377-12-41.
49. Li X, Sundquist J, Sundquist K. Subsequent risks of Parkinson disease in patients with autoimmune and related disorders: a nationwide epidemiological study from Sweden. Neurodegener Dis. 2012;10(1–4):277–84. https://doi.org/10.1159/000333222.
50. Hemminki K, Liu X, Ji J, Sundquist J, Sundquist K. Effect of autoimmune diseases on mortality and survival in subsequent digestive tract cancers. Ann Oncol. 2012;23(8):2179–84. https://doi.org/10.1093/annonc/mdr590.
51. Hemminki K, Liu X, Ji J, Forsti A, Sundquist J, Sundquist K. Effect of autoimmune diseases on risk and survival in female cancers. Gynecol Oncol. 2012;127(1):180–5. https://doi.org/10.1016/j.ygyno.2012.07.100.
52. Zöller B, Li X, Sundquist J, Sundquist K. Risk of subsequent coronary heart disease in patients hospitalized for immune-mediated diseases: a nationwide follow-up study from Sweden. PLoS One. 2012;7(3):1–8. https://doi.org/10.1371/journal.pone.0033442.
53. Hemminki K, Li X, Sundquist J, Sundquist K. Risk of asthma and autoimmune diseases and related conditions in patients hospitalized for obesity. Ann Med. 2012;44(3):289–95.
54. Hemminki K, Liu X, Forsti A, Ji J, Sundquist J, Sundquist K. Effect of autoimmune diseases on incidence and survival in subsequent multiple myeloma. J Hematol Oncol. 2012;5:59.
55. Fallah M, Liu X, Ji J, Forsti A, Sundquist K, Hemminki K. Hodgkin lymphoma after autoimmune diseases by age at diagnosis and histological subtype. Ann Oncol. 2014;25(7):1397–404. https://doi.org/10.1093/annonc/mdu144.
56. Fallah M, Liu X, Ji J, Forsti A, Sundquist K, Hemminki K. Autoimmune diseases associated with non-Hodgkin lymphoma: a nationwide cohort study. Ann Oncol. 2014;25:2025–30. https://doi.org/10.1093/annonc/mdu365.
57. Muller S, Hider SLS, Belcher J, Helliwell T, Mallen CD. Is cancer associated with polymyalgia rheumatica? A cohort study in the General Practice Research Database. Ann Rheum Dis. 2014;73:1769–73. https://doi.org/10.1136/annrheumdis-2013-203465.
58. Hancock AT, Mallen CD, Muller S, et al. Risk of vascular events in patients with polymyalgia rheumatica. Can Med Assoc J. 2014;186(13):495–501.
59. Pfeifer EC, Crowson CS, Major BT, Matteson EL. Polymyalgia Rheumatica and its Association with Cancer. Rheumatology (Sunnyvale). 2015;(Suppl 6):003. https://doi.org/10.4172/2161-1149.S6-003.Polymyalgia.
60. Pujades-Rodriguez M, Duyx B, Thomas SL, Stogiannis D, Smeeth L, Hemingway H. Associations between polymyalgia rheumatica and giant cell arteritis and 12 cardiovascular diseases. Heart. 2016;102(5):383–9.
61. Bellan M, Boggio E, Sola D, et al. Association between rheumatic diseases and cancer: results from a clinical practice cohort study. Intern Emerg Med. 2017;12(5):621-7. https://doi.org/10.1007/s11739-017-1626-8.
62. Askling J, Klareskog L, Hjalgrim H, Baecklund E, Bjorkholm M, Ekbom A. Do steroids increase lymphoma risk? A case-control study of lymphoma risk in polymyalgia rheumatica/giant cell arteritis. Ann Rheum Dis. 2005;64(12): 1765–8.
63. Anderson LA, Pfeiffer RM, Landgren O, Gadalla S, Berndt SI, Engels EA. Risks of myeloid malignancies in patients with autoimmune conditions. Br J Cancer. 2009;100(5):822–8.
64. Anderson LA, Gadalla S, Morton LM, et al. Population-based study of autoimmune conditions and the risk of specific lymphoid malignancies. Int J Cancer. 2009;125(2):398–405.
65. Lanoy E, Engels EA. Skin cancers associated with autoimmune conditions among elderly adults. Br J Cancer. 2010;103(1):112–4.
66. Kristinsson SY, Landgren O, Samuelsson J, Bjorkholm M, Goldin LR. Autoimmunity and the risk of myeloproliferative neoplasms. Haematologica. 2010;95(7):1216–20. https://doi.org/10.3324/haematol.2009.020412.
67. Anderson LA, Engels EA. Autoimmune conditions and hairy cell leukemia: an exploratory case-control study. J Hematol Oncol. 2010;3:35.
68. Lindqvist EK, Goldin LR, Landgren O, et al. Personal and family history of immune-related conditions increase the risk of plasma cell disorders: a population-based study. Blood. 2011;118(24):6284–91.
69. Chen SJ, Chao YL, Chen CY, et al. Prevalence of autoimmune diseases in in-patients with schizophrenia: nationwide population-based study. Br J Psychiatry. 2012;200:374–80. https://doi.org/10.1192/bjp.bp.111.092098.
70. Scrivo R, Gerardi MC, Rutigliano I, et al. Polymyalgia rheumatica and diverticular disease: just two distinct age-related disorders or more? Results from a case-control study. Clin Rheumatol. 2018;37(9):2573-7. https://doi.org/10.1007/s10067-018-4137-8.
71. Yates M, Graham K, Watts R, MacGregor A. The prevalence of giant cell arteritis and polymyalgia rheumatica in a UK primary care population. BMC Musculoskelet Disord. 2016;17:285.
72. Barraclough K, Liddell WG, du Toit J, et al. Polymyalgia rheumatica in primary care: a cohort study of the diagnostic criteria and outcome. Fam Pract. 2008;25(5):328–33.
73. Hellgren K, Baecklund E, Backlin C, Sundstrom C, Smedby KE, Askling J. Rheumatoid Arthritis and risk of malignant lymphoma: is the risk still increased? Arthritis Rheumatol. 2017;69(4):700–8. https://doi.org/10.1002/art.40017.
74. Floris A, Piga M, Cauli A, Salvarani C, Mathieu A. Polymyalgia rheumatica: zn autoinflammatory disorder? RMD Open. 2018;4(1):2–6. https://doi.org/10.1136/rmdopen-2018-000694.
75. Haut ER, Pronovost PJ. Surveillance bias in outcomes reporting. JAMA. 2011; 305(23):2462–3. https://doi.org/10.1001/jama.2011.822.
76. Piccirillo JF, Vlahiotis A, Barrett LB, Flood KL, Spitznagel EL, Steyerberg EW. The changing prevalence of comorbidity across the age spectrum. Crit Rev Oncol Hematol. 2008;67(2):124–32. https://doi.org/10.1016/j.critrevonc.2008.01.013.

6

Chemerin 156F, generated by chymase cleavage of prochemerin, is elevated in joint fluids of arthritis patients

Lei Zhao[1,3], Yasuto Yamaguchi[1,3], Xiaomei Ge[1,3], William H. Robinson[2,3,4], John Morser[1,3*] and Lawrence L. K. Leung[1,3]

Abstract

Background: Chemerin is a chemoattractant involved in immunity that also functions as an adipokine. Chemerin is secreted as an inactive precursor (chem163S), and its activation requires proteolytic cleavages at its C-terminus, involving proteases in coagulation, fibrinolysis, and inflammation. Previously, we found chem158K was the dominant chemerin form in synovial fluids from patients with arthritis. In this study, we aimed to characterize a distinct cleaved chemerin form, chem156F, in osteoarthritis (OA) and rheumatoid arthritis (RA).

Methods: Purified chem156F was produced in transfected CHO cells. To quantify chem156F in OA and RA samples, we developed a specific ELISA for chem156F using antibody raised against a peptide representing the C-terminus of chem156F.

Results: Ca^{2+} mobilization assays showed that the EC_{50} values for chem163S, chem156F, and chem157S were 252 ± 141 nM, 133 ± 41.5 nM, and 5.83 ± 2.48 nM, respectively. chem156F was more active than its precursor, chem163S, but very much less potent than chem157S, the most active chemerin form. Chymase was shown to be capable of cleaving chem163S at a relevant rate. Using the chem156F ELISA we found a substantial amount of chem156F present in synovial fluids from patients with OA and RA, 24.06 ± 5.51 ng/ml and 20.35 ± 5.19 ng/ml (mean ± SEM, n = 25) respectively, representing 20% of total chemerin in OA and 76.7% of chemerin in RA synovial fluids.

Conclusions: Our data show that chymase cleavage of chem163S to partially active chem156F can be found in synovial fluids where it can play a role in modulation of the inflammation in joints.

Keywords: Adipokine, Arthritis, Inflammation, Osteoarthritis, Serine protease

Background

Chemerin is involved in innate and adaptive immunity as a chemoattractant for natural killer (NK) cells, macrophages, and certain dendritic cell (DC) subsets [1, 2] but is also an adipokine [3–6]. Chemerin is well conserved across mammalian species with strong homology within its C-terminus. Human chemerin is expressed as a 163-amino-acid preproprotein containing a 20-amino-acid signal sequence, and is secreted as a 143-amino-acid precursor, prochemerin (chem163S) [2]. A characteristic of chemerin is that chem163S has low biological activity and requires precise extracellular C-terminal proteolytic processing to achieve its full functional activity. A variety of enzymes involved in blood coagulation, fibrinolysis, and inflammation—such as factor XIa, plasmin, carboxypeptidase B2 (also known as thrombin-activatable fibrinolysis inhibitor), elastase, or chymase—can proteolyze chemerin, leading to its activation or inactivation [7–10].

Rheumatoid arthritis (RA) and osteoarthritis (OA) are the most common forms of autoimmune and degenerative arthritis, respectively. Immune cell infiltrates are observed in synovial tissues in both diseases. We previously demonstrated that carboxypeptidase B2 (CPB2)

* Correspondence: jmorser@stanford.edu
[1]Department of Medicine, Division of Hematology, Stanford University School of Medicine, Stanford, CA 94305, USA
[3]Veterans Affairs Palo Alto Health Care System, Room A4-131, Building 101, 3801 Miranda Avenue, Palo Alto, CA 94304, USA
Full list of author information is available at the end of the article

regulates inflammation and tissue destruction in human and/or mouse models of RA and OA [11, 12]. In this study we investigate the presence of the cleaved isoforms of chemerin in RA and OA synovial fluid samples.

In order to study the biology of chemerin in vivo, we had previously produced various recombinant chemerin forms and developed specific ELISAs for them. Cleavage of the last four amino acids from chem163S by either FXIa or plasmin, giving rise to chem158K, represents a major step in prochemerin activation in vivo [13, 14]. Removal of the C-terminal lysine from chem158K, by either carboxypeptidase N (CPN) or CPB2, results in chem157S, the most potent chemerin form. On the other hand, chem155A is functionally inert [15]. A chemerin C-terminal peptide that represented chem156F is functionally active in vitro. In this article, we report the purification and characterization of chem156F, the generation of an anti-chem156F antibody, and the subsequent development of a specific ELISA for chem156F that we used to demonstrate the presence of chem156F in synovial fluid samples from patients with OA and RA.

Methods

Generation of CHO-S stable cell clones expressing human chem156F

A cDNA clone encoding human chemerin (NM_002889) was obtained from Open Biosystems (Huntsville, AL, USA). A cDNA fragment encoding chem156F was amplified by PCR using Platinum Pfx DNA polymerase (Invitrogen, Carlsbad, CA, USA) with termination codons inserted into the primers (CHEM-5 Ngo Primer 5′-AGCCGGCCACCATGCGACGGCTGCTGAT used as sense primer, and hCHEM-3 Nhe-F Primer 5′-AGCTAGCTTAGAAGGCGAACTGTCCAGGGA used as anti-sense primer) [13]. The cDNA encoding chem156F was cloned into a ubiquitous chromatin opening element (UCOE) vector, pCET-1019AS-puro, provided by Millipore. The plasmid encoding chem156F was transfected into CHO-S cells and subsequent selection was performed as described previously [15]. Plasmids encoding cDNAs for mouse chemerin forms, homologous to human chem156F (mouse mchem155F) and human chem157S (mouse chem156S), were produced in a similar fashion.

Protein production

The selected CHO-S clone expressing chem156F was grown in suspension culture in CD Opti-CHO medium. To avoid cleavage of chemerin, the CHO-S cells were expanded in 225-cm^2 T-flasks for 3 days before switching to CD-CHO medium. Static culture was then used to produce chem156F in 225-cm^2 T-flasks for 3 days at 37 °C and purified as described previously [15]. The purified protein was characterized by SDS-PAGE. Mouse mchem156S and mchem155F were produced, purified, and characterized by the same methods.

Calcium mobilization assays

L1.2 cells stably expressing human CMKLR1 were provided by Dr Brian Zabel and Dr Eugene C. Butcher (Stanford University School of Medicine and Veterans Affairs Palo Alto Health Care System) and cultured in RPMI 1640 with 10% FBS and 1 mg/ml geneticin [15]. Cells were labeled with Quest Fluo-8 AM dye, and then stimulated with recombinant chemerin forms in a 96-well plate calcium mobilization assay [15]. Each assay was repeated at least three times for each protein or peptide.

Antibody preparation

Anti-human chemerin 156F (anti-chem156F) IgY was raised in chickens against the peptide sequence CZ^{151}PGQFAF^{156} conjugated to KLH (Aves Labs, Tigard, OR, USA) and anti-chem156F IgY from eggs was purified by affinity chromatography to its cognate peptide bound to sepharose. To eliminate cross-reactivity with the chem157S form, negative selection affinity chromatography was performed by adsorption on an amino-linked (AminoLink kit; Thermo Scientific, Rockford, IL, USA) column coupled with the noncognate chemerin peptide KC^{152}GQFAFS^{157}. Rabbit polyclonal anti-human chemerin 163S (anti-chem163S), anti-human chemerin 158 K (anti-chem158K), anti-human chemerin 157S (anti-chem157S), and chicken polyclonal anti-human chemerin 155A (anti-chem155A) were prepared as described previously [14].

Western blot analysis of the specificity of anti-human chem156F IgY

Purified recombinant chem163S, chem158K, chem157S, chem156F, and chem155A (200 ng each) were separated by SDS-PAGE under reducing conditions followed by western blot analysis with 500 ng/ml of the purified anti-chem156F IgY. The blot was developed with peroxidase-conjugated goat anti-chicken IgY antibody (100 ng/ml; Aves Labs) and detected using ECL (GE Healthcare, Sunnyvale, CA, USA).

Specific ELISAs for chemerin forms

A rat monoclonal anti-human chemerin antibody (4 μg/ml; R&D Systems, Minneapolis, MN, USA) in PBS buffer was coated onto 96-well ELISA plates, and nonspecific binding sites were blocked with 1% BSA in PBS for 1 h before sample addition. Purified recombinant chem163S, chem158K, chem157S, chem156F, and chem155A were used as standards to construct calibration curves. Samples and standards were diluted with 1% BSA in PBS and incubated in the wells for 2 h. After washing with 0.05% Tween 20 in PBS, the samples were incubated with specific cognate antibodies (500 ng/ml) in PBS with 1% BSA for 1 h. In the case of anti-chem163S, chem158K peptide (10 μg/ml) was added to remove residual cross-reactivity with chem158K. In the case of anti-chem158K, chem163S peptide (10 μg/ml) was added to remove residual cross-reactivity with chem163S. In the case of anti-chem156F, chem155A peptide (10 μg/ml) was added to remove residual cross-reactivity with chem155A. For anti-chem155A, 10 μg/ml each of chem157S and chem158K peptides was added to remove the residual cross-reactivity with chem157S and chem158K. After washing with 0.05% Tween 20 in PBS, the samples were incubated with peroxidase-conjugated goat anti-rabbit IgG antibody (100 ng/ml) or peroxidase-conjugated goat anti-chicken IgY antibody (100 ng/ml) in PBS with 1% BSA for 1 h. After washing, tetramethylbenzidine substrate (Alpha Diagnostic International, San Antonio, TX, USA) was incubated for 10 min followed by the addition of Stop Solution (Alpha Diagnostic International) and absorbance at 450 nm measured. The concentrations of human chemerin forms were calculated from the calibration curves of the purified chemerin standards.

Determination of chemerin forms in synovial fluid samples

Human synovial fluid samples were obtained under a protocol for discarded specimens approved by Stanford University School of Medicine or Partners Healthcare Institutional Review Boards. The samples were stored frozen at − 80 °C until the time of analysis. After thawing, 30 μl of a synovial fluid sample diluted to 400 μl with PBS was mixed with 50 μl of heparin-agarose (Sigma, St. Louis, MO, USA) and Complete Protease Inhibitor (Roche Applied Science, Pleasanton, CA, USA) [14], and the eluates were assayed by the specific ELISAs.

Determination of chymase level in synovial fluid samples

Thawed synovial fluid samples were diluted 2-fold to 5-fold and assayed by human CMA1/Mast Cell Chymase ELISA kit (Life Span Biosciences Inc., Seattle, WA, USA).

Kinetics of chymase cleavage of chem163S

Peptides (1–3 μM) representing the C-terminus of chem163S (chem163S-15mer) and chem156F (chem156F-8mer) were treated with chymase (30 nM) in PBS for 30 min at 37 °C before terminating the reaction with 100 nM PPACK. Then 100 μl of each reaction mixture was loaded onto a Zorbax Eclipse Plus C18 (4.6 mm × 150 mm) column (Agilent, Santa Clara, CA, USA) and separated with a 0–40% acetonitrile gradient in 0.1% trifluoroacetic acid (v/v) by HPLC. The concentration of peptides present in the reaction mixture was determined from the area under the curve for that peptide by comparison to a standard curve (1 μM–3 mM) of that peptide. The values for K_M and k_{cat} were determined by fitting to the Michaelis–Menten equation by nonlinear regression analysis using Prism v6 (Graphpad, San Diego, CA, USA). The experiments were performed three times independently, and the data were pooled for analysis.

Statistics

Comparison of two samples was by Student's t test; multigroup comparisons were by ANOVA followed by post hoc Kruskal–Wallis analysis. The analysis was carried out using Prism v7 (GraphPad, La Jolla, CA, USA). $p < 0.05$ was considered significant.

Results

Expression and purification of recombinant chem156F

DNA encoding chem156F was cloned into a plasmid, pCET-1019AS-puro, that has a UCOE element upstream of a guinea pig CMV promoter before transfection into CHO-S cells [15]. Two days after transfection, stable clones were selected by limiting dilution in 10 μg/ml puromycin, and 90 clones were screened for production of chem156F. A clone was identified that produced chem156F with a productivity of 4.74 pg/cell per day. Recombinant chem156F was purified by single-step cation exchange chromatography (Additional file 1: Figure S1A) and its C-terminus was confirmed by mass spectroscopy as described for purification and characterization of other recombinant chemerin forms [15]. The purified chem156F together with other purified recombinant human chemerins, chem163S, chem158K, chem157S, and chem155A, were shown to be > 95% pure by SDS-PAGE (Additional file 1: Figure S1B). Antibody raised against chem156F reacted only with chem156F (Additional file 1: Figure S1C).

Functional characterization of chem156F

We evaluated the potency of the purified chem156F in induction of calcium mobilization using CMKLR1-transfected L1.2 cells. Purified chem163S and chem157S were used as controls (Fig. 1a). The EC_{50} values for chem163S and chem156F were 252 ± 141 nM and 133 ± 41.5 nM respectively, while the EC_{50} value of chem157S was 5.83 ± 2.48 nM which is > 20-fold more potent than chem156F and > 40-fold more potent than chem163S. Thus, chem156F was about twice as active as the precursor, chem163S, but very much less active than chem157S, the most active form of chemerin based on the CMKLR1-transfected cell assay. The relative potencies of chem163S,

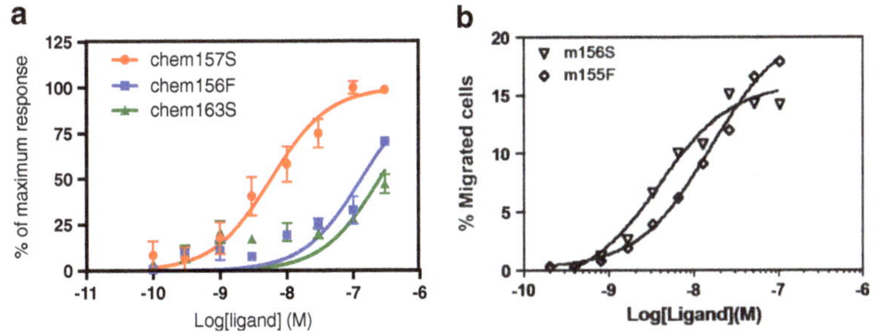

Fig. 1 Biological activities of human chem156F and mouse mchem155F on CMKLR1. **a** Calcium flux in L1.2 cells transfected with human CMKLR1 in response to indicated concentration of chem156F (blue) and control recombinant proteins chem163S (green) and chem157S (red). **b** Indicated concentrations of mouse mchem156S (m156S, triangles) and mouse mchem156F (m155F, diamonds) assayed for their chemotactic activity on human CMKLR1/L1.2 cells using Transwell chemotaxis assay

chem156F, and chem157S were similar to that of their equivalent C-terminal peptides [15].

Unlike in mouse where mouse mchem156S, the homolog of human chem157S, and mouse mchem155F, the homolog of human chem156F, have approximately the same activity (data not shown), in humans chem156F is significantly less potent than chem157S. One explanation is that species differences between human and mouse CMKLR1 lead to chem156F being active on mouse but much less so on human CMKLR1. We tested this possibility by determining the potency of mouse mchem156S and mouse mchem155F in chemotaxis on L1.2 cells transfected with human CMKLR1. As on the L1.2 cells transfected with mouse CMKLR1, mouse mchem156S and mchem155F were equipotent showing that the difference in potency is not due to species-specific activity of chemerin on CMKLR1 cells (Fig. 1b).

Generation and characterization of antibody specific for chem156F

In order to specifically detect chem156F in human samples, we prepared chicken anti-chemerin 156F (anti-chem156F) by immunization with a peptide representing the C-terminal sequence of chem156F. The specificity of the affinity-purified anti-chem156F IgY was demonstrated by western blot analysis in which anti-chem156F IgY only recognized its cognate protein but not the other four chemerin forms (Additional file 1: Figure S1C).

Development of ELISAs specific for different human chemerin forms

Antibodies directed against the different forms of chemerin were used to develop sandwich ELISAs specific for the different chemerins, chem163S, chem158K, chem157S , chem156F, and chem155A. Recombinant chem163S, but not recombinant chem158K, chem157S, chem156F, or chem155A, was specifically detected in a dose-dependent manner by anti-chem163S, with a lower limit of detection of 0.5 ng/ml (Fig. 2). Likewise, anti-chem158K specifically recognized recombinant chem158K and not the other forms, whereas anti-chem157S and anti-chem155A specifically recognized recombinant chem157S and chem155A, respectively (Fig. 2). Anti-chem156F recognized recombinant chem156F, with some cross-reactivity against recombinant chem157S (Fig. 2). In order to measure chem156F accurately, taking into account the antibody's cross-reactivity with chem157S, we used the signal from the chem156F ELISA to give the total concentration of [chem156F + chem157S] from which we then subtracted the chem157S concentration, as measured by the specific chem157S ELISA, to give the

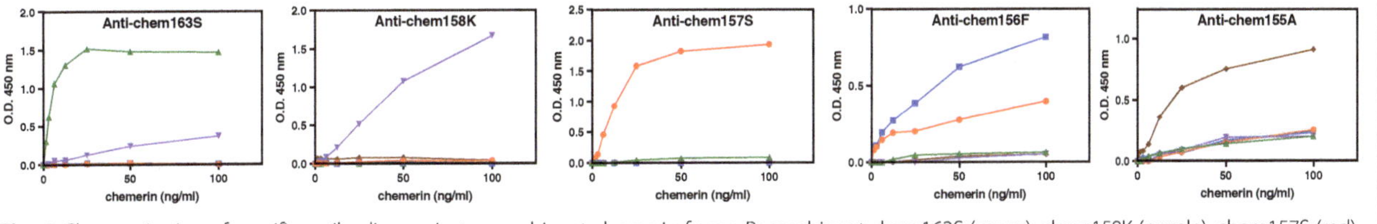

Fig. 2 Characterization of specific antibodies against recombinant chemerin forms. Recombinant chem163S (green), chem158K (purple), chem157S (red), chem156F (blue), and chem155A (brown) by anti-chem163S, anti-chem158K, anti-chem157S, anti-chem156F, and anti-chem155A detected using specific ELISAs as described under "Methods". O.D. optical density

concentration of chem156F. Using this panel of ELISAs, the levels of different forms of human chemerin can be determined specifically.

Detection of chemerin forms in the synovial fluid from arthritis

We have previously observed extensive proteolytic cleavage of chemerin (~ 75%) in synovial fluid samples from inflammatory arthritis patients and shown that chem158K is the dominant form [14]. To determine whether chem156F is present in the synovial fluid of arthritis patients, we investigated the levels of the five chemerin forms in synovial fluid samples from 25 patients with OA and 25 patients with RA. In OA synovial fluid samples, the levels of chem163S, chem158K, chem157S, chem156F, and chem155A were 24.28 ± 4.85 ng/ml, 77.04 ± 12.25 ng/ml, 1.31 ± 0.77 ng/ml, 24.06 ± 5.51 ng/ml, and 0.57 ± 0.43 ng/ml (mean ± SEM, $n = 25$) respectively (Fig. 3a). In RA synovial fluid samples, the corresponding levels were 3.06 ± 0.97 ng/ml, 40.57 ± 10.47 ng/ml, 0.29 ± 0.29 ng/ml, 20.35 ± 5.19 ng/ml, and 0 ± 0 ng/ml (mean ± SEM, $n = 25$) (Fig. 3b). In OA synovial fluid samples, when the fractions of individual chemerins from the sum of chemerin forms of each sample were averaged, 52% was chem158K, 20% was chem156F, while uncleaved chem163S was 23% (Fig. 3c). In RA joint fluid samples, the majority of chemerin was found to be chem156F (76.7%), with another 21.3% of chemerin presented as chem158K (Fig. 3c). The fraction of cleaved chemerins (chem158K + chem157S + chem156F + chem155A) was 75% in OA synovial fluid samples and 100% in RA synovial fluid samples (Fig. 3d), demonstrating that significant cleavage and processing of chemerin occurs in this extravascular compartment. Only minimal levels of chem157S and chem155A were detected in synovial fluids from either type of arthritis.

Detection of chymase in synovial fluid from arthritis patients

One enzyme that might generate chem156F from chem163S is chymase [8]. Therefore, we investigated chymase levels in OA and RA synovial fluid samples of arthritis patients. In OA and RA synovial fluid samples, the levels of chymase were 349.7 ± 200.2 pg/ml ($n = 10$) and 942.6 ± 366.8 pg/ml ($n = 8$) (mean ± SEM), respectively (Fig. 4a).

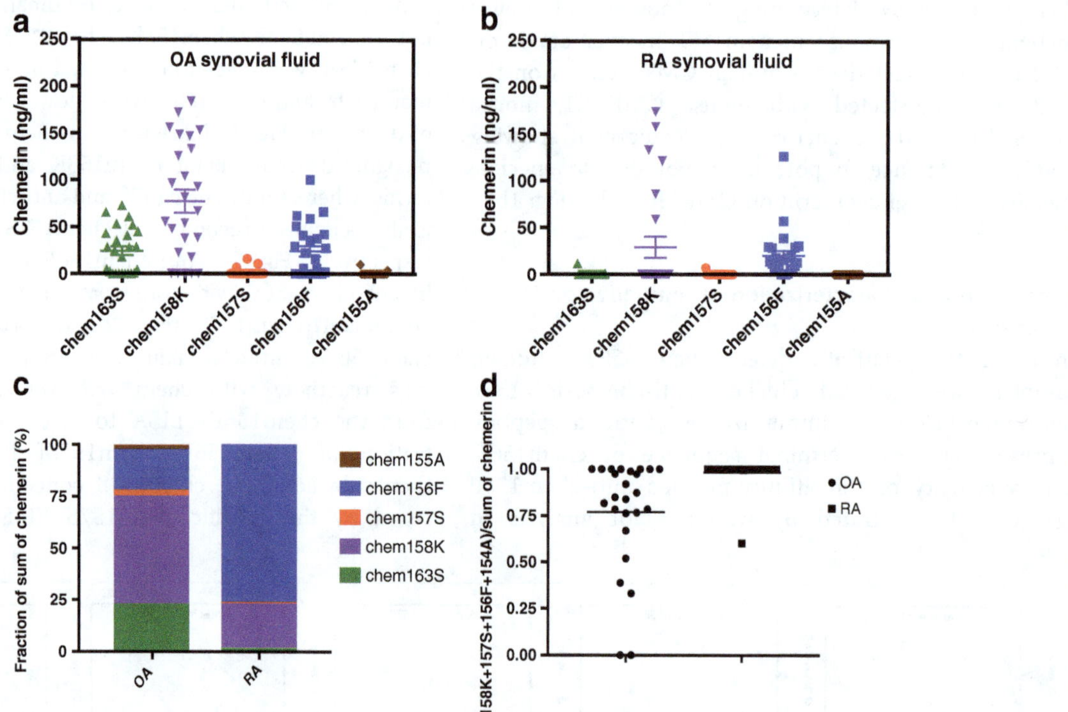

Fig. 3 Levels of chemerin forms in synovial fluid of patients with RA and OA. **a, b** chem163S (▲), chem158K (▼), chem157S (●), chem156F (■), and chem155A (◆) levels in synovial fluid of patients with **a** OA ($n = 25$) and **b** RA ($n = 25$) determined using specific ELISAs as described under "Methods". Horizontal lines show mean ± SEM. **c** Chemerin forms in synovial fluid of OA and RA presented as percentage of sum of five specific ELISAs. **d** Ratio of cleaved chemerin levels (sum of chem158K, chem157S, chem156F, and chem155A) to sum of five chemerin forms in synovial fluid of OA and RA. OA osteoarthritis, RA rheumatoid arthritis

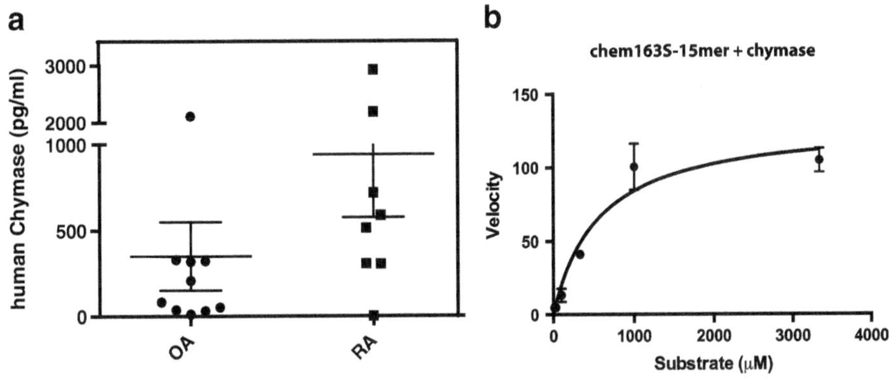

Fig. 4 Chymase in synovial fluid of patients with RA and OA and its cleavage of chemerin. **a** Chymase levels in synovial fluid of patients with OA ($n = 10$) and RA ($n = 8$) determined using human chymase ELISA as described under "Methods". **b** chem163S-15mer incubated with 10 nM chymase for 30 min before analysis by HPLC. Product concentration calculated by interpolation from standard curve, and velocities of product generation determined. OA osteoarthritis, RA rheumatoid arthritis

Characterization of chem163S cleavage by chymase

To determine the kinetic constants for cleavage of chem163S by chymase, chem163S peptides consisting of the last 15 amino acids of the C-terminus of chemerin (chem163S-15mer) were subjected to chymase cleavage followed by HPLC analysis. Hydrolysis of chem163S-15mer by chymase showed K_M of 556.1 ± 174 μM, k_{cat} of 436.4 ± 44.96/min (mean ± SEM), and k_{cat}/K_M of 0.78/μM/min (Fig. 4b and Table 1).

Discussion

In this study, we demonstrate that human chem156F is a distinct cleaved chemerin form. We show that chem156F is ~ 20-fold less potent than chem157S, the most potent form of active chemerin. Peptides representing the C-terminus of chem156F induced calcium mobilization and chemotaxis of CMKLR1/L1.2 cells to a similar degree to that observed with recombinant proteins [15], confirming that chem156F is not as potent as chem157S. This finding is different from that observed in the mouse where the corresponding mouse homologs mchem156S and mchem155F are equipotent (Zhao et al., PLoS One, submitted). The fact that these two mouse chemerins are also equipotent using the human CMKLR1-transfected cells indicates that the difference in potency is most likely not at the level of CMKLR1, the chemerin receptor. Instead, it implies that the difference resides in the proteins and peptides. As the chem156F peptide has similar potency to the chem156F protein, this shows that it must be a sequence difference within the C-terminal tail that leads to the differences in activity. The c-terminal sequence for human chem156F is AGEDPH**S**-**FYF**PGQFAF and for mouse mchem155F is AGEDPH-**GYFL**PGQFAF (amino acids in bold representing substitutions). Thus, mouse mchem155F may present the C-terminus in a better conformation for binding to CMKLR1 than does human chem156F.

In both OA and RA joint fluid samples, there is evidence of extensive activation and cleavage of prochemerin, with chem158K being the dominant form and minimal levels of chem157S [14]. Here we extend that observation by showing that there is a substantial amount of chem156F present in both OA and RA samples, with a strong trend toward increased chem156F in RA as compared to OA synovial fluids. The differential expression levels observed correlate with the lower degree of synovial inflammation in OA as compared to RA [16]. The expression, cleavage, and activation of chemerin in synovial tissues could contribute to the trafficking and activation of immune cells in RA and OA. Circulating chemerin levels in RA have been associated with endothelial cell activation and atherosclerosis [17].

There is immunohistological evidence for expression of prochemerin on endothelial cells and synovial lining in the synovium and its expression on fibroblast-like synoviocytes is upregulated by TNF-α and IFN-γ [18]. Human synovial fibroblasts from patients with RA and OA express both chemerin and its receptor

Table 1 Hydrolysis of chem163S peptides by chymase

Enzyme	Substrate	K_M (μM)	k_{cat} (/min)	k_{cat}/K_M (/M/min)
Chymase	chem163S-15mer	556.1 ± 174	436.4 ± 44.96	7.8×10^5

Substrates were digested with chymase as described in "Methods". The values for K_M, k_{cat}, and k_{cat}/K_M were compared between peptides derived from chem163S. Data are mean ± SEM ($n = 3$).

CMKLR1, and chemerin upregulates CCL2 in synovial fibroblasts [15]. Human chondrocytes express both chemerin and CMKLR1, and when treated with chemerin respond by producing inflammatory cytokines such as IL-1β [19], while chondrocytes increase chemerin production upon IL-1β treatment [20]. This suggests that chemerin may play a role in cartilage damage by increasing local inflammation.

A relationship has been found between disease severity and chemerin levels in OA [21, 22] and in patients with temperomandibular disorders [23], supporting a role for chemerin in OA. In RA, synovial fluid contains chemerin [24]. In none of these studies was the chemerin characterized in terms of the presence of different forms.

Based on the differences between plasma chemerin species and those found in the synovium [13, 14], enzymatic cleavage of prochemerin is probably occurring locally within the joint space. Mast cell chymase is detectable within the same joint fluid samples in which chem156F was found and it cleaves prochemerin chem163S into chem156F with kinetic constants similar to those of other substrates [25, 26]. Mast cells accumulate in arthritic joint tissues of RA patients [27], and mice deficient in either mast cell protease-4 (mMCP-4) or mMCP-5, the two mouse chymases that are the closest functional and structural homologs to the single human chymase, display significantly reduced inflammation in immune arthritis models [28, 29].

Chemerin is also an adipokine and activated chemerin can be found in adipose tissues [30, 31]. Mast cells are also present in adipose tissues and have been shown to release chymase [32, 33], suggesting that mast-cell-derived chymase may be contributing to the activation of chemerin in adipose tissue.

The other dominant form of chemerin in synovial fluids of arthritis, chem158K, can be generated by FXIa, plasmin, or tryptase cleavage of chem163S and is modestly active [14, 15, 30]. The chem158K levels present in the synovial fluid samples may be sufficient to contribute a significant amount of chemerin activity without further processing, or may be further cleaved to chem157S or chem156F. We have previously shown that fibroblast-like synoviocytes express procarboxypeptidase B2 (proCPB2) and there is functional thrombomodulin on these cells that supports thrombin activation of proCPB2 to active CPB2 [34]. CPB2 should convert chem158K into chem157S [13], but minimal chem157S was detected in the RA and OA joint fluid samples (Fig. 3), similar to our previous observation [14]. It is likely that chem157S is further proteolyzed, possibly to chem155A but since chem155A is present at a very low level this

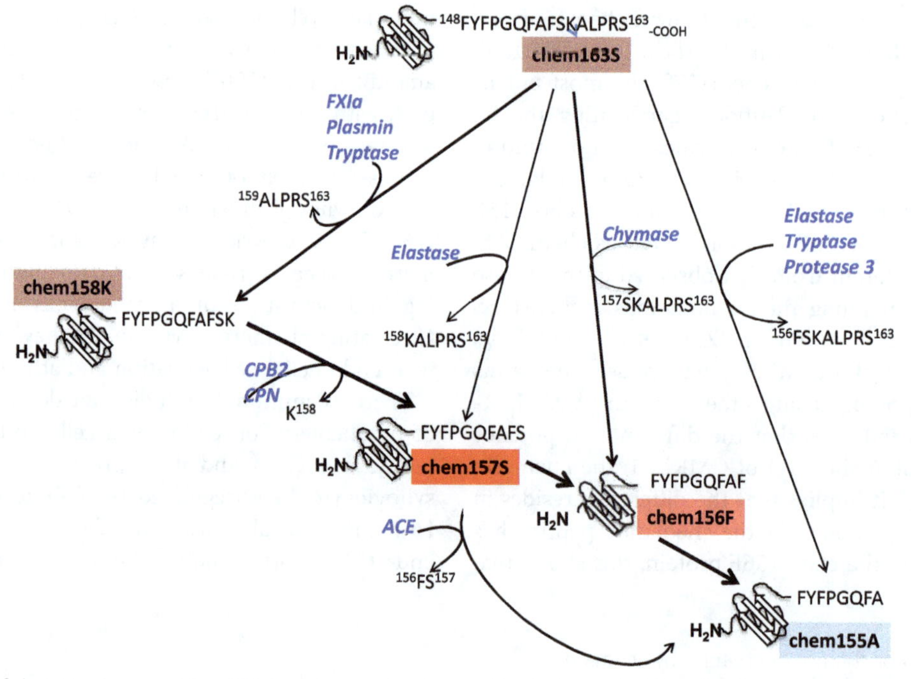

Fig. 5 Schematic of chemerin cleavages. Chem163S (pink box) can be cleaved either by factor XIa (FXIa), Plasmin, or Tryptase generating chem158K (pink box), by elastase generating a mixture of chem157S (red box) and chem155A (blue box), by chymase generating chem156F (dark pink box), or by proteinase 3 and Tryptase generating chem155A. chem158K can then be cleaved by carboxypeptidase B2 (CPB2) or carboxypeptidase N (CPN) to form active chem157S, which is subsequently inactivated by angiotensin-converting enzyme (ACE) forming inactive chem155A

may be unlikely, but also to other degraded forms, such as those found in the plasma of patients undergoing bariatric surgery [30].

Prochemerin (chem163S) can be cleaved in its C-terminal domain by different serine and cysteine proteases in vitro, generating a series of chemerin forms with different levels of activity (Fig. 5). The pathway(s) by which chemerin is activated and inactivated may depend on the location with plasma being different from tissues such as synovial fluid and adipose tissue [13, 30].

Conclusions

In this study, we produced and purified chem156F, and demonstrated its presence in synovial fluids of arthritis patients. This chemerin form and the specific antibody generated will enable further characterization of the proteolytic cleavages of prochemerin. Taken together with other studies of chemerin, these data suggest that in vivo in both humans and mice different proteolytic cleavage pathways occur in different tissue compartments to regulate prochemerin activation and inactivation [13, 30]. Our findings identify a new cleaved form of chemerin, chem156F, that could promote inflammation and tissue destruction in RA and OA. Future studies are needed to further define the potential mechanistic role of chem156F and other isoforms of chemerin in RA and OA.

Additional file

Additional file 1: Figure S1. Purification and characterization of chem156F. Following centrifugation and filtration, conditioned cell culture medium applied to an anion exchange column equilibrated with PBS (pH 7.4) and then chem156F protein eluted by a gradient of increasing ionic strength. **A** Absorbance at 280 nm (mAU, blue line), NaCl gradient from 150 to 500 mM (green), and conductivity (brown) of purification of hchem156F. **B** Coomassie Blue stained SDS-PAGE of purified recombinant chem163S (lane 1), chem158K (lane 2), chem157S (lane 3), chem156F (lane 4), and chem155A (lane 5). **C** Anti-chem156F specific for chem156F characterized by western blot analysis of recombinant chem163S (lane 1), chem158K (lane 2), chem157S (lane 3), chem156F (lane 4), and chem155A (lane 5), as described under "Methods". Molecular mass markers shown on left.

Abbreviations

CMKLR1: Chemokine-like receptor 1; CPB2: Carboxypeptidase B2; CPN: Carboxypeptidase N; mMCP: Mouse mast cell protease; OA: Osteoarthritis; proCPB2: Procarboxypeptidase B2; RA: Rheumatoid arthritis; UCOE: Universal chromosome opening element

Funding

This study was supported by grants from the National Institutes of Health (1RO1 HL57530) and the Department of Veterans Affairs (I01BX001959) (both to LLKL). WHR was supported by grants from the National Institute of Health (R01 AR06367604, U19 AI11049103) and the Department of Veterans Affairs (I01 BX002345, I01RX000588). XG was supported by a National Institutes of Health fellowship training grant (5T32HL120824).

Authors' contributions

JM and LLKL designed the experiments. LZ, YY, and XG carried out the experiments. WHR provided the synovial fluid samples. LZ and JM wrote the article. All authors reviewed the final version. All authors read and approved the final manuscript.

Competing interests

The authors declare that they have no competing interests.

Author details

[1]Department of Medicine, Division of Hematology, Stanford University School of Medicine, Stanford, CA 94305, USA. [2]Department of Medicine, Division of Endocrinology, Stanford University School of Medicine, Stanford, CA 94305, USA. [3]Veterans Affairs Palo Alto Health Care System, Room A4-131, Building 101, 3801 Miranda Avenue, Palo Alto, CA 94304, USA. [4]Department of Medicine, Division of Immunology and Rheumatology, Stanford University School of Medicine, Stanford, CA 94305, USA.

References

1. Wittamer V, Franssen JD, Vulcano M, Mirjolet JF, Le Poul E, Migeotte I, Brezillon S, Tyldesley R, Blanpain C, Detheux M, et al. Specific recruitment of antigen-presenting cells by chemerin, a novel processed ligand from human inflammatory fluids. J Exp Med. 2003;198(7):977–85.
2. Meder W, Wendland M, Busmann A, Kutzleb C, Spodsberg N, John H, Richter R, Schleuder D, Meyer M, Forssmann WG. Characterization of human circulating TIG2 as a ligand for the orphan receptor ChemR23. FEBS Lett. 2003;555(3):495–9.
3. Roh SG, Song SH, Choi KC, Katoh K, Wittamer V, Parmentier M, Sasaki S. Chemerin—a new adipokine that modulates adipogenesis via its own receptor. Biochem Biophys Res Commun. 2007;362(4):1013–8.
4. Bozaoglu K, Bolton K, McMillan J, Zimmet P, Jowett J, Collier G, Walder K, Segal D. Chemerin is a novel adipokine associated with obesity and metabolic syndrome. Endocrinology. 2007;148(10):4687–94.
5. Goralski KB, McCarthy TC, Hanniman EA, Zabel BA, Butcher EC, Parlee SD, Muruganandan S, Sinal CJ. Chemerin, a novel adipokine that regulates adipogenesis and adipocyte metabolism. J Biol Chem. 2007; 282(38):28175–88.
6. Takahashi M, Takahashi Y, Takahashi K, Zolotaryov FN, Hong KS, Kitazawa R, Iida K, Okimura Y, Kaji H, Kitazawa S, et al. Chemerin enhances insulin signaling and potentiates insulin-stimulated glucose uptake in 3T3-L1 adipocytes. FEBS Lett. 2008;582(5):573–8.
7. Du XY, Zabel BA, Myles T, Allen SJ, Handel TM, Lee PP, Butcher EC, Leung LL. Regulation of chemerin bioactivity by plasma carboxypeptidase N, carboxypeptidase B (activated thrombin-activable fibrinolysis inhibitor), and platelets. J Biol Chem. 2009;284(2):751–8.
8. Guillabert A, Wittamer V, Bondue B, Godot V, Imbault V, Parmentier M, Communi D. Role of neutrophil proteinase 3 and mast cell chymase in chemerin proteolytic regulation. J Leukoc Biol. 2008;84(6):1530–8.
9. Schultz S, Saalbach A, Heiker JT, Meier R, Zellmann T, Simon JC, Beck-Sickinger AG. Proteolytic activation of prochemerin by kallikrein 7 breaks an ionic linkage and results in C-terminal rearrangement. Biochem J. 2013; 452(2):271–80.
10. Zabel BA, Silverio AM, Butcher EC. Chemokine-like receptor 1 expression and chemerin-directed chemotaxis distinguish plasmacytoid from myeloid dendritic cells in human blood. J Immunol. 2005;174(1):244–51.
11. Lepus CM, Song JJ, Wang Q, Wagner CA, Lindstrom TM, Chu CR, Sokolove J, Leung LL, Robinson WH. Brief report: carboxypeptidase B serves as a protective mediator in osteoarthritis. Arthritis Rheumatol. 2014;66(1):101–6.
12. Song JJ, Hwang I, Cho KH, Garcia MA, Kim AJ, Wang TH, Lindstrom TM, Lee AT, Nishimura T, Zhao L, et al. Plasma carboxypeptidase B downregulates inflammatory responses in autoimmune arthritis. J Clin Invest. 2011;121(9): 3517–27.
13. Ge X, Yamaguchi Y, Zhao L, Bury L, Gresele P, Berube C, Leung LL, Morser J. Prochemerin cleavage by Factor XIa links coagulation and inflammation. Blood. 2018;131(3):353-64.
14. Zhao L, Yamaguchi Y, Sharif S, Du XY, Song JJ, Lee DM, Recht LD, Robinson WH, Morser J, Leung LL. Chemerin158K protein is the dominant chemerin isoform in synovial and cerebrospinal fluids but not in plasma. J Biol Chem. 2011;286(45):39520–7.

15. Yamaguchi Y, Du XY, Zhao L, Morser J, Leung LL. Proteolytic cleavage of chemerin protein is necessary for activation to the active form, Chem157S, which functions as a signaling molecule in glioblastoma. J Biol Chem. 2011; 286(45):39510–9.
16. Robinson WH, Lepus CM, Wang Q, Raghu H, Mao R, Lindstrom TM, Sokolove J. Low-grade inflammation as a key mediator of the pathogenesis of osteoarthritis. Nat Rev Rheumatol. 2016;12(10):580–92.
17. Dessein PH, Tsang L, Woodiwiss AJ, Norton GR, Solomon A. Circulating concentrations of the novel adipokine chemerin are associated with cardiovascular disease risk in rheumatoid arthritis. J Rheumatol. 2014;41(9): 1746–54.
18. Kaneko K, Miyabe Y, Takayasu A, Fukuda S, Miyabe C, Ebisawa M, Yokoyama W, Watanabe K, Imai T, Muramoto K, et al. Chemerin activates fibroblast-like synoviocytes in patients with rheumatoid arthritis. Arthritis Res Ther. 2011; 13(5):R158.
19. Berg V, Sveinbjornsson B, Bendiksen S, Brox J, Meknas K, Figenschau Y. Human articular chondrocytes express ChemR23 and chemerin; ChemR23 promotes inflammatory signalling upon binding the ligand chemerin(21-157). Arthritis Res Ther. 2010;12(6):R228.
20. Conde J, Gomez R, Bianco G, Scotece M, Lear P, Dieguez C, Gomez-Reino J, Lago F, Gualillo O. Expanding the adipokine network in cartilage: identification and regulation of novel factors in human and murine chondrocytes. Ann Rheum Dis. 2011;70(3):551–9.
21. Huang K, Du G, Li L, Liang H, Zhang B. Association of chemerin levels in synovial fluid with the severity of knee osteoarthritis. Biomarkers. 2012;17(1):16–20.
22. Ma J, Niu DS, Wan NJ, Qin Y, Guo CJ. Elevated chemerin levels in synovial fluid and synovial membrane from patients with knee osteoarthritis. Int J Clin Exp Pathol. 2015;8(10):13393–8.
23. Kaya SG, Yavuz YG, Kızıltunç A. Expression of chemerin in the synovial fluid of patients with temporomandibular joint disorders. J Oral Rehabil. 2018; 45(4);289-94.
24. Valcamonica E, Chighizola CB, Comi D, De Lucia O, Pisoni L, Murgo A, Salvi V, Sozzani S, Meroni PL. Levels of chemerin and interleukin 8 in the synovial fluid of patients with inflammatory arthritides and osteoarthritis. Clin Exp Rheumatol. 2014;32(2):243–50.
25. Kinoshita A, Urata H, Bumpus FM, Husain A. Multiple determinants for the high substrate specificity of an angiotensin II-forming chymase from the human heart. J Biol Chem. 1991;266(29):19192–7.
26. Sanker S, Chandrasekharan UM, Wilk D, Glynias MJ, Karnik SS, Husain A. Distinct multisite synergistic interactions determine substrate specificities of human chymase and rat chymase-1 for angiotensin II formation and degradation. J Biol Chem. 1997;272(5):2963–8.
27. Maruotti N, Crivellato E, Cantatore FP, Vacca A, Ribatti D. Mast cells in rheumatoid arthritis. Clin Rheumatol. 2007;26(1):1–4.
28. Magnusson SE, Pejler G, Kleinau S, Abrink M. Mast cell chymase contributes to the antibody response and the severity of autoimmune arthritis. FASEB J. 2009;23(3):875–82.
29. Stevens RL, McNeil HP, Wensing LA, Shin K, Wong GW, Hansbro PM, Krilis SA. Experimental arthritis is dependent on mouse mast cell protease-5. J Biol Chem. 2017;292(13):5392–404.
30. Chang SS, Eisenberg D, Zhao L, Adams C, Leib R, Morser J, Leung L. Chemerin activation in human obesity. Obesity. 2016;24(7):1522–9.
31. Roman AA, Parlee SD, Sinal CJ. Chemerin: a potential endocrine link between obesity and type 2 diabetes. Endocrine. 2012;42(2):243–51.
32. Divoux A, Moutel S, Poitou C, Lacasa D, Veyrie N, Aissat A, Arock M, Guerre-Millo M, Clement K. Mast cells in human adipose tissue: link with morbid obesity, inflammatory status, and diabetes. J Clin Endocrinol Metab. 2012; 97(9):E1677–85.
33. Zhang J, Shi GP. Mast cells and metabolic syndrome. Biochim Biophys Acta. 2012;1822(1):14–20.
34. Sharif SA, Du X, Myles T, Song JJ, Price E, Lee DM, Goodman SB, Nagashima M, Morser J, Robinson WH, Leung LLK. Thrombin-activatable carboxypeptidase B-cleavage of osteopontin regulates neutrophil survival and synoviocyte binding in rheumatoid arthritis. Arthritis Rheum. 2009; 60(10):2902–12.

7

Fcγ receptor-mediated influx of S100A8/A9-producing neutrophils as inducer of bone erosion during antigen-induced arthritis

Irene Di Ceglie[1], Giuliana Ascone[1], Niels A. J. Cremers[1], Annet W. Sloetjes[1], Birgitte Walgreen[1], Thomas Vogl[2], Johannes Roth[2], J. Sjef Verbeek[3], Fons A. J. van de Loo[1], Marije I. Koenders[1], Peter M. van der Kraan[1], Arjen B. Blom[1], Martijn H. J. van den Bosch[1] and Peter L. E. M. van Lent[1*]

Abstract

Background: Osteoclast-mediated bone erosion is a central feature of rheumatoid arthritis (RA). Immune complexes, present in a large percentage of patients, bind to Fcγ receptors (FcγRs), thereby modulating the activity of immune cells. In this study, we investigated the contribution of FcγRs, and FcγRIV in particular, during antigen-induced arthritis (AIA).

Methods: AIA was induced in knee joints of wild-type (WT), FcγRI,II,III$^{-/-}$, and FcγRI,II,III,IV$^{-/-}$ mice. Bone destruction, numbers of tartrate-resistant acid phosphatase-positive (TRAP^{+}) osteoclasts, and inflammation were evaluated using histology; expression of the macrophage marker F4/80, neutrophil marker NIMPR14, and alarmin S100A8 was evaluated using immunohistochemistry. The percentage of osteoclast precursors in the bone marrow was determined using flow cytometry. In vitro osteoclastogenesis was evaluated with TRAP staining, and gene expression was assessed using real-time PCR.

Results: FcγRI,II,III,IV$^{-/-}$ mice showed decreased bone erosion compared with WT mice during AIA, whereas both the humoral and cellular immune responses against methylated bovine serum albumin were not impaired in FcγRI,II,III,IV$^{-/-}$ mice. The percentage of osteoclast precursors in the bone marrow of arthritic mice and their ability to differentiate into osteoclasts in vitro were comparable between FcγRI,II,III,IV$^{-/-}$ and WT mice. In line with these observations, numbers of TRAP^{+} osteoclasts on the bone surface during AIA were comparable between the two groups. Inflammation, a process that strongly activates osteoclast activity, was reduced in FcγRI,II,III,IV$^{-/-}$ mice, and of note, mainly decreased numbers of neutrophils were present in the joint. In contrast to FcγRI,II,III,IV$^{-/-}$ mice, AIA induction in knee joints of FcγRI,II,III$^{-/-}$ mice resulted in increased bone erosion, inflammation, and numbers of neutrophils, suggesting a crucial role for FcγRIV in the joint pathology by the recruitment of neutrophils. Finally, significant correlations were found between bone erosion and the number of neutrophils present in the joint as well as between bone erosion and the number of S100A8-positive cells, with S100A8 being an alarmin strongly produced by neutrophils that stimulates osteoclast resorbing activity.

Conclusions: FcγRs play a crucial role in the development of bone erosion during AIA by inducing inflammation. In particular, FcγRIV mediates bone erosion in AIA by inducing the influx of S100A8/A9-producing neutrophils into the arthritic joint.

Keywords: Experimental arthritis, Bone erosion, Osteoclast, Immune complexes, FcγRs, Neutrophils, S100A8

* Correspondence: peter.vanlent@radboudumc.nl
[1]Experimental Rheumatology, Radboud university medical center, Geert Grooteplein Zuid 28, 6525 GA Nijmegen, the Netherlands
Full list of author information is available at the end of the article

Background

Rheumatoid arthritis (RA) is a chronic and systemic autoimmune disease that primarily affects the joints [1]. Along with inflammation, excessive bone erosion is one of the central hallmarks of this disease [2, 3]. Next to generalized osteoporosis, severe focal bone erosions are observed at the interface between the inflamed synovium and the bone. Osteoclasts, which differentiate from myeloid precursor cells under the influence of macrophage colony-stimulating factor (M-CSF) and receptor activator of nuclear factor-κB ligand (RANKL), are the cells responsible for this deleterious process [4–6]. Therefore, a deeper understanding of how the inflammatory response increases bone erosion in this disease is likely to be helpful in identifying new therapeutic targets.

Autoantibodies such as rheumatoid factor (RF) and anticitrullinated protein antibodies are present in the serum and synovial fluid of a large percentage of patients with RA [1]. Of note, in patients with RA the presence of autoantibodies predates disease onset and correlates with disease progression and severity [7–9]. Immunoglobulin G (IgG) antibodies can form immune complexes (ICs) with their cognate antigens and subsequently bind to Fcγ receptors (FcγRs), thereby modulating the activity of the FcγR-bearing immune cells [10].

In mice, four different FcγRs have been identified, of which the activating FcγRI, FcγRIII, and FcγRIV stimulate the cell via the activation motif immunoreceptor tyrosine-based activation motif (ITAM), leading to effector functions such as phagocytosis, antigen presentation, and cytokine secretion. In contrast, FcγRIIb is an inhibitory receptor, and its intracellular domain contains an immunoreceptor tyrosine-based inhibitory motif (ITIM) that counteracts the signaling of the activating FcγRs [10–12]. Alterations in the expression of FcγRs have been described in circulating monocytes and synovial tissue of patients with RA, suggesting their involvement in the pathogenesis of RA [13–18]. Moreover, the crucial pathogenic role of FcγRs has been proven in a multitude of experimental arthritis models, such as collagen-induced arthritis (CIA), glucose-6-phosphate isomerase-induced arthritis, collagen type II antibody-induced arthritis, the K/B×N serum transfer model, IC arthritis, and antigen-induced arthritis (AIA) models. Overall, despite some differences between the various experimental models, activating FcγRs stimulate innate immune cells, leading to deleterious effects. On the contrary, FcγRIIb induces negative feedback in the production of autoantibodies, thereby protecting the joint from the development and progression of the disease [19–28]. However, the function of the various FcγRs and their exact mechanism of action in the modulation of bone erosion remain to be elucidated.

In the AIA experimental RA model, the injection of methylated bovine serum albumin (mBSA) into the knee joints of previously immunized mice results in a strong local accumulation of ICs that, via activation of the immune system, are responsible for the degradation of both bone and cartilage. In previous studies using this model, we determined the relationship between synovial inflammation and bone destruction using knockout mouse strains for various (combinations of) FcγRs. We found that there was a link between FcγR-mediated inflammation and bone erosion [29]. Whereas FcγRs are expressed on osteoclasts and may thus be involved in their differentiation and activation, a central role in IC-mediated inflammation has been attributed to the FcγR-mediated activation of macrophages during AIA [30]. Their IC-mediated activation leads to the production of a plethora of mediators, such as chemotactic factors, responsible for the recruitment of, among others, neutrophils into the joint. However, which FcγR is particularly involved in regulating this cell influx and which cell is dominant in mediating bone destruction is still a matter of debate.

The importance of neutrophils in arthritis development has been shown in the K/B×N serum transfer experimental RA model, in which depletion of neutrophils leads to complete protection from disease development [31]. In agreement with this finding, high numbers of neutrophils are present in the joints of patients with active RA [32, 33]. Two factors produced by neutrophils in high quantities are the alarmins S100A8 and S100A9, which make up roughly 40% of all cytosolic proteins [34]. S100A8/A9 are small calcium-binding proteins that, upon cell stress, are released into the extracellular environment, where they function as potent inducers of the immune system [35, 36]. High levels of S100A8/A9 are present in the synovial fluid of patients with RA [37, 38]. Moreover, it has been shown that S100A8 is able to directly stimulate osteoclast activity via TLR4, suggesting a possible mechanism through which the IC-activated innate immunity can regulate bone erosion in RA [39].

In the present work, we investigated the involvement of FcγRs, and of FcγRIV in particular, in the regulation of osteoclast-mediated bone resorption. We induced AIA in mice deficient in all four FcγRs (FcγRI,II,III,IV$^{-/-}$ mice) and in their wild-type (WT) controls. The role of FcγRIV in particular was studied by comparing the development of AIA in FcγRI,II,III,IV$^{-/-}$ and FcγRI,II,III$^{-/-}$mice.

Methods

Animals

FcγRI,II,III,IV$^{-/-}$ mice in a C57BL/6 background were developed by Dr. S. Verbeek (Leiden University Medical Center, Leiden, the Netherlands) (Dr.J.Sjef Verbeek personal communication, January 2016). Control C57BL/6 mice were purchased from Janvier Labs (Le Genest Saint Isle, France). FcγRI,II,III$^{-/-}$ mice and their controls were generated as previously described [29]. Mice were housed under standard conditions in filter-top cages and fed a standard diet with food and tap water ad libitum. All animal studies were carried out according to the Dutch law and approved by the local animal experimentation committee (RU-DEC 2012-209).

Induction of AIA

Mice were immunized with 100 μg of mBSA (Sigma-Aldrich, St. Louis, MO, USA) emulsified in complete Freund's adjuvant (CFA; Difco Laboratories, Detroit, MI, USA). Heat-killed *Bordetella pertussis* was administrated intraperitoneally as an additional adjuvant. One week later, two subcutaneous injections in the neck region with a total of 50 μg of mBSA/CFA were administered as a booster. Three weeks after the immunization, arthritis was induced in both knee joints by intra-articular injection of 60 μg of mBSA in 6 μl of saline.

Serum collection and antibody titer determination in serum

At day 7 and day 21 after AIA induction, blood was drawn from the retro-orbital plexus in MiniCollect tubes (Greiner Bio-One, Monroe, NC, USA), and subsequently serum was obtained by centrifugation. Anti-mBSA-specific antibodies (total IgG, IgG1, IgG2a, IgG2b) were measured in sera with an enzyme-linked immunosorbent assay. mBSA was coated on plates (Nunc; Thermo Fisher Scientific, Rochester, NY, USA) at a concentration of 100 μg/ml. Antibody concentrations were assessed by two-fold serial dilution of the sera, followed by detection of bound mouse IgG with peroxidase-conjugated rabbit antimouse IgG (SouthernBiotech, Birmingham, AL, USA). 5-Aminosalicylic acid was used as a substrate. Absorbance was measured at 450 nm. Antibody titers were determined at 50% of the maximum absorption.

Lymphocyte stimulation test

Spleens were collected from mice at day 21 after AIA induction and homogenized through a cell strainer. Erythrocytes were lysed with lysis buffer (155 mM NH_4Cl, 12 mM $KHCO_3$, 0.1 mM ethylenediaminetetraacetic acid, pH 7.3). Cells were seeded into flasks, and after 1 hour at 37 °C, nonadherent cells were harvested and seeded into 96-well plates (1×10^5 cells/well). mBSA was added at final concentrations of 50, 25, 12.5, 6.25, 3.12, and 1.56 μg/ml. Concanavalin A and ovalbumin were used as positive and negative controls, respectively. Cultures were maintained for 4 days. [3H]Thymidine was added for the last 16 hours of culture, and its incorporation was determined as a measure of T-cell proliferation.

Histological analysis

Total knee joints were isolated, fixed in 4% phosphate-buffered formalin, decalcified in 5% formic acid, embedded in paraffin, and 7-μm coronal sections of various depths of the joint were made. Sections were stained with H&E for histological analysis. Inflammation (infiltrate and exudate) was arbitrarily scored on a scale from 0 (no inflammation) to 3 (severe inflammation). Bone destruction was evaluated in 13 well-defined areas of the knee joint (as depicted in the scheme in Additional file 1a) with a score ranging from 0 (no erosion) to 3 (connection between joint cavity and bone marrow). For the evaluation of proteoglycan (PG) depletion as a measure of cartilage destruction, joint sections were stained with Safranin O and Fast Green. PG depletion was evaluated at both the patellofemoral and the tibiofemoral areas as the amount of red staining present, using an arbitrary score ranging from 0 (absence of PG depletion) to 3 (complete PG depletion). For quantification of the number of osteoclasts, total knee joint sections were stained for tartrate-resistant acid phosphatase (TRAP), using the Leukocyte Acid Phosphatase Kit (Sigma-Aldrich) according to the manufacturer's protocol. The number of TRAP$^+$ cells present along the external bone surface was counted. For quantification of periarticular bone, the percentage of noncartilage collagenous tissue (blue staining) in the complete femur and tibia of joint sections stained with Safranin O and Fast Green was quantified using Leica Application Suite software (Leica Microsystems, Buffalo Grove, IL, USA).

Immunohistochemistry

To visualize S100A8-, NIMPR14-, and F4/80-expressing cells, knee joint sections were incubated with specific primary antibodies against S100A8 (made in our facilities), NIMPR14 (kindly provided by Dr. M. Strath, London, UK) and F4/80 (Thermo Fisher Scientific). Afterward, sections were incubated with horseradish peroxidase-conjugated or biotinylated secondary antibodies followed by avidin-biotin complex peroxidase (VECTASTAIN Elite Kit; Vector Laboratories, Burlingame, CA, USA). Antibody binding was visualized using diaminobenzidine. S100A8 staining was arbitrarily scored using a scale from 0 to 3. For quantification of NIMPR14- and F4/80-positive cells, pictures (original magnification ×100) of five specific areas of the joint were taken (two in the area adjacent to the patella and two in the area adjacent to the medial and lateral femur for the evaluation of infiltrate, and one in the area of the joint cavity between the patella and femur for evaluation of the exudate). The amount of cells in the infiltrate was measured as the positive area above a fixed threshold using Leica Application Suite software (Leica Microsystems). The number of positive cells in the exudate was counted using the cell counter plugin of ImageJ software (National Institutes of Health, Bethesda, MD, USA).

Flow cytometric analysis

Bone marrow was isolated from femurs and tibias of mice by flushing the marrow cavity with medium and passing the cell suspension through a cell strainer. After lysis of erythrocytes, bone marrow cells were incubated with Fc-blocking antibody (BD Pharmingen antimouse CD16/CD32, clone 2.4G2; BD Biosciences, San Jose, CA, USA), followed by staining with the following mix of antibodies: CD11b-fluorescein isothiocyanate, CD90.2-phycoerythrin (PE), CD45R/B220-PE, CD49b-PE, NK1.1-PE, Ly6G-PE, Ly6C-allophycocyanin-cyanine 7 (all BD Biosciences). Samples were acquired with a CyAn flow cytometer (Beckman Coulter Life Sciences, Indianapolis, IN, USA), and data analysis was performed with Kaluza Analysis Software (Beckman Coulter Life Sciences). The gating strategy we used is depicted in Additional file 2.

Bone marrow-derived osteoclast differentiation

Bone marrow was isolated from femurs and tibias of mice. Total bone marrow cells were seeded into 96-well plates at a density of 10^5 cells/well in 150 µl of α-minimum essential medium (Thermo Fisher Scientific), supplemented with 5% FCS, penicillin/streptomycin, 30 ng/ml recombinant mouse (rm)M-CSF, and 20 ng/ml rmRANKL (R&D Systems, Minneapolis, MN, USA). Culture medium was refreshed after 3 days.

Measurement of TRAP activity in the supernatants

Cell supernatants were collected after 5 days of differentiation, and TRAP activity was measured with a colorimetric assay. In short, *p*-nitrophenyl phosphate (New England Biolabs, Ipswich, MA, USA) was diluted in buffer containing 420 mM acetic acid (Sigma-Aldrich) and 160 mM tartrate solution (Merck, Kenilworth, NJ, USA) and added 1:1 to culture supernatant. After 1 hour, the reaction was stopped with 0.5 M NaOH (Sigma-Aldrich) , and the absorbance at 405 nm was determined using a spectrophotometric plate reader (Bio-Rad Laboratories, Hercules, CA, USA).

RNA isolation and qRT-PCR

Well-defined synovial samples were isolated from the inflamed murine knee joints as previously described [40]. Tissue samples were homogenized using the MagNA Lyser Instrument (Roche Diagnostics, Indianapolis, IN, USA). Total RNA was isolated using the RNeasy Fibrous Tissue Mini Kit (Qiagen, Hilden, Germany). RNA from osteoclast cultures was isolated with TRIzol reagent (Sigma-Aldrich). RNA was subsequently reverse-transcribed into complementary DNA. qRT-PCR was performed using the Applied Biosystems StepOnePlus RT-PCR System (Thermo Fisher Scientific, Foster City, CA, USA). Primer sequences are listed in Table 1 (primers obtained from Biolegio, Nijmegen, the Netherlands). Glyceraldehyde 3-phosphate dehydrogenase (*Gapdh*) was used as the reference gene. Samples were normalized for the expression of *Gapdh* by calculating the comparative threshold: $-\Delta C_t = -$ (C_t gene of interest $-$ C_t *Gapdh*).

Statistical analysis

Statistical differences between two groups were calculated using Student's *t* test for parametric variables (messenger RNA [mRNA] expression, IgG titer) or the Mann-Whitney *U* test for nonparametric variables (lymphocyte stimulation test/arbitrary score of inflammation, PG depletion, and S100A8 staining/percentage of osteoclast precursors/number of TRAP-positive cells in vivo/TRAP activity in the supernatant/quantification of NIMPR14- and F4/80-positive cells/percentage of noncartilage calcified tissue). For comparison of multiple groups in the quantification of in vivo bone erosion and TRAP$^+$ cells after in vitro differentiation, two-way analysis of variance was used. Spearman's rank correlation coefficients (r_S) were calculated for correlation analysis. All analyses were performed using Prism version 5.03 software (GraphPad Software, La Jolla, CA, USA), and *P* values less than 0.05 were considered significant.

Results

Decreased bone erosion in FcγRI,II,III,IV$^{-/-}$ mice compared with WT controls

First, to determine the effect of the absence of FcγRs on bone resorption during experimental arthritis, we scored bone erosion after induction of AIA in FcγRI,II,III,IV$^{-/-}$ mice and their WT controls. At both day 7 and day 21 after AIA induction, we observed significantly decreased bone

Table 1

Gene	Primer sequences (5′-3′)
Gapdh	Forward: GGCAAATTCAACGGCACA Reverse: GTTAGTGGGGTCTCGCTCCTG
Nfatc1	Forward: ATGCGAGCCATCATCGA Reverse: GGGATGTGAACTCGGAAGAC
Acp5	Forward: GACAAGAGGTTCCAGGAG ACC Reverse: GGGCTGGGGAAGTTCCAG
Calcr	Forward: CGTTCTTTATTACCTGGCTCTTGTG Reverse: TCTGGCAGCTAAGGTTCTTGA AA
Mmp9	Forward: GGAACTCACACGACATCTTCCA Reverse: GAAACTCACACGCCAGAAGAATTT
Ca2	Forward: GCTGCAGAGCTTCACTTGGT Reverse: AAACAGCCAATCCATCCGGT
Oscar	Forward: TGGTCATCAGTTTCGAAGGTTCT Reverse: CAGCCCCAAACGGATGAG
Dcstamp	Forward: TGTATCGGC TCATCTCCTCCAT Reverse: GACTCCTTGGGTTCCTTGCTT
Clcn7	Forward: AGCCTGGACTATGACAACAGC Reverse: GGAAAGCCGTGTGGTTGATT
Ctsk	Forward: GAAGCAGTATAACAGCAAGGTGGAT Reverse: TGTCTCCCAAGTGGTTCATGG

erosion in the FcγRI,II,III,IV$^{-/-}$ mice as compared with their WT controls, highlighting the importance of FcγRs in this process (Fig. 1). However, although the bone erosion was significantly decreased in the FcγRI,II,III,IV$^{-/-}$ mice compared with their WT controls, scores were not reduced to the same level of in naive mice. To investigate a possible basal phenotype due to the absence of FcγRs, we determined the bone erosion in knee joints of WT and FcγRI,II,III,IV$^{-/-}$ mice without AIA. This showed comparable basal levels of bone erosion in these naive knee joints (Fig. 1b). In addition, no differences were found in the surface area of noncartilage collagenous tissue present in the femur and tibia (Additional file 1b). Together, these findings suggest that the decreased bone resorption that was observed in the FcγRI,II,III,IV$^{-/-}$ mice after induction of experimental arthritis could not be explained by an underlying basal bone phenotype. As an additional readout of joint damage, we evaluated PG depletion as a measure of inflammation-induced cartilage destruction at the patello-femoral and tibiofemoral regions. In line with the decreased bone damage, we observed decreased PG depletion in FcγRI,II,III,IV$^{-/-}$ mice compared with their WT controls at day 7 and day 21 after AIA induction, particularly in the tibiofemoral area (Additional file 1c).

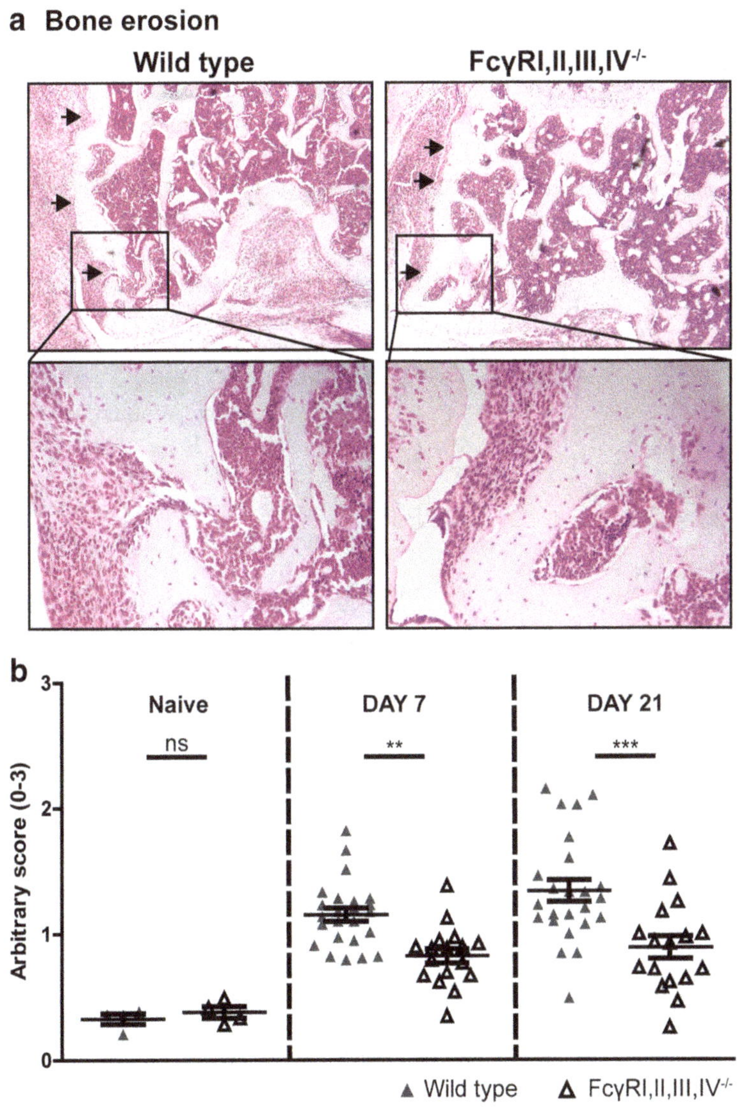

Fig. 1 Fcγ receptor (FcγR)I,II,III,IV$^{-/-}$ mice have decreased bone erosion compared with wild-type (WT) control mice. **a** Bone erosion (*black arrows*) is present in the joints of FcγRI,II,III,IV$^{-/-}$ and WT mice after induction of antigen-induced arthritis (AIA), as determined by using H&E-stained sections. Original magnification ×50 and ×200. **b** Quantification of bone erosion showed significantly decreased resorption in the joints of FcγRI,II,III,IV$^{-/-}$ mice compared with their WT controls ($n = 17$ and 24 joints per group respectively) at both 7 and 21 days after AIA induction. No basal differences in bone erosion could be observed in the joints of naive mice. Scatterplots are shown, with *horizontal* and *vertical lines* representing mean ± SEM values. *ns* Not significant. ** $P < 0.01$, *** $P < 0.001$ versus WT controls

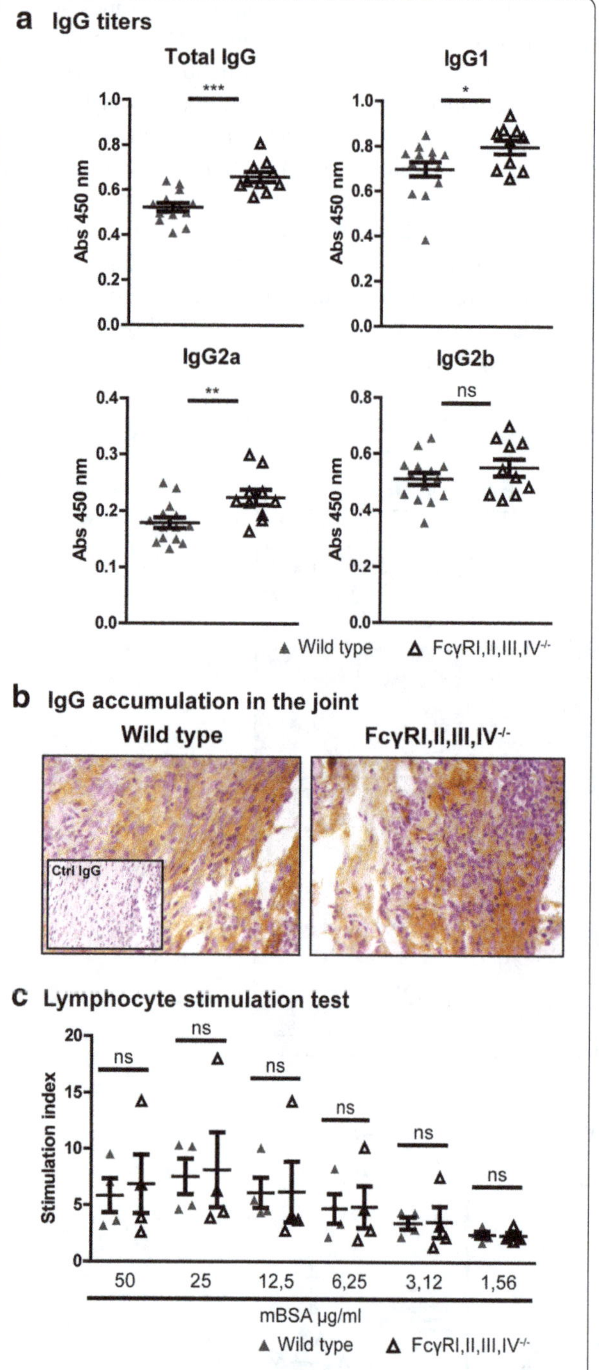

Fig. 2 Fcγ receptor (FcγR)I,II,III,IV deficiency does not impair the humoral and cellular immune responses against methylated bovine serum albumin (mBSA). **a** Significantly increased anti-mBSA total immunoglobulin G (IgG), IgG1, and Ig2a titers were measured in the serum of FcγRI,II,III,IV$^{-/-}$ mice compared with those of wild-type (WT) mice, whereas IgG2b titers were not significantly different (WT, $n = 14$; FcγRI,II,III,IV$^{-/-}$, $n = 10$; combined from day 7 and day 21). **b** Accumulation of IgG was present in the knee joints of both WT and FcγRI,II,III,IV$^{-/-}$ mice 7 days after induction of antigen-induced arthritis as determined by immunolocalization. Original magnification ×400. **c** The cellular anti-mBSA immune response, as determined by T-cell proliferation, was comparable between WT and FcγRI,II,III,IV$^{-/-}$ mice. Results are expressed as stimulation index (ratio of stimulation with/without antigen) ($n = 4$ mice/group). Scatterplots are shown, with *horizontal* and *vertical lines* representing mean ± SEM values. *ns* Not significant. * $P < 0.05$, ** $P < 0.01$, *** $P < 0.001$

Comparable immune response against mBSA in WT and FcγRI,II,III,IV$^{-/-}$ mice

Because the induction of the AIA model is highly dependent on the immune response against the mBSA antigen, we set out to determine whether the humoral and cellular immune responses against mBSA were affected by the absence of FcγRI,II,III,IV. Therefore, we determined anti-mBSA IgG titers in the serum of mice with AIA. We found increased titers of total IgG, IgG1, and IgG2a, but a comparable titer of IgG2b, in FcγRI,II,III,IV$^{-/-}$ mice as compared with WT mice (Fig. 2a). Moreover, using immunostaining against IgG in the joint, we showed IgG accumulation in both WT and FcγRI,II,III,IV$^{-/-}$ mice (Fig. 2b). Finally, we observed comparable mBSA-induced proliferation of T cells obtained from FcγRI,II,III,IV$^{-/-}$ and WT mice (Fig. 2c).

Absence of Fcγ receptors does not affect the number of osteoclast precursors

In the next set of experiments, we aimed at elucidating the mechanism underlying the decreased bone erosion observed in the absence of FcγRs. We first determined whether the FcγRI,II,III,IV$^{-/-}$ mice had a different percentage of osteoclast precursors in their bone marrow after induction of AIA. The percentage of CD11b^{pos}Ly6C^{high} and CD11b$^{low/neg}$Ly6C^{high} cells, both of which have been shown to differentiate into osteoclasts [41, 42], were comparable between FcγRI,II,III,IV$^{-/-}$ and WT mice (Fig. 3a). These data suggest that the observed decrease in bone erosion does not originate from differences in osteoclast precursor populations.

Absence of Fcγ receptors does not affect the osteoclastogenic potential and the number of osteoclasts on the bone surface during AIA

Next, we determined whether the osteoclast progenitors from FcγRI,II,III,IV$^{-/-}$ mice have the same osteoclastogenic potential as WT cells. After in vitro differentiation of bone marrow cells into osteoclasts with M-CSF and RANKL, we

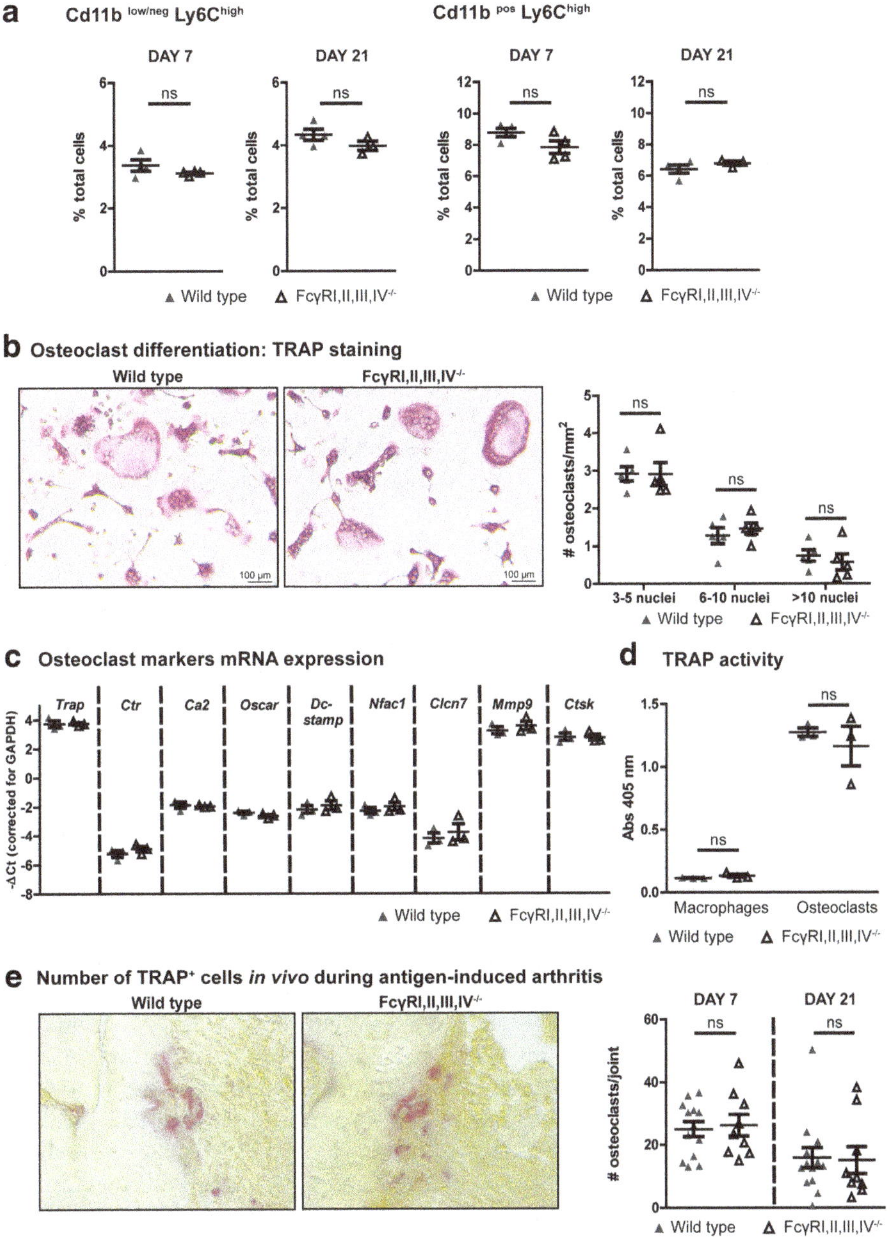

Fig. 3 Absence of Fcγ receptor (FcγR)I,II,III,IV does not affect the percentage of osteoclast precursors and their osteoclastogenic potential. **a** Comparable percentages of CD11b^{pos}Ly6C^{high} and CD11b$^{low/neg}$Ly6C^{high} osteoclast precursors were present in the bone marrow of wild-type (WT) and FcγRI,II,III,IV$^{-/-}$ mice at days 7 and 21 of antigen-induced arthritis (AIA) ($n = 3$ or 4 mice/group). **b** Images of tartrate-resistant acid phosphatase (TRAP) staining of osteoclasts after 5 days of in vitro differentiation. Quantification showed comparable numbers of osteoclasts obtained from WT and FcγRI,II,III,IV$^{-/-}$ bone marrow cells ($n = 5$ mice/group). **c** Moreover, comparable messenger RNA expression levels of various osteoclast markers were determined in WT and FcγRI,II,III,IV$^{-/-}$ osteoclasts ($n = 3$ mice/group). **d** Finally, TRAP activity in the culture supernatant of WT and FcγR I,II,III,IV$^{-/-}$ macrophages and osteoclasts was comparable ($n = 3$ mice/group). **e** Representative photomicrographs of TRAP staining and quantification of the number of positive cells along the bone surface in total knee joint sections of WT and FcγRI,II,III,IV$^{-/-}$ mice at days 7 and 21 after induction of AIA ($n = 14$ and $n = 10$ per time point for WT and FcγRI,II,III,IV$^{-/-}$ mice, respectively). Scatterplots are shown, with *horizontal* and *vertical lines* representing mean ± SEM values. *ns* Not significant

observed comparable numbers of multinucleated TRAP$^+$ cells in the cultures with WT and FcγRI,II,III,IV$^{-/-}$ cells (Fig. 3b). In agreement with this finding, we found comparable mRNA expression levels of key osteoclast differentiation markers, such as nuclear factor of activated T-cells, cytoplasmic 1 (*Nfatc1*), *TRAP*, dendritic cell-specific transmembrane protein (*Dcstamp*), calcitonin receptor (*Ctr*), and osteoclast-associated immunoglobulin-like receptor (*Oscar*), as well as comparable mRNA expression levels of activation markers, such as chloride channel 7 (*Clcn7*), carbonic anhydrase II (*Ca2*), matrix metallopeptidase 9 (*Mmp9*), and cathepsin K (*Ctsk*) (Fig. 3c). Moreover, the TRAP enzyme activity as measured in the supernatant of the osteoclast cultures was comparable (Fig. 3d). Together, these findings show that the absence of FcγRs does not affect the osteoclastogenic potential of precursor cells. Finally, because in vivo osteoclastogenesis is a complex process that can be influenced by many factors, we determined the number of osteoclasts on the bone surface of FcγRI,II,III,IV$^{-/-}$ and WT mice during AIA using TRAP staining. Interestingly, in line with their comparable osteoclastogenic potential in vitro, the number of TRAP^{+} cells along the bone surface did not differ between FcγRI,II,III,IV$^{-/-}$ and WT mice both at day 7 and day 21 after AIA induction (Fig. 3e).

FcγRs differentially regulate the influx of neutrophils present in the joint

Because proinflammatory cells and their products can strongly increase the resorbing activity of osteoclasts, we evaluated the severity of inflammation in the arthritic knee joints. The degree of both infiltrate and exudate was significantly decreased in the knee joints of FcγRI,II,III,IV$^{-/-}$ mice at day 7 after AIA induction (Fig. 4). At day 21 after induction, the degree of inflammation was decreased in both strains, and no significant difference could be observed between FcγRI,II,III,IV$^{-/-}$ and WT mice anymore. The early phase of inflammation (day 7) during AIA is particularly characterized by an abundant presence of neutrophils in the exudate and infiltrate in the knee joint. Interestingly, we observed significantly decreased numbers of NIMPR14-positive neutrophils in the exudate, and the NIMPR14-positive area in the infiltrate was significantly lower in FcγRI,II,III,IV$^{-/-}$ mice than in WT mice (Fig. 5a). In contrast, numbers of F4/80-positive monocytes/macrophages in both the exudate and infiltrate were comparable between FcγRI,II,III,IV$^{-/-}$ and WT mice (Fig. 5b), and a trend toward an increased percentage of F4/80 cells in the infiltrate of FcγRI,II,III,IV$^{-/-}$ mice was observed. Previous data developed at our laboratory showed that in contrast to the decreased inflammation and bone resorption in FcγRI,II,III,IV$^{-/-}$ mice that we describe in the present work, FcγRI,II,III$^{-/-}$ mice showed increased bone resorption, together with more inflammation, compared with their WT controls after induction of AIA [29]. Of note, we observed a significant increase and a trend toward an increase in the numbers of neutrophils present in the infiltrate and exudate, respectively, of these FcγRI,II,III$^{-/-}$ mice (Fig. 5c). However, in agreement with our findings in the FcγRI,II,III,IV$^{-/-}$ mice, the number of F4/80-positive monocytes/ macrophages cells was not significantly different between FcγRI,II,III$^{-/-}$ and WT mice, and the percentage of F4/80-positive area was decreased in FcγRI,II,III$^{-/-}$ mice (Fig. 5d). Representative photomicrographs are shown in Additional files 3 and 4. Together, these findings suggest that FcγRIV might be of particular importance in the recruitment of neutrophils into the arthritic joint and that these neutrophils likely contribute to the bone erosion process.

Numbers of S100A8/A9-producing neutrophils strongly correlate with the amount of bone erosion

In line with the decreased numbers of neutrophils present in their joints, lower expression levels of S100A8, at both the mRNA and protein levels, were observed in FcγRI,II,III,IV$^{-/-}$ than in WT mice (Fig. 6a and b). Moreover, in agreement with the higher numbers of neutrophils observed in the joints of FcγRI,II,III$^{-/-}$ mice, increased expression of S100A8 was previously described by researchers at our laboratory [24]. Supporting our idea that the S100A8 produced by neutrophils plays an important role in the observed bone erosion, we found that the number of neutrophils in both the infiltrate and exudate, as well as their production of S100A8, strongly and significantly correlated with the severity of bone erosion (Fig. 6c and d).

Discussion

In the present study, we show that FcγRs are crucially involved in bone erosion during AIA. Moreover, we show that the absence of all FcγRs does not affect the number of osteoclast precursors or their osteoclastogenic potential, but that it decreases the subsequent bone erosion during experimental arthritis via a reduction of inflammation. The comparison of development of AIA in FcγRI,II,III,IV$^{-/-}$ and FcγRI,II,III$^{-/-}$ mice suggested a possible crucial role of FcγRIV in mediating neutrophil inflammation during AIA.

We observed that mice lacking all FcγRs had decreased inflammation at day 7 and decreased bone erosion at both day 7 and day 21 after induction of the disease. This is in agreement with a previous study by Hobday and colleagues, which showed that FcγRI,II,III,IV$^{-/-}$ mice were completely protected from serum-transferred arthritis at a macroscopic level [43]. However, in contrast to this serum transfer model, the AIA model is characterized by clear T-cell involvement, which is probably FcγR-independent. This might explain why we did not observe complete protection in FcγRI,II,III,IV$^{-/-}$ mice. In another study, in line with what we observed in FcγRI,II,III,IV-/- mice, γ-chain/FcγRIIb -/- mice lacking signaling of both activating and inhibitory FcγRs, as well as of other receptors using the γ-chain, were completely protected from development of CIA, although bone erosion data were not reported [44].

The induction of the AIA experimental RA model is highly dependent on the binding of mBSA/anti-mBSA-containing ICs to FcγRs, thereby potently

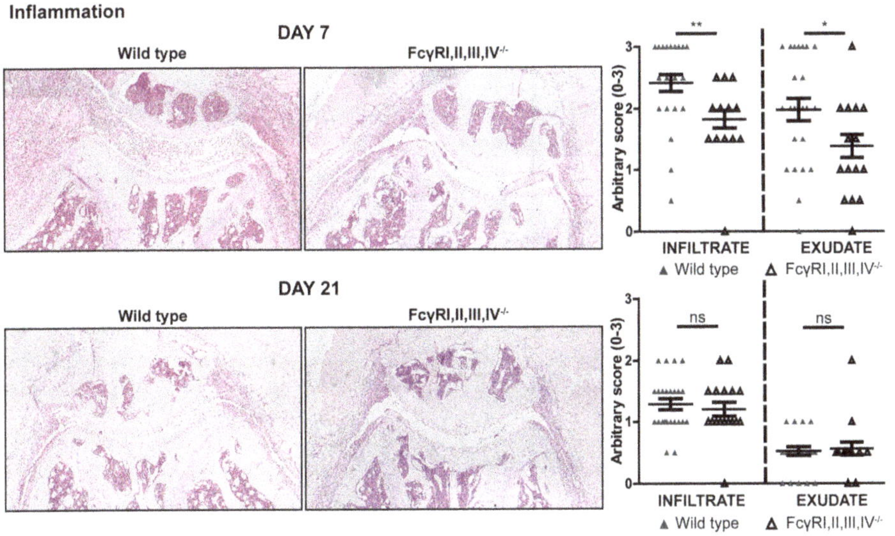

Fig. 4 Fcγ receptor (FcγR)I,II,III,IV$^{-/-}$ mice have decreased inflammation in arthritic joints. Photomicrographs of H&E staining showing the infiltrate and exudate in knee joints of wild-type (WT) and FcγRI,II,III,IV$^{-/-}$ mice at days 7 and 21 of antigen-induced arthritis (AIA). Original magnification ×100. Quantification showed decreased infiltrate and exudate in the knee joints of FcγRI,II,III,IV$^{-/-}$ mice compared with WT controls at day 7 of AIA. In contrast, no differences were observed at day 21 ($n = 24$ and $n = 17$ joints per time point for WT and FcγRI,II,III,IV$^{-/-}$ mice, respectively). Scatterplots are shown, with *horizontal* and *vertical lines* representing mean ± SEM values. *ns* Not significant. * $P < 0.05$, ** $P < 0.01$

activating the cell, and on the activation of T-cell responses against mBSA. However, we observed comparable T-cell responses against the mBSA antigen in FcγRI,II,III,IV$^{-/-}$ and WT animals, which shows that their contribution to the induction of the model was not affected by the absence of the FcγRs. This is consistent with previous studies in which normal T-cell responses were found in the absence of either activating or inhibitory FcγRs after the induction of the AIA [27, 28]. Together, these findings suggest that the development of the T-cell immune response is FcγR-independent.

It has previously been shown that the absence of FcγRIIb often leads to increased IgG titers in mice owing to a lack of negative feedback on the production of IgGs by plasma cells, which results in enhanced stimulation of the immune response [28, 45]. In line with these findings, the FcγRI,II,III,IV$^{-/-}$ mice used in this study, which also lack FcγRIIb, showed increased IgG titers (total IgG, IgG1, IgG2a) compared with their WT controls. Moreover, accumulation of IgG was present in the joints of FcγRI,II,III,IV$^{-/-}$ mice. Together, these data showing a normal T-cell response against mBSA and increased IgG titers in FcγRI,II,III,IV$^{-/-}$ mice suggest that the observed decrease in bone pathology cannot be the result of an insufficient immune response against mBSA after induction of the AIA model.

Osteoclasts are the main cells responsible for the degradation of bone tissue during RA. Although it is known that osteoclasts differentiate from bone marrow-derived myeloid precursors under the influence of M-CSF and RANKL, a strictly defined osteoclast precursor set has not yet been identified [4]. CD11b^{pos}Ly6C^{high} bone marrow monocytes have been reported to differentiate into osteoclasts when stimulated with M-CSF and RANKL in vitro, and depletion of Ly6C^{high} cells in vivo results in decreased osteoclast formation and subsequent bone resorption in the K/B×N serum transfer model [41]. Moreover, Charles and colleagues recently identified the CD11b$^{low/neg}$Ly6C^{hi} bone marrow population as having osteoclastogenic potential both in vitro and in vivo [42]. In the present study, we did not observe differences in the relative percentages of both the Ly6C^{high} and CD11b$^{low/neg}$Ly6C^{high} osteoclast precursor populations between FcγRI,II,III,IV$^{-/-}$ and WT mice, which allowed us to exclude the possibility that decreased bone erosion in the FcγRI,II,III,IV$^{-/-}$ mice was merely the result of decreased numbers of osteoclast precursors.

Next to M-CSF and RANKL signaling, a costimulatory signal via the activation of the ITAM domain, which is present in the γ-chain and in DNAX activation protein of 12 kDa (DAP-12), is required for the activation of NFATc1, which is the transcription factor essential for osteoclast differentiation [46, 47]. Because activating FcγRI, FcγRIII, and FcγRIV are expressed by osteoclasts and are associated with the ITAM-containing γ-chain, they potentially can affect osteoclast differentiation. However, in the present study, we found that the absence of all four FcγRs does not impact the differentiation of osteoclasts from their precursors in vitro. Underlining our findings, Negishi-Koga and colleagues

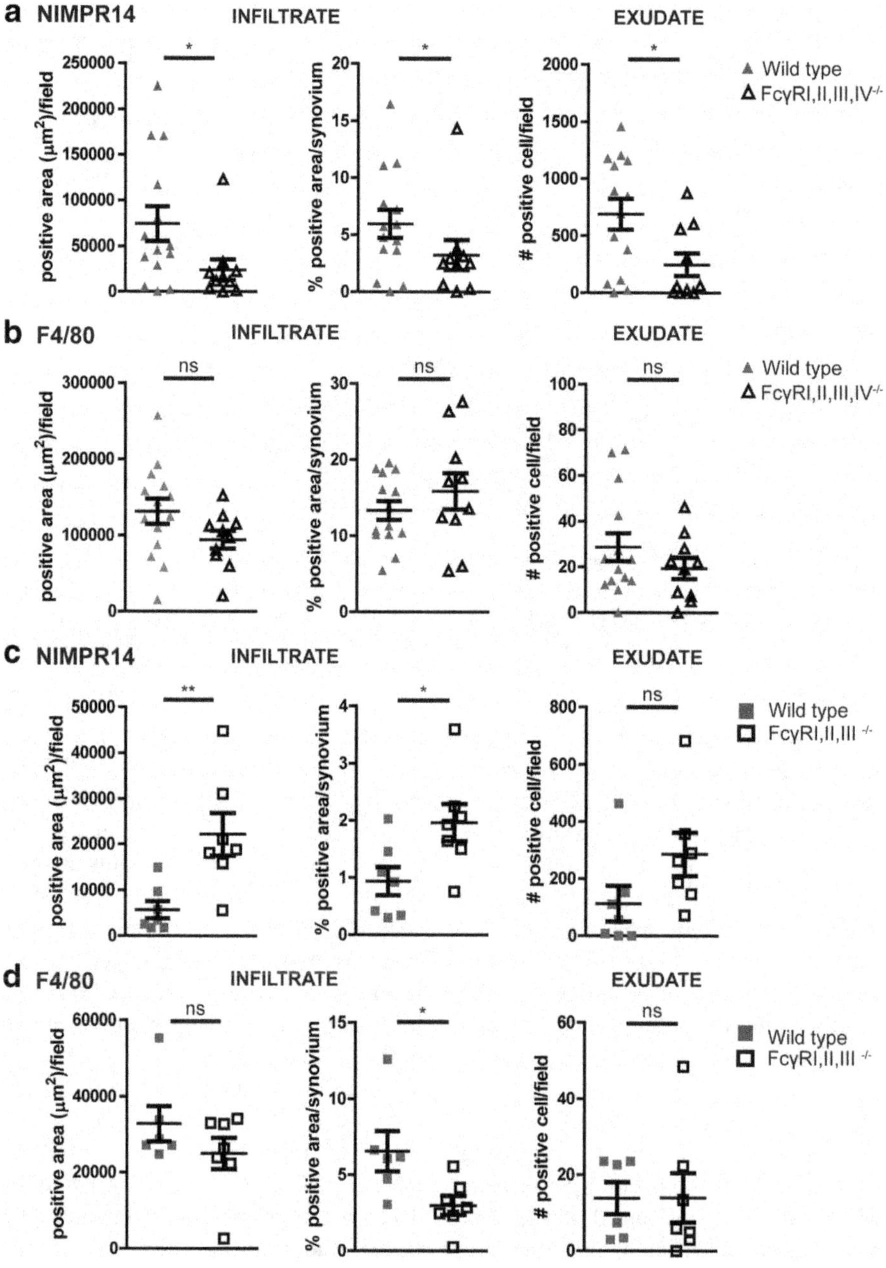

Fig. 5 Prominent role for Fcγ receptor (FcγR)IV in regulating the influx of neutrophils into the joint. **a** NIMPR14-positive area, percentage of NIMPR14-positive area in the infiltrate, and number of NIMPR14-positive cells in the exudate are decreased in FcγRI,II,III,IV$^{-/-}$ mice compared with wild-type (WT) mice in day 7 antigen-induced arthritis (AIA). **b** Comparable numbers of F4/80-positive cells are present in the joints of FcγRI,II,III,IV$^{-/-}$ mice compared with their WT controls at day 7 AIA. **c** In contrast to FcγRI,II,III,IV$^{-/-}$ mice, the total NIMPR14-positive area, percentage of NIMPR14-positive area in the infiltrate, and number of NIMPR14-positive cells in the exudate are increased in FcγR I,II,III$^{-/-}$ mice. **d** Comparable numbers and reduced percentage of F4/80-positive cells in the joint of FcγR I,II,III$^{-/-}$ mice compared with their WT controls at day 7 of AIA. Scatterplots are shown, with *horizontal* and *vertical lines* representing mean ± SEM values of at least six mice per group. *ns* Not significant. * $P < 0.05$, ** $P < 0.01$

showed that FcγRIIb$^{-/-}$/γ-chain$^{-/-}$ cells, which lack signaling of both activating and inhibitory FcγRs, did not show alterations in osteoclast differentiation. However, varying results have previously been described concerning the effects of FcγRs on osteoclastogenesis. Surprisingly, Negishi-Koga and colleagues reported that FcγRIII$^{-/-}$ mice have an osteoporotic phenotype that was associated with increased numbers of osteoclasts. These authors also demonstrated increased in vitro osteoclast differentiation of FcγRIII$^{-/-}$ bone marrow cells, together suggesting an inhibitory role for FcγRIII in osteoclastogenesis [48]. They stated that the mechanistic

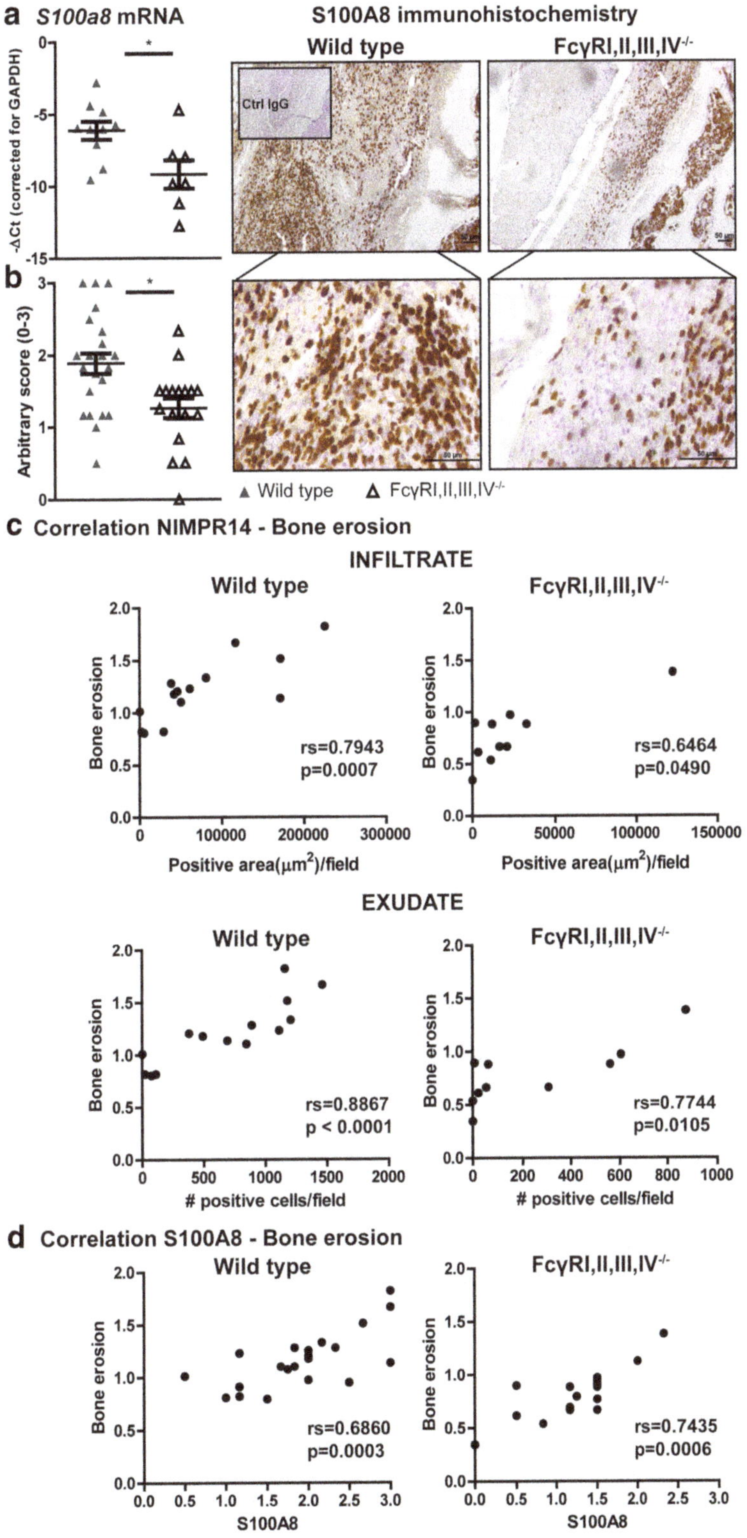

Fig. 6 (See legend on next page.)

(See figure on previous page.)

Fig. 6 The number of S100A8-producing neutrophils correlates with the severity of bone erosion during antigen-induced arthritis. **a** *S100a8* messenger RNA levels in the synovium of Fcγ receptor (FcγR)I,II,III,IV$^{-/-}$ mice are decreased compared with wild-type (WT) mice at day 7 of antigen-induced arthritis (AIA). **b** Representative photomicrographs show S100A8 staining in knee joint sections of WT and FcγRI,II,III,IV$^{-/-}$ mice at day 7 of AIA. Original magnification ×100 and ×400. Quantification showed a decreased number of S100A8-positive cells in FcγRI,II,III,IV$^{-/-}$ mice compared with their WT controls. **c** A significant correlation was observed between the number of neutrophils (NIMPR14-positive cells) in the infiltrate and exudate in the joint and bone erosion in both WT and FcγRI,II,III,IV$^{-/-}$ mice at day 7 of AIA. **d** A significant correlation between the number of S100A8-positive cells in the joint and the severity of bone erosion in both WT and FcγRI,II,III,IV $^{-/-}$ mice at day 7 of AIA was found. * $P < 0.05$. rs = Spearman's rank correlation coefficient

basis for this surprising finding could be the sequestration of the γ-chain by FcγRIII. Therefore, in the absence of FcγRIII, more γ-chain is available for other proteins, such as osteoclast-associated immunoglobulin-like receptor (OSCAR) and paired immunoglobulin-like receptor A (PIR-A), which both act as costimulatory factors during osteoclastogenesis via their association with the γ-chain. In addition, the same research group showed that FcγRIIb$^{-/-}$ cells, which lack the ITIM domain that inhibits pro-osteoclastogenic ITAM signaling, showed increased osteoclastogenic potential. Therefore, in the present study, where we show that FcγRI,II,III,IV$^{-/-}$ cells have normal in vitro osteoclastogenic potential, we cannot rule out a compensatory effect on osteoclast differentiation via γ-chain-dependent costimulatory pathways, such as via OSCAR or PIR-A signaling, or via triggering receptor expressed on myeloid cells 2 (TREM2), which depends on the ITAM-domain containing DAP12 protein for its signaling. In line with this possibility, it has been shown that DAP12 is primarily responsible for in vitro M-CSF- and RANKL-induced osteoclastogenesis because γ-chain$^{-/-}$ cells show normal differentiation. However, in the absence of DAP12, the γ-chain can compensate for its absence, acting via $\alpha_v\beta_3$ integrin [49].

Finally, underlining the normal osteoclast differentiation that we observed in vitro, nonarthritic FcγRI,II,III,IV$^{-/-}$ mice had no basal bone phenotype in their knee joints, measured as the amount of subchondral calcified tissue in the femur and tibia, and we observed comparable numbers of TRAP$^+$ osteoclasts along the bone surface after AIA induction. Together, these findings imply that the absence of all FcγRs does not impair the ability of cells to differentiate into mature osteoclasts, suggesting that a difference in osteoclast activity, rather than differences in osteoclast numbers, must underlie the decreased erosion in FcγRI,II,III,IV$^{-/-}$ mice in the studied AIA model.

It has been shown that inflammation plays a critical role in the activation of osteoclasts in vivo by the production of a plethora of factors that in this way lead to bone erosion. In this study, we found that inflammation (both infiltrate and exudate) was decreased in FcγRI,II,III,IV$^{-/-}$ mice compared with WT controls at day 7, but not at day 21, after AIA induction. This suggests that FcγRs are probably most involved in the early inflammatory response of the AIA model, which still resulted in significantly decreased bone erosion in the FcγRI,II,III,IV$^{-/-}$ mice at day 21 after induction.

It has been shown that the four FcγRs in mice are differentially expressed on immune cells and that the individual FcγRs are known to bind the various IgG subclasses with different affinities [10]. The activity of IgG1 is dependent mainly on FcγRIII, and IgG2a binds with high affinity to FcγRI and with low affinity to FcγRIII and IV, whereas IgG2b bind with the highest affinity to FcγRIV. This implies that the absence of one or more FcγRs and the cellular composition might facilitate the binding of IgGs to other FcγRs more than normally would occur, possibly leading to abnormal intracellular signaling. Previous researchers have investigated the role of FcγRs in AIA using mice deficient in one or more FcγRs. Induction of AIA in FcγRIIb$^{-/-}$ mice resulted in increased inflammation, most probably because of the absence of both FcγRIIb-mediated IgG clearance and a negative feedback loop on IgG production by B cells [28, 29]. In contrast, the inflammation in FcγRI$^{-/-}$ or FcγRIII$^{-/-}$ mice was not affected [28], suggesting that either these receptors can compensate for each other's absence or that FcγRIV is the dominant FcγR in both cases. However, the combined absence of FcγRI and FcγRIII [24] led to reduced inflammation. Interestingly, when combined with the absence of the IgG-clearing FcγRIIb, resulting in FcγRI,II,III$^{-/-}$ mice, stronger accumulation of ICs is present, which results in increased inflammation, probably via binding of ICs to FcγRIV [29]. The important function of FcγRIV in this situation is substantiated by the finding that the inflammation is reduced when, in addition to FcγRI, FcγRII, and FcγRIII, FcγRIV is also absent. Although our results indicate an important role for FcγRIV in the pathology of AIA, definitive proof should come from AIA induction in an FcγRIV single-knockout. Consistent with our findings in the AIA model, the fact that 35–40% of FcγRI,II,III$^{-/-}$ mice developed CIA, whereas γ-chain$^{-/-}$/FcγRIIb$^{-/-}$mice that also lack functional FcγRIV were protected from disease development, further supports the role of FcγRIV in this arthritis model [44]. Moreover, a clear confirmation for the crucial involvement of

FcγRIV in K/B×N comes from a study by Seeling and colleagues in which FcγRIV$^{-/-}$ animals showed significantly decreased inflammation and bone erosion [41]. Finally, arthritis development can be prevented using a blocking antibody against FcγRIV in mice lacking all FcγRs except for FcγRIV [50].

Together, these studies and the data reported in the present article show that an important role can likely be attributed to FcγRIV in experimental RA models. Interestingly, a polymorphism in FcγRIIIA, which is the human ortholog of the murine FcγRIV, has been associated with increased susceptibility to RA development. This polymorphism, in which a phenylalanine is substituted for a valine at amino acid position 158 (158 V/F), located at the immunoglobulin-binding domain, results in an increased affinity of the receptor for IgG1 and IgG3 antibodies [51–53]. Although these associations could not be reproduced in all populations, these data support a possible important role for the human ortholog of murine FcγRIV in RA development and further support the importance of additional studies to investigate the role of FcγRs in RA [54].

In our present study, we describe a clear increase in the numbers of neutrophils in both the infiltrate and exudate in FcγRI,II,III$^{-/-}$ mice, whereas decreased neutrophil numbers were observed in FcγRI,II,III,IV$^{-/-}$ mice. This suggests that particularly FcγRIV is responsible for the presence of neutrophils to the joint. The importance of neutrophils in RA development has been shown in the K/B×N experimental RA model [31]. Moreover, in agreement with this role for neutrophils in experimental RA models, high numbers of neutrophils are present in the joints of patients with active RA [32, 33]. We show a strong and significant correlation between the number of neutrophils present in the joint and the amount of bone erosion. Because in the AIA model ICs are produced locally in the joint, we propose that ICs can stimulate synovial macrophages via FcγRIV to release chemotactic factors such as complement components and keratinocyte-derived chemochine, thereby inducing the recruitment of neutrophils into the joint. Neutrophils are strong producers of the alarmin S100A8/A9, which has been shown to directly induce osteoclast activity in vitro via TLR4 signaling [39]. This suggests a mechanism through which infiltrated neutrophils can regulate bone erosion in RA. Indeed, we observed lower expression levels of S100A8 coinciding with lower neutrophil numbers in the joints of FcγRI,II,III,IV$^{-/-}$ mice than in WT mice. Moreover, we observed that the production of S100A8 by neutrophils strongly and significantly correlated with the severity of bone erosion. In agreement with these findings, our laboratory previously showed that FcγRI,II,III$^{-/-}$ mice, which have increased numbers of neutrophils in their joints after AIA induction, showed increased S100A8 expression. S100A8/A9 has been shown to be strongly upregulated in the synovial fluid of patients with RA [37, 38], and its levels are linked to joint inflammation and damage [55–58]. Together, these data support the idea that FcγRIV mediates bone erosion in AIA by modulating the influx of S100A8/A9-producing neutrophils into the arthritic joint, although an additional direct effect of ICs on osteoclasts cannot be completely ruled out.

Conclusions

Our present study adds important new data to the existing body of knowledge concerning the involvement of FcγRs in inducing bone erosion and particularly highlights, for the first time to our knowledge, the role of FcγRIV in neutrophil-mediated bone erosion during AIA.

Additional files

Additional file 1: Graphical representation of bone erosion scoring method and quantification of noncartilage collagenous tissue and proteoglycan (PG) depletion. **a** Graphical representation of the 13 locations along the patella, femur, tibia, and cruciate ligament where bone erosion was scored. **b** Quantification of the noncartilage collagenous tissue (blue staining in Safranin O/Fast Green staining) in femur and tibia showed no differences between naive FcγRI,II,III,IV$^{-/-}$ and wild-type (WT) mice. *ns* Not significant. **c** Quantification of PG depletion showed a significant decrease at the tibiofemoral area in the joints of FcγRI,II,III,IV$^{-/-}$ mice as compared with their WT controls ($n = 10$ and 14 joints per group, respectively) at both 7 and 21 days after AIA induction. Scatterplots are shown, with horizontal and vertical lines showing mean ± SEM values. *ns* Not significant. * $P < 0.05$, ** $P < 0.01$ versus WT controls. (PDF 437 kb)

Additional file 2: Gating strategy for flow cytometric analysis. Gating strategy for flow cytometric analysis used to identify CD11b^{pos}Ly6C^{high} and CD11b$^{low/neg}$Ly6C^{high} osteoclast precursor populations. First, single cells were selected. For identification of CD11b^{pos}Ly6C^{high} monocytes, cells negative for CD90.2, CD45R/B220, CD49b, NK1.1, and Ly6G and positive for CD11b were selected (gate A). Subsequently, cells were back-gated for side scatter and forward scatter to exclude cells with high granulosity (gate B), and finally Ly6C^{high} cells were selected (gate C). For identification of CD11b$^{low/neg}$Ly6C^{high}, after exclusion of CD90.2-, CD45R/B220-, CD49b-, NK1.1-, Ly6G-positive cells (gate D), cells were gated for their expression of CD11b and Ly6C (CD11B$^{low/neg}$Ly6C^{high}) (gate E). (PDF 299 kb)

Additional file 3: NIMPR14- and F4/80-positive cells in the infiltrate and in the exudate in the joints of FcγRI,II,III,IV$^{-/-}$ mice and their WT controls. Representative photomicrographs of (**a**) NIMPR14 and (**b**) F4/80 staining showing neutrophils and macrophages in the infiltrate and exudate of the knee joints of FcγRI,II,III,IV$^{-/-}$ mice and their WT controls at day 7 after induction of antigen-induced arthritis. Original magnification ×400 for infiltrate and ×200 and ×400 for exudate. (PDF 422 kb)

Additional file 4: NIMPR14- and F4/80-positive cells in the infiltrate and exudate in the joints of FcγRI,II,III$^{-/-}$ mice and their WT controls. Representative photomicrographs of (**a**) NIMPR14 and (**b**) F4/80 staining showing neutrophils and macrophages in the infiltrate and exudate of the knee joints of FcγRI,II,III$^{-/-}$ mice and their WT controls at day 7 after induction of antigen-induced arthritis. Original magnification ×400 for infiltrate and ×200 and ×400 for exudate. (PDF 401 kb)

Abbreviations

AIA: Antigen-induced arthritis; CFA: Complete Freund's adjuvant; CIA: Collagen-induced arthritis; DAP-12: DNAX activation protein of 12 kDa; FcγR: Fcγ receptor; *Gapdh*: Glyceraldehyde 3-phosphate dehydrogenase; IC: Immune complex; IgG: Immunoglobulin G; ITAM: Activation motif immunoreceptor tyrosine-based activation motif; ITIM: Immunoreceptor tyrosine-based inhibitory motif; mBSA: Methylated bovine serum albumin; M-CSF: Macrophage colony-stimulating factor; mRNA: Messenger RNA; ns: Not significant; OSCAR: Osteoclast-associated immunoglobulin-like receptor; PE: Phycoerythrin; PG: Proteoglycan; PIR-A: Paired immunoglobulin-like receptor A; RA: Rheumatoid arthritis; RANKL: Receptor activator of nuclear factor-κB ligand; RF: Rheumatoid factor; TRAP: Tartrate-resistant acid phosphatase; TREM2: Triggering receptor expressed on myeloid cells 2; WT: Wild type

Acknowledgements

We gratefully acknowledge financial support from the Seventh Framework Programme of the European Union, Project Osteoimmune (grant 289150).

Funding

This project was funded by the Seventh Framework Programme of the European Union, Project Osteoimmune (grant 289150).

Authors' contributions

IDC, GA, MHJvdB, ABB, and PLEMvL conceived of, designed, and coordinated the study. IDC, GA, MHJvdB, and BW conducted the animal experiments. IDC performed in vitro experiments. IDC, NAJC, and AWS performed immunohistochemistry. JSV generated and provided FcγRI,II,III$^{-/-}$ and FcγRI,II,III,IV$^{-/-}$ mice. TV and JR provided materials, reagents, and analytical tools. IDC, GA, ABB, MHJvdB, and PLEMvL analyzed and interpreted the data. IDC drafted the manuscript. GA, MHJvdB, ABB, and PLEMvL helped with drafting the manuscript. GA, TV, JR, JSV, FAJvdL, MIK, PMvdK, ABB, MHJvdB, and PLEMvL provided critical revision of the manuscript. All the authors read and approved the final manuscript.

Competing interests

The authors declare that they have no competing interests.

Author details

[1]Experimental Rheumatology, Radboud university medical center, Geert Grooteplein Zuid 28, 6525 GA Nijmegen, the Netherlands. [2]Institute of Immunology, University of Münster, Münster, Germany. [3]Human Genetics, Leiden University Medical Center, Leiden, the Netherlands.

References

1. Andersson AK, Li C, Brennan FM. Recent developments in the immunobiology of rheumatoid arthritis. Arthritis Res Ther. 2008;10(2):204.
2. Schett G, Gravallese E. Bone erosion in rheumatoid arthritis: mechanisms, diagnosis and treatment. Nat Rev Rheumatol. 2012;8(11):656–64.
3. Goldring SR, Gravallese EM. Pathogenesis of bone erosions in rheumatoid arthritis. Curr Opin Rheumatol. 2000;12(3):195–9.
4. Boyle WJ, Simonet WS, Lacey DL. Osteoclast differentiation and activation. Nature, 2003;423(6937): 337-342.
5. Leisen JC, et al. The erosive front: a topographic study of the junction between the pannus and the subchondral plate in the macerated rheumatoid metacarpal head. J Rheumatol. 1988;15(1):17–22.
6. Gravallese EM, et al. Identification of cell types responsible for bone resorption in rheumatoid arthritis and juvenile rheumatoid arthritis. Am J Pathol. 1998;152(4):943–51.
7. Berglin E, et al. Radiological outcome in rheumatoid arthritis is predicted by presence of antibodies against cyclic citrullinated peptide before and at disease onset, and by IgA-RF at disease onset. Ann Rheum Dis. 2006;65(4):453–8.
8. Forslind K, et al. Prediction of radiological outcome in early rheumatoid arthritis in clinical practice: role of antibodies to citrullinated peptides (anti-CCP). Ann Rheum Dis. 2004;63(9):1090–5.
9. Lindqvist E, et al. Prognostic laboratory markers of joint damage in rheumatoid arthritis. Ann Rheum Dis. 2005;64(2):196–201.
10. Nimmerjahn F, Ravetch JV. FcγRs in health and disease. Curr Top Microbiol Immunol. 2011;350:105–25.
11. Karsten CM, Kohl J. The immunoglobulin, IgG Fc receptor and complement triangle in autoimmune diseases. Immunobiology. 2012;217(11):1067–79.
12. Nimmerjahn F, Ravetch JV. Fcγ receptors: old friends and new family members. Immunity 2006;24(1):19-28.
13. Kawanaka N, et al. CD14$^+$,CD16$^+$ blood monocytes and joint inflammation in rheumatoid arthritis. Arthritis Rheum. 2002;46(10):2578–86.
14. Wijngaarden S, et al. Fcγ receptor expression levels on monocytes are elevated in rheumatoid arthritis patients with high erythrocyte sedimentation rate who do not use anti-rheumatic drugs. Rheumatology (Oxford). 2003;42(5):681–8.
15. Hepburn AL, Mason JC, Davies KA. Expression of Fcγ and complement receptors on peripheral blood monocytes in systemic lupus erythematosus and rheumatoid arthritis. Rheumatology (Oxford). 2004;43(5):547–54.
16. Bunescu A, et al. Enhanced Fcγ receptor I, αMβ2 integrin receptor expression by monocytes and neutrophils in rheumatoid arthritis: interaction with platelets. J Rheumatol. 2004;31(12):2347–55.
17. Magnusson SE, et al. High synovial expression of the inhibitory FcγRIIb in rheumatoid arthritis. Arthritis Res Ther. 2007;9(3):R51.
18. Blom AB, et al. Increased expression of Fcγ receptors II and III on macrophages of rheumatoid arthritis patients results in higher production of tumor necrosis factor α and matrix metalloproteinase. Arthritis Rheum. 2003;48(4):1002–14.
19. Yuasa T, et al. Deletion of Fcγ receptor IIB renders H-2^b mice susceptible to collagen-induced arthritis. J Exp Med. 1999;189(1):187–94.
20. Diaz de Stahl T, et al. Expression of FcγRIII is required for development of collagen-induced arthritis. Eur J Immunol. 2002;32(10):2915–22.
21. Schubert D, et al. Immunization with glucose-6-phosphate isomerase induces T cell-dependent peripheral polyarthritis in genetically unaltered mice. J Immunol. 2004;172(7):4503–9.
22. Nandakumar KS, et al. Induction of arthritis by single monoclonal IgG anti-collagen type II antibodies and enhancement of arthritis in mice lacking inhibitory FcγRIIB. Eur J Immunol. 2003;33(8):2269–77.
23. Corr M, Crain B. The role of FcγR signaling in the K/B × N serum transfer model of arthritis. J Immunol. 2002;169(11):6604–9.
24. van Lent P, et al. The inhibitory receptor FcγRII reduces joint inflammation and destruction in experimental immune complex-mediated arthritides not only by inhibition of FcγRI/III but also by efficient clearance and endocytosis of immune complexes. Am J Pathol. 2003;163(5):1839–48.
25. Blom AB, et al. FcγR expression on macrophages is related to severity and chronicity of synovial inflammation and cartilage destruction during experimental immune-complex-mediated arthritis (ICA). Arthritis Res. 2000; 2(6):489–503.
26. Nabbe KC, et al. Coordinate expression of activating Fcγ receptors I and III and inhibiting Fcγ receptor type II in the determination of joint inflammation and cartilage destruction during immune complex-mediated arthritis. Arthritis Rheum. 2003;48(1):255–65.
27. van Lent PL, et al. Role of Fc receptor γ chain in inflammation and cartilage damage during experimental antigen-induced arthritis. Arthritis Rheum. 2000;43(4):740–52.
28. van Lent PL, et al. Role of activatory FcγRI and FcγRIII and inhibitory FcγRII in inflammation and cartilage destruction during experimental antigen-induced arthritis. Am J Pathol. 2001;159(6):2309–20.
29. van Lent PL, et al. Fcγ receptors directly mediate cartilage, but not bone, destruction in murine antigen-induced arthritis: uncoupling of cartilage damage from bone erosion and joint inflammation. Arthritis Rheum. 2006; 54(12):3868–77.
30. van Lent PL, et al. Phagocytic synovial lining cells regulate acute and chronic joint inflammation after antigenic exacerbation of smouldering experimental murine arthritis. J Rheumatol. 1998;25(6):1135–45.
31. Wipke BT, Allen PM. Essential role of neutrophils in the initiation and progression of a murine model of rheumatoid arthritis. J Immunol. 2001; 167(3):1601–8.
32. Kitsis E, Weissmann G. The role of the neutrophil in rheumatoid arthritis. Clin Orthop Relat Res. 1991;265:63–72.
33. Mohr W, Westerhellweg H, Wessinghage D. Polymorphonuclear granulocytes in rheumatic tissue destruction: III. An electron microscopic study of PMNs at the pannus-cartilage junction in rheumatoid arthritis. Ann Rheum Dis. 1981;40(4):396–9.
34. Nacken W, et al. S100A9/S100A8: myeloid representatives of the S100 protein family as prominent players in innate immunity. Microsc Res Tech. 2003;60(6):569–80.
35. Ehrchen JM, et al. The endogenous Toll-like receptor 4 agonist S100A8/S100A9 (calprotectin) as innate amplifier of infection, autoimmunity, and cancer. J Leukoc Biol. 2009;86(3):557–66.

36. Pruenster M, et al. S100A8/A9: From basic science to clinical application. Pharmacol Ther. 2016;167:120–31.
37. Uchida T, et al. Application of a novel protein biochip technology for detection and identification of rheumatoid arthritis biomarkers in synovial fluid. J Proteome Res. 2002;1(6):495–9.
38. Baillet A, et al. Synovial fluid proteomic fingerprint: S100A8, S100A9 and S100A12 proteins discriminate rheumatoid arthritis from other inflammatory joint diseases. Rheumatology (Oxford). 2010;49(4):671–82.
39. Grevers LC, et al. S100A8 enhances osteoclastic bone resorption in vitro through activation of Toll-like receptor 4: implications for bone destruction in murine antigen-induced arthritis. Arthritis Rheum. 2011;63(5):1365–75.
40. Van Meurs JB, et al. Quantification of mRNA levels in joint capsule and articular cartilage of the murine knee joint by RT-PCR: kinetics of stromelysin and IL-1 mRNA levels during arthritis. Rheumatol Int. 1997;16(5):197–205.
41. Seeling M, et al. Inflammatory monocytes and Fcγ receptor IV on osteoclasts are critical for bone destruction during inflammatory arthritis in mice. Proc Natl Acad Sci U S A. 2013;110(26):10729–34.
42. Charles JF, et al. Inflammatory arthritis increases mouse osteoclast precursors with myeloid suppressor function. J Clin Invest. 2012;122(12): 4592–605.
43. Hobday PM, et al. Fcγ receptor III and Fcγ receptor IV on macrophages drive autoimmune valvular carditis in mice. Arthritis Rheumatol. 2014;66(4):852–62.
44. Boross P, et al. Destructive arthritis in the absence of both FcγRI and FcγRIII. J Immunol. 2008;180(7):5083–91.
45. Kleinau S, Martinsson P, Heyman B. Induction and suppression of collagen-induced arthritis is dependent on distinct Fcγ receptors. J Exp Med. 2000; 191(9):1611–6.
46. Koga T, et al. Costimulatory signals mediated by the ITAM motif cooperate with RANKL for bone homeostasis. Nature. 2004;428(6984):758–63.
47. Mocsai A, et al. The immunomodulatory adapter proteins DAP12 and Fc receptor γ-chain (FcRγ) regulate development of functional osteoclasts through the Syk tyrosine kinase. Proc Natl Acad Sci U S A. 2004;101(16):6158–63.
48. Negishi-Koga T, et al. Immune complexes regulate bone metabolism through FcRγ signalling. Nat Commun. 2015;6:6637.
49. Zou W, Teitelbaum SL. Absence of Dap12 and the $\alpha_v\beta_3$ integrin causes severe osteopetrosis. J Cell Biol. 2015;208(1):125–36.
50. Mancardi DA, et al. Cutting edge: The murine high-affinity IgG receptor FcγRIV is sufficient for autoantibody-induced arthritis. J Immunol. 2011; 186(4):1899–903.
51. Koene HR, et al. FcγRIIIa-158V/F polymorphism influences the binding of IgG by natural killer cell FcγRIIIa, independently of the FcγRIIIa-48L/R/H phenotype. Blood. 1997;90(3):1109–14.
52. Morgan AW, et al. Fcγ receptor type IIIA is associated with rheumatoid arthritis in two distinct ethnic groups. Arthritis Rheum. 2000;43(10):2328–34.
53. Morgan AW, et al. FcγRIIIA-158V and rheumatoid arthritis: a confirmation study. Rheumatology (Oxford). 2003;42(4):528–33.
54. Milicic A, et al. The F158V polymorphism in FcγRIIIA shows disparate associations with rheumatoid arthritis in two genetically distinct populations. Ann Rheum Dis. 2002;61(11):1021–3.
55. Hammer HB, et al. Calprotectin (a major leucocyte protein) is strongly and independently correlated with joint inflammation and damage in rheumatoid arthritis. Ann Rheum Dis. 2007;66(8):1093–7.
56. Hammer HB, et al. Calprotectin (a major S100 leucocyte protein) predicts 10-year radiographic progression in patients with rheumatoid arthritis. Ann Rheum Dis. 2010;69(1):150–4.
57. Kang KY, Woo JW, Park SH. S100A8/A9 as a biomarker for synovial inflammation and joint damage in patients with rheumatoid arthritis. Korean J Intern Med. 2014;29(1):12–9.
58. Choi IY et al. MRP8/14 serum levels as a strong predictor of response to biological treatments in patients with rheumatoid arthritis. Ann Rheum Dis 2015;74(3):499-505.

8

Endothelial injury in rheumatoid arthritis: a crosstalk between dimethylarginines and systemic inflammation

Theodoros Dimitroulas[1,2*], James Hodson[3], Aamer Sandoo[4], Jacqueline Smith[2] and George D. Kitas[5]

Abstract

Background: Symmetric (SDMA) and asymmetric (ADMA) dimethylarginines have emerged as novel biomarkers of cardiovascular disease (CVD) in several disease settings associated with atherosclerosis. Rheumatoid arthritis (RA) is a chronic systemic inflammatory disease characterized by high CVD mortality and morbidity. ADMA and SDMA levels are abnormal in RA patients, but their correlation with assessments of endothelial function and structure remains unknown. We aimed to investigate whether SDMA and ADMA are associated with carotid intima media thickness (cIMT) and arterial stiffness as well as non-invasive assessments of in vivo micro- and macrovascular endothelial function in RA patients with high systemic inflammatory load.

Method: ADMA and SDMA levels were measured using immunoassays in 197 RA individuals. Twenty-six of these [23 (86.4%) females, median age 70, quartiles (60, 73)] were identified as having high inflammatory markers [erythrocyte sedimentation rate (ESR) >25 mm/hr and C-reactive protein (CRP) > 5 mg/L], and were compared to the remainder of the cohort. Patients underwent assessments of microvascular endothelium-dependent and endothelium-independent function [laser Doppler imaging with iontophoresis of acetylcholine (Ach) and sodium-nitroprusside (SNP) respectively], macrovascular endothelium-dependent and endothelium-independent function (flow-mediated dilatation and glyceryl-trinitrate-mediated dilation respectively), and vascular morphology [pulse wave analysis, and carotid intima media thickness (cIMT)].

Results: Significant interactions with inflammation were detected in the associations between ACh and both SDMA ($p = 0.014$) and ADMA:SDMA ratio ($p = 0.027$), as well as between SNP and SDMA ($p = 0.042$) and between arterial stiffness and ADMA:SDMA ($p = 0.036$), with the associations being stronger in the patients with high inflammatory markers in each case.

Conclusions: Besides their emerging role as markers of endothelial dysfunction SDMA and ADMA may promote endothelial injury in RA as mediators of the adverse effects of systemic inflammation on micro- and macrovasculature respectively in patients with active disease.

Keywords: ADMA, SDMA, Rheumatoid arthritis, cIMT, Inflammation

* Correspondence: dimitroul@hotmail.com
[1]4th Department of Internal Medicine, Hippokration Hospital, School of Medicine, Aristotle University of Thessaloniki, Thessaloniki, Greece
[2]Department of Rheumatology, Russells Hall Hospital, Dudley Group NHS FT, Pensnett Road, DY1 2HQ Dudley, UK
Full list of author information is available at the end of the article

Background

Patients with rheumatoid arthritis (RA) have an increased risk for cardiovascular disease (CVD), which appears to be of equal frequency and severity to those with diabetes mellitus of similar duration [1]. This elevated CVD risk is only partially explained by the higher prevalence of traditional CVD risk factors in RA [2] and accounts for almost 40–50% of all deaths resulting in premature mortality and reduced life expectancy amongst RA patients compared to the general population [3]. The precise pathogenic mechanisms of CVD remain partially understood. It appears that inflammation-induced accelerated atherosclerosis is the main contributor to the excess CVD risk in RA, as inflammatory processes in rheumatoid synovia and atherosclerotic plaque share striking similarities [4].

Derangement of endothelial function is a key early step in the initiation of vascular injury leading to accelerated atherosclerosis and the development of plaque. Nitric oxide (NO) is the main endothelium-derived regulator of vascular homeostasis with vasodilatory, anti-proliferative and anti-atherogenic properties [5]. Reduced NO synthesis and bioavailability can lead to endothelial dysfunction through several mechanisms such as loss of basal vasodilator tone, enhanced blood cell migration and raised local chemokine and/or cytokine release. In RA, systemic inflammation is a pivotal player in the disruption of the equilibrium between the production of NO and other vasoactive agents and the ensuing imbalance initiates platelet activation, abnormal fibrinolytic activity, lipid and glucose metabolism disorders as well as oxidative stress, all of which contribute to impaired vascular patency and a hypercoagulable state [6–8]. There is a continuous need for the investigation of potential pathogenetic pathways that may shed more light in the complex interrelations between vascular dysfunction and systemic inflammation in RA.

Recently, interest has shifted towards the identification of molecules associated with suppression of NO synthase activity, the enzyme responsible for NO synthesis. Asymmetric (ADMA) and symmetric (SDMA) dimethylarginines are analogues of L-arginine - the precursor of NO - naturally liberated in biological fluids following proteolysis. They inhibit NO synthesis by competing with L-arginine at the active site of NO synthase. Regulation of ADMA metabolism depends on the enzymatic activity of dimethylarginine dimethylaminohydrolase whilst SDMA is mainly cleaved by kidneys, with ADMA:SDMA ratio suggested as an index of dimethylarginine dimethylaminohydrolase activity [9]. Dimethylarginines have emerged as novel markers of endothelial dysfunction and CVD risk in several conditions associated with severe vascular disease, such as coronary artery disease [10], renal failure [11], diabetes mellitus [12] as well as in the general population [13]. A recent meta-analysis of 22 prospective studies suggested that ADMA is strongly associated with CVD outcomes in a broad range of circumstances [14], confirming previous reports and illustrating a role for dimethylarginines in the assessment of CVD risk in high-risk populations. In RA, we and others have demonstrated abnormal circulating levels of ADMA and SDMA and established robust correlations with other indices of atherosclerotic burden, namely insulin resistance and cumulative systemic inflammatory load [15–18]. In RA, ADMA has been associated with morphological markers of subclinical atherosclerosis, such as carotid intima-media thickness (cIMT) in some [19] but not all studies [15, 20]. Published data employing non-invasive techniques of endothelium-dependent and endothelium-independent peripheral micro- and macrovascular function and pulse wave analysis have failed to establish relationships between dimethylargines and measurements of vascular morphology [21]. However, most of these studies included unselected RA patients with a mixture of high, moderate, low and/or minimal disease activity. Although endothelial function and structure are affected in patients with RA [22], no clear association between vascular abnormalities and systemic inflammation has been demonstrated [23].

The aim of the current study was to address whether dimethylarginine levels correlate with structural and functional markers of atherosclerosis specifically in RA patients with high systemic inflammatory load.

Methods

Patient characteristics

One hundred and ninety-seven consecutive patients were recruited from the Dudley Rheumatoid Arthritis Co-morbidity Cohort (DRACCO), a prospective study examining CV burden in RA. Detailed characteristics of the participants have been described previously [17]. Exclusion criteria included confirmed acute coronary syndrome, evidence of chronic kidney disease or serious psychiatric disorders. The study received ethics approval from The Black Country Research Ethics Committee and all participants gave their written informed consent according to the Declaration of Helsinki. In the present study, RA patients with high inflammatory markers defined as erythrocyte sedimentation rate (ESR) > 25 mm/hr and C-reactive protein (CRP) > 5 mg/L were identified and analysed as a distinct group. Comparisons were performed between the two subgroups of RA patients: the one with high inflammatory markers and the remaining patients with normal values of ESR and CRP.

Protocol

All patients reported to a thermoregulated (22 ± 0.9 °C) vascular laboratory after a 12-hour overnight fast. They were asked to refrain from exercise 24 hours before the session, and from smoking 12 hours before the session.

Drug regimens were not interrupted. All participants underwent a detailed clinical examination and demographic information was collected by questionnaire. A blood sample was also obtained on the same day, for the assessments of routine hematologic and biochemistry, lipid profile, fasting glucose, fasting insulin, and acute phase response. ESR was measured using the Starrsed Auto Compact blood sedimentation instrument, which automatically carries out the erythrocyte sedimentation analysis according to the Westergren reference method. CRP was measured using the VITROS™ 5,1 FS Chemistry System (Ortho-Clinical Diagnostics, Raritan, NJ, USA). This is an immunoturbidimetric method. The antibody in the reagent combines with CRP in the specimen thereby increasing turbidity in the solution. This is measured as an increase in absorbance at 340 nm. The identification of patients with high/abnormal inflammatory markers (ESR > 25 mm/hr and CRP > 5 mg/L) was performed on the basis of the upper limits of normal as provided by the lab. All biochemical tests were carried out in the Biochemistry Laboratory at Russells Hall Hospital, The Dudley Group NHS Foundation Trust, UK.

Microvascular endothelial function

Endothelial function of the microvasculature was assessed non-invasively using laser Doppler imaging (LDI) (Moor laser Doppler imager, Moor Instruments Ltd, Axminster, UK) with iontophoresis of 1% acetylcholine (ACh, endothelium-dependent, Miochol-E, Novartis, Camberley, UK) and 1% sodium-nitroprusside (SNP, endothelium-independent, Nitroprussiat Fides, Rottapharm, Barcelona, Spain) in 2.5 ml solution containing 0.5% saline by a single observer (AS). This technique has an intra-observer co-efficient of variation for ACh and SNP of 6.5% and 5.9% respectively for AS [24].

Macrovascular endothelial function

Assessment of macrovascular endothelium-dependent function was performed using flow-mediated dilatation (FMD) with high-resolution ultrasonography of the brachial artery (Acuson Antares ultrasound system, Siemens PLC, Camberley, UK) according to previously established guidelines [25]. The intra-observer co-efficient of variation for the study ultrasonographer (AS) was 10.7% for flow-mediated dilatation (FMD) and 11.8% for glyceryl-trinitrate-mediated dilatation (GTN) assessments respectively. For all vascular tests, endothelial function was expressed as the percentage increase in perfusion or diameter from baseline, and all analysis was carried out offline by AS, who was blinded to the identity of the patient.

Carotid atherosclerosis

High-resolution ultrasonography of the carotid artery was performed by an experienced ultrasonographer (AS) according to previously established guidelines [26]. The cIMT was defined by determining the thickness between the lines of Pignoli; with the first echogenic line representing the lumen-intima interface, and the second line representing the media-adventitia interface [27]. Assessments of cIMT were performed in the far wall, 1 cm proximal to the carotid bulb, at sites free of plaque in both the right and left common carotid arteries, using the longitudinal scanning plane. Three measurements were taken on each side, and these were averaged to give the mean cIMT for the right and left carotid arteries separately. The cIMT from both sides were further averaged to give the overall cIMT. The intra-observer co-efficient of variation was 8.6%.

Pulse wave analysis

Pulse wave analysis (SphygmoCor Px Pulse Wave Analysis, ScanMed Medical Instruments, Moreton-in-Marsh, UK) was used to determine subendocardial viability ratio (SEVR) and augmentation index (AIx) as described previously [28]. Briefly, an applanation tonometer was positioned over the radial artery with enough pressure to flatten (but not occlude) the patient's artery. The applanation tonometer detects the pulse pressure wave, which is calibrated against the standard brachial blood pressure and gives the maximum (systolic) and minimum (diastolic) points of the pressure wave. The pressure waveform is then mathematically transformed into a central aortic waveform, which contains the first (peak flow) and second (peak pressure) systolic peaks and displays information on ejection duration. SEVR is calculated by utilising the ejection duration, which is automatically measured by the Sphygmocor system, and dividing the area under the diastolic curve (coronary perfusion) by the area under the systolic curve (cardiac workload). In normal conditions, SEVR can be anywhere between 130% and 200%. Values that are below unity (100%) reflect poor perfusion of the subendocardium.

Measurement of ADMA and SDMA

ADMA levels were measured in serum samples by using a commercial enzyme immunoassay ELISA kit (Immundiagnostik, Bensheim, Germany) as previously described [17]. The intra-assay coefficient of variation was 7.6%.

The SDMA assay is based on the method of competitive enzyme-linked immunoassays. The sample preparation includes the addition of a derivatization reagent for SDMA coupling. During the incubation period, the target SDMA in the sample competes with the SDMA derivative (tracer) immobilised on the wall of the microtiter plates for the binding of the polyclonal antibodies. The SDMA in the sample displaces the antibodies out of the binding to the tracer. Therefore, the concentration of the tracer-bound antibody is inversely proportional to the SDMA concentration in the sample. The absorbance is measured at 450 nm and patient samples are read from a standard curve. The intra-assay standard deviation was 7.5% and inter-assay was 6%. The lowest amount detected was 0.05 µmol/L.

Statistical analysis

Prior to the analysis, the distributions of all variables being considered were assessed. Log_2-transfomations were applied to any variables found to be skewed, in order to normalise the distributions and improve model fit. For variables with negative values, a constant was added to all cases before the log_2-transfomation, to ensure that this was calculable in all cases. There were several clear outliers in the SDMA measurements, which were excluded from the main analysis, in order to produce reliable models for the remaining cases.

Patients with high levels of inflammation were compared to the group with normal inflammatory markers, using t tests for normally distributed (or log-transformed) variables, Mann–Whitney tests for variables that were not normally distributed, and Fisher's exact tests for dichotomous variables.

General linear models were then produced, in order to assess how the relationships between ADMA and/or SDMA and a range of factors differed by the degree of inflammation. A dichotomous variable indicating the inflammation group (normal or high) was added as an independent variable in each model, along with the factor being considered. An interaction term between these variables was also included, to test whether the gradient for the factor being considered differed between patients with normal and high levels of inflammation.

Where significant interactions were detected, the resulting models were plotted, in order to visualise how the relationships between ADMA and/or SDMA and the factor being considered differed by inflammation. The coefficients from these models were also anti-logged and converted into gradients, representing the percentage increase in ADMA and/or SDMA for a unit increase in the factor.

A sensitivity analysis was also performed, in order to assess whether excluding the outliers had biased the sample and influenced the conclusions. For the whole cohort, Spearman's correlation coefficients between the factors and outcomes were produced separately for the high and normal inflammation groups. The resulting coefficients were then compared, to highlight any cases where the relationships between variables differed by the level of inflammation.

All analyses were performed using IBM SPSS Statistics 22 (IBM Corp. Armonk, NY, USA). Missing data were excluded on a per analysis basis and $p < 0.05$ was deemed to be indicative of statistical significance.

Results

Patients, characteristics, outliers

Data were available for 197 RA individuals. After being log_2-transformed, SDMA was found to closely follow a normal distribution, with the exception of 11 (6%) patients with SDMA values >1. These outliers were excluded, in order to make parametric analysis valid, and to prevent them from becoming excessively influential in the analyses performed, leaving $N = 186$. Of these patients, 26 (14%) were identified as having high levels of inflammation, as defined above.

Comparisons between the high and normal inflammation groups are reported in Table 1. With the exception of disease activity score 28, which was found to be increased in the high inflammation group as expected, none of the other factors were found to differ significantly between the two groups. Table 2 reports the p values from the models used to test for interactions between inflammation and the factors being considered. Significant interactions with inflammation were detected in the associations between vasodilatory responses to acetylocholine (Ach) and both SDMA ($p = 0.014$) and ADMA:SDMA ratio ($p = 0.027$), as well as between vasodilatory responses to 1% sodium-nitroprusside (SNP) and SDMA ($p = 0.042$) and between augmentation index (AIx) and ADMA:SDMA ratio ($p = 0.036$). In each of these cases, it was found that the associations between the factors and SDMA or ADMA:SDMA ratio were stronger in the high inflammation group compared to the normal inflammation group (Table 3).

Microvascular function

For those patients with normal inflammatory markers, there was no significant association between ACh and SDMA ($p = 0.791$). However, a significant negative correlation was detected in patients with high levels of inflammation ($p = 0.006$) (Fig. 1a). In this cohort, a twofold increase in ACh was found to be associated with a 16% reduction in SDMA.

The relationship between ACh and ADMA:SDMA was also non-significant in patients with normal levels of inflammation ($p = 0.528$). However, in patients with high levels of inflammation, a twofold increase in ACh was associated with a significant ($p = 0.008$) increase of 26% in ADMA:SDMA (Fig. 1b).

SNP

No significant association between SNP and SDMA was detected in the group of patients with normal inflammation levels ($p = 0.778$). However, in the patients with high levels of inflammation, a significant negative correlation was detected ($p = 0.034$), with SDMA found to decline by 6.2% for each twofold increase in SNP (Fig. 2).

Table 1 Demographics and RA disease characteristics and surrogate markers of atherosclerosis and endothelial dysfunction in RA patients

Factor	N	All patients (N = 186)	Inflammation Normal (N = 160)	High (N = 26)	p value
Age (years)[b]	186	66 (59, 73)[b]	66 (58, 72)	70 (60, 73)	0.225
Female gender (%)[a]	186	144 (77.4%)	121 (75.6%)	23 (88.5%)	0.206
Disease duration (years)[b]	154	16 (11, 25)[b]	16 (11,25)	16 (12. 21)	0.692
RF (%)[a]	183	136 (74.3%)	114 (72.2%)	22 (88.0%)	0.137
Anti-CCP antibodies (%)[a]	181	115 (63.5%)	96 (61.5%)	19 (76.0%)	0.186
ESR (mm/h)[b]	181	11 (5, 22)[b]	9 (5, 16)	40 (30, 56)	-
CRP (mg/L)[b]	186	3.0 (2.9, 8.0)[b]	2.9 (2.9, 4.5)	21.0 (13.0, 31.0)	-
DAS 28[c]	181	3.14 (1.18)[c]	2.97 (1.10)	4.19 (1.12)	**<0.001**
ADMA (μmol/L)[d]	181	0.56 (0.54–0.58)[d]	0.55 (0.53–0.57)	0.59 (0.56–0.63)	0.136
SDMA (μmol/L)[d]	186	0.46 (0.44–0.47)[d]	0.46 (0.45–0.47)	0.45 (0.41–0.50)	0.812
ADMA:SDMA[d]	181	1.22 (1.17–1.27)[d]	1.20 (1.15–1.25)	1.30 (1.17–1.46)	0.167
Arterial stiffness[c]	165	33 (9)[c]	33 (9)	33 (8)	0.791
Microvascular endothelial dependent (ACh %)[d]	179	235 (207–265)[d]	244 (213–276)	184 (119–262)	0.145
Microvascular endothelial- independent (SNP %)[d]	179	116 (100–134)[d]	119 (102–138)	100 (60–159)	0.421
Macrovascular endothelial- dependent (FMD %)[d]	173	9.8 (8.8–10.8)[d]	9.9 (8.8–11.0)	9.0 (6.4–11.9)	0.554
Macrovascular endothelial- independent (GTN %)[d]	155	19.6 (18.2–21.1)[d]	19.7 (18.2–21.4)	18.9 (16.0–22.4)	0.715
cIMT (mm)[d]	157	0.68 (0.66–0.70)[d]	0.67 (0.65–0.70)	0.72 (0.67–0.79)	0.116

Bold p values are significant at $p < 0.05$

RA rheumatoid arthritis, *RF* rheumatoid factor, *anti-CCP* anti-citrullinated protein antibody, *ESR* erythrocyte sedimentation rate, *CRP* C-reactive protein, *DAS 28* disease activity score 28, *ADMA* asymmetric dimethylarginine, *SDMA* symmetric dimethylarginine, *ACh* acetylcholine, *SNP* sodium nitroprusside, *FMD* flow-mediated dilatation, *GTN* glyceryl-trinitrate mediated dilatation, *cIMT* intima media thickness

[a]N (%), with p values from Fisher's exact tests

[b]Median (quartiles), with p values from Mann–Whitney tests

[c]Mean (SD), with p values from t tests

[d]Geometric mean (95% CI), with p values from t tests on log-transformed data

Macrovascular function

No significant associations between dimethylarginines and assessments of macrovascular endothelial function were detected either in the group of patients with normal or in those with high levels of inflammatory markers.

Arterial stiffness

No significant association between AIX and ADMA:SDMA ratio was detected in the group of patients with normal inflammation levels ($p = 0.827$). However, in the patients with high levels of inflammation, a significant positive correlation was detected ($p = 0.033$),

Table 2 p values from general linear models

	ADMA			SDMA			ADMA:SDMA		
Factor	Main Eff.	Inflam.	Int.	Main Eff.	Inflam.	Int.	Main Eff.	Inflam.	Int.
Log_2ACh	0.390	0.954	0.636	**0.008**	**0.030**	**0.014**	**0.007**	0.093	**0.027**
Log_2SNP	0.702	0.989	0.824	0.074	0.056	**0.042**	0.100	0.151	0.087
Log_2FMD	0.363	0.767	0.677	0.420	0.097	0.092	0.174	0.138	0.110
Log_2GTN	0.754	0.702	0.823	0.799	0.812	0.868	0.959	0.607	0.737
Log_2cIMT	0.217	0.323	0.051	0.550	0.265	0.562	0.607	0.953	0.259
Log_2SEVR	0.876	0.727	0.706	**0.006**	**0.049**	0.052	0.058	0.252	0.268
AIx (HR 75)	0.204	0.367	0.246	0.205	0.221	0.127	0.050	0.097	**0.036**

p values from general linear models, with three terms included in each model: Main Eff. - the main effect of the factor being considered, Inflam. - a binary variable, stating whether a patient had high levels of inflammation (ESR > 25 and CRP > 5), Int. - an interaction term between Main Eff. and Inflam., testing whether the relationship between the factor and outcome differs by the degree of inflammation. Bold p values are significant at $p < 0.05$

ADMA asymmetric dimethylarginine, *SDMA* symmetric dimethylarginine, *ACh* acetylcholine, *SNP* sodium nitroprusside, *FMD* flow-mediated dilatation, *GTN* glyceryl-trinitrate mediated dilatation, *cIMT* intima media thickness, *SEVR* subendocardial viability ratio, *AIx* augmentation index, *HR* heart rate

Table 3 Results from general linear models for factors with significant interaction terms

		Normal inflammation		High inflammation	
Outcome	Factor	Gradient	*p* value	Gradient	*p* value
SDMA	Log_2ACh	−0.7% (−5.6%, 4.5%)	0.791	−16.3% (−26.3%, −5.0%)	**0.006**
ADMA:SDMA	Log_2ACh	2.2% (−4.5%, 9.4%)	0.528	25.6% (6.1%, 48.7%)	**0.008**
SDMA	Log_2SNP	0.4% (−2.4%, 3.3%)	0.778	−6.2% (−11.5%, −0.5%)	**0.034**
ADMA:SDMA	AIx (HR 75)	−0.1% (−0.5%, 0.4%)	0.827	1.6% (0.1%, 3.1%)	**0.033**

Results are from the models reported in Table 2. Since the outcome variables of SDMA and ADMA:SDMA had been log-transformed prior to analysis, the resulting coefficients were anti-logged, and converted into gradients representing the percentage increase in the outcome for a one unit increase in the factor. For the log-transformed factors, this is equivalent to the change associated with a twofold increase in the untransformed factor. Bold *p* values are significant at $p < 0.05$
SDMA symmetric dimethylarginine, *ACh* acetylcholine, *ADMA* asymmetric dimethylarginine, *SNP* sodium nitroprusside, *AIx* augmentation index, *HR* heart rate

with ADMA:SDMA ratio found to increase by 1.6% for each unit increase in AIx (Fig. 3).

Sensitivity analysis

A sensitivity analysis was performed on the whole cohort without exclusions ($N = 197$, 28 [14%] with high levels of inflammation). Since the outliers were now being included in the data, it was not possible to produce valid regression models, so a non-parametric approach was used. Patients were split into normal and high inflammation groups, and Spearman's correlation coefficients produced to assess the level of correlation between variables (Table 4).

The results were consistent with the main analysis, with significant negative correlations detected between SDMA and both ACh and SNP in patients with high inflammation that were not observed in those with normal inflammation. ADMA:SDMA ratio was found to be significantly positively correlated with ACh and AIx in patients with high inflammation, but not in those with normal inflammation, as in the main analysis. The sensitivity analysis additionally identified a significant negative correlation between cIMT and ADMA in patients with high inflammation that was not present in those with normal inflammation. This effect was not found to be significant in the main analysis, although it only narrowly missed significance, with $p = 0.051$.

Discussion

The main finding of our study is the establishment of statistically significant relationships between circulating dimethylargines and assessments of microvascular function and arterial stiffness in RA patients with high levels of systemic inflammatory activity. To the best of our knowledge, this is the first time that such associations are reported in this population and our results may provide further insights in the complex interrelations between functional vascular changes, atherosclerosis and inflammation in RA.

Several non-invasive techniques for the assessment of endothelial morphology and function in micro- and macrovasculature can examine the development of premature atherosclerosis and provide useful information regarding an individual's CVD risk status, particularly in clinical settings associated with excess CVD risk, such as RA [29]. In this study, we utilized a broad range of assessments to ensure the global evaluation of vascular function and morphology and investigate potential relationships between indices of vascular health and surrogate markers of endothelial dysfunction and systemic inflammation.

Our findings suggest that dimethylarginines represent not only biomarkers of endothelial dysfunction, but may themselves be important mediators of disruption of vascular homeostasis in RA. Besides their inhibitory properties on NO synthesis, dysregulated ADMA and SDMA metabolism may affect endothelial function through other mechanisms independent of NO synthase inhibition such as inflammation [30]. Under these circumstances, dimethylarginines contribute to the precipitation of oxidative stress by altering endothelial NO synthase activity, switching it to a superoxide synthase [31, 32] and acting as amplifiers, promoting vascular injury. This is in line with previous observations, demonstrating links between derangement of NO/ADMA pathway, oxidative stress and inflammation in RA individuals [17, 33, 34].

The inverse correlation between SDMA and microvascular function demonstrated in our study may look at first glance fundamentally counterintuitive. However, SDMA levels are lower in RA subjects compared to controls [16] similarly to what occurs in diabetes mellitus and insulin-resistant patients [35, 36]. It appears that common mechanisms affecting intracellular migration of endogenous dimethylarginines in RA and insulin resistance are associated with atherosclerosis in both conditions [1]. Given that SDMA competitively inhibits ADMA for entry into the cells, increased SDMA cellular uptake induced by decreased insulin sensitivity [37] indirectly contributes to raised serum ADMA levels and progression of vascular disease. This intriguing interaction could explain how lower SDMA levels are associated with microvascular endothelium dysfunction. Finally, the establishment of associations with both endothelium-dependent and endothelium-independent microvascular function suggests that particularly SDMA

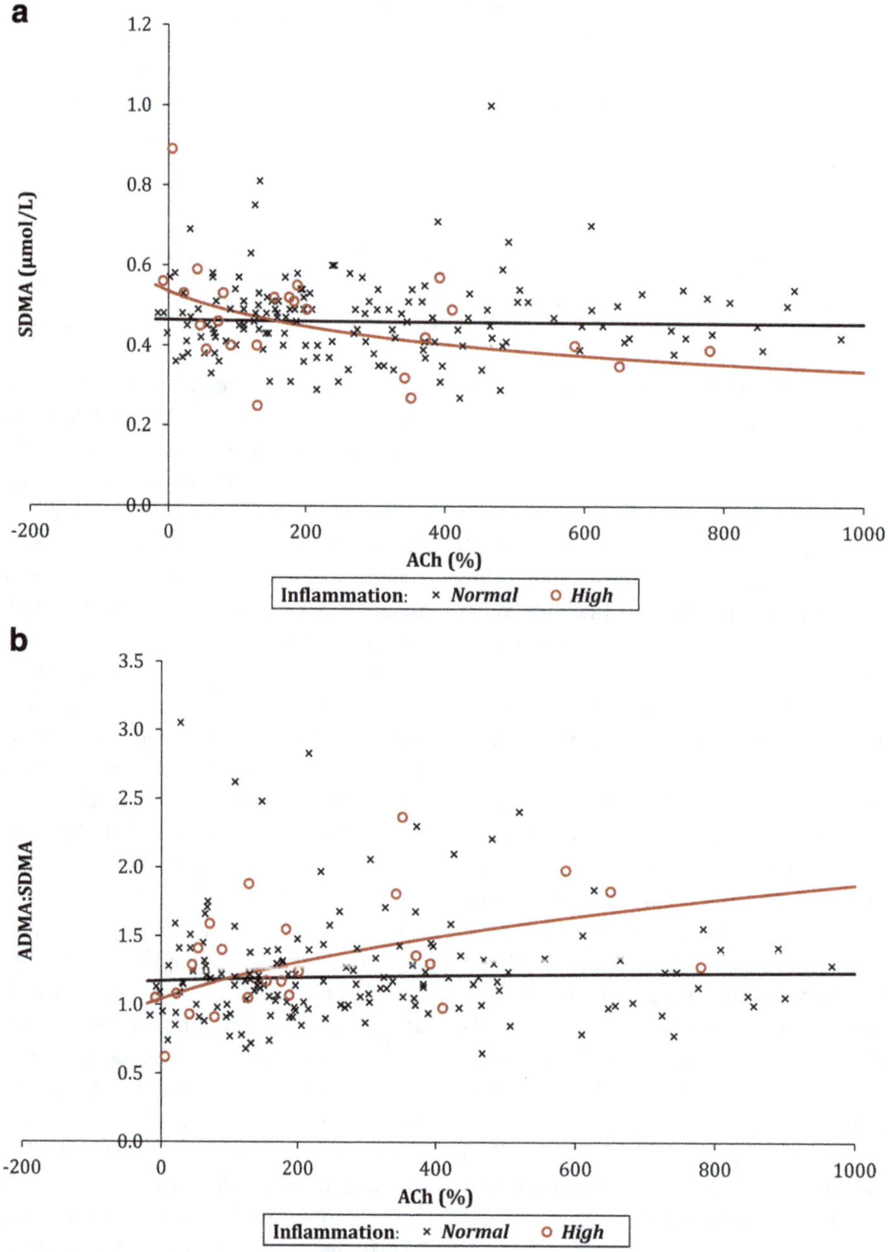

Fig. 1 a The relationship between ACh and SDMA. **b** The relationship between ACh and ADMA:SDMA. *ACh* acetylcholine, *ADMA* asymmetric dimethylarginine, *SDMA* symmetric dimethylarginine

induces NO depletion through NO synthase-dependent and NO synthase -independent pathways.

Cross-sectional studies have indicated a possible time lag between endothelial injury and structural wall damage, as impairment of endothelial function occurs differently and in different vascular beds with microvascular function affected earlier than the macrovascular one in RA individuals [38–40]. Despite the cross-sectional design of these studies, which cannot confirm temporal relationships, it can be speculated that the reported associations between SDMA only with microvascular function may underscore the role of dimethylarginines in initiating endothelial damage under conditions where high systemic inflammatory markers are present. On the other hand, the correlations between ADMA and cIMT indicate a role for endogenous NO synthase inhibitors in the development of later stages of atherosclerosis in individuals with high levels of systemic inflammation, which concurs with reports linking elevated CRP with cIMT in RA population [41].

It is worth noting that, in the modern era, 'Treat to Target' strategies and biologic regimens have considerably

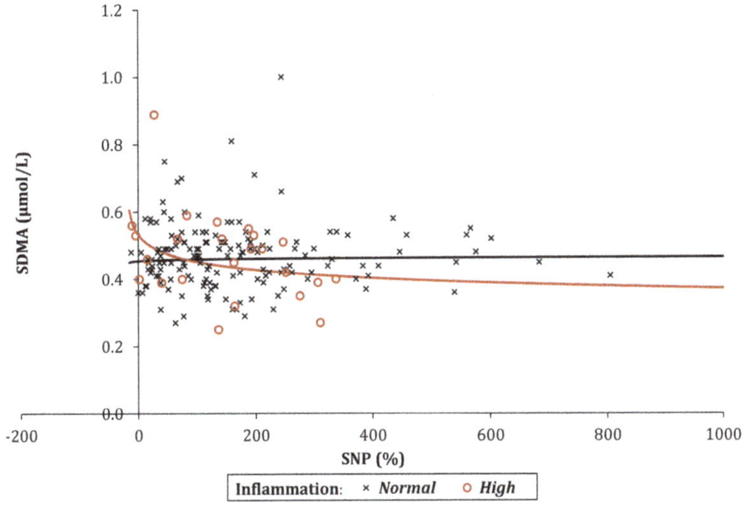

Fig. 2 The relationship between SNP and SDMA. *SNP* sodium nitroprusside, *SDMA* symmetric dimethylarginine

reduced the proportion of patients with high disease activity, to the point that only about 10% of the individuals in our cohort presented with high levels of systemic inflammation and only seven with disease activity score 28 > 5.1. The results of our study indicate that subpopulations analysis may unfold mechanisms more prominent in specific subgroups of patients, for example those with high systemic inflammation. Once more, these findings confirm the effect of active disease on vasculature and emphasize the need for more aggressive management of CVD risk in this subpopulation. The clinical relevance of interventions specifically targeting ADMA- and SDMA-related pathways in RA patients with high inflammatory activity remains to be evaluated in future large studies focusing on specific end points. A recent double-blind randomized study demonstrated that supplementation of oral tetrahydrobiopterin - a cofactor for the production of NO down-regulated by oxidative stress - improved FMD in a small cohort of RA patients [42], providing the rationale for further research.

The strengths and limitations of our study merit consideration. Since the number of patients with high inflammation was small, the analyses performed had relatively low statistical power, particularly for the interaction term in the model, which was the main focus of the study. As a result, small but genuine differences between the two groups may have been missed. For these reasons, it would be preferable to validate the findings from this analysis in an external cohort, in order to ensure reliability of the conclusions. The other limitation

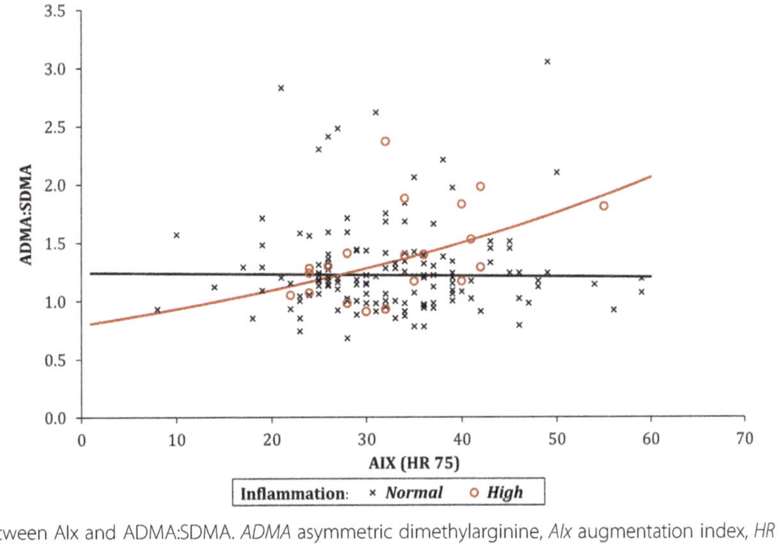

Fig. 3 The relationship between AIx and ADMA:SDMA. *ADMA* asymmetric dimethylarginine, *AIx* augmentation index, *HR* heart rate, *SDMA* symmetric dimethylarginine

Table 4 Sensitivity analysis

	ADMA		SDMA		ADMA:SDMA	
Inflammation	Normal	High	Normal	High	Normal	High
Ach%	0.067 ($p = 0.397$)	0.251 ($p = 0.216$)	−0.077 ($p = 0.325$)	**−0.401 ($p = 0.042$)**	0.128 ($p = 0.108$)	**0.406 ($p = 0.040$)**
SNP%	0.016 ($p = 0.840$)	0.173 ($p = 0.397$)	−0.018 ($p = 0.816$)	**−0.404 ($p = 0.040$)**	0.023 ($p = 0.776$)	0.384 ($p = 0.053$)
FMD%	−0.002 ($p = 0.976$)	0.185 ($p = 0.365$)	0.099 ($p = 0.220$)	−0.165 ($p = 0.421$)	−0.076 ($p = 0.353$)	0.280 ($p = 0.165$)
GTN%	−0.023 ($p = 0.782$)	−0.090 ($p = 0.698$)	−0.052 ($p = 0.540$)	0.007 ($p = 0.978$)	0.033 ($p = 0.698$)	−0.090 ($p = 0.697$)
cIMT	0.100 ($p = 0.247$)	**−0.482 ($p = 0.017$)**	0.005 ($p = 0.958$)	−0.231 ($p = 0.278$)	0.064 ($p = 0.466$)	−0.101 ($p = 0.637$)
SEVR	−0.013 ($p = 0.869$)	0.039 ($p = 0.865$)	0.124 ($p = 0.121$)	0.255 ($p = 0.251$)	−0.091 ($p = 0.264$)	−0.303 ($p = 0.170$)
AIx (HR75)	−0.011 ($p = 0.893$)	0.272 ($p = 0.222$)	0.069 ($p = 0.398$)	−0.287 ($p = 0.195$)	−0.065 ($p = 0.434$)	**0.527 ($p = 0.012$)**

Values are quoted as Spearman's correlation coefficients with p values. Bold coefficients/p values are significant at $p < 0.05$
ADMA asymmetric dimethylarginine, *SDMA* symmetric dimethylarginine, *ACh* acetylcholine, *SNP* sodium nitroprusside, *FMD* flow-mediated dilatation, *GTN* glyceryl-trinitrate-mediated dilatation, *cIMT* intima media thickness, *SEVR* subendocardial viability ratio, *AIx* augmentation index, *HR* heart rate

was the requirement to exclude those patients with high SDMA levels from the main analysis. Leaving these cases in the data meant that they became influential outliers in the models produced, resulting in poor model fit and breaking the assumption of normally distributed residuals. However, the sensitivity analysis performed on the data returned consistent results, implying that any bias introduced by excluding these patients had not fundamentally affected the conclusions of the study. Nevertheless, our study contains adequate functional assessments and morphological measurements of vasculature in a real-life population representative of 'average' RA patients attending routine rheumatology clinics.

Conclusions

In conclusion, we demonstrated that microvascular function, arterial stiffness and cIMT are associated with circulating ADMA and SDMA levels in RA patients with high inflammatory markers. Although CVD represents an unresolved issue throughout the whole RA population, it appears that high systemic uncontrolled inflammatory activity poses the higher risk for CVD events in RA subjects in the short and long term. In that respect, the present study suggests a possible pathway through which high systemic inflammatory load exerts its deleterious effects on vascular wall by precipitating the interaction between dimethylarginines, and endothelial cells and diminishing NO production directly or indirectly. Dimethylarginines therefore, can be considered important mediators of endothelial dysfunction contributing to the oxidative stress burden in the vasculature and the development of CVD in this population.

Abbreviations

ACh: Acetylcholine; ADMA: Asymmetric dimethylarginine; AIx: Augmentation index; cIMT: Carotid intima media thickness; CRP: C-reactive protein; CVD: cardiovascular disease; ESR: Erythrocyte sedimentation rate; FMD: Flow-mediated dilatation; NO: Nitric oxide; RA: Rheumatoid arthritis; SDMA: -Symmetric dimethylarginine; SEVR: Subendocardial viability ratio; SNP: 1% sodium-nitroprusside

Acknowledgements

Not applicable.

Funding

Not applicable.

Authors' contributions

TD, AS and GK contributed to the conception and design of the study. TD drafted the manuscript. JH performed the analysis of the data and considerably contributed to the drafting of the manuscript. AS performed the assessments of vascular function and morphology. JS performed the laboratory part of the study. GK substantially contributed to revising the manuscript critically for important intellectual content and gave approval of the final manuscript. All authors read and approved the final manuscript.

Competing interests

The authors declare that they have no competing interests.

Author details

[1]4th Department of Internal Medicine, Hippokration Hospital, School of Medicine, Aristotle University of Thessaloniki, Thessaloniki, Greece. [2]Department of Rheumatology, Russells Hall Hospital, Dudley Group NHS FT, Pensnett Road, DY1 2HQ Dudley, UK. [3]Institute of Translational Medicine, University Hospital Birmingham NHS Foundation Trust, Queen Elizabeth Hospital Birmingham, Mindelsohn Way, Birmingham B15 2WB, UK. [4]School of Sport, Health and Exercise Sciences, Bangor University, George Building, Bangor, Gwynedd, Wales LL57 2PZ, UK. [5]Arthritis Research UK Epidemiology Unit, University of Manchester, Oxford Road, Manchester M13 9PT, UK.

References

1. Mavrogeni S, Dimitroulas T, Bucciarelli-Ducci C, Ardoin S, Sfikakis PP, Kolovou G, et al. Rheumatoid arthritis: an autoimmune disease with female preponderance and cardiovascular risk equivalent to diabetes mellitus: role of cardiovascular magnetic resonance. Inflamm Allergy Drug Targets. 2014; 13:81–93.
2. Nurmohamed MT, Heslinga M, Kitas GD. Cardiovascular comorbidity in rheumatic diseases. Nat Rev Rheumatol. 2015;11:693–704.
3. Avina-Zubieta JA, Thomas J, Sadatsafavi M, Lehman AJ, Lacaille D. Risk of incident cardiovascular events in patients with rheumatoid arthritis: a meta-analysis of observational studies. Ann Rheum Dis. 2012;71:1524–29.
4. Full LE, Ruisanchez C, Monaco C. The inextricable link between atherosclerosis and prototypical inflammatory diseases rheumatoid arthritis and systemic lupus erythematosus. Arthritis Res Ther. 2009;11:217.

5. Sandoo A, Veldhuijzen Van Zanten JJ, Metsios GS, Carroll D, Kitas GD. The endothelium and its role in regulating vascular tone. Open Cardiovasc Med J. 2010;4:302–12.
6. Dimitroulas T, Douglas KM, Panoulas VF, Toms T, Smith JP, Treharne GJ, Nightingale P, Hodson J, Kitas GD. Derangement of hemostasis in rheumatoid arthritis: association with demographic, inflammatory and metabolic factors. Clin Rheumatol. 2013;32:1357–64.
7. Yang X, Chang Y, Wei W. Endothelial dysfunction and inflammation: immunity in rheumatoid arthritis. Mediat Inflamm. 2016;2016:6813016.
8. Chimenti MS, Triggianese P, Conigliaro P, Candi E, Melino G, Perricone R. The interplay between inflammation and metabolism in rheumatoid arthritis. Cell Death Dis. 2015;6:e1887.
9. Valtonen P, Punnonen K, Saarelainen H, Heiskanen N, Raitakari OT, Juonala M, et al. ADMA concentration changes across the menstrual cycle and during oral contraceptive use: the cardiovascular risk in young Finns study. Eur J Endocrinol. 2010;162:259–65.
10. Mangiacapra F, Conte M, Demartini C, Muller O, Delrue L, et al. Relationship of asymmetric dimethylarginine (ADMA) with extent and functional severity of coronary atherosclerosis. Int J Cardiol. 2016;220:629–33.
11. Fleck C, Schweitzer F, Karge E, Busch M, Stein G. Serum concentrations of asymmetric (ADMA) and symmetric (SDMA) dimethylarginine in patients with chronic kidney diseases. Clin Chim Acta. 2003;336:1–12.
12. Zsuga J, Török J, Magyar MT, Valikovics A, Gesztelyi R, Lenkei A, et al. Dimethylarginines at the crossroad of insulin resistance and atherosclerosis. Metabolism. 2007;56:394–99.
13. Kiechl S, Lee T, Santer P, Thompson G, Tsimikas S, Egger G, et al. Asymmetric and symmetric dimethylarginines are of similar predictive value for cardiovascular risk in the general population. Atherosclerosis. 2009;205:261–5.
14. Willeit P, Freitag DF, Laukkanen JA, Chowdhury S, Gobin R, Mayr M, et al. Asymmetric dimethylarginine and cardiovascular risk: systematic review and meta-analysis of 22 prospective studies. J Am Heart Assoc. 2015;4:e001833.
15. Sandoo A, Dimitroulas T, van Zanten JJ V, Smith JP, Metsios GS, Nightingale P, et al. Lack of association between asymmetric dimethylarginine and in vivo microvascular and macrovascular endothelial function in patients with rheumatoid arthritis. Clin Exp Rheumatol. 2012;30:388–96.
16. Dimitroulas T, Hodson J, Sandoo A, Smith J, Kitas GD. Symmetric dimethylarginine (SDMA) serum levels in rheumatoid arthritis: correlations with insulin resistance and disease activity scores. Amino Acids. 2015;47:1995–2004.
17. Sandoo A, Dimitroulas T, Hodson J, Smith JP, Douglas KM, Kitas GD. Cumulative inflammation associates with asymmetric dimethylarginine in rheumatoid arthritis: a 6 year follow-up study. Rheumatology (Oxford). 2015; 54:1145–52.
18. Klimek E, Skalska A, Kwaśny-Krochin B, Surdacki A, Sulicka J, Korkosz M, et al. Differential associations of inflammatory and endothelial biomarkers with disease activity in rheumatoid arthritis of short duration. Mediat Inflamm. 2014;2014:681635.
19. Surdacki A, Martens-Lobenhoffer J, Wloch A, Marewicz E, Rakowski T, et al. Elevated plasma asymmetric dimethyl-L-arginine levels are linked to endothelial progenitor cell depletion and carotid atherosclerosis in rheumatoid arthritis. Arthritis Rheum. 2007;56:809–19.
20. Karaoğlan B, Öztürk GT, Özdoğan V, Cumaoğlu A, Oktar S, et al. Investigation of the correlation between ADMA levels and carotid artery intima-media thickness in rheumatoid arthritis patients. Turk J Phys Med Rehab. 2011;57:114–8.
21. Dimitroulas T, Sandoo A, Hodson J, Smith JP, Kitas GD. In vivo microvascular and macrovascular endothelial function is not associated with circulating dimethylarginines in patients with rheumatoid arthritis: a prospective analysis of the DRACCO cohort. Scand J Clin Lab Invest. 2016;76:331–7.
22. Di Minno MN, Ambrosino P, Lupoli R, Di Minno A, Tasso M, Peluso R, et al. Clinical assessment of endothelial function in patients with rheumatoid arthritis: a meta-analysis of literature studies. Eur J Intern Med. 2015;26:835–42.
23. Sandoo A, van Zanten JJ V, Metsios GS, Carroll D, Kitas GD. Vascular function and morphology in rheumatoid arthritis: a systematic review. Rheumatology. 2011;50:2125–39.
24. Sandoo A, Kitas GD. A methodological approach to non-invasive assessments of vascular function and morphology. J Vis Exp. 2015;7:96.
25. Corretti MC, Anderson TJ, Benjamin EJ, Celermajer D, Charbonneau F, Creager MA, et al. International Brachial Artery Reactivity Task Force. Guidelines for the ultrasound assessment of endothelial-dependent flow mediated vasodilation of the brachial artery: a report of the international brachial artery reactivity task force. J Am Coll Cardiol. 2002;39:257–65.
26. Touboul PJ, Hennerici MG, Meairs S, Adams H, Amarenco P, Bornstein N, et al. Mannheim Carotid Intima-Media Thickness and Plaque Consensus (2004-2006-2011). An update on behalf of the advisory board of the 3rd, 4th and 5th watching the risk symposia, at the 13th, 15th and 20th European Stroke Conferences, Mannheim, Germany, 2004, Brussels, Belgium, 2006, and Hamburg, Germany, 2011. Cerebrovasc Dis. 2012;34:290–6.
27. Pignoli P, Tremoli E, Poli A, Oreste P, Paoletti R. Intimal plus medial thickness of the arterial wall: a direct measurement with ultrasound imaging. Circulation. 1986;74:1399–406.
28. Klocke R, Cockcroft JR, Taylor GY, Hall IR, Blake DR. Arterial stiffness and central blood pressure, as determined by pulse wave analysis, in rheumatoid arthritis. Ann Rheum Dis. 2003;62:414–8.
29. Khan F, Galarraga B, Belch JJ. The role of endothelial function and its assessment in rheumatoid arthritis. Nat Rev Rheumatol. 2010;6:253–61.
30. Wang Z, Tang WH, Cho L, Brennan DM, Hazen SL. Targeted metabolomic evaluation of arginine methylation and cardiovascular risks: potential mechanisms beyond nitric oxide synthase inhibition. Arterioscler Thromb Vasc Biol. 2009;29:1383–91.
31. Karbach S, Wenzel P, Waisman A, Münzel T, Daiber A. eNOS uncoupling in cardiovascular diseases - the role of oxidative stress and inflammation. Curr Pharm Des. 2014;20:3579–94.
32. Feliers D, Lee DY, Gorin Y, Kasinath BS. Symmetric dimethylarginine alters endothelial nitric oxide activity in glomerular endothelial cells. Cell Signal. 2015;27:1–5.
33. Bunjevacki V, Maksimovic N, Jekic B, Milic V, Lukovic L, Novakovic I, et al. Polymorphisms of the eNOS gene are associated with disease activity in rheumatoid arthritis. Rheumatol Int. 2016;36:597–602.
34. Kwaśny-Krochin B, Głuszko P, Undas A. Plasma asymmetric dimethylarginine in active rheumatoid arthritis: links with oxidative stress and inflammation. Pol Arch Med Wewn. 2012;122:270–6.
35. Schutte AE, Schutte R, Huisman HW, van Rooyen JM, Fourie CM, Malan L, et al. Dimethylarginines: their vascular and metabolic roles in Africans and Caucasians. Eur J Endocrinol. 2010;162:525–33.
36. Anderssohn M, Schwedhelm E, Lüneburg N, Vasan RS, Böger RH. Asymmetric dimethylarginine as a mediator of vascular dysfunction and a marker of cardiovascular disease and mortality: an intriguing interaction with diabetes mellitus. Diab Vasc Dis Res. 2010;7:105–18.
37. González M, Flores C, Pearson JD, Casanello P, Sobrevia L. Cell signalling-mediating insulin increase of mRNA expression for cationic amino acid transporters-1 and −2 and membrane hyperpolarization in human umbilical vein endothelial cells. Pflugers Arch. 2004;448:383–94.
38. Sandoo A, Hodson J, Douglas KM, Smith JP, Kitas GD. The association between functional and morphological assessments of endothelial function in patients with rheumatoid arthritis: a cross-sectional study. Arthritis Res Ther. 2013;15:R107.
39. Toutouzas K, Sfikakis PP, Karanasos A, Aggeli C, Felekos I, Kitas G, et al. Myocardial ischaemia without obstructive coronary artery disease in rheumatoid arthritis: hypothesis-generating insights from a cross-sectional study. Rheumatology (Oxford). 2013;52:76–80.
40. Sandoo A, Carroll D, Metsios GS, Kitas GD, van Zanten JJ V. The association between microvascular and macrovascular endothelial function in patients with rheumatoid arthritis: a cross-sectional study. Arthritis Res Ther. 2011;13:R99.
41. Gonzalez-Gay MA, Gonzalez-Juanatey C, Piñeiro A, Garcia-Porrua C, Testa A, Llorca J. High-grade C-reactive protein elevation correlates with accelerated atherogenesis in patients with rheumatoid arthritis. J Rheumatol. 2005;32:1219–23.
42. Mäki-Petäjä KM, Day L, Cheriyan J, Hall FC, Östör AJ, Shenker N, Wilkinson IB. Tetrahydrobiopterin supplementation improves endothelial function but does not alter aortic stiffness in patients with rheumatoid arthritis. J Am Heart Assoc. 2016;5:e002762.

The impact of arthritis and joint pain on individual healthcare expenditures: findings from the Medical Expenditure Panel Survey (MEPS), 2011

Edith M. Williams[1,2], Rebekah J. Walker[2,3,4], Trevor Faith[1] and Leonard E. Egede[2,3,4*]

Abstract

Background: Joint pain, including back pain, and arthritis are common conditions in the United States, affecting more than 100 million individuals and costing upwards of $200 billion each year. Although activity limitations associated with these disorders impose a substantial economic burden, this relationship has not been explored in a large U.S. cohort.

Methods: In this study, we used the Medical Expenditures Panel Survey to investigate whether functional limitations explain the difference in medical expenditures between patients with arthritis and joint pain and those without. We used sequential explanatory linear models to investigate this relationship and accounted for various covariates.

Results: Unadjusted mean expenditures were $10,587 for those with joint pain or arthritis, compared with $3813 for those without. In a fully adjusted model accounting also for functional limitations, those with joint pain or arthritis paid $1638 more than those without, a statistically significant difference.

Conclusions: The growing economic and public health burden of arthritis and joint pain, as well as the corresponding complications of functional, activity, and sensory limitations, calls for an interdisciplinary approach and heightened awareness among providers to identify strategies that meet the needs of high-risk patients in order to prevent and delay disease progression.

Keywords: Joint pain, Arthritis, Healthcare cost, Medical expenditures, MEPS, Functional limitations

Background

Joint pain (including back pain) and arthritis (osteoarthritis, rheumatoid arthritis) are some of the most common and costly conditions in the United States, affecting more than 100 million individuals and costing more than $200 billion per year [1]. Compared with the general population, those with diseases characterized by arthritis/rheumatism and chronic joint pain experience high rates of functional limitation [1–7]. Functional limitations include those related to limitations in mobility, self-care, daily activities, and pain [1, 3]. Researchers have observed significant impacts to the individual patient as a result of functional limitations, as well as a quantifiable burden to society. One example is the impact of functional limitation on mental health. Turner and Turner [8] examined the relationships among physical disability, mental health, and unemployment. They found that the three factors were closely related and suggested that this combination could lead to a unique pattern of disadvantage for these individuals. They observed that those with disabilities were five times more likely to be involuntarily unemployed and that rates of depression were higher for all individuals with physical limitations, but the trend was more pronounced for those without a job [8]. These unique and compounding factors may

* Correspondence: legede@musc.edu; egedel@musc.edu
[2]Center for Health Disparities Research, Medical University of South Carolina, 135 Rutledge Avenue, Room 280H, Charleston, SC 29425, USA
[3]Division of General Internal Medicine and Geriatrics, Department of Medicine, Medical University of South Carolina, 96 Jonathan Lucas Street, Suite 803, Charleston, SC 29425, USA
Full list of author information is available at the end of the article

significantly increase both healthcare use and associated costs.

Annual direct costs have been estimated on the basis of reported ambulatory care visits, hospitalizations, diagnostic tests, medications, assistive devices, nonallopathic treatments, travel to visits, and paid household help [9]. In other studies focused on specific disorders (i.e., gout, ankylosing spondylitis), researchers have explored costs of illness to the patient and found that functional limitations contribute to such costs and in some cases are the most important predictor of total costs in patients [10, 11].

Indirect costs have been estimated from missed work days or, for retirees and homemakers, the number of days of activity limitation, as well as employment, household income, and receipt of supplemental security income for disability [9, 10, 12]. One investigation revealed that employers lost 28.2 million workdays annually ($4.95 billion in lost income) due to functional limitation caused by chronic diseases, including arthritis [3]. Additionally, 5.3% of the entire U.S. working population experiences work limitations attributable to arthritis [1]. The monetary cost of these work-specific limitations is not yet known, but the prevalence at which these limitations occur may have a significant impact on workplace productivity, especially in physically demanding fields.

Although activity limitations associated with musculoskeletal disorders impose a substantial economic burden on American society, this relationship has not been explored in a large U.S. cohort. As a result, in this study, we used the Medical Expenditures Panel Survey (MEPS) to investigate whether functional limitations explain the difference in medical expenditures between patients with any type or degree of arthritis and/or joint pain and those without.

Methods

Sample population

Using the MEPS consolidated file for 2011, we analyzed data from 35,313 adults (ages 18 years and older). Of this sample, 3793 adults self-reported arthritis or joint pain of some type. MEPS is an ongoing national household survey for the civilian noninstitutionalized U.S. population, with oversampling for blacks and Hispanics [13]. The data are collected through in-person interviews and include detailed information on demographic characteristics, self-reported health conditions, health status, use of medical services, charges and sources of payment, access to care, satisfaction with care, health insurance coverage, income, and employment for each person in the household [13]. The complex survey design provides weights to account for sampling and stratification, and it allows generalization to the U.S. population [14, 15]. Use of the complex survey design enables the 35,313 adults in the sample population to represent 311,125,758 individuals living in the United States in 2011. In addition, it allows generalization from the 3793 adults with self-reported arthritis and/or joint pain in the MEPS sample to represent the 150,378,648 population of adults in the United States with arthritis or joint pain.

Dependent variable

The dependent variable was total healthcare expenditures, defined as the sum of direct payments for office-based medical, hospital inpatient (including zero night stays) and outpatient, emergency department, pharmacy, dental, home health, and other medical care. Total healthcare expenditures represent annual expenditures for the year of reporting (2011) for each individual. Expenditures represent direct payments, not charges, for care provided during 2011 and are collected through both self-report via the household component and through provider reporting via the medical provider component of the survey. The medical provider component is used to verify information collected at the household level, as well as to collect information not known by the household [13].

Independent variable

The primary independent variable was any self-reported diagnosis with arthritis or joint pain. *Joint pain* and *arthritis* are used here as overarching terms; however, they include any diagnosis of this nature, including various rheumatic conditions as well as back pain. We were also interested in the independent variable "any limitation," which summarizes whether a person has any limitations in instrumental activities of daily living, activities of daily living, function (walking), activity, or sensory (any visual or hearing impairment). The presence of any limitation was defined as a positive response to any of these components.

Covariates

Additional covariates were included on the basis of the Anderson model for healthcare use, and we categorized them as predisposing, enabling, and need factors [16]. Predisposing factors included age, race/ethnicity, gender, region, and metropolitan statistical area (MSA). Age was categorized into four groups of 18–34 years, 35–44 years, 45–64 years, and 65+ years. Race/ethnicity was grouped into four categories of non-Hispanic white (NHW), non-Hispanic black, non-Hispanic other (including both Asian and other categories), and Hispanic. Gender was dichotomized. Region was categorized as Northeast, Midwest, South, and West. MSA was dichotomized as MSA (urban) vs. non-MSA (rural).

Enabling factors included household income, employment status, education, insurance, and marital status. Household income was categorized into four groups:

<\$25,000, \$25,000–\$49,999, \$50,000–\$74,999, and > \$75,000. Employment was dichotomized. Education was categorized into four groups as less than high school, high school, college, and graduate school. Insurance was categorized into three categories of private, public, and uninsured. Marital status was categorized into three groups of never married, separated/divorced/widowed, and married.

Need factors included health status, body mass index (BMI), and comorbidities. Comorbidities included chronic bronchitis, asthma, cancer, coronary heart disease, myocardial infarction, other heart disease, angina, diabetes, emphysema, high blood pressure, high cholesterol, depression, and stroke. Health status was self-reported into five categories of excellent, very good, good, fair, and poor. BMI was categorized into four groups of underweight, normal, overweight, and obese. Binary indicators of comorbidities were based on a positive response to a question, "Have you ever been diagnosed with ___?," for each diagnosis.

Statistical analysis

We used sequential explanatory linear models to investigate whether functional limitations explain the difference in medical expenditures between patients with arthritis and joint pain and those without. For each model, we ran a generalized linear model (GLM) using gamma distribution with total expenditures as the dependent variable and reporting joint pain or arthritis as the main independent variable. We then added variables in blocks according to the Anderson model for healthcare use categories of predisposing variables, enabling variables, and need variables. Finally, we ran a final fully adjusted model and added any functional limitation. After each GLM, we determined the marginal effects using the margins command in Stata 14.0 statistical software (StataCorp, College Station, TX, USA). In order to generalize our study findings to the U.S. population, the complex sampling design of the MEPS dataset was taken into account by using sampling weight, variance estimation stratum, and primary sampling unit in all regression models and sample demographic estimates.

Results

Table 1 shows the characteristics for U.S. adults with and without arthritis or joint pain. Of the 3793 adults who self-reported any arthritis and/or joint pain, 63% reported any limitations, compared with 18% of individuals not reporting arthritis or joint pain. Unadjusted mean expenditures were \$10,587 for those reporting joint pain or arthritis, compared with \$3813 for those without. Most (87.7%) of U.S. adults reporting arthritis or joint pain are older than 45 years of age, and they are predominantly NHW (75.6%) and female (63.1%). The

Table 1 Sample characteristics of U.S. adults with self-reported arthritis or joint pain (sample = 3791; population = 311,125,758)

	U.S. adults reporting arthritis or joint pain	U.S. adults in sample with no reported arthritis or joint pain
Limitations, %		
Any limitations	62.86	18.18
IADL	9.16	1.80
ADL	5.68	1.03
Walk limitations	39.01	6.12
Mean total expenditure ± SD	\$10,587 ± \$504	\$3813 ± \$119
Predisposing factors, %		
Age, years		
18–24	0.77	15.36
25–44	11.54	39.19
45–64	45.85	32.72
65+	41.85	12.72
Race		
Non-Hispanic white	75.64	64.76
Non-Hispanic black	11.66	11.42
Non-Hispanic other	4.77	7.58
Hispanic	7.93	16.24
Sex		
Male	36.86	50.49
Female	63.14	49.51
Region		
Northeast	18.29	18.28
Midwest	23.24	21.07
South	38.48	36.75
West	19.99	23.91
MSA		
Rural	19.17	14.72
Urban	80.83	85.28
Enabling factors, %		
Income		
< \$25,000	48.59	42.88
\$25,000–\$49,999	29.33	29.80
\$50,000-\$74,999	12.38	14.70
> \$75,000	9.70	12.62
Employment		
Not employed	58.05	28.73
Employed	41.95	71.27
Education		
Less than high school	17.34	14.66
High school	31.44	27.70
College	40.87	45.59

Table 1 Sample characteristics of U.S. adults with self-reported arthritis or joint pain (sample = 3791; population = 311,125,758) *(Continued)*

Graduate school	10.35	12.05
Insurance		
Any private	63.09	68.99
Public only	30.46	14.67
No insurance	6.45	16.35
Marital status		
Never married	10.48	31.04
Separated/divorced/ widowed	35.30	16.61
Married	54.22	52.34
Need factors, %		
Asthma	15.21	7.80
Diabetes	20.11	7.19
Emphysema	7.12	1.21
High blood pressure	63.28	26.05
High cholesterol	55.75	25.01
Stroke	9.89	2.14
Depression	17.32	6.98
CVD	32.32	9.91
BMI		
Underweight	1.45	1.96
Normal	23.80	37.05
Overweight	32.17	34.29
Obese	42.58	26.70

Abbreviations: ADL Activities of daily living, *BMI* Body mass index, *CVD* Cardiovascular disease, *IADL* Instrumental activities of daily living, *MSA* Metropolitan statistical area

majority are not employed (58.1%) and have private insurance (63.1%). The most common comorbidities are high blood pressure (63.3%) and high cholesterol (55.8%), and the majority are overweight (32.2%) or obese (42.6%).

As shown in Table 2, adults with self-reported arthritis or joint pain pay, on average, $6773 more in medical expenditures than those not reporting arthritis or joint pain. Adjustment decreased the marginal difference to $4427 when accounting for predisposing factors; $3980 when accounting for predisposing and enabling; and $2764 when accounting for predisposing, enabling, and need factors. Finally, in a fully adjusted model accounting also for functional limitations, those reporting joint pain or arthritis paid $1638 more than those without. Those with functional limitations regardless of comorbidity paid $3308 more than those without functional limitations, which was a higher marginal impact than any other comorbidity included in the model.

Discussion

Our analyses showed that individuals self-reporting any diagnosis of arthritis and/or joint pain had substantially higher mean total healthcare expenditures ($6773) than individuals without either. In addition, whereas accounting for predisposing, enabling, and need variables lowered this marginal difference in expenditures, it did not remove the significance. Adjusting for functional limitations further decreased the difference in healthcare expenditures to $1638, but it did not remove significance. The marginal decrease resulting from adding functional limitations into the model was similar in size to the marginal decrease resulting from adding all other comorbidities.

This study emphasizes the need for aggressive measures and strategies for the prevention, early recognition, and treatment of functional limitations in populations with arthritis and joint pain because they have significant impact on differences in medical expenditures. In an investigation of risk factors for work disability, Allaire et al. [17] found that two of the most common indicators of work cessation were severity of disease condition and physical limitations in arthritis and other rheumatic conditions. Work cessation is especially important to populations with chronic conditions, often manifested in two primary concerns. First, loss of employment means loss of income, and for a population that experiences disproportionately high healthcare costs, losing the primary source of income could lead many individuals to financial ruin. Second, according to the Henry J. Kaiser Family Foundation, 49% of the U.S. adult population obtain health insurance through their employers [18]. Thus, many individuals with arthritis or joint pain who cease working because of functional limitations will lose their health insurance and have to pay significant out-of-pocket expenses or be forced to purchase private insurance, which may be more expensive and/or provide less coverage.

Our findings are consistent with existing literature that estimates annual costs associated with some rheumatic conditions to be $10,000–$50,000 more per patient than those for the general population [19–22]. Major cost drivers include inpatient hospitalizations [23], poor physical and mental health, and low education and employment levels. Significant functional and emotional challenges resulting from symptoms, side effects, and complications may also include anxiety, depression, mood disorders, and decreased health-related quality of life [24–27], which further increase service use costs. In another study, Ozaras et al. [28] observed that in patients with ankylosing spondylitis and psoriatic arthritis, disease activity (self-reported pain and symptoms) was associated with greater physical limitation. Given the direct relationships observed between disease activity,

Table 2 Sequential explanatory model for marginal total healthcare expenditures in those with self-reported joint pain and/or arthritis

Variable	Model 1	Model 2	Model 3	Model 4	Model 5
No reported joint pain and/or arthritis (reference)	–	–	–	–	–
Self-reported joint pain and/or arthritis	\$6773*	\$4427*	\$3980*	\$2764*	\$1638*
Predisposing factors					
Age, years					
18–24 (reference)		–	–	–	–
25–44		\$1571*	\$1873*	\$2381*	\$2372*
45–64		\$3633*	\$3717*	\$3224*	\$3038*
65+		\$6150*	\$3510*	\$2087*	\$1607*
Race					
Non-Hispanic white (reference)		–	–	–	–
Non-Hispanic black		−\$883**	−\$1053**	−\$1325**	−\$1287*
Non-Hispanic other		−\$543	−\$448	−\$741	−\$136
Hispanic		−\$2196*	−\$1960*	−\$1845*	−\$1683*
Sex					
Male (reference)		–	–	–	–
Female		\$1053*	\$929*	\$1272*	\$1383*
Region					
Northeast (reference)		–	–	–	–
Midwest		−\$149	\$78	−\$101	−\$168.78
South		−\$514	−\$69	−\$458	−\$325.85
West		\$272	\$489	\$610	\$746.14
MSA					
Rural (reference)		–	–	–	–
Urban		\$797**	\$1124*	\$1216*	\$1241*
Enabling factors					
Income					
< \$25,000 (reference)			–	–	–
\$25,000–\$49,999			−\$414	−\$293	−\$44
\$50,000–\$74,999			\$3	\$444	\$817
> \$75,000			\$364	\$1487***	\$1761**
Employment					
Not employed (reference)			–	–	–
Employed			−\$3239	−\$2654*	−\$2018*
Education					
Less than high school (reference)			–	–	–
High school			\$849***	\$1566**	\$1634*
College			\$709	\$1242*	\$1305*
Graduate school			\$1515**	\$2493*	\$2457*
Insurance					
Any private (reference)			–	–	–
Public only			\$1526***	\$1639***	\$947
No insurance			−\$3615*	−\$3875*	−\$3943*

Table 2 Sequential explanatory model for marginal total healthcare expenditures in those with self-reported joint pain and/or arthritis *(Continued)*

Marital status			
Married (reference)	–	–	–
Separated/divorced/widowed	$63	$34	–$131
Never married	–$55	$79	–$172
Need factors****			
Asthma		$2428*	$2001*
Diabetes		$3001*	$2669*
Emphysema		$2476***	$1559***
High blood pressure		$938*	$876*
High cholesterol		$1149*	$1194*
Stroke		$2683*	$1727***
Depression		$3182*	$1939*
CVD		$2814*	$2375*
BMI			
Underweight (reference)		–	–
Normal		$726	$1200
Overweight		$388	$732
Obese		$534	$824
Risk factor of interest****			
Any limitations			$3308*
IADL			$2488***
ADL			$2284***
Walk limitations			$253

Abbreviations: ADL Activities of daily living, *BMI* Body mass index, *CVD* Cardiovascular disease, *IADL* Instrumental activities of daily living, *MSA* Metropolitan statistical area

Sequential linear models were used, with each column representing a separate generalized linear model using gamma distribution

*$p < 0.001$

**$p < 0.01$

***$p < 0.05$

****Reference groups compared with those without need factor or risk factor

comorbidities, and limitations [17, 28–31], the provision of optimal care to individuals with arthritis and joint pain is critical. This ultimately results in control of disease and slows the progression of related complications such as functional, activity, and sensory limitations.

Though the present study had a number of strengths, including the generalizability of results to the U.S. population, it has some limitations. First, diagnoses were based on self-report, which may differ from physician diagnosis. Second, though we attempted to include factors that could affect the relationship based on a theoretical framework, there are additional factors not in the dataset, including social determinants such as social support and emotional distress. Additionally, self-reports are subject to recall bias, which can introduce random error into the data. Finally, the data are cross-sectional in nature, which precludes commentary on causation or direction of the association.

Conclusions

Our study shows that self-reported arthritis and/or joint pain of any type is associated with higher total healthcare expenditures, and though accounting for functional limitations decreases this difference, the difference remains significant. The growing economic and public health burden of arthritis and joint pain [17, 32, 33], as well as the corresponding complications of functional, activity, and sensory limitations, calls for an interdisciplinary approach and heightened awareness among providers to identify strategies that meet the needs of high-risk patients in order to prevent and delay disease progression. This study provides an estimate for potential savings from future interventions geared toward reduction of any limitations in patients with arthritis and joint pain. Future researchers may benefit from this analysis and expand upon it by examining specifically where these increased costs are coming from, such as whether the increased cost is due to a greater number of visits to health professionals, in-hospital treatments, medications, or other causes. Enumerating the breakdown of these expenditures would allow future development of solutions to target specific areas with disproportionately high costs.

Abbreviations

ADL: Activities of daily living; BMI: Body mass index; CVD: Cardiovascular disease; GLM: Generalized linear model; IADL: Instrumental activities of daily living; MEPS: Medical Expenditures Panel Survey; MSA: Metropolitan statistical area; NHW: Non-Hispanic white

Funding

This study was supported by the National Institute of Diabetes and Digestive and Kidney Diseases (grant K24DK093699 [to principal investigator LEE]).

Authors' contributions

LEE was involved in conception of the study and statistical design, participated in data analysis, and oversaw manuscript development. RJW carried out the data analysis, drafted the Methods and Results sections of the manuscript, and revised the manuscript. EW conceived of and designed the study, drafted the manuscript, and helped to revise the manuscript. TF participated in drafting and helping to revise the manuscript. All authors revised the article critically for important intellectual content and approved the final manuscript.

Competing interests

The authors declare that they have no competing interests.

Author details

[1]Department of Public Health Sciences, Medical University of South Carolina, 135 Cannon Street, Suite CS303, Charleston, SC 29425, USA. [2]Center for Health Disparities Research, Medical University of South Carolina, 135 Rutledge Avenue, Room 280H, Charleston, SC 29425, USA. [3]Division of General Internal Medicine and Geriatrics, Department of Medicine, Medical University of South Carolina, 96 Jonathan Lucas Street, Suite 803, Charleston, SC 29425, USA. [4]Health Equity and Rural Outreach Innovation Center (HEROIC), Ralph H. Johnson Veterans Affairs Medical Center, 109 Bee Street, Charleston, SC 29401, USA.

References

1. Ma VY, Chan L, Carruthers KJ. Incidence, prevalence, costs, and impact on disability of common conditions requiring rehabilitation in the United States: stroke, spinal cord injury, traumatic brain injury, multiple sclerosis, osteoarthritis, rheumatoid arthritis, limb loss, and back pain. Arch Phys Med Rehabil. 2014;95(5):986–95.
2. Spaetgens B, Tran-Duy A, Wijnands JM, van der Linden S, Boonen A. Health and utilities in patients with gout under the care of a rheumatologist. Arthritis Care Res (Hoboken). 2015;67(8):1128–36.
3. Vuong TD, Wei F, Beverly CJ. Absenteeism due to functional limitations caused by seven common chronic diseases in US workers. J Occup Environ Med. 2015;57(7):779–84.
4. Theis KA, Murphy L, Hootman JM, Wilkie R. Social participation restriction among US adults with arthritis: a population-based study using the International Classification of Functioning, Disability and Health. Arthritis Care Res (Hoboken). 2013;65(7):1059–69.
5. Durcan L, Wilson F, Conway R, Cunnane G, O'Shea FD. Increased body mass index in ankylosing spondylitis is associated with greater burden of symptoms and poor perceptions of the benefits of exercise. J Rheumatol. 2012;39(12):2310–4.
6. Iqbal I, Dasgupta B, Taylor P, Heron L, Pilling C. Elicitation of health state utilities associated with differing durations of morning stiffness in rheumatoid arthritis. J Med Econ. 2012;15(6):1192–200.
7. Nuñez DE, Keller C, Ananian CD. A review of the efficacy of the self-management model on health outcomes in community-residing older adults with arthritis. Worldviews Evid Based Nurs. 2009;6(3):130–48.
8. Turner J, Turner R. Physical disability, unemployment, and mental health. Rehabil Psych. 2004;49(3):241–9.
9. Ward MM. Functional disability predicts total costs in patients with ankylosing spondylitis. Arthritis Rheum. 2002;46(1):223–31.
10. Dall TM, Gallo P, Koenig L, Gu Q, Ruiz D. Modeling the indirect economic implications of musculoskeletal disorders and treatment. Cost Eff Resour Alloc. 2013;11(1):5.
11. Spaetgens B, Wijnands JM, van Durme C, van der Linden S, Boonen A. Cost of illness and determinants of costs among patients with gout. J Rheumatol. 2015;42(2):335–44.
12. Wolfe F, Michaud K, Choi HK, Williams R. Household income and earnings losses among 6,396 persons with rheumatoid arthritis. J Rheumatol. 2005;32(10):1875–83.
13. Agency for Healthcare Research and Quality (AHRQ). MEPS HC-147: 2011 full year consolidated data file. Rockville: AHRQ; 2013. http://meps.ahrq.gov/mepsweb/data_stats/download_data/pufs/h147/h147doc.pdf. Accessed 5 Apr 2014.
14. Agency for Healthcare Research and Quality (AHRQ). MEPS HC-036: 1996¯2011 pooled linkage variance estimation file. Rockville: AHRQ; 2013. http://meps.ahrq.gov/data_stats/download_data/pufs/h36/h36u11doc.shtml. Accessed 18 Aug 2014.
15. Agency for Healthcare Research and Quality (AHRQb). Medical Expenditure Panel Survey. 2011 Full year consolidated data file 2013c, Available from http://meps.ahrq.gov/mepsweb/data_stats/download_data_files.jsp.
16. Aday LA, Andersen R. A framework for the study of access to medical care. Health Serv Res. 1974;9(3):208–20.
17. Allaire SJ, AlHeresh R, Keysor JJ. Risk factors for work disability associated with arthritis and other rheumatic conditions. Work. 2013;45(4):499–503.
18. Henry J, Kaiser Family Foundation (KFF). Health insurance coverage of the total population. Menlo Park: KFF; 2015.
19. Kan HJ, Song X, Johnson BH, Bechtel B, O'Sullivan D, Molta CT. Healthcare utilization and costs of systemic lupus erythematosus in Medicaid. Biomed Res Int. 2013;2013:808391.
20. Panopalis P, Yazdany J, Gillis JZ, Julian L, Trupin L, Hersh AO, et al. Health care costs and costs associated with changes in work productivity among persons with systemic lupus erythematosus. Arthritis Rheum. 2008;59(12):1788–95.
21. Panopalis P, Clarke AE, Yelin E. The economic burden of systemic lupus erythematosus. Best Pract Res Clin Rheumatol. 2012;26(5):695–704.
22. Birnbaum H, Pike C, Kaufman R, Marynchenko M, Kidolezi Y, Cifaldi M. Societal cost of rheumatoid arthritis patients in the US. Curr Med Res Opin. 2010;26(1):77–90.
23. Garris C, Jhingran P, Bass D, Engel-Nitz N, Riedel A, Dennis G. Healthcare utilization and cost of systemic lupus erythematosus in a US managed care health plan. J Med Econ. 2013;16(5):667–77.
24. Jolly M. How does quality of life of patients with systemic lupus erythematosus compare with that of other common chronic illnesses? J Rheumatol. 2005;32(9):1706–8.
25. Da Costa D, Dobkin PL, Fitzcharles MA, Fortin PR, Beaulieu A, Zummer M, et al. Determinants of health status in fibromyalgia: a comparative study with systemic lupus erythematosus. J Rheumatol. 2000;27(2):365–72.
26. Greco C, Rudy T, Manzi S. Adaptation to chronic pain in systemic lupus erythematosus: applicability of the multidimensional pain inventory. Pain Med. 2003;4(1):39–50.
27. Cornwell C, Schmitt M. Perceived health status, self-esteem and body image in women with rheumatoid arthritis or systemic lupus erythematosus. Res Nurs Health. 1990;13(2):99–107.
28. Ozaras N, Havan N, Poyraz E, Rezvani A, Aydin T. Functional limitations due to foot involvement in spondyloarthritis. J Phys Ther Sci. 2016;28(7):2005–8.

29. Omariba DWR. Gender differences in functional limitations among Canadians with arthritis: the role of disease duration and comorbidity. Health Rep. 2011;22(4):7–14.
30. Marques WV, Cruz VA, Rego J, Silva NA. The impact of comorbidities on the physical function in patients with rheumatoid arthritis. Rev Bras Reumatol Engl Ed. 2016;56(1):14–21.
31. Shih VC, Song J, Chang RW, Dunlop DD. Racial differences in activities of daily living limitation onset in older adults with arthritis: a national cohort study. Arch Phys Med Rehab. 2005;86(8):1521–6.
32. Drenkard C, Bao G, Dennis G, Kan HJ, Jhingran PM, Molta CT, et al. Burden of systemic lupus erythematosus on employment and work productivity: data from a large cohort in the southeastern United States. Arthritis Care Res (Hoboken). 2014;66(6):878–87.
33. Looper KJ, Mustafa SS, Zelkowitz P, Purden M, Baron M, McGill Early Arthritis Research Group. Work instability and financial loss in early inflammatory arthritis. Int J Rheum Dis. 2012;15(6):546–53.

10

The 23-valent pneumococcal polysaccharide vaccine in patients with rheumatoid arthritis

Yasumori Izumi[1], Manabu Akazawa[2], Yukihiro Akeda[3], Shigeto Tohma[1], Fuminori Hirano[1], Haruko Ideguchi[1], Ryutaro Matsumura[1], Tomoya Miyamura[1], Shunsuke Mori[1], Takahiro Fukui[1], Nozomi Iwanaga[1], Yuka Jiuchi[1], Hideko Kozuru[1], Hiroshi Tsutani[1], Kouichirou Saisyo[1], Takao Sugiyama[1], Yasuo Suenaga[1], Yasumasa Okada[1], Masao Katayama[1], Kenji Ichikawa[1], Hiroshi Furukawa[1], Kenji Kawakami[1], Kazunori Oishi[4] and Kiyoshi Migita[1,5*]

Abstract

Background: Pneumococcal pneumonia is the most frequent form of pneumonia. We herein assessed the effectiveness of the 23-valent pneumococcal polysaccharide vaccine (PPSV23) in the prevention of pneumonia overall in rheumatoid arthritis (RA) patients at risk for infections. We hypothesized that PPSV23 vaccination is superior in preventing pneumococcal pneumonia compared with placebo in RA patients.

Methods: A prospective, multicenter, double-blinded, randomized, placebo-controlled (1:1) trial was conducted across departments of rheumatology in Japanese National Hospital Organization hospitals. RA patients ($n = 900$) who had been treated with biological or immunosuppressive agents were randomly assigned PPSV23 or placebo (sodium chloride). The primary endpoints were the incidences of all-cause pneumonia and pneumococcal pneumonia. The secondary endpoint was death from pneumococcal pneumonia, all-cause pneumonia, or other causes. Cox regression models were used to estimate the risk of pneumonia overall for the placebo group compared with the vaccine group.

Results: Seventeen (3.7%) of 464 patients in the vaccine group and 15 (3.4%) of 436 patients in the placebo group developed pneumonia. There was no difference in the rates of pneumonia between the two study groups. The overall rate of pneumonia was 21.8 per 1000 person-years for patients with RA. The presence of interstitial pneumonia (hazard ratio: 3.601, 95% confidence interval: 1.547–8.380) was associated with an increased risk of pneumonia in RA patients.

Conclusion: PPSV23 does not prevent against pneumonia overall in RA patients at relative risk for infections. Our results also confirm that the presence of interstitial lung disease is associated with pneumonia in Japanese patients with RA.

Keywords: Interstitial lung disease, Pneumococcal polysaccharide vaccine, Pneumonia, Rheumatoid arthritis

* Correspondence: migita@fmu.ac.jp
[1]Japanese National Hospital Organization (NHO) (Evidence-based Medicine Study Group), Higashigaoka 2-5-23, Meguro, Tokyo 152-8621, Japan
[5]Department of Rheumatology, Fukushima Medical University, Hikarigaoka 1, Fukushima 960-1295, Japan
Full list of author information is available at the end of the article

Background

Patients with rheumatoid arthritis (RA) are at increased risk of serious infections. Although a newer class of biologic disease-modifying antirheumatic drugs (bDMARDs) has significantly advanced the treatment of RA, these drugs are associated with an increased risk of several types of infections [1, 2]. Pneumonia is also one of the major causes of mortality in patients with RA [3]. Influenza and pneumococcal infections are two vaccine-preventable infectious diseases that have been associated with high morbidity in patients with RA caused by immunosuppressive treatments [4, 5]. In view of these data highlighting the increased risk of infectious diseases in RA patients receiving immunosuppressive treatments and the awareness and performance of vaccinations, clear recommendations for vaccinations under the use of biological agents is needed.

Streptococcus pneumoniae is the most common cause of community-acquired pneumonia [6]. Recent randomized controlled trials (RCTs) demonstrated that the 23-valent pneumococcal polysaccharide vaccine (PPSV23) is effective in the prevention of invasive pneumococcal disease among high-risk older populations [7]. However, the vaccine's protective efficacy against pneumococcal pneumonia in immunosuppressed people including patients with autoimmune diseases remains unknown [8]. PPSV23 was licensed more than 30 years ago and is recommended as the standard intervention for the older population (>60 years of age) and adults with underlying diseases [9]. PPSV23 is also strongly recommended for patients with autoimmune inflammatory rheumatic diseases [10]. However, data regarding efficacy of pneumococcal vaccines in patients with RA receiving immunotherapy including biological agents are rare and often conflicting. We therefore conducted a prospective, multicenter, double-blinded, randomized, placebo-controlled trial to determine the efficacy of PPSV23 in patients with RA receiving immunosuppressive treatments. Our primary objective was to assess the effectiveness of PPSV23 in the prevention of pneumococcal pneumonia and pneumonia overall in RA patients at risk of pneumonia.

Methods

Study design and patient population

We performed a double-blinded, randomized, placebo-controlled trial. Patients with clinically diagnosed RA were recruited in National Hospital Organization (NHO) hospitals throughout Japan (the trial was conducted in NHO 32 hospitals) from September 2010 to December 2012 [11]. The risk of infections was reported to be associated with their comorbidity and treatments in RA patients [12]. Eligible patients were therefore divided into the following groups: patients with rheumatoid lung disease ($n = 144$), patients treated with biological agents ($n = 510$; TNF inhibitors = 336, toclizumab = 124, abatacept = 50), patients treated with immunosuppressive agents ($n = 144$), patients receiving more than 5 mg/day of prednisone ($n = 241$), and patients classified as Steinbrocker stage 3 or 4 ($n = 485$). Almost all patients (>93%) initiated biologics >3 months prior to study entry. Patients were excluded if they had previously received pneumococcal vaccination. Eligible RA patients were assigned randomly to the vaccine group or the placebo group. A statistician who was not on the study team performed the randomization using a random number table and numbered the containers accordingly.

The following parameters were analyzed when the patient was first admitted to the study: swollen joint count, tender joint count, patient global assessment of disease activity, physician global assessment of disease activity, Health Assessment Questionnaire Disability Index score, serum levels of C-reactive protein (CRP), and Disease Activity Score 28-joint assessment with CRP [13]. This study was registered in UMIN-CTR (www.umin.ac.jp/ctr/UMIN-CTR; UMIN000009566).

Intervention

Investigators in each NHO hospital registered patient information to the NHO's central data center through an online system. According to the predetermined allocation code book, either vaccine or placebo (1:1) was simply allocated in the order of registration. Patients were randomly assigned to receive either 0.5 ml (25 μg) of PPSV23 (Pneumovax NP; Merck Sharp & Dohme Corp., Tokyo, Japan) or 0.5 ml of placebo (sodium chloride) subcutaneously in the upper arm. The placebo medication was identical in color. The vaccines were prepared in a masked fashion for those who administered it, blinding both the administrator of the vaccine and the patient to the type of vaccine given. Vaccine and placebo were presented in identical, single-dose syringes and needle combinations that were labeled with sequential study numbers only. A statistician who was not on the study team performed the randomization using a random number table and numbered the containers accordingly.

Patients were instructed to record local reactions (e.g., redness, swelling, and tenderness) and systemic reactions (e.g., fever, nausea, and vomiting). Patients were also monitored for 12 months after enrollment to follow the development of pneumonia, including that stemming from pneumococcal disease.

Outcome measures and definitions

The primary effectiveness endpoint was the prevention of overall pneumonia using an intention-to-treat (ITT) approach. The primary endpoints were pneumonia and pneumococcal pneumonia. Pneumonia was diagnosed by the medical staff of the respiratory unit at the affiliated hospital according to the presence of clinical symptoms and a new infiltrate on chest radiography. Pneumococcal pneumonia was diagnosed from a positive blood, pleural fluid, or sputum culture or from a positive pneumococcal antigen test result using a urine sample. Information on fatal cases was obtained from a provincial registry, which is based on death certificates written by the attending physicians. During the study period, the patient was instructed to contact the local doctor responsible for the study if he or she developed a fever of 38 °C or greater for more than 3 days, with or without respiratory tract symptoms, or if he or she had any other cause to suspect recurrent pneumonia. Chest radiography was performed upon clinical suspicion of pneumonia. If pneumonia was confirmed, blood, sputum, and urine samples were obtained from the patient, if possible, for etiological diagnosis. Blood testing was performed using routine procedures and quantitative sputum cultures were tested using purulent samples. The secondary effectiveness endpoint was all cases of death.

Statistical analyses

Data are expressed as the mean (standard deviation) and analyzed using the SPSS software program. For univariate analyses, the χ^2 test or Fisher's exact test was used for categorical data and the Mann–Whitney U test for continuous variables. The primary or secondary effectiveness endpoint was evaluated by χ^2 test or Fisher's exact test. Logistic regression analysis was used to estimate the effectiveness of PPSV23 in preventing pneumococcal pneumonia, nonpneumococcal pneumonia, and all-cause pneumonia. Kaplan–Meier methods were used to calculate the survival curves. The log-rank test was used for time to event analyses and Cox regression models were used to calculate hazard ratios. P values are two-tailed, with $P < 0.05$ considered statistically significant. All data processing and analyses were performed using the Statistical Analysis System (SAS) and SPSS version 18 software (SPSS, Chicago, IL, USA). According to the sample size calculation, 1600 evaluable patients were required (800 in each group). We assumed that the risk of pneumonia among RA patients was 2 cases per 100 patient-years and vaccine efficacy was 50% according to previous clinical studies and epidemiology data available in Japan (references). Also, a type I error probability of 0.05 (two-sided) and a statistical power of 80% were selected.

Results

Consecutive eligible patients between December 2012 and March 2014 were reviewed for inclusion. Of 989 patients, 59 patients were excluded (Fig. 1). The reasons for exclusion included inability to obtain the informed consent ($n = 41$) and conflict with the exclusion criteria ($n = 18$), including previous PPSV23 vaccination ($n = 2$). Among the remaining 930 patients, 18 patients withdrew consent after randomization. Thus, 912 patients were ultimately included; 472 were randomly assigned vaccine and 440 placebo.

The trial was conducted in accordance with the original protocol and there was no change in the outcome

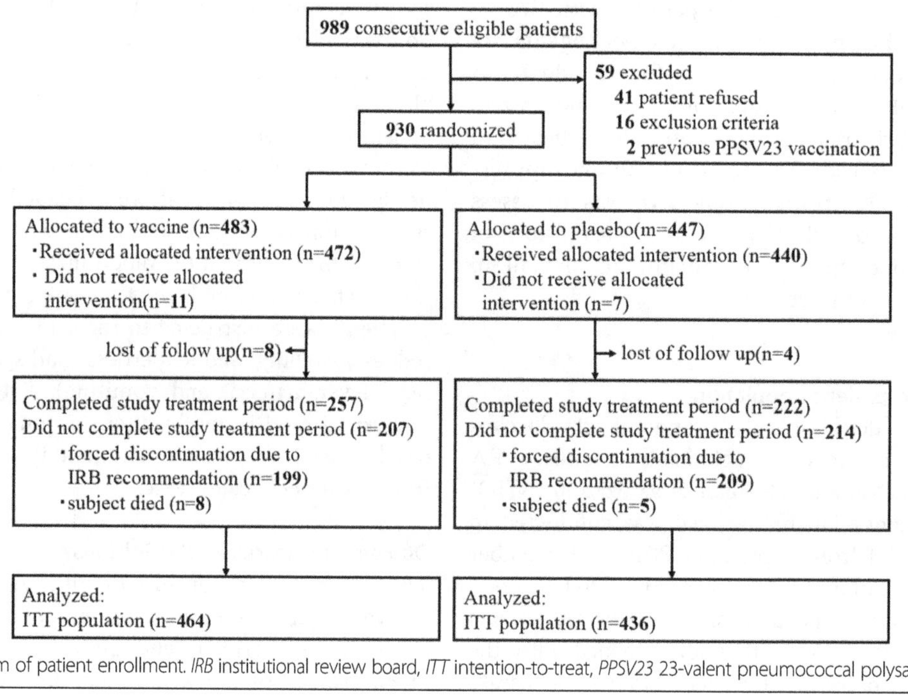

Fig. 1 Flow diagram of patient enrollment. *IRB* institutional review board, *ITT* intention-to-treat, *PPSV23* 23-valent pneumococcal polysaccharide vaccine

Table 1 Baseline characteristics of 900 rheumatoid arthritis patients at randomization to PPSV23 or placebo

	Vaccine group (n = 464)	Placebo group (n = 436)	P value
Demographics			
Age (years)	63.3 ± 12.1	62.7 ± 11.8	0.529
Gender, male/female	90 (19.4%)/374 (80.6%)	106 (24.3%)/330 (75.7%)	0.074
Smoking history	90 (19.4%)	116 (26.6%)	0.010
Laboratory data			
CRP (mg/dl)	0.49 ± 1.11	0.51 ± 0.99	0.298
Serum albumin (g/dl)	4.06 ± 0.38	4.06 ± 0.37	0.926
Serum creatinine (mg/dl)	0.68 ± 0.36	0.68 ± 0.22	0.934
RA characteristics			
RA duration (years)	12.1 ± 10.4	11.6 ± 9.7	0.747
HAQ	0.66 ± 0.74	0.67 ± 0.75	0.918
DAS28 (CRP)	2.43 ± 1.10	2.51 ± 1.15	0.324
SDAI	8.00 ± 7.72	8.73 ± 8.55	0.252
CDAI	7.50 ± 7.38	8.24 ± 8.33	0.257
Comorbidity			
Cardiovascular disease	127 (27.4%)	131 (30.0%)	0.375
CVA	14 (3.0%)	10 (2.3%)	0.501
Ischemic heart disease	9 (1.9%)	9 (2.1%)	0.894
Hypertension	109 (23.5%)	116 (26.6%)	0.281
Arrythmia	6 (1.3%)	5 (1.1%)	0.842
Cardiac failure	6 (1.3%)	4 (0.9%)	0.415
Metabolic disease	111 (23.9%)	96 (22.0%)	0.498
Hyperlipidemia	72 (15.5%)	56 (12.8%)	0.251
Hyperuricemia	0	9 (2.1%)	0.001
Diabetes	48 (10.3%)	45 (10.3%)	0.991
CKD	17 (3.7%)	18 (4.1%)	0.719
Autoimmune disease	23 (5.0%)	14 (3.2%)	0.187
Rheumatoid lung	81 (17.5%)	71 (16.3%)	0.890
Interstitial pneumonia	56 (12.1%)	46 (10.6%)	0.473
Bronchial lesion	19 (4.1%)	19 (4.4%)	0.845
Pleural lesion	6 (1.3%)	6 (1.4%)	0.914
COPD	11 (2.4%)	16 (3.7%)	0.254
NTM	7 (1.5%)	8 (1.8%)	0.702
Treatment			
PSL	242 (52.2%)	214 (49.1%)	0.357
Dose of PSL (mg/day)	4.54 ± 2.79	4.71 ± 2.84	0.530
PSL ≥ 5 mg/day	130 (28.0%)	117 (26.8%)	0.691
MTX	300 (64.7%)	304 (69.7%)	0.106
Dose of MTX (mg/week)	8.01 ± 2.75	8.33 ± 2.85	0.227
MTX alone	40 (8.6%)	47 (10.8%)	0.273
MTX + PSL	54 (11.6%)	49 (11.2%)	0.851
MTX + biologics	103 (22.2%)	107 (24.5%)	0.406
TAC	60 (12.9%)	60 (13.8%)	0.714
Biologics	257 (55.4%)	253 (58.0%)	0.425

Data presented as number (percentage) or mean ± standard deviation
PPSV23 23-valent pneumococcal polysaccharide vaccine, *CRP* C-reactive protein, *RA* rheumatoid arthritis, *HAQ* Health Assessment Questionnaire Disability Index score, *DAS28* Disease Activity Score 28, *SDAI* simplified disease activity index, *CDAI* clinical disease activity index, *CVA* cerebrovascular accident, *CKD* chronic kidney disease, *COPD* chronic obstructive pulmonary disease, *NTM* nontuberculous mycobacteria, *PSL* prednisolone, *MTX* methotrexate, *TAC* tacrolimus

measures. In November 2014, however, the Committee on Immunization Practices of the Ministry of Health, Labour and Welfare in Japan stated that all adults ≥65 years of age should receive PPSV23 and began promoting routine vaccination with PPSV23. In response to this public comment, the NHO central IRB recommended stopping this trial continuation and vaccination with PPSV23 for all subjects receiving placebo after being keyed "open". We decided trial discontinuation before the interim analysis according to this recommendation. Participants aged ≥65 years receiving placebo were thus assigned to receive PPSV23 vaccination and forced into discontinuation of follow-up until December 31, 2014.

In this study, participants in the forced discontinuation groups were keyed "open" and received PPSV23 even when they were assigned to receive placebo (Fig. 1). The primary endpoint was assessed in the ITT population, which included all randomized patients regardless of the forced discontinuation. Of 912 patients who were randomized to PPSV23 (n = 483) or placebo (n = 447), 12 patients lost to follow-up were excluded from the ITT analysis. The ITT population therefore included 900 patients (Fig. 1).

Demographic data for the two groups are presented in Table 1. The exposure time was 765.7 person-years (mean 1.7 years) in the vaccine group and 703.7 (mean 1.6 years) person-years in the placebo group. Patient characteristics were similar in both groups. During the follow-up period, pneumonia was diagnosed in 32 (3.6%) of the 900 patients; pneumonia was diagnosed in 15 (3.4%) of the 436 patients in the placebo group and in 17 (3.7%) of the 464 patients in the vaccine group. The incidence of pneumonia per 1000 person-years was 21.3 and 22.2 in the placebo and vaccine groups, respectively. The incidence rate for pneumonia in the vaccine group did not differ from that in the placebo group (P = 0.856).

Sputum cultures and blood cultures were obtained in 18 and 14 episodes of pneumonia and urine samples for pneumococcal antigen detection were obtained in 21 episodes of pneumonia. An etiological diagnosis was obtained in 10 (15.6%) of the 64 episodes of pneumonia.

Table 2 Incidence of primary endpoints in rheumatoid arthritis patients assigned to PPSV23 or placebo

	Vaccine group ($n = 464$)		Placebo group ($n = 436$)		
	Incidence rate per 1000 patient-years (*n*)	95% CI	Incidence rate per 1000 patient-years (*n*)	95% CI	*P* value
Pneumococcal pneumonia	2.6 (2)	0.7–9.5	1.4 (1)	0.3–8.0	0.523
Nonpneumococcal pneumonia	19.6 (15)	11.9–32.3	19.9 (14)	11.9–33.4	0.985
All-cause pneumonia	22.2 (17)	13.9–35.6	21.3 (15)	12.9–35.2	0.856

PPSV23 23-valent pneumococcal polysaccharide vaccine, *CI* confidence interval

Causative pathogens were identified in 12 (37.5%) of the 32 participants. Pneumococcal pneumonia was diagnosed in two participants in the vaccine group (2/17, 11.8%) and one participant in the placebo group (1/15, 6.7%). The causative agents of nonpneumococcal pneumonia were *Staphylococcus aureus* ($n = 2$), *Pseudomonas aeruginosa* ($n = 2$), *Klebsiella pneumoniae* ($n = 1$), *Haemophilus influenzae* ($n = 1$), *Escherichia coli* ($n = 1$), *Moraxella catarrhalis* ($n = 1$), and *Neisseria* sp. ($n = 1$). The incidence rate of pneumococcal pneumonia was not significantly different between the vaccine and placebo groups (Table 2). One adverse event (bronchial asthma) in the placebo group and three adverse events (interstitial pneumonia, mycoplasma pneumonia, heart failure) in the vaccine group were documented during the follow-up period.

Kaplan–Meier survival curves were plotted for the pneumonia-free survival between the vaccine and placebo groups (Fig. 2). The pneumonia free-survival rates were not significantly different between the vaccine and placebo groups.

For stratified analyses based on risk for developing respiratory infections, patients were divided into the following groups: patients with rheumatoid lung disease, patients receiving biologics, patients receiving immunosuppressants (tacrolimus, mizoribine, and cyclosporine A), patients receiving more than 5 mg/day of prednisone, and patients classified as Steinbrocker stage 3 or 4. However, there was no significant difference in the number of pneumonia cases between the vaccine and placebo groups in each subgroup (Table 3). Also, as we planned, stratified analyses based on risk for developing respiratory infections were conducted according to the following groups: patients with rheumatoid lung disease, patients with RA treated with biological agents, patients with RA treated with immunosuppressive agents, patients receiving more than 5 mg/day of prednisone, and patients classified as Steinbrocker stage 3 or 4. However, there was no significant difference in the number of pneumonia cases between the vaccine and placebo groups in each subgroup (Table 3). Age categories were not considered because most of the study population were 65 years or older because of eligibility for pneumococcal vaccines in Japan.

Finally, we compared baseline data between patients with or without pneumonia in the total subjects. A few of the demographic and clinical variables were associated with risk of pneumonia, as shown in Table 4. Older age and the presence of interstitial pneumonia were found to be predictive factors for pneumonia. The effect of treatment variables on the risk of pneumonia was analyzed using univariate analyses (Table 5); however, no treatment variable was identified as a risk factor for pneumonia. A multivariate analysis of all variables is presented in Table 6. The presence of interstitial pneumonia remained a significant risk factor for pneumonia in RA patients. Kaplan–Meier curves stratified by the

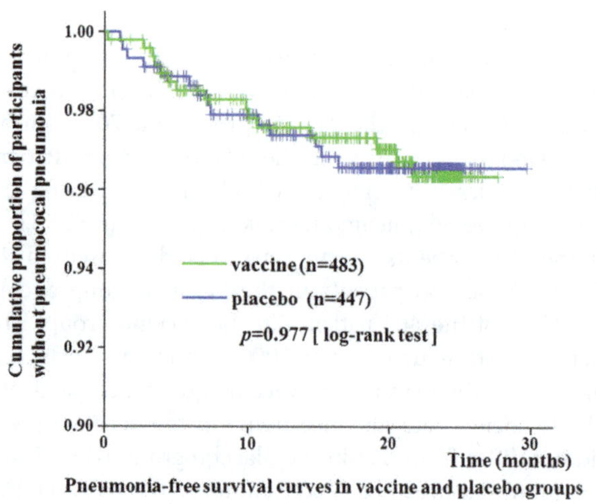

Fig. 2 Pneumonia-free survival curves of RA patients receiving PPSV23 and placebo. Statistically significant difference was not observed between patients receiving PPSV23 and placebo ($P = 0.084$, log-rank test)

Table 3 Primary endpoint (pneumonia) in each subgroup

Subgroup	PPSV23	Placebo	*P* value
With rheumatoid lung	12.3% (10/81)	5.6% (4/71)	0.1534
Receiving biologics	3.1% (8/257)	2.4% (6/253)	0.6085
Receiving immunosuppressants	4.1% (3/74)	2.9% (2/70)	0.6950
Receiving steroid (>5 mg/day of prednisolone)	3.9% (5/130)	2.6% (3/117)	0.5698
With advanced stage	3.7% (9/246)	3.8% (9/239)	0.9502

Data presented as percentage (number)
PPSV23 23-valent pneumococcal polysaccharide vaccine

Table 4 Baseline clinical and demographic data between RA patients with or without pneumonia

	Pneumonia (*n* = 32)	Without pneumonia (*n* = 868)	*P* value
Demographics			
Age (years)	68.6 ± 10.8	62.8 ± 11.9	0.010
Gender, male/female	7 (21.9%)/25 (78.1%)	189 (21.8%)/679 (78.2%)	0.989
Smoking history	7 (21.9%)	199 (22.9%)	0.889
Laboratory data			
CRP (mg/dl)	1.14 ± 2.29	0.48 ± 0.97	0.023
Serum albumin (g/dl)	3.95 ± 0.44	4.07 ± 0.37	0.210
Serum creatinine (mg/dl)	0.70 ± 0.21	0.68 ± 0.31	0.248
RA characteristics			
RA duration (years)	12.3 ± 8.3	11.9 ± 10.1	0.378
HAQ	0.78 ± 0.81	0.66 ± 0.74	0.564
DAS28 (CRP)	2.32 ± 0.97	2.48 ± 1.13	0.548
SDAI	6.72 ± 6.11	8.41 ± 8.20	0.237
CDAI	5.64 ± 4.76	7.94 ± 7.94	0.123
Comorbidity			
Cardiovascular disease	13 (40.6%)	245 (28.2%)	0.128
CVA	2 (6.3%)	22 (2.5%)	0.209
Ischemic heart disease	1 (3.1%)	17 (2.0%)	0.482
Hypertension	10 (31.3%)	215 (24.8%)	0.406
Arrythmia	2 (6.3%)	9 (1.0%)	0.055
Cardiac failure	2 (6.3%)	8 (0.9%)	0.046
Metabolic disease	10 (31.3%)	197 (22.7%)	0.259
Hyperlipidemia	6 (18.8%)	122 (14.1%)	0.297
Hyperuricemia	0	9 (1.0%)	0.721
Diabetes	5 (15.6%)	88 (10.1%)	0.229
CKD	2 (6.3%)	33 (3.8%)	0.356
Autoimmune disease	1 (3.1%)	36 (4.1%)	0.617
Rheumatoid lung	14 (43.8%)	138 (15.9%)	<0.0001
Interstitial pneumonia	11 (34.4%)	91 (10.5%)	<0.0001
Bronchial lesion	3 (9.4%)	35 (4.0%)	0.148
Pleural lesion	1 (3.1%)	11 (1.3%)	0.354
COPD	0	27 (3.1%)	0.371
NTM	1 (3.1%)	14 (1.6%)	0.422
PPSV23 vaccination	17 (53.1%)	447 (51.5%)	0.856
Treatment			
PSL	18 (56.3%)	438 (50.5%)	0.520
Dose of prednisolone (mg/day)	5.61 ± 4.90	4.58 ± 2.69	0.521
MTX	20 (62.5%)	584 (67.3%)	0.572
Dose of MTX (mg/week)	7.90 ± 2.38	8.18 ± 2.82	0.660
TAC	4 (12.5%)	116 (13.4%)	0.573
Biologics	14 (43.8%)	496 (57.1%)	0.133

Data presented as number (percentage) or mean ± standard deviation
PPSV23 23-valent pneumococcal polysaccharide vaccine, *CRP* C-reactive protein, *RA* rheumatoid arthritis, *HAQ* Health Assessment Questionnaire Disability Index score, *DAS28* Disease Activity Score 28, *SDAI* simplified disease activity index, *CDAI* clinical disease activity index, *CVA* cerebrovascular accident, *CKD* chronic kidney disease, *COPD* chronic obstructive pulmonary disease, *NTM* nontuberculous mycobacteria, *PSL* prednisolone, *MTX* methotrexate, *TAC* tacrolimus

presence of interstitial pneumonia showed a significant difference between RA patients with or without interstitial pneumonia. Additionally, the presence of interstitial pneumonia significantly affected the pneumonia-free survival rates of RA patients (Fig. 3).

Discussion

The effectiveness of PPSV23 in preventing pneumococcal pneumonia remains controversial, especially in high-risk individuals [14]. Although several studies have demonstrated the effectiveness of PPSV23 [15], few studies have focused on patients with autoimmune diseases. To our knowledge, this is the first RCT to evaluate this concern in patients with RA. We demonstrated previously that PPSV23 vaccination induced the serotype-specific IgG and functional opsonization index responses were not impaired even in RA patients receiving immunosuppressive treatments [11]. However, we were unable to show that PPSV23 was effective in the prevention of pneumonia overall or pneumococcal pneumonia. This might be because of lack of power and shortened follow-up periods. The fundamental difficulty in obtaining a definitive pathological cause of pneumonia may also be related to these negative data. Definitive pneumococcal pneumonia (positive blood or sputum culture) is the most specific outcome to evaluate vaccine effectiveness; however, it has a low sensitivity. Therefore, we used the BinaxNOW® *S. pneumoniae* Antigen Card test for diagnosis [16]. However, 13 of 34 pneumonia cases did not receive this urinary antigen test and only a fraction of pneumonia cases caused by *S. pneumoniae* were included in our analysis. A Cochrane review also failed to show any protective efficacy of PPSV23 in patients with chronic pulmonary diseases [17]. Further high-quality trials with sufficient sample size would be useful to confirm our findings. Pneumococcal conjugate vaccines offer an alternative approach to prevent pneumococcal disease. The seven-valent pneumococcal conjugate has been shown to protect HIV-infected adults from recurrent pneumococcal infection [18]. The effectiveness of PPSV23 preventing

Table 5 Predictors of pneumonia in RA patients by the Cox-hazard model (univariate analysis)

	Hazard ratio	*P* value	95% CI
Demographics			
Age (years)	1.058	0.002	1.021–1.095
Gender, male	1.073	0.870	0.464–2.480
Laboratory data			
CRP (mg/dl)	1.321	<0.0001	1.140–1.531
Serum albumin (g/dl)	0.414	0.051	0.171–1.004
Serum creatinine (mg/dl)	1.358	0.413	0.652–2.828
RA characteristics			
RA duration (years)	1.002	0.927	0.968–1.036
HAQ	1.219	0.366	0.794–1.871
DAS28 (CRP)	0.894	0.498	0.646–1.237
SDAI	0.970	0.281	0.919–1.025
CDAI	0.949	0.115	0.890–1.013
Comorbidity			
Smoking history	0.936	0.877	0.405–2.165
Cardiovascular disease	1.745	0.122	0.862–3.533
Metabolic disease	1.612	0.211	0.763–3.405
CKD	1.814	0.415	0.433–7.592
Autoimmune disease	0.723	0.750	0.099–5.299
Interstitial pneumonia	4.449	<0.0001	2.143–9.237
PPSV23 vaccination	1.048	0.894	0.523–2.099
Treatment			
PSL	1.314	0.443	0.654–2.643
Dose of prednisolone (mg/day)	1.117	0.102	0.978–1.276
MTX	0.778	0.493	0.381–1.593
Dose of MTX (mg/week)	0.962	0.634	0.821–1.128
TAC	0.956	0.934	0.335–2.727
Biologics	0.544	0.088	0.270–1.094

PPSV23 23-valent pneumococcal polysaccharide vaccine, *CRP* C-reactive protein, *RA* rheumatoid arthritis, *HAQ* Health Assessment Questionnaire Disability Index score, *DAS28* Disease Activity Score 28, *SDAI* simplified disease activity index, *CDAI* clinical disease activity index, *CKD* chronic kidney disease, *PSL* prednisolone, *MTX* methotrexate, *TAC* tacrolimus, *CI* confidence interval

Table 6 Predictors of pneumonia in RA patients by the Cox-hazard model (Multivariate analysis)

	Hazard ratio	*P* value	95% CI
Demographics			
Age (years)	1.039	0.068	0.997–1.083
Gender, male	0.580	0.317	0.200–1.686
Smoking history	1.247	0.670	0.452–3.443
Laboratory data			
CRP (mg/dl)	1.384	0.268	0.779–2.459
Serum albumin (g/dl)	0.917	0.877	0.305–2.758
Serum creatinine (mg/dl)	1.550	0.366	0.599–4.005
RA characteristics			
RA duration (years)	1.010	0.582	0.974–1.048
HAQ	1.202	0.506	0.699–2.067
DAS28 (CRP)	1.026	0.936	0.545–1.933
SDAI	0.945	0.845	0.534–1.670
CDAI	0.944	0.851	0.517–1.723
Comorbidity			
Cardiovascular disease	1.138	0.749	0.515–2.518
Metabolic disease	1.283	0.542	0.576–2.856
CKD	1.402	0.689	0.268–7.344
Autoimmune disease	0.468	0.494	0.053–4.137
Interstitial pneumonia	3.611	0.003	1.553–8.399
PPSV23 vaccination	0.849	0.656	0.414–1.743
Treatment			
PSL	1.081	0.846	0.492–2.375
MTX	1.431	0.390	0.632–3.240
TAC	0.712	0.552	0.232–2.182
Biologics	0.664	0.307	0.302–1.458

PPSV23 23-valent pneumococcal polysaccharide vaccine, *CRP* C-reactive protein, *RA* rheumatoid arthritis, *HAQ* Health Assessment Questionnaire Disability Index score, *DAS28* Disease Activity Score 28, *SDAI* simplified disease activity index, *CDAI* clinical disease activity index, *CKD* chronic kidney disease, *PSL* prednisolone, *MTX* methotrexate, *TAC* tacrolimus, *CI* confidence interval

pneumococcal infections among patients with chronic pulmonary diseases is unclear [19]. However, the efficacy and cost-effectiveness of PPSV23 in preventing IPD among the general population had been demonstrated [20]. Based on the new guidelines, the sequential administration of conjugate and polysaccharide pneumococcal vaccines has recently been the most appropriate approach for the prevention of pneumonia in the general population [21]. Our study confirmed that polysaccharide vaccine alone is not effective for prevention of pneumonia. Therefore, sequential administration of PCV13 and PPSV23 could also be an appropriate approach for the prevention for pneumonia in RA patients receiving immunosuppresssive treatments.

Pneumonia is the most common type of infection in RA [22]. Previous studies demonstrated increased frequencies of pneumonia with higher mortality in RA patients [23]. Our data showed that the incidence of pneumonia was 2.14 per 100 person-years in RA patients with a relatively high risk for infections. Glucocorticoid use was also shown to increase the risk of serious infections in a dose-dependent manner in RA patients [24]. The magnitude of the risk of infection associated with prednisolone dose > 10 mg/day was similar to that associated with TNF-α antagonists [25]. However, neither glucocorticoid dosage nor bDMARD use was demonstrated to be a predictor of pneumonia risk in our study. Of note, we found no evidence for increased rates of pneumonia associated with bDMARD use. However, our data are inconsistent with a recent meta-analysis of

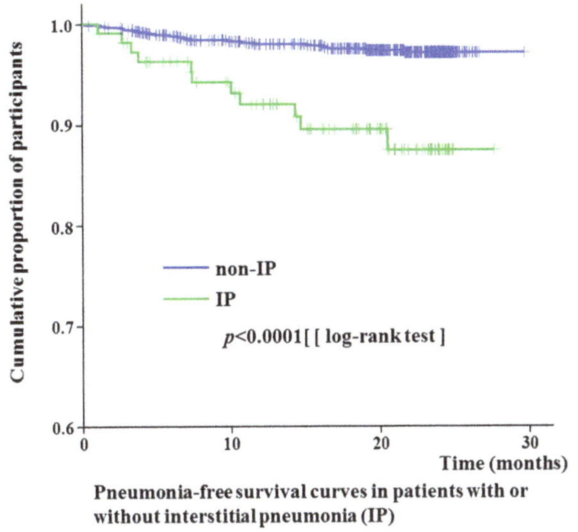

Fig. 3 Pneumonia-free survival curves of RA patients with or without interstitial lung disease (ILD). Curves are stratified by the presence or absence of ILD. Statistically significant differences were observed between patients with or without ILD ($P < 0.0001$, log-rank test)

RCTs of RA patients who received bDMARDs [26]. Nevertheless, the included patients and analytical methods in previous studies differed significantly from those in this study. Additionally, the relatively lower corticosteroid dosage prescribed to our RA patients may have influenced the association between glucocorticoid dosage and the occurrence of pneumonia.

As reported for RA patients, older age and pulmonary disease were found to be independently associated with bacterial infection. Among variables, preexisting interstitial pneumonia and older age were demonstrated to be associated with the risk of pneumonia [27]. Among the extra-articular manifestations of RA, there has been renewed interest in pulmonary complications directly associated with RA, which manifest as a variety of clinical signs such as pleural disease, pulmonary nodules, interstitial lung disease (ILD), and airway disease [28]. A large observational cohort study in Japan showed that the presence of ILD is one of the factors associated with increased mortality in RA patients [29]. Our data are consistent with these previous studies. Although the pathophysiologic mechanism for this finding has not been elucidated, decreased ciliary and respiratory epithelial function seen in patients with interstitial pneumonia may contribute to the higher frequency of pneumonia [30].

There are several limitations associated with this study. First, the forced discontinuation of follow-up is unusual and the disconfirmation rates were high. Thus, potential bias introduced by the discontinuation group (≥65 years of age) should be considered. Second, our sample size was limited. For sample size calculation, we assumed, from previously published data on RA patients under biologic treatment [31], a rate of pneumonia of 2.5/100 patient-years. Based on these assumptions, we primarily calculated that we needed 714 patients receiving PPSV23 and 714 patients receiving placebo to confirm 50% reduction of pneumonia occurrence during 2 years of follow-up at an α error of 0.10 and a β error of 0.80. However, we could not reserve sufficient sample size, and the possibility of an underpowered study cannot be denied. Third, our RA population consisted of groups at high risk for infections, and thus our results may not be generalizable to other RA populations. Fourth, we cannot rule out the imprecision of our complete data due to unreliability in the diagnosis of pneumonia.

The strengths of our study include examination of an RA patient cohort using data captured from the largest NHO data center. Laboratory results and physician notes are available in this data resource and allow for examination of potential risk factors that are not typically available when using only administrative claims data. Our study represents the most comprehensive, hospital-based study with the outcomes in all enrolled patients followed completely. The participants in this study, in contrast to those in many clinical trials, were similar demographically to general RA patients. Our data can therefore provide a great deal of useful information about generalizability.

Conclusions

Our data showed that PPSV23 vaccination was not effective in preventing pneumonia. While PPSV23 vaccination is recommended for adults ≥65 years of age, our results suggested uncertainty regarding its effectiveness for pneumonia in RA patients at high risk for infections. Clinicians should keep in mind the patient's age and the presence of interstitial pneumonia because such patients are at an increased risk of developing pneumonia.

Abbreviations

ILD: Interstitial lung disease; NHO: Japanese National Hospital Organization; PCV: Pneumococcal conjugate vaccine; PPV23: 23-Valent pneumococcal polysaccharide vaccine; RA: Rheumatoid arthritis

Acknowledgements

This study could not have been accomplished without the effective and dedicated participation of each of the following contributors: Takao Yamanaka, MD (NHO Minami-Okayama Medical Center); Shiro Ohshima, MD (NHO Osaka Minami Medical Center); Yojiro Kawabe, MD (NHO Ureshino Medical Center); Akira Okamoto, MD (NHO Himeji Medical Center); Hisaji Ohshima, MD (NHO Tokyo Medical Center); Naoya Mori, MD (NHO Shinshu Ueda Medical Center); Akinori Matsumori, MD (NHO Kochi National Hospital); Tetsuo Ozawa, MD (NHO Niigata National Hospital); Koichiro Takahi, MD (NHO Toneyama National Hospital); Kiyoki Kitagawa, MD (NHO Kanazawa Medical Center); Norikazu Hamada, MD (NHO Kure Medical Center); Shigeru Yoshizawa, MD (NHO Fukuoka Hospital); Kyoichi Nakajima, MD (NHO East Saitama National Hospital); Norio Tamura, MD (NHO Sendai Nishitaga National Hospital); Itou Jun, MD (NHO Hachinohe National Hospital); Hideaki Nagai, MD (NHO Tokyo National Hospital); Yasuhiro Komiya, MD (NHO Shigaraki Hospital); Masaharu Kawabata, MD (NHO Minami Kyushu National hospital).

Funding
This study was supported by a grant from the Japanese National Hospital Organization (NHO)-Evidence-based Medicine (EBM) study group.

Authors' contributions
YI, YA, HF, KK, KO, and KM carried out the molecular genetic studies, participated in the sequence alignment, and drafted the manuscript. YA and KM carried out the immunoassays and revised the manuscript. YI, ST, FH, HI, RM, TM, SM, TF, NI, HT, KS, TS, YS, YO, MK, and KI participated in the sequence alignment and drafted the manuscript. MA, YJ, and HK participated in the design of the study, performed the statistical analysis, and helped to revise the manuscript. YI, MA, and KM conceived of the study, participated in its design and coordination, and helped to draft the manuscript. All authors read and approved the final manuscript.

Competing interests
The authors declare that they have no competing interests.

Author details
[1]Japanese National Hospital Organization (NHO) (Evidence-based Medicine Study Group), Higashigaoka 2-5-23, Meguro, Tokyo 152-8621, Japan. [2]Department of Public Health and Epidemiology, Meiji Pharmaceutical University, Noshio 2-522-1, Kiyose, Tokyo 204-8588, Japan. [3]Research Institute for Microbial Diseases, Osaka University, Yamadaoka 3-1, Suita, Osaka 565-8563, Japan. [4]Infectious Diseases Surveillance Center, National Institute of Infectious Diseases, Toyama 1-23-1, Shinjuku, Tokyo 162-8640, Japan. [5]Department of Rheumatology, Fukushima Medical University, Hikarigaoka 1, Fukushima 960-1295, Japan.

References

1. Doran MF, Crowson CS, Pond GR, O'Fallon WM, Gabriel SE. Frequency of infection in patients with rheumatoid arthritis compared with controls: a population-based study. Arthritis Rheum. 2002;46:2287–93.
2. Bongartz T, Sutton AJ, Sweeting MJ, Buchan I, Matteson EL, Montori V. Anti-TNF antibody therapy in rheumatoid arthritis and the risk of serious infections and malignancies: systematic review and meta-analysis of rare harmful effects in randomized controlled trials. JAMA. 2006;295:2275–85.
3. Naz SM, Symmons DP. Mortality in established rheumatoid arthritis. Best Pract Res Clin Rheumatol. 2007;21:871–83.
4. van Assen S, Elkayam O, Agmon-Levin N, Cervera R, Doran MF, Dougados M, et al. Vaccination in adult patients with auto-immune inflammatory rheumatic diseases: a systematic literature review for the European League Against Rheumatism evidence-based recommendations for vaccination in adult patients with auto-immune inflammatory rheumatic diseases. Autoimmun Rev. 2011;10:341–52.
5. van Assen S, Agmon-Levin N, Elkayam O, Cervera R, Doran MF, Dougados M, et al. EULAR recommendations for vaccination in adult patients with autoimmune inflammatory rheumatic diseases. Ann Rheum Dis. 2011;70:414–22.
6. Diao WQ, Shen N, Yu PX, Liu BB, He B. Efficacy of 23-valent pneumococcal polysaccharide vaccine in preventing community-acquired pneumonia among immunocompetent adults: a systematic review and meta-analysis of randomized trials. Vaccine. 2016;34:1496–503.
7. Maruyama T, Taguchi O, Niederman MS, Morser J, Kobayashi H, Kobayashi T, et al. Efficacy of 23-valent pneumococcal vaccine in preventing pneumonia and improving survival in nursing home residents: double blind, randomised and placebo controlled trial. BMJ. 2010;340:c1004.
8. Glück T, Müller-Ladner U. Vaccination in patients with chronic rheumatic or autoimmune diseases. Clin Infect Dis. 2008;46:1459–65.
9. Moberley S, Holden J, Tatham DP, Andrews RM. Vaccines for preventing pneumococcal infection in adults. Cochrane Database Syst Rev. 2013;1, CD000422.
10. Perry LM, Winthrop KL, Curtis JR. Vaccinations for rheumatoid arthritis. Curr Rheumatol Rep. 2014;16:431.
11. Migita K, Akeda Y, Akazawa M, Tohma S, Hirano F, Ideguchi H, et al. Pneumococcal polysaccharide vaccination in rheumatoid arthritis patients receiving tacrolimus. Arthritis Res Ther. 2015;17:149.
12. Listing J, Gerhold K, Zink A. The risk of infections associated with rheumatoid arthritis, with its comorbidity and treatment. Rheumatology. 2013;52:53.
13. Matsui T, Kuga Y, Kaneko A, Nishino J, Eto Y, Chiba N, et al. Disease Activity Score 28 (DAS28) using C-reactive protein underestimates disease activity and overestimates EULAR response criteria compared with DAS28 using erythrocyte sedimentation rate in a large observational cohort of rheumatoid arthritis patients in Japan. Ann Rheum Dis. 2007;66:1221–6.
14. Wiemken TL, Carrico RM, Klein SL, Jonsson CB, Peyrani P, Kelley RR, et al. The effectiveness of the polysaccharide pneumococcal vaccine for the prevention of hospitalizations due to Streptococcus pneumoniae community-acquired pneumonia in the elderly differs between the sexes: results from the Community-Acquired Pneumonia Organization (CAPO) international cohort study. Vaccine. 2014;32:2198–203.
15. Ochoa-Gondar O, Vila-Corcoles A, Rodriguez-Blanco T, Gomez-Bertomeu F, Figuerola-Massana E, Raga-Luria X, et al. Effectiveness of the 23-valent pneumococcal polysaccharide vaccine against community-acquired pneumonia in the general population aged ≥ 60 years: 3 years of follow-up in the CAPAMIS study. Clin Infect Dis. 2014;58:909–17.
16. Sinclair A, Xie X, Teltscher M, Dendukuri N. Systematic review and meta-analysis of a urine-based pneumococcal antigen test for diagnosis of community-acquired pneumonia caused by Streptococcus pneumoniae. J Clin Microbiol. 2013;51:2303–10.
17. Walters JA, Smith S, Poole P, Granger RH, Wood-Baker R. Injectable vaccines for preventing pneumococcal infection in patients with chronic obstructive pulmonary disease. Cochrane Database Syst Rev. 2010;(11):CD001390.
18. French N, Gordon SB, Mwalukomo T, White SA, Mwafulirwa G, Longwe H, et al. A trial of a 7-valent pneumococcal conjugate vaccine in HIV-infected adults. N Engl J Med. 2010;362:812–22.
19. Vila-Corcoles A, Ochoa-Gondar O, Rodriguez-Blanco T, Gutierrez-Perez A, Vila-Rovira A. Clinical effectiveness of 23-valent pneumococcal polysaccharide vaccine against pneumonia in patients with chronic pulmonary diseases: a matched case-control study. Hum Vaccin Immunother. 2012;8:639.
20. Moberley SA, Holden J, Tatham DP, Andrews RM. Vaccines for preventing pneumococcal infection in adults. Cochrane Database Syst Rev. 2008;23, CD000422.
21. Pilishvili T, Bennett NM. Pneumococcal disease prevention among adults. strategies for the use of pneumococcal vaccines. Vaccine. 2015;33 Suppl 4:D60–5.
22. Doran MF, Crowson CS, Pond GR, O'Fallon WM, Gabriel SE. Predictors of infection in rheumatoid arthritis. Arthritis Rheum. 2002;46:2294–300.
23. Nakajima A, Inoue E, Tanaka E, Singh G, Sato E, Hoshi D, et al. Mortality and cause of death in Japanese patients with rheumatoid arthritis based on a large observational cohort, IORRA. Scand J Rheumatol. 2010;39:360-7.
24. Dixon WG, Suissa S, Hudson M. The association between systemic glucocorticoid therapy and the risk of infection in patients with rheumatoid arthritis: systematic review and meta-analyses. Arthritis Res Ther. 2011;13:R139.
25. Listing J, Gerhold K, Zink A. The risk of infections associated with rheumatoid arthritis, with its comorbidity and treatment. Rheumatology (Oxford). 2013;52:53–61.
26. Singh JA, Cameron C, Noorbaloochi S, Cullis T, Tucker M, Christensen R, et al. Risk of serious infection in biological treatment of patients with rheumatoid arthritis: a systematic review and meta-analysis. Lancet. 2015;386:258–65.
27. Crowson CS, Hoganson DD, Fitz-Gibbon PD, Matteson EL. Development and validation of a risk score for serious infection in patients with rheumatoid arthritis. Arthritis Rheum. 2012;64:2847–55.
28. Kelly CA, Saravanan V, Nisar M, Arthanari S, Woodhead FA, Price-Forbes AN, et al. Rheumatoid arthritis-related interstitial lung disease: associations, prognostic factors and physiological and radiological characteristics—a large multicentre UK study. Rheumatology (Oxford). 2014;53:1676–82.
29. Solomon JJ, Ryu JH, Tazelaar HD, Myers JL, Tuder R, Cool CD, et al. Fibrosing interstitial pneumonia predicts survival in patients with rheumatoid arthritis-associated interstitial lung disease (RA-ILD). Respir Med. 2013;107:1247–52.
30. Lake F, Proudman S. Rheumatoid arthritis and lung disease: from mechanisms to a practical approach. Semin Respir Crit Care Med. 2014;35:222–38.
31. Yun H, Xie F, Delzell E, Levitan EB, Chen L, Lewis JD, et al. Comparative risk of hospitalized infection associated with biologic agents in rheumatoid arthritis patients enrolled in Medicare. Arthritis Rheum. 2016;68:56–66.

11

Establishment of age- and sex-adjusted reference data for hand bone mass and investigation of hand bone loss in patients with rheumatoid arthritis treated in clinical practice: an observational study from the DANBIO registry and the Copenhagen Osteoarthritis Study

Lykke Midtbøll Ørnbjerg[1,2*], Mikkel Østergaard[1,2], Trine Jensen[3], Lars Hyldstrup[3], Pernille Bach-Mortensen[3], Pernille Bøyesen[4], Anja Thormann[1], Ulrik Tarp[5], Wolfgang Peter Bøhme[6], Hanne Lindegaard[7], Uta Engling Poulsen[8], Anette Schlemmer[9], Niels Graudal[10], Anne Rødgaard[11], Jakob Espesen[12], Gina Birgitte Kollerup[13], Bente Glintborg[14], Ole Rintek Madsen[15], Dorte Vendelbo Jensen[16] and Merete Lund Hetland[1,2]

Abstract

Background: Rheumatoid arthritis is characterised by progressive joint destruction and loss of periarticular bone mass. Hand bone loss (HBL) has therefore been proposed as an outcome measure for treatment efficacy. A definition of increased HBL adjusted for age- and sex-related bone loss is lacking. In this study, we aimed to: 1) establish reference values for normal hand bone mass (bone mineral density measured by digital x-ray radiogrammetry (DXR-BMD)); and 2) examine whether HBL is normalised in rheumatoid arthritis patients during treatment with tumour necrosis factor alpha inhibitors (TNFI).

Methods: DXR-BMD was measured from hand x-rays in a reference cohort (1485 men/2541 women) without arthritis randomly selected from an urban Danish population. Sex- and age-related HBL/year was estimated. DXR-BMD was measured in rheumatoid arthritis patients (n = 350: at start of TNFI, and ~2 years after TNFI start), of which 135 patients had three x-rays (~2 years prior to TNFI, at start of TNFI, and ~2 years after TNFI start). Individual HBL/year prior to and during TNFI was calculated and compared to reference values.

(Continued on next page)

* Correspondence: lykke@oernbjerg.dk
[1]DANBIO registry and Copenhagen Center for Arthritis Research, Center for Rheumatology and Spine Diseases, Centre of Head and Orthopedics, Ndr. Ringvej 57, DK-2600 Glostrup, Denmark
[2]Rigshospitalet, Department of Clinical Medicine, Faculty of Health and Medical Sciences, University of Copenhagen, Copenhagen, Denmark
Full list of author information is available at the end of the article

(Continued from previous page)

Results: Estimated HBL/year varied strongly with age and sex. Compared to the reference values, 75 % of 135 patients had increased HBL prior to TNFI treatment and 59 % had increased HBL during TNFI treatment ($p = 0.17$, Chi-squared). In 38 % (38/101) of patients with increased HBL, HBL was normalised during TNFI treatment, whereas 47 % (16/34) of patients with normal HBL prior to TNFI had increased HBL during TNFI treatment. In the 350 patients, increased HBL during TNFI was associated with time-averaged 28-joint disease activity score (odds ratio 1.69 (95 % Confidence Interval 1.34-2.15)/unit increase, $p < 0.001$), and patients in time-averaged remission had lower HBL than patients without remission (0.0032 vs. 0.0058 g/cm^2/year; $p < 0.001$, Mann-Whitney).

Conclusions: We established age- and sex-specific reference values for DXR-BMD in a large cohort without arthritis. HBL was increased in the majority of rheumatoid arthritis patients initiating TNFI in clinical practice, and only normalised in a minority during TNFI.

Keywords: Rheumatoid arthritis, Bone mineral density, Anti-TNF

Background

Bone involvement in rheumatoid arthritis (RA) has three hallmarks: localised destruction of joint bone, periarticular bone loss and generalised bone loss. The two former features are visible on x-rays as erosions and periarticular osteoporosis and are suggested to be caused by the same pathophysiologic pathway [1, 2]. Increased hand bone loss (HBL) measured by digital x-ray radiogrammetry (DXR) may precede the development of erosions, takes place throughout the disease course, and occurs in patients with no progression of radiographic joint damage [3–5]. Thus, HBL has been proposed as a more sensitive outcome measure for monitoring disease progression and treatment effect than the traditional evaluation of radiographs [5].

A common definition of increased HBL has not yet been established, which limits the clinical value of HBL and comparison between studies. Attempts to define increased HBL include HBL above the median in the study population, and the smallest detectable difference of HBL or cut-off values provided by the manufacturer based on the distribution of HBL in two early RA cohorts [6–10]. However, the normal HBL in healthy persons, shown to vary considerably with sex and age, has so far not been included in the definition of increased HBL [11, 12].

Impact of tumour necrosis factor alpha inhibitors (TNFI) on HBL in RA patients has been investigated in the PREMIER and BEST randomised controlled trials (RCTs) in early RA, where patients treated with TNFI in combination with methotrexate (MTX) had a significantly lower HBL compared with MTX monotherapy [5, 13]. No studies have analysed whether HBL is normalised during TNFI treatment.

The primary aims of the present study were: 1) to establish a large reference material for hand bone mass measured by DXR in order to estimate sex- and age-related HBL/year; and 2) to determine whether HBL in RA patients treated in clinical practice normalises during treatment with TNFI when switched from conventional synthetic disease-modifying anti-rheumatic drugs (csDMARDs) due to an unsatisfactory clinical response.

Secondarily, in RA patients treated in clinical practice, we aimed to: 3) investigate the association between HBL and radiographic progression during treatment with csDMARDs and TNFI; 4) investigate the association between HBL and inflammatory activity during TNFI; and 5) identify predictors of increased HBL during TNFI.

Methods

Reference cohort

The Copenhagen City Heart Study is a health survey of an adult urban Danish population selected by a random social security number algorithm. From 1991 to 1994, 10,135 participants were included and from this main cohort 1533 men and 2618 women without inflammatory joint disease had x-rays of the pelvis, knees, lumbar spine, hands and wrists performed once (Copenhagen Osteoarthritis Study) [14]. Age, sex and hand x-ray films were used in the present study.

Patients with RA

In the Danish DANBIO registry, disease outcomes are reported prospectively in RA patients treated in clinical practice. DANBIO covers >90 % of TNFI treated RA patients [15].

We included all RA patients in DANBIO who: 1) were TNFI naïve; 2) started treatment with adalimumab, etanercept or infliximab before 1 July 2007; and 3) had at least two relevant hand x-rays (baseline and follow-up). A baseline x-ray had to precede the initiation of TNFI by less than 3 months, while the follow-up x-ray had to be obtained >6 months after the baseline x-ray. If available, a pre-baseline x-ray, which preceded both TNFI start and baseline x-ray with >6 months was collected. Five hundred and seventeen patients had three available x-rays, while 930 patients had two x-rays (baseline and follow-up) [16, 17].

Ethical approval and patient consent

The individuals in the reference cohort signed an informed consent form. The Danish ethics committee for the City of Copenhagen and Frederiksberg approved the Copenhagen City Heart Study (100.2039/91).

The data from the patient cohort originates from the nationwide Danish DANBIO registry. DANBIO has been approved by The Danish Data Registry since the year 2000 (j. nr. 2007-58-0014 and j.nr. 2007-58-0006), and since October 2006 as a national quality registry by the National Board of Health (j. nr. 7-201-03-12/1). According to Danish law, informed consent and ethical approval were not required for the present study.

Radiographic assessment of patient radiographs

Patient x-rays were available and collected as x-ray films or digital images. To facilitate reading, x-ray films were scanned and converted to a digital format. Reading was performed by an experienced reader, blinded to patient identity and image sequence, according to the modified Sharp method [18].

Annual radiographic progression rates prior to baseline (csDMARD period) and during TNFI treatment (TNFI period) were calculated [16]. Radiographic progression was defined as: a) a change in total Sharp score (TSS) >0; and b) a change in TSS greater than the smallest detectable change (SDC) [19]. Intra-observer intra-class correlation coefficient (one-way random effects model) (ICC) for baseline TSS was 0.96 and for TSS change was 0.35 [20]. SDC was 3.9 TSS units/year [17, 21].

DXR-BMD

DXR is a computerized version of the traditional radiogrammetry, previously described in detail [22]. Software automatically detects regions of interest in the three middle metacarpal bones and estimates the bone mineral density (DXR-BMD) based on cortical thickness. Short-term coefficient of variation has been shown to be 0.28 % and smallest detectable difference 0.0046 g/cm [7, 23].

X-ray films from the reference cohort were analysed with the Pronosco X-posure™ v. 2.0 equipment (Sectra, Sweden). DXR-BMD of both hands were obtained and the mean used for analyses (available in 1485/2541 men/women as 48 men and 77 women were excluded due to missing or unsuitable x-rays). Patient x-rays in a digital format were analysed with the DXR-online system (Sectra, Sweden). The same algorithm was used for calculating DXR-BMD with the Pronosco X-posure™ and DXR-online systems [24].

As indicated in Fig. 1, DXR-BMD analysis or HBL calculation was not possible in a substantial number of patient x-rays due to methodological or disease-related issues. Both hands were measured if possible and the mean used for analyses. If a patient only had DXR-BMD of one hand at any one time point, all analyses were based on that hand (applicable in 38 patients). Three DXR-BMD measurements were available in 135 patients (csDMARD-to-TNFI cohort), while 350 patients had two DXR-BMD measurements (baseline and follow-up; TNFI cohort).

Clinical data

Health assessment questionnaire (HAQ) score and disease activity score in 28 joints based on three variables (DAS28) including C-reactive protein (CRP) were obtained from DANBIO at three visits. For the 135 patients included in the csDMARD-to-TNFI cohort, the three visits were selected to be: closest in time to the pre-baseline x-ray (pre-baseline), closest to the date of TNFI initiation (baseline) and closest in time to the follow-up x-ray (follow-up). For the 215 additional patients included in the TNFI cohort, the baseline and follow-up visits were selected in a similar manner, while the pre-baseline visit was the visit closest to 2 years prior to TNFI.

Patient files were reviewed and data on csDMARD and glucocorticoid treatment in the csDMARD and TNFI period registered.

To provide an estimate of inflammatory burden time-averaged CRP (available in 344 patients, median (interquartile range (IQR)) number of measurements 13 (7–20)), time-averaged DAS28, 28 swollen joint count (28SJC) and 28 tender joint count (28TJC) were calculated (available in 335 patients, based on 7 (5–11) measurements) [25].

Statistical analyses

All analyses were performed with R (version 2.15.3) [26]. Analyses were two-sided with a significance level of 0.05.

Reference cohort

Linear regression models for the relation between age and DXR-BMD were fitted for men and women separately. Model fits were compared with the Akaike information criterion (AIC) for non-nested models and analysis of variance (ANOVA) for nested models. Standard graphical tests of model assumptions were performed (plots inspected for linearity, homoscedasticity and normally distributed residuals). From the final models estimated mean annual change in DXR-BMD were calculated for all years of ages from 18 to 89 in both sexes. These estimates constitute reference values for normal HBL/year in the present study.

Patients with RA

HBL is presented as annual absolute (g/cm^2) and relative (%) change in DXR-BMD. Increased HBL in an individual patient was defined as a negative HBL/year exceeding the lower 95 % confidence interval (CI) of the normal HBL/year for the matching sex and year of age. For example, a female patient of 54 years would be said to have increased HBL if her HBL/year was lower than –

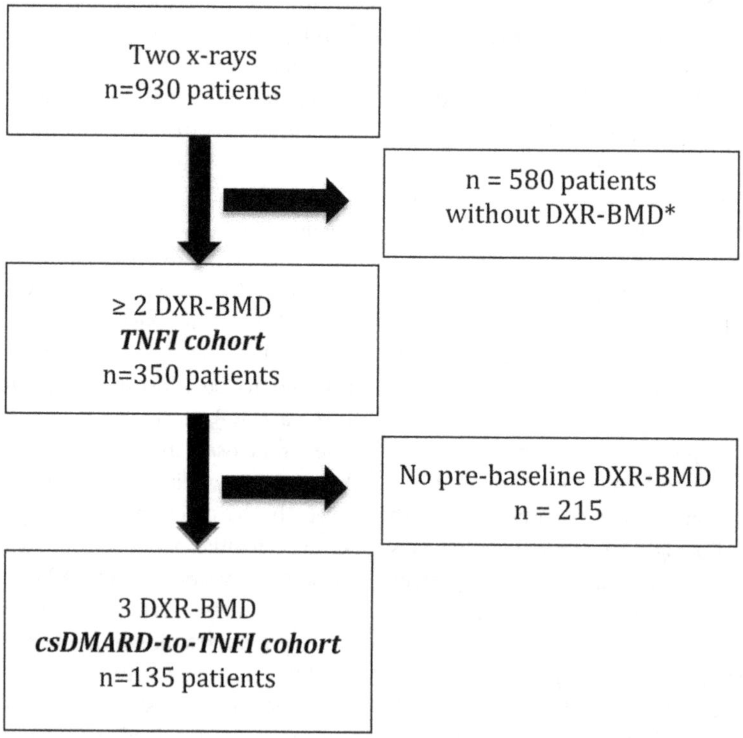

Fig. 1 Patient disposition. *Patients were excluded if: a) DXR-BMD could not be analysed due to technical problems (insufficient exposure of x-rays, insufficient positioning of hands) or disease-related factors (prostheses, severe bone damage); or b) DXR-BMD change (i.e. hand bone loss) could not be calculated due to change in acquisition modality between original x-rays (e.g. x-ray film at baseline and digital image at follow-up) or large change in digital image post-processing between x-rays (edge enhancement and change in x-ray resolution). *csDMARD* Conventional synthetic disease-modifying anti-rheumatic drug, *DXR-BMD* Bone mineral density estimated by digital x-ray radiogrammetry, *TNFI* Tumour necrosis factor alpha inhibitors

0.0051 g/cm^2 (Additional file 1: supplementary table). HBL was compared between csDMARD and TNFI periods by non-parametric analyses due to a skewed distribution of HBL.

Univariate logistic and linear regression were used to analyse the association between inflammatory activity (assessed with time-averaged CRP, DAS28, 28SJC and 28TJC) and increased and absolute HBL, respectively.

Correlation between HBL and radiographic progression was analysed with Spearman's rho.

Possible predictors for increased HBL were analysed with univariate logistic regression, and significant variables ($p < 0.10$) included in a multiple logistic regression analysis with backward selection.

Results

Reference cohort

Distribution of DXR-BMD in women and men in the reference cohort is presented in Fig. 2. In women, the best fitting model was DXR-BMD = 0.020 × age − 0.00040 × age^2 + 0.0000021 × age^3 (R^2 = 0.54); in men, DXR-BMD = 0.0018 × age − 0.0000371 × age^2 (R^2 = 0.27). Estimated mean annual changes in DXR-BMD (i.e. normal HBL/year) in men and women derived from the models are presented in Additional file 1. Table 1 presents normal HBL/year averaged over 5-year age intervals (10-year intervals in the lowest and highest age groups). In men, the model estimated an increasing HBL/year from 35 years of age onwards reaching a maximum of −0.0047 g/cm^2/−0.8 % per year at the age of 85. In women, an annual increase in DXR-BMD until 35 years of age was estimated, followed by a continuous HBL that accelerated between 55 and 70 years (greater than −0.0050/−1.0 %).

Patients with RA

A patient disposition is shown in Fig. 1, while demographic, clinical, treatment and radiographic characteristics of included RA patients are summarised in Table 2. Patients with x-rays unsuitable for DXR-BMD had longer disease duration and more radiographic damage than patients included in the TNFI cohort, but had less functional disability. Other characteristics were similar between cohorts. In the csDMARD-to-TNFI cohort, the median (range) number of days from pre-baseline x-ray to baseline (TNFI initiation) was 607 (180–2989) days, from baseline to baseline x-ray 11 (90–866) days, and from baseline to follow-up x-ray 687 (198–1812) days.

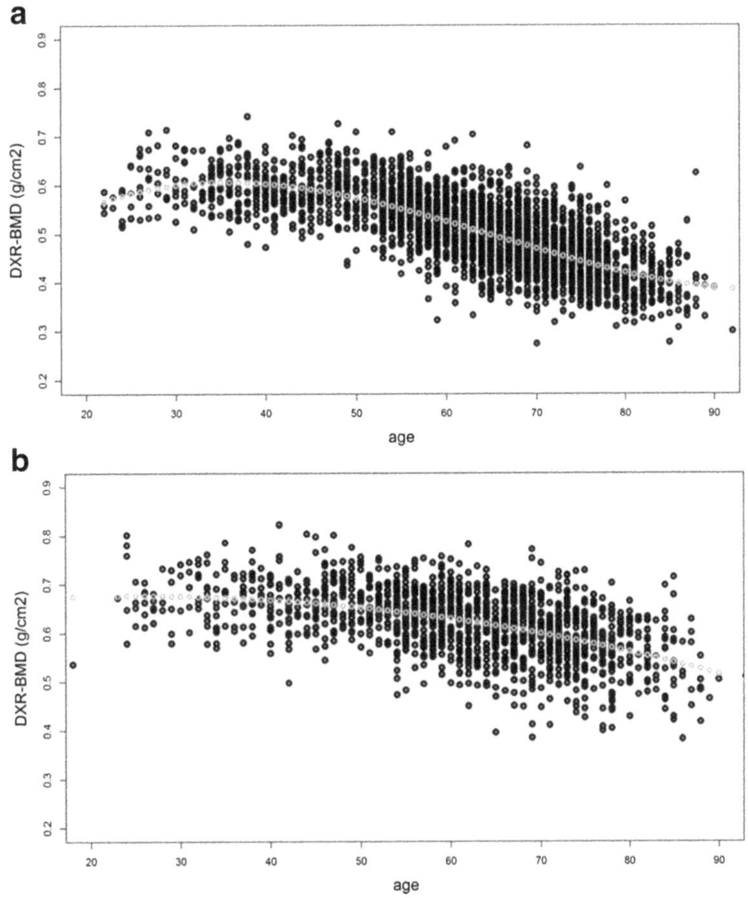

Fig. 2 Distribution of DXR-BMD (g/cm^2) in **a** 2541 Danish women and **b** 1485 Danish men. The *grey dotted* lines indicate regression lines fitted to the data from the reference cohort. *DXR-BMD* Bone mineral density estimated by digital x-ray radiogrammetry

HBL in the csDMARD-to-TNFI cohort

In the 135 patients in the csDMARD-to-TNF cohort, pre-baseline median (IQR) DXR-BMD was 0.545 (0.474–0.597) g/cm^2 decreasing to 0.516 (0.441–0.578) g/cm^2 at baseline ($p < 0.001$, Wilcoxon Signed Rank). At follow-up, DXR-BMD had further decreased to 0.504 (0.424–0.557) g/cm^2 ($p < 0.001$, Wilcoxon Signed Rank). In the csDMARD period, 101 (75 %) patients had increased HBL while increased HBL was found in 79 (59 %) patients in the TNFI period ($p = 0.004$, McNemars test). Thirty-eight patients had an increased HBL in the csDMARD period that normalised in the TNFI period, while 16 patients had a normal HBL in the DMARD period but increased HBL in the TNFI period. Of the latter 16 patients, 6 patients continued their first TNFI treatment throughout follow-up, while three and seven patients, respectively, withdrew from TNFI treatment or switched to a different biological drug. Corresponding numbers for the 38 patients with normalized HBL during TNFI were 26, 5 and 7.

HBL was significantly lower in the TNFI period (−0.0051 g/cm^2/year and −1.15 %/year) compared to the csDMARD period (−0.0082 g/cm^2/year and −1.55 %/year; $p < 0.001$ for both comparisons, Wilcoxon Signed Rank).

Figure 3 illustrates a probability plot for HBL in the csDMARD and TNFI periods.

HBL and inflammatory activity during TNFI treatment

In the TNFI cohort (n = 350), increased HBL during TNFI was associated with time-averaged DAS28 (odds ratio (OR) 1.69 (95 % Confidence Interval 1.34-2.15/unit increase) $p < 0.001$) and all of its components: time-averaged 28SJC (OR 1.29 (1.15–1.46/joint increase), $p < 0.001$), time-averaged 28TJC (OR 1.11 (1.05–1.19/joint increase), $p < 0.001$) and time-averaged CRP (OR 1.02 (1.005–1.04/(mg/L) increase), $p = 0.02$). Similarly, absolute HBL was associated with time-averaged DAS28 (β-coefficient −0.0032 (−0.0020 to −0.0041) g/cm^2, $p < 0.001$) and all of its components: time-averaged 28SJC (−0.0008 to −0.002) g/cm^2, $p < 0.001$), time-averaged 28TJC (−0.0004 (−0.00008 to 0.0007) g/cm^2, $p = 0.01$) and time-averaged CRP (−0.0003 (−0.0002 to −0.00004) g/cm^2, $p < 0.001$)) in linear regression analyses.

Table 1 DXR-BMD and estimated mean annual change in DXR-BMD (i.e. normal HBL/year) in 1485 Danish men and 2541 Danish women

			Absolute HBL/year		
Age (years)	n	BMD (g/cm^2) (mean (SD))	Estimate	95 % Confidence interval	Percentage HBL/year
Men					
18–29	32	0.666 (0.06)	−0.00012	−0.00095 to 0.00071	−0.02
30–34	35	0.671 (0.06)	−0.00060	−0.00128 to 0.00007	−0.09
35–39	45	0.679 (0.05)	−0.00098	−0.00153 to −0.00042	−0.1
40–44	71	0.660 (0.05)	−0.00135	−0.00179 to −0.00090	−0.2
45–49	98	0.668 (0.05)	−0.00172	−0.00206 to −0.00138	−0.3
50–54	133	0.653 (0.05)	−0.00202	−0.00235 to −0.00184	−0.3
55–59	209	0.636 (0.05)	−0.00247	−0.00269 to −0.00225	−0.4
60–64	198	0.623 (0.06)	−0.00284	−0.00309 to −0.00259	−0.5
65–69	211	0.602 (0.06)	−0.00321	−0.00354 to −0.00288	−0.5
70–74	213	0.594 (0.06)	−0.00358	−0.00401 to −0.00316	−0.6
75–79	140	0.572 (0.06)	−0.00396	−0.00450 to −0.00342	−0.7
80–84	68	0.563 (0.06)	−0.00432	−0.00499 to −0.00367	−0.8
85–93	32	0.534 (0.08)	−0.00470	−0.00548 to −0.00392	−0.8
Total	1485	0.619 (0.07)			
Women					
18–29	41	0.597 (0.05)	0.00416	0.00268 to 0.00564	0.7
30–34	51	0.599 (0.04)	0.00123	0.00031 to 0.00213	0.2
35–39	84	0.601 (0.05)	− 0.00066	−0.00122 to −0.00009	−0.1
40–44	116	0.589 (0.04)	− 0.00224	−0.00260 to −0.00189	−0.4
45–49	131	0.592 (0.05)	−0.00351	−0.00379 to −0.00323	−0.6
50–54	185	0.569 (0.05)	−0.00437	−0.00470 to −0.00411	−0.8
55–59	322	0.541 (0.05)	−0.00513	−0.00543 to 0.00483	−0.9
60–64	311	0.513 (0.06)	−0.00548	−0.00575 to −0.00521	−1.0
65–69	430	0.486 (0.06)	−0.00552	−0.00577 to −0.00527	−1.1
70–74	394	0.460 (0.05)	−0.00525	−0.00559 to −0.00492	−1.1
75–79	307	0.440 (0.05)	−0.00468	−0.00525 to −0.00410	−1.0
80–84	123	0.411 (0.05)	−0.00380	−0.00472 to −0.00288	−0.9
85–93	46	0.400 (0.06)	−0.00261	−0.00397 to −0.00124	−0.7
Total	2541	0.505 (0.08)			

BMD Bone mineral density, *DXR-BMD* Bone mineral density estimated by digital x-ray radiogrammetry, *HBL* hand bone loss, *SD* Standard deviation

During TNFI treatment, 81 patients were in time-averaged remission (time-averaged DAS28 < 2.6) and 42 (52 %) of these patients had a normal HBL. In contrast, 98 (39 %) of the 254 patients not in time-averaged remission had a normal HBL ($p = 0.04$, Chi squared). Patients in time-averaged remission had a lower HBL than patients who were not (−0.0032 vs. −0.0058 g/cm^2/year; $p = 0.003$, Mann-Whitney).

Time-averaged CRP was <10 mg/L during TNFI treatment in 174 patients and 84 (48 %) of these patients had a normal HBL, while 51 (36 %) of the 141 patients with a time-averaged CRP >10 mg/L had a normal HBL ($p = 0.04$, Chi squared).

HBL and radiographic progression

Median (IQR)/mean (standard deviation) rate of radiographic progression decreased from 0.6 (0.0–2.5)/1.9 (3.2) TSS units/year in the csDMARD period to 0.0 (0.0–0.8)/0.5 (1.7) TSS units/year in the TNFI period ($p < 0.001$, Wilcoxon Signed Rank, paired t-test). In the TNFI cohort the rate of radiographic progression was 0 (0–0)/0.5 (1.8) TSS units/year.

In the csDMARD-to-TNFI cohort (n = 135), 73 patients progressed radiographically (change in TSS >0) during csDMARD treatment and 56 (77 %) of these patients experienced increased HBL. Of the 62 patients who did not progress radiographically, 45 (72 %) had

Table 2 Demographic, clinical, treatment and radiographic characteristics of the patients included in the csDMARD-to-TNFI and TNFI cohorts

	csDMARD-to-TNFI cohort			TNFI cohort		Patients with radiographs unsuitable for DXR analysis	
Time point	Pre-baseline	Baseline	Follow-up	Baseline	Follow-up	Baseline	*p* value[a]
No. of patients	135	135	135	350	350	580	
Age (years)	55 (44–62)	57 (47–64)	59 (48–65)	56.5 (47–64)	58 (48–66)	57 (49–64)	0.44*
Women (%)	85	85	85	79	79	75	0.08**
Disease duration (years)	4.5 (1–10)	6 (4–12)	8 (5–14)	8 (4–14)	10 (6–15)	10 (5–18)	**0.004***
DAS28	4.3 (3.0–5.3)	5.3 (4.4–6.1)	3.1 (2.2–3.9)	5.3 (4.5–6.1)	3.0 (2.1–4.0)	5.4 (4.7–6.2)	0.24*
CRP (mg/l)	16 (8–33)	18 (8–40)	8 (4–14)	17 (8–35)	8 (3–14)	19 (8–42)	0.09*
IgM-RF positivity (%)	71	71	71	76	76	79	0.77**
Current smokers (%)	36	35	30	34	32	37	0.25**
HAQ score	NA	1.250 (0.750–1.750)	0.825 (0.250–1.375)	1.250 (0.750–1.750)	0.875 (0.250–1.375)	0.875 (0.250–1.500)	**<0.001***
Previous csDMARDs (n)	NA	3 (3–4)	–	3 (2–4)	–	3 (2–4)	0.26*
Length of TNFI period (days)	–	–	574 (405–759)	–	511 (381–695)	538 (397–761)	**0.03***
Concomitant MTX (%)	93	83	74	78	72	75	0.32**
Corticosteroid treatment (%)	–	88[c]	76[d]	71[c]	64[d]	57[d]	**0.03****
Prednisolone dosage (mg/day)[b]	–	1.32 (0.4–5.2)[c]	1.33 (0.4–3.8)[d]	1.8 (0.5–5.1)[c]	2.0 (0.5–4.6)[d]	2.7 (0.6–5.6)[d]	**0.02***
Type of TNFI (n (%))							
INF		101 (75)		218 (62)			
ETA		17 (12)		68 (20)			
ADA		18 (13)		64 (18)			
Treatment at follow-up (n (%))							
On first TNFI			79 (59)		216 (62)		
Switched from first TNFI			38 (27)		94 (27)		
Withdrawn from TNFI			18 (14)		40 (11)		
Sharp score (TSS units)	6 (0–21)	10 (1–29)	12 (2–31)	11 (2–34)	12 (3–35)	17 (3–53)	**0.001***
Sharp score (TSS units) (mean (SD))	16 (22)	19 (24)	20 (24.6)	22 (27)	23 (27)	36 (45)	**0.001*****
Erosive disease (%)	70	76	77	81	81	83	0.55**
DXR-BMD (g/cm^2) (mean (SD))	0.529 (0.09)	0.506 (0.10)	0.495 (0.10)	0.502 (0.10)	0.490 (0.10)	NA	

[a]Comparing TNFI cohort with the cohort of patients with radiographs unsuitable for DXR (values in bold are significant)

[b]All administered corticosteroids (peroral, intra-articular and intramuscular) were converted to a corresponding daily dosage of prednisolone in patients who had received corticosteroids at least once

[c]In the csDMARD period

[d] In the TNFI period. Medians (interquartile range) are presented unless otherwise indicated.

*Mann-Whitney

**Chi-square

***Students *t*-test

ADA Adalimumab, *CRP* C-reactive protein, *csDMARD* Conventional synthetic disease-modifying anti-rheumatic drug, *DAS28* Disease activity score in 28 joints based on three variables including CRP, *DXR* Digital x-ray radiogrammetry, *DXR-BMD* Bone mineral density measured by digital x-ray radiogrammetry, *ETA* Etanercept, *HAQ* Health assessment questionnaire, *IgM-RF* Immunoglobulin M rheumatoid factor, *INF* Infliximab, *NA* not available, *SD* Standard deviation, *TSS* Total Sharp Score, *MTX* Methotrexate, *TNFI* Tumour necrosis factor inhibitor

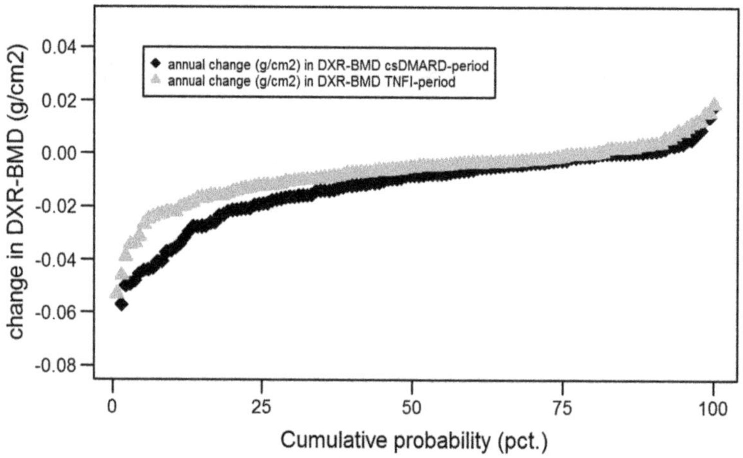

Fig. 3 Cumulative probability plot illustrating HBL in each individual patient in the csDMARD period and TNFI period. The csDMARD period is the period between the pre-baseline and baseline x-rays, while the TNFI period is the period between baseline and follow-up x-rays (see Patients and methods for details). *csDMARD* Conventional synthetic disease-modifying anti-rheumatic drug, *DXR-BMD* Bone mineral density measured by digital x-ray radiogrammetry, *TNFI* Tumour necrosis factor inhibitors

increased HBL (Chi squared = 0.72). In the TNFI period, 41 patients progressed radiographically and 28 of these patients (68 %) had increased HBL, while increased HBL was found in 51 of the 94 patients who did not progress radiographically (54 %; Chi squared = 0.18). Similarly, 64 % vs. 56 % of the patients who progressed/did not progress radiographically in the TNFI cohort (n = 350) had increased HBL (Chi squared = 0.18). Radiographic progression above the SDC (3.9) was found in 24 patients in the csDMARD-to-TNFI cohort in the csDMARD period, while six patients experienced progression in the TNFI period. As was the case for the cut-off of 0, no relation between increased HBL and radiographic progression above the SDC was found in either the csDMARD or the TNFI period (Chi squared = 0.7 and 0.4, respectively).

Correlations between TSS status scores and separate erosion score (ES) and joint space narrowing (JSN) scores with DXR-BMD were moderate, while correlations between TSS, JSN and ES changes with HBL were low (Table 3).

Predictors of HBL during TNFI treatment

In univariate analyses of the TNFI cohort, high baseline DXR-BMD, longer disease duration, immunoglobulin M rheumatoid factor positivity and high DAS28 were associated with increased HBL, while age, HAQ score, CRP, sex, smoking status, type of TNFI, calendar year of treatment initiation and concomitant treatment with prednisolone and MTX were not. In the multivariable model, DXR-BMD (OR 1.005/mg increase (95 % CI 1.003–1.008)) and DAS28 (OR 1.43/unit increase (95% CI 1.15–1.81)) were independently associated with increased HBL. Fraction of explained variation (Nagelkerkes R^2) was 0.12. In a model including time-averaged DAS28 during TNFI treatment, baseline DXR-BMD and DAS28 remained independent predictors of increased HBL (R^2 increased to 0.20).

Discussion

In this paper we have established reference values for hand bone mass measured by DXR-BMD. Based on this reference material we estimated sex- and age-related mean HBL/year and used this to define whether HBL was increased or not in individual RA patients. Our main finding was that the majority of patients initiating TNFI treatment in clinical practice had increased HBL and that normalisation of HBL during TNFI treatment was achieved only in a minority of patients.

Table 3 Correlations between DXR-BMD and radiographic scores in the csDMARD-to-TNFI cohort

	DXR-BMD status				Hand bone loss	
n =135	Pre-baseline	Baseline	Follow-up		csDMARD period	TNFI period
JSN	−0.42 (<0.001)	−0.41 (<0.001)	−0.37 (<0.001)	JSN change	−0.09 (0.27)	−0.18 (0.002)
ES	−0.46 (<0.001)	−0.48 (<0.001)	−0.47 (<0.001)	ES change	−0.19 (0.02)	−0.13 (0.01)
TSS	−0.47 (<0.001)	−0.47 (<0.001)	−0.45 (<0.001)	TSS change	−0.21 (0.01)	−0.25 (0.003)

p values from Spearmans rho are shown in parentheses
csDMARD Conventional synthetic disease-modifying anti-rheumatic drug, *DXR-BMD* Bone mineral density estimated by digital x-ray radiogrammetry, *ES* Erosion score, *JSN* Joint space narrowing, *TNFI* Tumour necrosis factor alpha inhibitors, *TSS* Total Sharp score

The large reference cohort (n = 4026) allows precise estimation of sex- and age-related mean HBL/year. The reference cohort was randomly recruited and excluded individuals with inflammatory joint diseases. Individuals with other diseases affecting BMD (osteoporosis, kidney disease, etc.) were not excluded. Theoretically, this could result in overestimation of HBL in the reference cohort. However, a smaller Danish reference cohort excluded such individuals and no systematic differences between DXR-BMD in the two cohorts were found (data not shown) [27].

Based on the distribution of HBL in two early RA cohorts (EURIDISS and BARFOT), the manufacturer of DXR (Sectra, Sweden) defines moderately increased HBL as a negative change in DXR-BMD >0.25 mg/cm^2/month and <2.5 mg/cm^2/month (>0.003 g/cm^2/year and <0.03 g/cm^2/year) and highly increased HBL as negative change in DXR-BMD >2.5 mg/cm^2/month (>0.03 g/cm^2/year) irrespective of age and sex [6, 7, 10]. According to our reference values, normal HBL in women >50 years of age and men >70 years is >0.003 g/cm^2/year (corresponding to moderately increased HBL according to the manufacturer), emphasizing the need for an improved definition of increased HBL. No data have demonstrated clinical relevance of the distinction between moderately and highly increased HBL, which is why we chose to simply dichotomise normal vs. increased HBL. The main limitation of our approach is the cross-sectional design of the reference cohort resulting in estimated mean values of HBL, not true HBL measured in individuals. This approach is an established method when no longitudinal studies are available, but should ideally be supplemented with longitudinal data [28]. Melton et al. compared rates of BMD loss by dual-energy x-ray absorptiometry (DEXA) estimated from cross-sectional baseline data with rates obtained from longitudinal assessment and found that cross-sectional data overestimated BMD loss in some skeletal sites (hip and spine) and underestimated the loss in others (radius and ulna) [29]. The background for these findings is unclear and the relevance for DXR is not known.

This study is the first to investigate HBL in established RA during csDMARD treatment and subsequent TNFI treatment. In the BEST and PREMIER trials, patients on MTX monotherapy had a relative HBL/year of −2.6 and −1.9 %, respectively, compared to −1.55 % in our cohort during csDMARD treatment [5, 13]. The higher HBL in the RCT monotherapy arms may be explained by frequent use of combination treatment and intra-articular injections in our cohort and the RCT inclusion criteria selecting patients with early and aggressive disease.

As expected, we observed a decrease in HBL (from −1.55 %/year to −1.15 %/year) after initiation of TNFI treatment. The latter is considerably higher than HBL in the combination treatment arms in BEST (−0.6 and −0.9 %/year), but lower than the −1.63 %/year in the combination arm of PREMIER, probably reflecting stricter inclusion criteria in PREMIER than in BEST and our observational study. An HBL of −0.45 %/year was found in 215 patients with established RA receiving different treatments in the Oslo RA register [3]. This considerably lower HBL may be explained by moderate baseline disease activity (DAS28 = 4.0) in contrast to high disease activity in our cohort (DAS28 = 5.3).

Baseline DAS28 was an independent predictor of increased HBL in our cohort in accordance with previous studies documenting a predictive value of baseline DAS28 for future HBL [3, 5, 13, 24]. Interestingly, baseline CRP was not predictive of increased HBL while time-averaged CRP during TNFI treatment was strongly associated with increased HBL. This suggests a key role of sustained inflammation in HBL supporting results from the BEST trial where differences in HBL between treatment groups disappeared after adjustment for changes in disease activity. A similar association is well established with regards to radiographic progression but has not previously been shown for HBL [17, 30].

Previously, older age (PREMIER) and postmenopausal status (BEST) has been shown to be predictive of HBL in linear regression analyses [5, 13]. In contrast, we found that older age was not associated with increased HBL. This difference stresses the importance of establishing reference data for normal HBL in different age groups and in both sexes.

In accordance with earlier studies, correlations between DXR-BMD and radiographic damage were moderate, and correlations between HBL and radiographic progression low [5–7, 22, 24]. Increased HBL was found in 110 patients with no radiographic progression during TNFI treatment, suggesting a higher sensitivity of HBL in detecting RA-related bone damage. However, we also identified 40 patients who progressed radiographically, but had normal HBL. This dissociation between the two types of bone damage was also seen in a study by Hoff et al. implying that the exact pathophysiological mechanisms may differ and that the traditional evaluation of x-rays cannot be substituted by DXR or vice versa [7, 31]. In our study, overall radiographic progression was low, reflected in a poor ICC for TSS change [32]. The SDC of 3.9 TSS units is comparable to SDCs reported in major RCTs of patients with established RA [33, 34].

A definite limitation of our study is that many patient x-rays could not be analysed. This is a general weakness of DXR, limiting generalisability of our findings as patients with the most advanced and aggressive disease were excluded. A potential limitation of our study is the timing of x-rays, as the selection criteria theoretically allow for a HBL during TNFI treatment to be calculated based on x-rays obtained 90 days prior to baseline and 90 days after baseline. This could lead to an underestimation of the effectiveness of TNFI treatment. However, only two patients in the csDMARD-to-TNFI cohort had a baseline x-ray that preceded TNFI start in combination with a follow-up x-ray less than 300 days after TNFI start, and this is why we consider this bias minimal.

A potential limitation was the lack of information on the use of anti-resorptive treatment in the cohorts. Since previous studies have found no influence of alendronate on HBL, and the more potent anti-resorptive treatments were only marketed in the last part of our study period, we consider this limitation to be of minor significance [9, 13].

Conclusions

In this study, we established a reference material for DXR-BMD in the general population and from this reference material we estimated normal sex- and age-related HBL/year. Applying these reference values we found increased HBL in the majority of RA patients in a cohort from clinical practice initiating TNFI treatment. HBL was only normalised in a few patients during TNFI treatment, and more often in patients who were in time-averaged remission.

Abbreviations

28SJC: 28 Swollen joint count; 28TJC: 28 Tender joint count; AIC: Akaike information criterion; ANOVA: Analysis of variance; BMD: Bone mineral density; CI: Confidence interval; CRP: C-reactive protein; csDMARD: Conventional synthetic disease-modifying anti-rheumatic drug; DAS28: Disease activity score in 28 joints based on three variables; DXR: Digital x-ray radiogrammetry; DXR-BMD: Bone mineral density estimated by digital x-ray radiogrammetry; ES: Erosion score; HAQ: Health assessment questionnaire; HBL: Hand bone loss; ICC: Intra-observer intra-class correlation coefficient; IQR: Interquartile range; JSN: Joint space narrowing; MTX: Methotrexate; Nagelkerkes R^2: Fraction of explained variation; OR: Odds ratio; RA: Rheumatoid arthritis; RCT: Randomised controlled trial; SDC: Smallest detectable change; TNFI: Tumour necrosis factor alpha inhibitors; TSS: Total Sharp score.

Competing interests

MØ received grants, personal fees and non-financial support from AbbVie; grants and personal fees from BMS; personal fees from Boehringer-Ingelheim; personal fees from Eli Lilly; personal fees and non-financial support from Janssen; grants, personal fees and non-financial support from Merck; personal fees and non-financial support from Pfizer; personal fees and non-financial support from Roche; grants, personal fees and non-financial support from UCB; personal fees from Celgene; personal fees from Sanofi; personal fees from Regeneron; and personal fees from Novartis. Outside the submitted work, MØ has no non-financial competing interests to declare. HL received personal fees from Berlin-Chemie Menarini; grants from Eli Lilly; grants from MSD; grants and personal fees from Roche; grants from Novartis; outside the submitted work, HL has no non-financial competing interests to declare. ORM has received research grants and/or consultancy/speaker fees from Abbott, BMS, MSD, Pfizer, Roche and UCB. Outside of the submitted work, ORM has no non-financial competing interests to declare. All other authors declare that they have no competing interests.

Authors' contributions

LMØ participated in the design and conception of the study, contributed to x-ray and clinical data collection in the RA cohort, performed the statistical analyses, interpreted the results and drafted the manuscript. MØ participated in the design and conception of the study, interpreted results and revised the manuscript. TJ participated in the design and conception of the study, performed DXR analyses of the reference cohort x-rays, and helped with interpretation of results and revision of the manuscript. LH contributed to collection and analyses of x-rays in the reference cohort and revised the manuscript. PBM collected reference cohort x-rays, performed DXR analyses of the reference cohort and revised the manuscript. PB read all patient x-rays and helped to revise the manuscript. AT contributed substantially with x-ray collection in the RA cohort and helped to revise the manuscript. UT contributed substantially with clinical and x-ray data collection in the RA cohort and helped to revise the manuscript. WB contributed substantially with clinical and x-ray data collection in the RA cohort and helped to revise the manuscript. HL contributed substantially with clinical and x-ray data collection in the RA cohort and helped to revise the manuscript. UEP contributed substantially with clinical and x-ray data collection in the RA cohort and helped to revise the manuscript. AS contributed substantially with clinical and x-ray data collection in the RA cohort and helped to revise the manuscript. NG contributed substantially with clinical and x-ray data collection in the RA cohort and helped to revise the manuscript. AR contributed substantially with clinical and x-ray data collection in the RA cohort and helped to revise the manuscript. JE contributed substantially with clinical and x-ray data collection in the RA cohort and helped to revise the manuscript. GK contributed substantially with clinical and x-ray data collection in the RA cohort and helped to revise the manuscript. BG contributed substantially with clinical and x-ray data collection in the RA cohort and helped to revise the manuscript. ORM contributed substantially with clinical and x-ray data collection in the RA cohort and helped to revise the manuscript. DVJ contributed substantially with clinical and x-ray data collection in the RA cohort and helped to revise the manuscript. MLH participated in the design and conception of the study, interpretation of results and revised the manuscript. All authors read and approved the final manuscript.

Acknowledgements

The DANBIO X-ray Study Group investigators: Glostrup: Lykke Midtbøll Ørnbjerg, Merete Lund Hetland, Mikkel Østergaard, Anja Thormann, Anne Rødgaard Andersen; Århus: Ulrik Tarp; Gråsten: Uta Engling Poulsen; Vejle: Jakob Espesen; Aalborg: Vibeke Stevenius Ringsdal, Anette Schlemmer; Rigshospitalet: Niels Graudal; Frederiksberg: Gina Kollerup; Helsingør: Dorte Vendelbo Jensen; Gentofte: Ole Rintek Madsen, Annette Hansen; Holbæk: Bente Glintborg, Randi Pelck; Slagelse: Torben Grube Christensen; Odense: Hanne Lindegaard; Esbjerg: Ditte Dencker, Wolfgang Bøhme. The DANBIO secretariat (Hanne Bagger Christiansen, Sandra Zbinden Pedersen, Cecilie Lindstrøm Egholm) is acknowledged for its assistance. Niels Steen Krogh, Zitelab Aps is acknowledged for data management. The Departments of Radiology at the study hospitals are acknowledged for their help in collecting analogue and digitised radiographs. The Copenhagen Osteoarthritis Study and the Copenhagen City Heart Study is acknowledged for the collection of x-rays in the reference cohort.

Funding

The work of LMØ was financed by a clinical Ph.d. grant from the University of Copenhagen. Danish Regions (i.e. the hospital owners) gave financial support to DANBIO. Janssen Biologics (formerly Centocor) supported the collection and scoring of x-rays with an unrestricted grant and Sectra performed the DXR-BMD analysis without costs. Abbott, Pfizer (formerly Wyeth) and MSD (formerly Schering-Plough) (since 2004), Bristol-Myers Squibb and Roche (since 2006), and UCB-Nordic (since 2007) have supported DANBIO with unrestricted grants. The sponsors have had no influence on data collection, analysis or publication.

Data sharing

Data are available upon request for academic researchers.

Author details

[1]DANBIO registry and Copenhagen Center for Arthritis Research, Center for Rheumatology and Spine Diseases, Centre of Head and Orthopedics, Ndr. Ringvej 57, DK-2600 Glostrup, Denmark. [2]Rigshospitalet, Department of Clinical Medicine, Faculty of Health and Medical Sciences, University of

Copenhagen, Copenhagen, Denmark. [3]Department of Endocrinology, Hvidovre Hospital, Hvidovre, Denmark. [4]Department of Rheumatology, Diakonhjemmet Hospital, Oslo, Norway. [5]Department of Rheumatology, Aarhus University Hospital, Aarhus, Denmark. [6]Department of Medicine, Hospital of South West Jutland, Esbjerg, Denmark. [7]Department of Rheumatology, Odense University Hospital, Odense, Denmark. [8]Rheumatism Hospital, University of Southern Denmark, Gråsten, Denmark. [9]Department of Rheumatology, Aalborg University Hospital, Aalborg, Denmark. [10]Department of Infectious Diseases and Rheumatology, Copenhagen University Hospital Rigshospitalet Blegdamsvej, Copenhagen, Denmark. [11]Center for Rheumatology and Spine Diseases, Rigshospitalet Glostrup, Glostrup, Denmark. [12]Department of Internal Medicine, Lillebælt Hospital, Vejle, Denmark. [13]Department of Rheumatology, Copenhagen University Hospital Bispebjerg and Frederiksberg, Copenhagen, Denmark. [14]Department of Internal Medicine, Holbæk Hospital, Holbæk, Denmark. [15]Department of Medicine and Rheumatology, Copenhagen University Hospital Gentofte, Gentofte, Denmark. [16]Department of Rheumatology, Nordsjællands Hospital, Hillerød, Denmark.

References

1. Arnett FC, Edworthy SM, Bloch DA, McShane DJ, Fries JF, Cooper NS, et al. The American Rheumatism Association 1987 revised criteria for the classification of rheumatoid arthritis. Arthritis Rheum. 1987;1988(31):315–24.
2. Schett G. Osteoimmunology in rheumatic diseases. Arthritis Res Ther. 2009;11:210.
3. Hoff M, Haugeberg G, Kvien TK. Hand bone loss as an outcome measure in established rheumatoid arthritis: 2-year observational study comparing cortical and total bone loss. Arthritis Res Ther. 2007;9:R81.
4. Sharp JT, Tsuji W, Ory P, Harper-Barek C, Wang H, Newmark R. Denosumab prevents metacarpal shaft cortical bone loss in patients with erosive rheumatoid arthritis. Arthritis Care Res (Hoboken). 2010;62:537–44.
5. Hoff M, Kvien TK, Kalvesten J, Elden A, Haugeberg G. Adalimumab therapy reduces hand bone loss in early rheumatoid arthritis: explorative analyses from the PREMIER study. Ann Rheum Dis. 2009;68:1171–6.
6. Forslind K, Boonen A, Albertsson K, Hafstrom I, Svensson B. Hand bone loss measured by digital X-ray radiogrammetry is a predictor of joint damage in early rheumatoid arthritis. ScandJ Rheumatol. 2009;38:431–8.
7. Hoff M, Haugeberg G, Odegard S, Syversen S, Landewe R, van der Heijde D, et al. Cortical hand bone loss after 1 year in early rheumatoid arthritis predicts radiographic hand joint damage at 5-year and 10-year follow-up. Ann Rheum Dis. 2009;68:324–9.
8. Kapetanovic MC, Lindqvist E, Algulin J, Jonsson K, Saxne T, Eberhardt K, et al. Early changes in bone mineral density measured by digital X-ray radiogrammetry predict up to 20 years radiological outcome in rheumatoid arthritis. Arthritis Res Ther. 2011;13:R31.
9. Jensen TW, Hansen MS, Horslev-Petersen K, Hyldstrup L, Abrahamsen B, Langdahl B, et al. Periarticular and generalised bone loss in patients with early rheumatoid arthritis: influence of alendronate and intra-articular glucocorticoid treatment. Post hoc analyses from the CIMESTRA trial. Ann Rheum Dis. 2014;73:1123–39.
10. de Rooy DP, Kalvesten J, Huizinga TW, van der Helm-van Mil AH. Loss of metacarpal bone density predicts RA development in recent-onset arthritis. Rheumatology (Oxford). 2012;51:1037–41.
11. Toledo VA, Jergas M. Age-related changes in cortical bone mass: data from a German female cohort. Eur Radiol. 2006;16:811–7.
12. Bottcher J, Pfeil A, Schafer ML, Petrovitch A, Seidl BE, Mentzel HJ, et al. Normative data for digital X-ray radiogrammetry from a female and male German cohort. J Clin Densitom. 2006;9:341–50.
13. Guler-Yuksel M, Allaart CF, Goekoop-Ruiterman YP, de Vries-Bouwstra JK, van Groenendael JH, Mallee C, et al. Changes in hand and generalised bone mineral density in patients with recent-onset rheumatoid arthritis. Ann Rheum Dis. 2009;68:330–6.
14. Laxafoss E, Jacobsen S, Gosvig KK, Sonne-Holm S. Case definitions of knee osteoarthritis in 4,151 unselected subjects: relevance for epidemiological studies: the Copenhagen Osteoarthritis Study. Skeletal Radiol. 2010;39:859–66.
15. Hetland ML. DANBIO—powerful research database and electronic patient record. Rheumatology (Oxford). 2011;50:69–77.
16. Ornbjerg LM, Ostergaard M, Boyesen P, Krogh NS, Thormann A, Tarp U, et al. Impact of tumour necrosis factor inhibitor treatment on radiographic progression in rheumatoid arthritis patients in clinical practice: results from the nationwide Danish DANBIO registry. Ann Rheum Dis. 2012;72:57–63.
17. Ornbjerg LM, Ostergaard M, Boyesen P, Krogh NS, Thormann A, Tarp U, et al. Which factors influence radiographic progression during treatment with tumor necrosis factor inhibitors in clinical practice? Results from 930 patients with rheumatoid arthritis in the nationwide Danish DANBIO registry. J Rheumatol. 2014;41:2352–60.
18. van der Heijde D. How to read radiographs according to the Sharp/van der Heijde method. J Rheumatol. 1999;26:743–5.
19. van der Heijde D, Simon L, Smolen J, Strand V, Sharp J, Boers M, et al. How to report radiographic data in randomized clinical trials in rheumatoid arthritis: guidelines from a roundtable discussion. Arthritis Rheum. 2002;47:215–8.
20. Rankin G, Stokes M. Reliability of assessment tools in rehabilitation: an illustration of appropriate statistical analyses. Clin Rehabil. 1998;12:187–99.
21. Bruynesteyn K, Boers M, Kostense P, van der Linden S, van der Heijde D. Deciding on progression of joint damage in paired films of individual patients: smallest detectable difference or change. Ann Rheum Dis. 2005;64:179–82.
22. Bottcher J, Pfeil A, Rosholm A, Schafer ML, Malich A, Petrovitch A, et al. Computerized digital imaging techniques provided by digital X-ray radiogrammetry as new diagnostic tool in rheumatoid arthritis. J Digit Imaging. 2006;19:279–88.
23. Hoff M, Dhainaut A, Kvien TK, Forslind K, Kalvesten J, Haugeberg G. Short-time in vitro and in vivo precision of direct digital X-ray radiogrammetry. J Clin Densitom. 2009;12:17–21.
24. Hoff M, Boyesen P, Haugeberg G, Vis M, Woolf AD, Havaardsholm EA, et al. High disease activity is a predictor of cortical hand bone loss in post-menopausal patients with established rheumatoid arthritis: a 5-year multicentre longitudinal study. Rheumatology (Oxford). 2010;49:1676–82.
25. Matthews JN, Altman DG, Campbell MJ, Royston P. Analysis of serial measurements in medical research. BMJ. 1990;300:230–5.
26. [http://www.r-project.org/]. Accessed 20 Feb 2015.
27. Rosholm A, Hyldstrup L, Backsgaard L, Grunkin M, Thodberg HH. Estimation of bone mineral density by digital X-ray radiogrammetry: theoretical background and clinical testing. Osteoporosis Int. 2001;12:961–9.
28. Berntsen GK, Fonnebo V, Tollan A, Sogaard AJ, Magnus JH. Forearm bone mineral density by age in 7,620 men and women: the Tromso study, a population-based study. Am J Epidemiol. 2001;153:465–73.
29. Melton 3rd LJ, Khosla S, Atkinson EJ, Oconnor MK, Ofallon WM, Riggs BL. Cross-sectional versus longitudinal evaluation of bone loss in men and women. Osteoporosis Int. 2000;11:592–9.
30. Welsing PM, Landewe RB, van Riel PL, Boers M, van Gestel AM, van der Linden S, et al. The relationship between disease activity and radiologic progression in patients with rheumatoid arthritis: a longitudinal analysis. Arthritis Rheum. 2004;50:2082–93.
31. Goldring SR. Periarticular bone changes in rheumatoid arthritis: pathophysiological implications and clinical utility. Ann Rheum Dis. 2009;68:297–9.
32. Lukas C, Braun J, van der Heijde D, Hermann KG, Rudwaleit M, Ostergaard M, et al. Scoring inflammatory activity of the spine by magnetic resonance imaging in ankylosing spondylitis: a multireader experiment. J Rheumatol. 2007;34:862–70.
33. Klareskog L, van der Heijde D, de Jager JP, Gough A, Kalden J, Malaise M, et al. Therapeutic effect of the combination of etanercept and methotrexate compared with each treatment alone in patients with rheumatoid arthritis: double-blind randomised controlled trial. Lancet. 2004;363:675–81.
34. Breedveld FC, Emery P, Keystone E, Patel K, Furst DE, Kalden JR, et al. Infliximab in active early rheumatoid arthritis. Ann Rheum Dis. 2004;63:149–55.

12

Early biomarkers of joint damage in rheumatoid and psoriatic arthritis

Angela Mc Ardle[1], Brian Flatley[1], Stephen R. Pennington[1*†] and Oliver FitzGerald[1,2*†]

Abstract

Joint destruction, as evidenced by radiographic findings, is a significant problem for patients suffering from rheumatoid arthritis and psoriatic arthritis. Inherently irreversible and frequently progressive, the process of joint damage begins at and even before the clinical onset of disease. However, rheumatoid and psoriatic arthropathies are heterogeneous in nature and not all patients progress to joint damage. It is therefore important to identify patients susceptible to joint destruction in order to initiate more aggressive treatment as soon as possible and thereby potentially prevent irreversible joint damage. At the same time, the high cost and potential side effects associated with aggressive treatment mean it is also important not to over treat patients and especially those who, even if left untreated, would not progress to joint destruction. It is therefore clear that a protein biomarker signature that could predict joint damage at an early stage would support more informed clinical decisions on the most appropriate treatment regimens for individual patients. Although many candidate biomarkers for rheumatoid and psoriatic arthritis have been reported in the literature, relatively few have reached clinical use and as a consequence the number of prognostic biomarkers used in rheumatology has remained relatively static for several years. It has become evident that a significant challenge in the transition of biomarker candidates to clinical diagnostic assays lies in the development of suitably robust biomarker assays, especially multiplexed assays, and their clinical validation in appropriate patient sample cohorts. Recent developments in mass spectrometry-based targeted quantitative protein measurements have transformed our ability to rapidly develop multiplexed protein biomarker assays. These advances are likely to have a significant impact on the validation of biomarkers in the future. In this review, we have comprehensively compiled a list of candidate biomarkers in rheumatoid and psoriatic arthritis, evaluated the evidence for their potential as biomarkers of bone (joint) damage, and outlined how mass spectrometry-based targeted and multiplexed measurement of candidate biomarker proteins is likely to accelerate their clinical validation and the development of clinical diagnostic tests.

Introduction

Rheumatoid arthritis (RA) and psoriatic arthritis (PsA) are the most prevalent forms of inflammatory arthritis affecting ~1 % and ~ 0.3 to 1 % of the population, respectively [1, 2]. Disease aetiology is unknown but it is thought that both genetic and environmental factors trigger the onset of these arthropathies [3]. The onset of RA and PsA is clinically recognised when a patient presents with symptoms fulfilling disease classification criteria, importantly the American College of Rheumatology criteria for RA and the Classification for Psoriatic Arthritis CASPAR criteria [4, 5]. However, it is recognised that disease onset may occur much earlier, even prior to symptom onset [6, 7]. Several disease-specific characteristics differentiate RA from PsA. For example, rheumatoid factor (RF) is present often at high titre in 80 % of RA patients whereas it is present at low titre in only 13 % of PsA patients. PsA is included among the spondylarthopathies because it shares both clinical features and association with HLAB27 with other spondylarthopathy members. The presence of psoriasis is a hallmark of PsA, although joint involvement may precede skin manifestations in ~10 % of patients. Asymmetric joint involvement is seen commonly in PsA whereas joint involvement in RA follows a symmetrical pattern. Dactylitis, enthesitis, sacroiliitis and interphalangeal joint involvement are also more common in PsA [3].

* Correspondence: Stephen.Pennington@ucd.ie; Oliver.Fitzgerald@ucd.ie
†Equal contributors
[1]Conway Institute of Biomedical Research, University College Dublin, Belfield, Dublin 4, Ireland
[2]Department of Rheumatology, St Vincent's University Hospital, Elm Park, Dublin 4, Ireland

At the cellular level, histological studies have revealed important differences between synovial tissue in RA and PsA [8]. Angiogenesis is dysregulated in both conditions and abnormal vessel morphology and function has been reported. Increased straight, branching vascularisation is a prominent feature observed in RA joints, whereas the formation of elongated, bushy, torturous blood vessels is a more marked feature of the PsA joint [8, 9]. In the RA joint there is increased macrophage infiltration and subsequent synovial invasion compared with that observed in PsA. As a result, lining layer hyperplasia observed in RA is more striking than that observed in PsA [3]. Conversely, PsA is characterised by more extensive infiltration of polymorphonuclear cells [8]. It has been reported that the extent of T-cell and B-cell infiltration is comparable in both conditions and the formation of germinal centres (zones of T-cell and B-cell proliferation) are observed in both PsA and RA joints [8, 10, 11]. The differences in synovitis in RA and PsA are illustrated in Fig. 1.

Radiographic progression

Radiographic progression is considered a consequence of synovial inflammation. However, at least for RA, the observations that bone loss can occur before clinical onset and at very early stages of disease have been widely acknowledged [6, 7]. These observations are surprising since synovitis requires some time to destroy bone to an extent that is clinically detectable. Synovitis might thus not be the exclusive cause of joint damage. An alternative

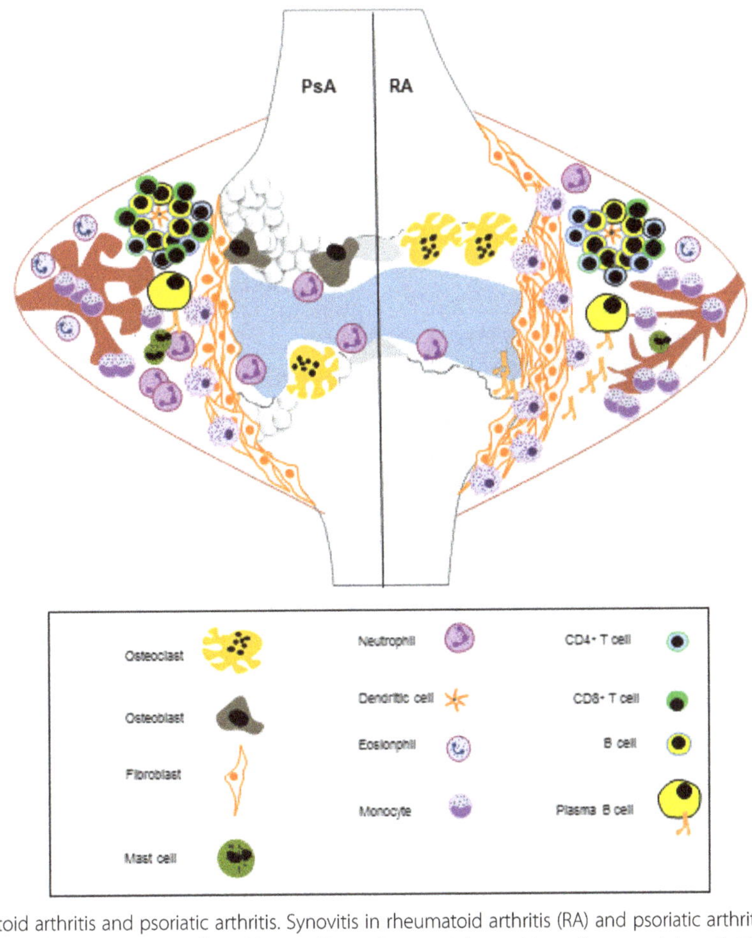

Fig. 1 Synovitis in rheumatoid arthritis and psoriatic arthritis. Synovitis in rheumatoid arthritis (RA) and psoriatic arthritis (PsA) is triggered by unknown event(s). It is thought that a genetic predisposition and/or environmental cues trigger inappropriate activation of synoviocytes, thereby promoting an autoimmune inflammatory response. Once activated, synoviocytes produce proinflammatory cytokines that in turn activate proximal cells, including endothelial cells that line the blood vessels supplying the joint. This results in dysregulated angiogenesis and the increased infiltration of leukocytes, including monocytes, macrophages, neutrophils, mast cells, eosinophils, B cells and T cells. Infiltrating cells produce cytokines that act in synergy to propagate the inflammatory response. Importantly, tumour necrosis factor alpha (TNFα) and interleukin (IL)-17 are cytokines with major implied roles in PsA and RA pathogenesis and represent important therapeutic targets. With the development of a chronic inflammatory response, the synovial lining becomes hyperplastic. Fibroblasts and macrophages form an invasive matrix (pannus) that promotes the destruction of cartilage and bone. Activation of osteoclast cells promotes bone resorption whereas activation of osteoblasts promotes bone proliferation

concept suggests that autoimmune processes begin years before the clinical onset of disease and that these processes promote joint destruction. Indeed, levels of anti-citrullinated protein antibodies (ACPA) can be detected in RA years before the clinical onset of disease. A comparative imaging study used micro computerised tomography to assess bone densities in healthy individuals that were either positive or negative for ACPA. The ACPA-positive individuals exhibited significant alterations in cortical bone architecture as compared with the ACPA-negative individuals. These findings support the theory that bone damage is not exclusively a consequence of synovitis [7].

Previously, PsA was believed to be a mild nonprogressive form of arthritis. However, it is now well understood that 47 % of PsA patients will develop erosions within 2 years of symptom onset, and that of the patients suffering from polyarticular PsA at least 20 % are at risk of progressing to a severe destructive phenotype (mutilans) comparable with that observed in RA [12]. What is more, bone changes observed in PsA are particularly heterogeneous both between and also within individual sufferers (Fig. 2). X-ray images are used in the clinic to follow radiographic progression and may be scored to measure the extent of joint damage. The Sharp–van der Heijde scoring method is most commonly used to measure joint damage in RA. This method provides separate scores for erosion and joint space narrowing in the hands, wrists and feet. A modified Sharp–van der Heijde score is used to measure radiographic progression in PsA where the distal interphalangeal joints of the hands are also included [13, 14].

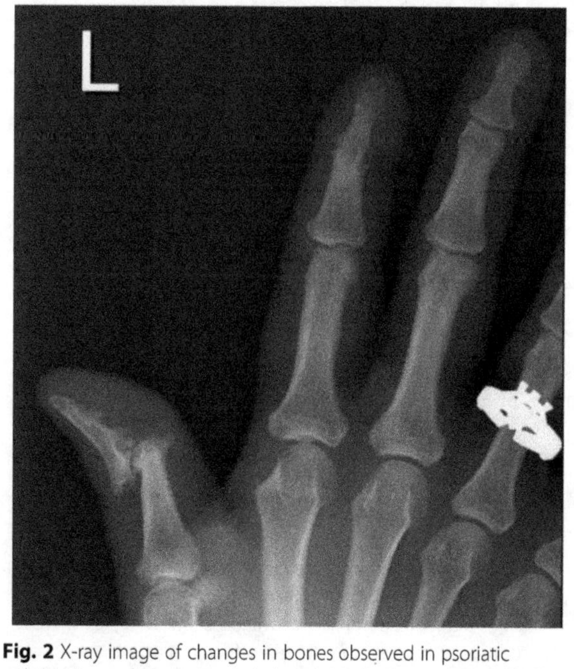

Fig. 2 X-ray image of changes in bones observed in psoriatic arthritis. Bone changes in psoriatic arthritis (PsA) patients may differ between patients and may also differ within the same patient. The heterogeneity observed within a PsA patient is illustrated. Left-hand radiograph from a PsA patient showing severe erosive disease and subluxation at the first distal interphalangeal (DIP) with fluffy periosteal new bone formation on the terminal phalange. Ankylosis of the second DIP joint is also demonstrated

While X-ray imaging is the best validated technique for detecting bone erosion, it is limited by its two-dimensional character. Additional imaging modalities such as magnetic resonance imaging, micro computerised tomography and ultrasound are utilised to identify distinguishing features between RA and PsA. Radiographic progression in RA and PsA is remarkably different. RA is a bone-resorbing, erosive disease whereas the pattern of radiographic progression in PsA is more complex. As in RA, bone resorption and erosion may be evident in PsA, but radiographic progression may also be marked by more severe resorption or osteolysis and commonly bony proliferation is prominent. To the best of our knowledge early protein biomarkers of bone proliferation have not yet been reported in the literature, but these markers will probably differ from biomarkers of erosion. Distinguishing patterns of disease progression in RA and PsA have been captured by different imaging modalities and are summarised in Table 1.

Biomarkers

Molecular events that drive joint damage may precede disease onset and can cause detrimental long-term effects such as disability [6, 7, 10, 15, 16]. It is therefore essential to begin therapy as soon as possible in order to prevent irreversible damage. Some of the therapies currently available are associated with high cost and potential for side effects. Additionally, up to 40 % of patients will not meet the primary outcome measure and, in those who do respond, levels of disease activity can remain significant. To add to the complexity, not all patients will develop a destructive form of disease. Aggressive treatment should thus be reserved for patients that will develop a more severe form of disease [17]. In light of this, the need to develop biomarker signatures predictive of joint damage in RA and PsA is of critical importance. Currently there is a major international effort driven by the Outcome Measures in Rheumatology Clinical Trials and the Group for Research and Assessment in Psoriasis and Psoriatic Arthritis well underway in RA and to start soon in PsA whereby biomarker samples are being prospectively collected in an effort to identify predictors of radiographic damage.

Biomarkers serve as objective molecular indicators of pathological processes such as the development of joint destruction. Owing to the heterogeneous nature of RA and PsA, identifying a single biomarker predictive of joint damage would be an onerous task. Indeed, no single biomarker has so far emerged as a reliable predictor

Table 1 Radiological features that distinguish between rheumatoid arthritis and psoriatic arthritis

Disease feature	Rheumatoid arthritis	Psoriatic arthritis	Imaging technique	Reference
Number of erosions	+++	+	X-ray	[18]
	+++	+++	μCT	[82]
Severity of erosions	+++	++	μCT	[83]
Shape of erosions				
Ʊ	+	+++	μCT	[83]
Tubule	+	+++	μCT	
U	+++	+	μCT	
Erosion distribution	Preponderance for radial sites	Evenly distributed	μCT	[83]
DIP joint erosion	–	+++	US, MRI, X-ray	[84]
Number of osteophytes	+	+++	μCT	[82]
Severity of osteophytes (size)	+	+++	μCT	[82]
Bone proliferation	+	+++	US, MRI, X-ray	[84]
Inflammatory changes				
Synovitis	+++	++	MRI, US	[84]
Tenosynovitis	+++	++	MRI, US	[84]
Enthesitis	+	+++	MRI, US	[85]
Dactylitis	–	+++	US, MRI	[86]
Mutilans (erosions on both sides of joints)		+	X-ray	[87]

Disease features present in RA and PsA and the radiological imaging technique used to measure the feature. The number of erosions observed in RA appears to be greater than that in PsA. However, more sophisticated higher resolution techniques reveal this is not accurate because erosions in PsA are generally smaller and their detection requires these more sensitive techniques. Hence, μCT reveals a comparable extent of bone erosion in RA and PsA. MRI and US capture differences in sites affected by inflammation in these disorders. In PsA it is the enthesis that are major sites of inflammation, whereas in RA the synovium becomes chronically inflamed. Inflammation of the tendons is also prevalent in both disorders although more severe in RA. Distinct features of PsA include bony proliferation, and dactylitis. DIP, distal interphalangeal; μCT, micro computational tomography; MRI, magnetic resonance imaging; PsA, psoriatic arthritis; RA, rheumatoid arthritis; US, ultrasound

of damage in RA [18–20]. Consequently there is great interest in identifying a panel of biomarkers that could be incorporated into a signature predictive of disease progression. Such a signature could be used as an indicator of joint destruction and thus facilitate clinicians in making more informed clinical decisions and help guide personalised medical approaches [18, 20]. It is important to recognise that joint destruction contributes significantly to disability in patients suffering from inflammatory arthritis, but it is not the sole cause of disability. Joint inflammation, swelling, pain and disability occur in the absence of joint destruction [21]. In PsA, for example, there are many debilitating phenotypes of disease but not all PsA phenotypes include bone erosion [22]. It would be useful to have a biomarker that distinguishes between different disease phenotypes (for example, progressors from nonprogressors). Such a biomarker would help inform the clinical decision of whether to treat symptoms only or to adopt a more aggressive treatment strategy in order to prevent radiographic progression.

The aim of this review is to identify previously published reports that include proteins predictive of joint damage at early disease time points. Joint damage is most definitively measured by radiographic progression. Hence this review is limited to observational prospective cohort studies that used radiographic progression as a measure of joint destruction and included patients with early-stage disease at baseline. Observational studies are considered inferior to randomised control trials due to the fact that results can be influenced by confounding factors such as a patient's response to therapy. Biomarkers predictive of joint damage at baseline in a treatment-naïve patient may not be predictive after initiation of therapy due to the suppressive effect of the pharmacological intervention on inflammatory mediators. However, evidence derived from well-designed prospective cohort studies that follow patients longitudinally and correct for confounding factors is considered important in the clinical decision-making process and is comparable with that provided by randomised control trials [23, 24]. Limiting this approach, there is a paucity of early cohort studies in PsA in which radiographic progression is measured. As disease activity and changes in tissue organisation may serve as surrogate measures of joint damage, we have included soluble biomarkers that correlated with these disease parameters in the PsA studies reviewed. In addition, the potential opportunities afforded by new mass spectrometry-based protein measurement approaches will be highlighted. These methods are reaching clinical diagnostics application and have the potential to change dramatically the landscape of protein biomarkers.

Biomarkers of joint damage in rheumatoid arthritis

Markers of the acute phase response

Inflammation in the synovium is reflected by a systemic inflammatory response. Increased erythrocyte sedimentation rate (ESR) and hepatocyte production of acute phase proteins including C-reactive protein (CRP) and acute phase serum amyloid A (A-SAA) are surrogate markers of this process. The acute phase response has been considered important in the context of RA as it mirrors synovial inflammation. CRP and the ESR have been shown to correlate with radiographic progression and these indices have been incorporated into composite scores typically used to predict damage. However, these are general markers of inflammation; they are not disease specific. Furthermore, CRP and the ESR remain normal in a proportion of RA patients that may progress – and thus additional and more sensitive predictors are required. One RA cohort study which incorporated patients with a range of disease durations showed that A-SAA correlated with radiographic progression. It would be interesting to investigate the correlation of A-SAA with joint damage in an early cohort as this protein reflects not only systemic but also local inflammation [25].

Auto-antibodies

Auto-antibodies such as RF and ACPA are very useful prognostic markers in RA. It has previously been reported that patients positive for ACPA or RF are more likely to develop erosions compared with those who are negative for both. Additionally it was reported that those who were positive for ACPA and negative for RF were more likely to progress to a severe disease state compared with those who were RF-positive but ACPA-negative. Furthermore it was noted that patients positive for both ACPA and RF were at greatest risk of disease progression [26–28]. ACPA emerge as the most useful indicator of joint damage. Indeed, RF is quite limited in its ability to predict damage because this antibody is not disease specific. Moreover RF is considered useful only at early disease time points, and its predictive power is lost as disease progresses. In contrast, in addition to being more sensitive, ACPA are more disease specific and useful at both early and later disease time points [26, 29]. There exist, however, subgroups of patients who are susceptible to joint damage but who test negative for both RF and ACPA. Since RF and ACPA have been proven very useful indicators of damage, the identification of novel auto-antibodies may prove advantageous especially in patients who lack RF and ACPA. It was reported recently that a distinct family of auto-antibodies which recognise carbamylated antigens, the anti-carbamylated protein antibodies, are predictive of a severe disease course in early RA patients even after correction for RF and ACPA. It was demonstrated that patients who were positive for immunoglobulin G anti-carbamylated protein antibodies but negative for ACPA developed a more severe disease course compared with patients who were ACPA-positive only. Those who were positive for both anti-carbamylated protein antibodies and ACPA were comparable in severity [30]. Anti-carbamylated protein antibodies might thus prove a useful biomarker in RA, and their ability to predict joint damage warrants further research.

Cytokines and chemokines

Cytokines play a major role in promoting joint damage and their association with radiographic progression has been investigated in several early RA cohort studies. It has been reported separately that elevated levels of interleukin (IL)-6, IL-16, IL-22, IL-33, chemokine ligand (CCL)11 and chemokine (C-X-C) motif ligand (CXCL)13 are predictive of radiographic progression [31–35]. The finding that IL-6 was associated with joint damage is controversial, however, and contradictory findings have been reported. Klein-Wieringa and colleagues demonstrated that elevated levels of IL-6 were not significantly correlated with radiographic progression in an early RA cohort [36]. This is in disagreement with Knudsen and colleagues, who demonstrated that IL-6 was a strong independent predictor of radiographic progression [31]. These controversial findings might be explained in part by differences in study design. Klein-Wieringa and colleagues measured serum levels of IL-6 in a large RA cohort consisting of 253 patients. Patients enrolled in this study received three different treatment strategies. Radiographic progression was assessed over 4 years using the Sharp–van der Heijde scoring method. Multivariate regression analysis was used to find an association between levels of IL-6 and disease progression. This model corrected for confounding factors including therapeutic intervention. In contrast, Knudsen and colleagues measured plasma levels of IL-6 in a smaller RA cohort consisting of 51 patients and treatment change was permitted over the duration of the study. Radiographic progression was measured using the Larsen method. Levels of IL-6 were measured 13 times over 2 years and the mean concentration (area under the curve) of IL-6 measurements over 24 months were used to associate levels of IL-6 with bone erosions observed at 12 and 24 months [31, 36]. Conversely, a study by van Leeuwen and colleagues demonstrated that elevated levels of plasma IL-6 were not predictive of damage [37]. However, the IL-6 assay used during this study was less sensitive than that used by

Knudsen and colleagues [31]. The differential findings in relation to IL-6 highlight the impact of study design on reported findings in the literature. Single reports provide evidence that IL-16, IL-22, IL-33, CCL11 and CXCL13 retain prognostic capacity in early RA. It was interesting to note that CCL11 was associated with reduced radiographic progression and thus may have a protective role during pathogenesis [33]. Additional studies should be carried out to validate the finding that the aforementioned molecules independently correlate with radiographic progression.

Adipokines

Adipokines are cytokines produced by fat cells. These proteins are elevated in patients with RA, where they are thought to have potent immunomodulatory effects. A study by Rho and colleagues demonstrated that adiponectin, visfatin and leptin correlated with measures of radiographic progression. Adiponectin and visfatin were shown to correlate with increased radiographic progression, whereas leptin was associated with reduced progression [38]. Klein-Wieringa and colleagues confirmed the finding that adiponectin is predictive of radiographic progression in patients with early RA [36].

Calprotectin

Calprotectin is released from activated leukocytes that derive mainly from the inflamed synovium in RA patients. A recent cohort study by Hammer and colleagues demonstrated that RA patients with higher baseline levels of calprotectin developed more severe radiographic damage after 10 years compared with patients with lower levels of calprotectin. Furthermore, calprotectin levels measured at baseline and at 10 years significantly correlated with radiographic damage after 10 years. The correlation observed for calprotectin was similar to that observed for CRP and ESR [39]. Taken together these results can lead to the conclusion that calprotectin is more specific and just as sensitive at predicting joint damage as CRP and may provide valuable information in the context of a biomarker signature predictive of joint damage.

Markers of angiogenesis

Angiogenesis is central to the development of RA synovitis and thus assessing levels of angiogenic markers in RA patients may prove useful for predicting joint damage. Vascular endothelial growth factor (VEGF) is thought to be the most important mediator of angiogenesis and there is good evidence to suggest that this molecule should be considered a candidate marker of joint damage in RA [40, 41]. A study by Ballara and colleagues demonstrated in early RA that elevated VEGF levels at inclusion significantly correlated with radiographic progression after 1 year [41]. Clavel and colleagues confirmed the finding that VEGF was predictive of joint damage in early RA patients. Additional analysis revealed that VEGF levels at inclusion were correlated with initial Sharp scores and Sharp scores measured after 1 year. It was also demonstrated that levels of angiopoeitin-1 (a marker of angiogenesis) were predictive of damage at inclusion and after 1 year. This finding suggests that VEGF and angiopotietin-1 remain predicative at later disease stages after initiation of therapy [40].

Products of collagen degradation

Fragments released as a result of type I and type II collagen degradation – including C-terminal telopeptide of collagen (CTX)I and CTXII, collagen type II degradation product epitopes C2C and C1,2C as well as matrix proteins such as cartilage oligomatrix protein (COMP) – are reflective of bone and cartilage damage. Several studies have investigated the association of these molecules with radiographic progression in early RA patients. Three authors reported that elevated levels of CTXI and CTXII are associated with long-term radiographic progression in early RA patients [42–44]. What is more, Garnero and colleagues reported that CTXI and CTXII were even more predictive of joint damage compared with CRP and ESR [42]. Bakker and colleagues found that elevated baseline levels of C1,2C were associated with radiographic progression after 1 year of treatment [45]. Additionally Verstappen and colleagues demonstrated that C2C significantly correlated with radiographic progression after 1 year and importantly remained predictive the following year [46]. Andersson and colleagues demonstrated that increments in COMP levels during a 3-month period following diagnosis were predictive of joint damage at 1-year, 2-year and 5-year follow-up [47]. The culmination of positive findings makes these degradation products attractive candidates for a biomarker panel predictive of joint damage.

Enzyme mediators of destruction

The association of matrix metalloproteinase (MMPs), proteases that promote cartilage breakdown, with joint damage has also been investigated. Previous early RA cohort studies demonstrated that elevated levels of MMP-3 at baseline correlate significantly with radiographic progression [48–50]. However, another study documented that serial, longitudinal measurements of MMP-3 fail to correlate with measures of joint damage [51]. It can thus be speculated that MMP-3 may be a useful predictive marker of joint destruction at disease onset prior to treatment. MMP-1 might also have prognostic utility and its association with joint damage has been assessed. Previously, elevated baseline levels of MMP-1 were demonstrated to significantly correlate with radiographic progression observed at 12 months [49]. It has also been reported that serial measurements of MMP-1 over a period of 18 months correlate significantly with measures of joint damage [51]. In contrast, Young-Min and colleagues found no correlation between levels of MMP-1 and joint damage in early RA patients [50]. It is certainly possible that differences in study design and data analysis gave rise to these discrepancies, and the relationship between MMP-1 and joint damage warrants further investigation.

Biomarkers of joint damage in psoriatic arthritis

Cytokines

The cytokine expression profile in the PsA synovium is relatively similar to that observed in RA [8]. IL-17 has emerged as an important cytokine in autoimmune diseases and this protein in synergy with tumour necrosis factor alpha contributes to pathogenesis in RA and PsA. It has previously been demonstrated that, compared with osteoarthritic controls, levels of IL-17 are elevated in the synovial tissue of patients with PsA and RA (no significant difference between the two). It was also demonstrated that in vitro stimulation of synovial tissue with IL-17 induced proteins involved in matrix turnover and cartilage destruction [52].

There are very few studies reporting the association of soluble cytokines with joint damage in PsA. However, cytokines that segregate patients with polyarthritis from those with oligoarticular disease have been identified. In an early PsA cohort, elevated levels of IL-1 were detected in the synovial fluid of polyarthritic patients compared with those with monoarthritis, suggesting that this protein is a marker of disease progression [53]. A Norwegian cohort found that elevated levels of IL-12p40, interferon alpha, IL-15 and CCL3 could segregate PsA patients with polyarticular disease from those with oligoarticular disease [54]. Since patients with polyarthritis have more severe joint involvement, these molecules might drive progression and would be interesting to investigate in the context of early PsA.

Calgranulin (S100A8/S100A9)

A study by Kane and colleagues demonstrated that elevated levels of calgranulin (S100A8/S100A9) correlated with measures of disease activity and markers of intra-articular inflammation (white blood cell counts). The study further demonstrated that treatment with methotrexate resulted in a significant decrease in S100A8/S100A9 levels. A significant reduction in swollen joint count, Richie articular index and Disease Activity Score was also observed after treatment, suggesting that S100A8/S100A9 may also correlate with joint damage in PsA [55]. Additional evidence reporting an association between S100A8/S100A9 with progressive disease exists. A study by Aochi and colleagues demonstrated that S100A8/S100A9 levels in PsA patients (disease duration not specified) with more than 10 affected joints were higher compared with levels in those who had less than 10 affected joints [56]. These results together suggest that S100A8/S100A9 may be associated with joint damage and that this marker might provide additional information in the context of a biomarker signature.

Markers of angiogenesis

The ability of angiogenic markers to predict joint damage in RA has been reported [41, 57]. Abnormalities in angiogenesis are more pronounced in PsA compared with RA and levels of VEGF and angiopotietin-2 have been reported to be higher during PsA relative to RA [56]. It is thus logical to conclude that these molecules could act as early markers of radiographic progression, but there is a lack of data in the literature to validate this hypothesis. Interestingly, the association of VEGF with active versus inactive disease and with changes in synovial vascular morphology has been described [56–58].

Molecules that regulate bone turnover

Dalbeth and colleagues examined the association between soluble mediators of bone remodelling (receptor activator of nuclear factor-κB ligand, osteoprotegerin, wnt signalling pathway inhibitor-1, macrophage colony-stimulating factor) with radiographic progression in PsA patients with established disease duration. A positive correlation between macrophage colony-stimulating factor and receptor activator of nuclear factor-κB ligand concentrations with radiographic progression was described [59]. Connolly and colleagues found that baseline levels of A-SAA were independently associated with 1-year radiographic progression in PsA patients with long disease duration. A-SAA promotes the production of MMPs by fibroblast-like synoviocytes. A-SAA levels were demonstrated to correlate with MMP-1, MMP-3, MMP-13 and MMP/tissue inhibitor of matrix metalloproteinases [25]. Since it has been demonstrated previously that MMP-1 and MMP-3 are associated with radiographic progression in early RA, it could be speculated that an association between A-SAA and MMPs might correlate with radiographic progression in early PsA – this warrants further research.

An emerging mass spectrometry technology

The development of a protein biomarker identified in discovery experiments for clinical assay is both long and challenging [60]. The clinical validation of candidate biomarkers has traditionally relied on the development of antibody-based assays. Enzyme-linked immunosorbent assays (ELISAs) are one of the most widely used methods for clinical diagnostic protein biomarker measurements [61, 62].

Large numbers of candidate biomarkers are emerging and it has become apparent that an alternative technology is required to evaluate them in a time- and cost-effective manner [63, 64]. The relatively recent introduction of a multiple reaction monitoring (MRM) mass spectrometry platform for the measurement of peptides has provided the opportunity to develop multiplexed assays for simultaneously measuring multiple candidate biomarkers and to progress them through the biomarker development pipeline [65]. There are a number of key drivers for the adoption of MRM as a viable alternative to the traditional antibody-based approach. The economics of MRM analysis far outweigh methods requiring antibodies (western blot or ELISA). Good antibodies are relatively expensive and in some cases not always available for the proteins of interest. Even for proteins for which antibodies are available, the length of time needed to optimise an assay using MRM mass spectrometry is much shorter relative to that using antibody-based protein detection [63, 64].

MRM assays are developed for peptides released from proteolytically cleaved proteins. A peptide that is unique to the protein of interest (a proteotypic peptide, generally ranging from 7 to 25 amino acids in length) and that is routinely observed by the mass spectrometer is crucial to guaranteeing accurate detection of specific proteins [66]. By measuring only selected proteotypic peptides, the abundance of selected proteins can be definitively established [65, 67, 68]. In MRM mode, only those peptides of interest pass through the mass spectrometer by setting the first quadrupole to filter based on the known mass/charge ratio of the peptide. In the second quadrupole the peptides are then fragmented and will produce fragments of known size. The third quadrupole is then used to filter these fragments, allowing them to pass to a detector. The prior knowledge of peptide sequences is used to direct the mass spectrometry in MRM mode. The triple-quadrupole mass spectrometer can be set to filter hundreds of peptides in the first quadrupole and thousands of peptide fragments (transitions) in the third quadrupole, thereby enabling many proteins to be measured. Therefore, for example, in a typical analytical run (<30 minutes) it is possible to measure hundreds of peptides [69, 70], which is analogous to performing hundreds of western blot analyses or ELISAs within a 30-minute timeframe. Indeed the MRM approach has been implemented in several large-scale biomarker studies over the past couple of years. These assays have so far proved particularly useful in the field of toxicology and oncology [71–73]. This technique has not yet been exploited to its full potential in rheumatology, but evidence supporting its potential utility does exist. For example, an MRM assay was developed for CRP and this assay was then used to distinguish progressive from nonprogressive arthritic patients [74]. More recently, Ademowo and colleagues developed an MRM assay for a panel of 57 synovial tissue proteins. This assay was then used to predict PsA patients who responded well to therapy compared with those who did not respond [75].

Luminex technology is another example of a multiplex platform for biomarker validation. This technology is based on polystyrene beads that are coated with specific capture antibodies and impregnated with dyes of different intensities. Interrogation of the beads with lasers results in the identification of a bead and hence an analyte due to its unique spectral properties [76]. The luminex is cable of measuring proteins that span a low dynamic range ($<10^3$) which would not be detected by MRM. In addition to being a high-throughput assay, the sensitivity and specificity of the luminex technique is comparable with the ELISA [77, 78]. This technology is limited, however, by availability of antibodies against proteins of interest, high cost and the quantity of sample required for analysis [78].

Conclusions

In relation to what has been shown to date, considerably more candidate biomarkers have been identified in RA compared with PsA (Table 2). No single biomarker has been validated as a potent predictor of joint damage and it is well recognised that a multi-biomarker panel is needed to compensate for the heterogeneity between individuals. A multi-biomarker panel incorporating 12 serum proteins has been shown to accurately reflect disease activity in RA [18]. This panel of proteins may be measured using a blood-based test referred to as a multi-biomarker disease activity (MBDA) test. Concentrations of the 12 biomarkers are incorporated into an algorithm that provides a low, moderate or high disease activity score as an output [18]. A recent study has shown that the MBDA test correlates well with measures of CRP, but there may also be discordance between levels of CRP and the MBDA test. In patients with both low levels of CRP and a low MBDA score, radiographic progression is infrequent. In contrast, in patients with low levels of CRP but a high MBDA score, a significant proportion developed radiographic progression during 1 year of follow-up. Levels of the multi-biomarker panel (which include CRP) thus better predict radiographic progression than CRP alone [79]. In a further study the MBDA test has been shown to predict risk of radiographic progression and outperform CRP as a predictive biomarker in the SWEFOT cohort trial. In this trial, only patients with a high MBDA score were at risk of developing radiographic progression. In contrast, a substantial proportion of patients with low, moderate and high levels of CRP were at risk of developing joint damage [80]. Finally, the ability of the MBDA score to predict joint damage has been demonstrated in an additional trial that included 163 patients from the Leiden Early Arthritis Cohort. The MBDA score and the Disease

Table 2 Candidate biomarkers of joint damage in rheumatoid arthritis and psoriatic arthritis

Candidate biomarker	Evidence for role in inflammatory arthritis	Use
Inflammatory proteins		
C-reactive protein	Opsonisation and compliment activation	RA
Calprotectin (S100A12)	Ca^{2+} binding protein released upon phagocyte activation, important intracellular and extracellular roles	RA/PsA
Calgranulin (S100A8/S100A9)	Ca^{2+} binding protein with pleotropic effects. Regulates myeloid derived cells	PsA
A-SAA	Promotes the production of MMPs	RA/PsA
Cytokines		
IL-1	Promotes activation of keratocytes, endothelial cells, chondrocytes and osteoclasts. Promotes the production of proinflammatory cytokines	PsA
IL-6	Promotes neutrophil chemotaxis and production of proinflammatory cytokines, induces an acute phase response	RA
IL-13	Promotes antibody production by B cells	RA
IL-15	Induces T cell proliferation and B cell differentiation. Recruits memory T cells to the synovium and induces TNFα production	PsA
IL-16	Promotes chemotaxis of $CD4^{+}$ T cells, monocytes and eosinophils. Modulates T-cell activation	RA
IL-22	Induces proliferation of fibroblasts and production of MCP-1 (monocyte chemokine)	RA
IL-33	Promotes chronic inflammatory response	RA
Chemokines		
CCL3	Lymphocyte, monocyte, basophil, eosinophil chemoattractant	PsA
CCL11	Eosinophil chemoattractant	PsA
CXCL13	B-cell chemoattractant	RA
Adipokines		
Adiponectin	Induces IL-6 and MMP-1 production by SLFs. Promotes IL-6, TNFα and MCP-1 production in chondrocytes	RA
Visfatin	Role unclear, thought to modulate inflammation	RA
Markers of angiogenesis		
VEGF	Potent inducer of angiogenesis and vascular permeability	RA/PsA
Angiopotietin-1	Promotes angiogenesis (growth of new blood vessels)	RA
Angiopotietin-2	Promotes angiogenesis	PsA
Auto-antibodies		
Rheumatoid factor	Forms immune complexes, promotes complement activation and formation of rheumatoid nodules	RA
Anti-CCP	Promotes complement activation	RA
Anti-Carp	Bind homocitrulline containing proteins	RA
Enzyme mediators of destruction		
MMP-1	Degrades collagen	RA
MMP-3	Degrades collagen	RA
Regulators of bone remodelling		
RANKL	Induces osteoclast bone destruction	PsA
M-CSF	Induces aggressive phenotype in macrophages	PsA
Products of collagen degradation		
COMP	Cartilage oligomatrix protein	RA
CTXI	C-terminal telopeptide of collagen type I	RA
CTXII	C-terminal telopeptide of collagen type I	RA
C1,2C	Collagen type II degradation product	RA
C2C	Collagen type II degradation product	RA

Candidate biomarkers predictive of joint damage in RA and PsA have been identified in the literature. These include inflammatory proteins, cytokines, chemokines, adipokines, markers of angiogenesis, auto-antibodies, enzyme mediators of destruction, molecules that regulate bone turnover and products of collagen degradation. For references see text. A-SAA acute-phase serum amyloid A; anti-Carp, anti-carbamylated protein antibodies; CCL, chemokine ligand; CCP, cyclic citrullinated peptide; CXCL, chemokine (C-X-C) motif ligand; IL, interleukin; M-CSF, macrophage colony stimulating factor; MCP-1, monocyte chemoattractant protein-1; MMP, matrix metalloproteinase; RA, rheumatoid arthritis; PsA, psoriatic arthritis; RANKL, receptor activator of nuclear factor-κB ligand; SLF, synovium-like fibroblasts; TNFα, tumour necrosis factor alpha; VEGF, vascular endothelial growth factor

Activity Score in 28 joints–CRP score were assessed as predictors of radiographic progression. The study found that patients with low MBDA had significantly less radiographic progression than patients who meet Disease Activity Score in 28 joints–CRP European League Against Rheumatism defined remission. It was also shown that patients with a high MBDA score were six times more likely to develop radiographic progression compared with patients with a high Disease Activity Score in 28 joints–CRP score, who were only twice as likely to progress [81].

In conclusion, the MBDA panel has been shown to be a reliable predictor of joint damage across clinical trials. It is tempting to speculate that the incorporation of additional serum proteins into this panel might increase its predictive power. Given the utility of a multi-biomarker panel demonstrated in RA it is also logical to suggest that such a panel might prove clinically useful in PsA. From this literature search it is evident that markers of angiogenesis and bone remodelling represent strong candidates. The predictive ability of such markers might be enhanced if incorporated into a panel with other newly identified molecules. It is interesting to note some markers have been identified exclusively in RA and PsA (Table 2). This identification suggests that distinct pathological mechanisms underpin joint destruction in these disorders. However, this might in part be a consequence of the lag in PsA research. The identification of additional biomarkers, particularly in PsA, should not only provide us with valuable prognostic information but also with a greater mechanistic insight into disease processes. Finally, identifying markers exclusive to one disease condition would also facilitate the development of diagnostic assays.

We suggest that the development of MRM assays for the candidate proteins identified here could be usefully developed to support the evaluation of multiplexed protein signatures that could predict joint damage. These assays could be developed into clinical diagnostic assays and used routinely in a daily practice and this should have a significant positive impact on patient care.

Abbreviations

ACPA: Anti-citrullinated protein antibodies; A-SAA: Acute phase serum amyloid A; CCL: Chemokine ligand; COMP: Cartilage oligomatrix protein; CRP: C-reactive protein; CTX: C-terminal telopeptide of collagen; CXCL: Chemokine (C-X-C) motif ligand; ELISA: Enzyme-linked immunosorbent assay; ESR: Erythrocyte sedimentation rate; IL: Interleukin; MBDA: Multi-biomarker disease activity; MMP: Matrix metalloproteinase; MRM: Multiple reaction monitoring; PsA: Psoriatic arthritis; RA: Rheumatoid arthritis; RF: Rheumatoid factor; VEGF: Vascular endothelial growth factor.

Competing interests

The authors declare that they have no competing interests.

Acknowledgements

The authors acknowledge support from the European Commissions under the EU FP7 Programme 'MIAMI'. The UCD Conway Institute and Proteome Research Centre is funded by the Programme for Research in Third level Institutions, as administered by the Higher Education Authority of Ireland. The authors appreciate the technical support from Aisha Q Butt while the manuscript was being completed.

References

1. Firestein GS. Evolving concepts of rheumatoid arthritis. Nature. 2003;423:356–61.
2. Leung YY, Tam LS, Kun EW, Li EK. Psoriatic arthritis as a distinct disease entity. J Postgrad Med. 2007;53:63–71.
3. Veale DJ, FitzGerald O. Psoriatic arthritis – pathogenesis and epidemiology. Clin Exp Rheumatol. 2002;20:S27–33.
4. Kay J, Upchurch KS. ACR/EULAR 2010 rheumatoid arthritis classification criteria. Rheumatology. 2012;51:vi5–9.
5. Tillett W, Costa L, Jadon D, Wallis D, Cavill C, McHugh J, et al. The ClASsification for Psoriatic ARthritis (CASPAR) criteria – a retrospective feasibility, sensitivity, and specificity study. J Rheumatol. 2012;39:154–6.
6. de Rooy DP, Kalvesten J, Huizinga TW, van der Helm-van Mil AH. Loss of metacarpal bone density predicts RA development in recent-onset arthritis. Rheumatology. 2012;51:1037–41.
7. Kleyer A, Finzel S, Rech J, Manger B, Krieter M, Faustini F, et al. Bone loss before the clinical onset of rheumatoid arthritis in subjects with anticitrullinated protein antibodies. Ann Rheum Dis. 2014;73:854–60.
8. van Kuijk AW, Tak PP. Synovitis in psoriatic arthritis: immunohistochemistry, comparisons with rheumatoid arthritis, and effects of therapy. Curr Rheumatol Rep. 2011;13:353–9.
9. Reece RJ, Canete JD, Parsons WJ, Emery P, Veale DJ. Distinct vascular patterns of early synovitis in psoriatic, reactive, and rheumatoid arthritis. Arthritis Rheum. 1999;42:1481–4.
10. Veale DJ, Ritchlin C, FitzGerald O. Immunopathology of psoriasis and psoriatic arthritis. Ann Rheum Dis. 2005;64:ii26–9.
11. Veale D, Yanni G, Rogers S, Barnes L, Bresnihan B, Fitzgerald O. Reduced synovial membrane macrophage numbers, ELAM-1 expression, and lining layer hyperplasia in psoriatic arthritis as compared with rheumatoid arthritis. Arthritis Rheum. 1993;36:893–900.
12. Kane D, Stafford L, Bresnihan B, FitzGerald O. A prospective, clinical and radiological study of early psoriatic arthritis: an early synovitis clinic experience. Rheumatology. 2003;42:1460–8.
13. Sokka T. Radiographic scoring in rheumatoid arthritis: a short introduction to the methods. Bull NYU Hosp Jt Dis. 2008;66:166–8.
14. Ravindran J, Cavill C, Balakrishnan C, Jones SM, Korendowych E, McHugh NJ. A modified Sharp score demonstrates disease progression in established psoriatic arthritis. Arthritis Care Res. 2010;62:86–91.
15. Gent YY, Ter Wee MM, Ahmadi N, van Kuijk C, Voskuyl AE, van der Laken CJ, et al. Three-year clinical outcome following baseline magnetic resonance imaging in anti-citrullinated protein antibody-positive arthralgia patients: an exploratory study. Arthritis Rheumatol. 2014;66:2909–10.
16. van Schaardenburg D, Nielen MM, Lems WF, Twisk JW, Reesink HW, van de Stadt RJ, et al. Bone metabolism is altered in preclinical rheumatoid arthritis. Ann Rheum Dis. 2011;70:1173–4.
17. Plant D, Bowes J, Potter C, Hyrich KL, Morgan AW, Wilson AG, et al. Genome-wide association study of genetic predictors of anti-tumor necrosis factor treatment efficacy in rheumatoid arthritis identifies associations with polymorphisms at seven loci. Arthritis Rheum. 2011;63:645–53.
18. Eastman PS, Manning WC, Qureshi F, Haney D, Cavet G, Alexander C, et al. Characterization of a multiplex, 12-biomarker test for rheumatoid arthritis. J Pharm Biomed Anal. 2012;70:415–24.
19. Robinson WH, Lindstrom TM, Cheung RK, Sokolove J. Mechanistic biomarkers for clinical decision making in rheumatic diseases. Nat Rev Rheumatol. 2013;9:267–76.
20. Gibson DS, Rooney ME, Finnegan S, Qiu J, Thompson DC, Labaer J, et al. Biomarkers in rheumatology, now and in the future. Rheumatology. 2012;51:423–33.
21. Scott DL, Smith C, Kingsley G. Joint damage and disability in rheumatoid arthritis: an updated systematic review. Clin Exp Rheumatol. 2003;21:S20–7.
22. Haroon M, Winchester R, Giles JT, Heffernan E, FitzGerald O. Certain class I HLA alleles and haplotypes implicated in susceptibility play a role in

determining specific features of the psoriatic arthritis phenotype. Ann Rheum Dis. 2014 doi:10.1136/annrheumdis-2014-205461.

23. Song JW, Chung KC. Observational studies: cohort and case–control studies. Plastic Reconstruct Surg. 2010;126:2234–42.
24. Langham S, Langham J, Goertez HP, Ratcliffe M. Large-scale, prospective, observational studies in patinets with psorisis and psoriatic arthritis: a systematic and critical review. BMC Med Res Methodol. 2011;11:32.
25. Connolly M, Mullan RH, McCormick J, Matthews C, Sullivan O, Kennedy A, et al. Acute-phase serum amyloid A regulates tumor necrosis factor alpha and matrix turnover and predicts disease progression in patients with inflammatory arthritis before and after biologic therapy. Arthritis Rheum. 2012;64:1035–45.
26. Syversen SW, Gaarder PI, Goll GL, Odegard S, Haavardsholm EA, Mowinckel P, et al. High anti-cyclic citrullinated peptide levels and an algorithm of four variables predict radiographic progression in patients with rheumatoid arthritis: results from a 10-year longitudinal study. Ann Rheum Dis. 2008;67:212–7.
27. Meyer O, Nicaise-Roland P, Santos MD, Labarre C, Dougados M, Goupille P, et al. Serial determination of cyclic citrullinated peptide autoantibodies predicted five-year radiological outcomes in a prospective cohort of patients with early rheumatoid arthritis. Arthritis Res Ther. 2006;8:R40.
28. Forslind K, Ahlmen M, Eberhardt K, Hafstrom I, Svensson B, Group BS. Prediction of radiological outcome in early rheumatoid arthritis in clinical practice: role of antibodies to citrullinated peptides (anti-CCP). Ann Rheum Dis. 2004;63:1090–5.
29. Nell VP, Machold KP, Stamm TA, Eberl G, Heinzl H, Uffmann M, et al. Autoantibody profiling as early diagnostic and prognostic tool for rheumatoid arthritis. Ann Rheum Dis. 2005;64:1731–6.
30. Trouw LA, Mahler M. Closing the serological gap: promising novel biomarkers for the early diagnosis of rheumatoid arthritis. Autoimmun Rev. 2012;12:318–22.
31. Knudsen LS, Klarlund M, Skjodt H, Jensen T, Ostergaard M, Jensen KE, et al. Biomarkers of inflammation in patients with unclassified polyarthritis and early rheumatoid arthritis. Relationship to disease activity and radiographic outcome. J Rheumatol. 2008;35:1277–87.
32. Syversen SW, Goll GL, Haavardsholm EA, Boyesen P, Lea T, Kvien TK. A high serum level of eotaxin (CCL 11) is associated with less radiographic progression in early rheumatoid arthritis patients. Arthritis Res Ther. 2008;10:R28.
33. Lard LR, Roep BO, Toes RE, Huizinga TW. Enhanced concentrations of interleukin 16 are associated with joint destruction in patients with rheumatoid arthritis. J Rheumatol. 2004;31:35–9.
34. Leipe J, Schramm MA, Grunke M, Baeuerle M, Dechant C, Nigg AP, et al. Interleukin 22 serum levels are associated with radiographic progression in rheumatoid arthritis. Ann Rheum Dis. 2011;70:1453–7.
35. Talabot-Ayer D, McKee T, Gindre P, Bas S, Baeten DL, Gabay C, et al. Distinct serum and synovial fluid interleukin (IL)-33 levels in rheumatoid arthritis, psoriatic arthritis and osteoarthritis. Joint Bone Spine. 2012;79:32–7.
36. Klein-Wieringa IR, van der Linden MP, Knevel R, Kwekkeboom JC, van Beelen E, Huizinga TW, et al. Baseline serum adipokine levels predict radiographic progression in early rheumatoid arthritis. Arthritis Rheum. 2011;63:2567–74.
37. van Leeuwen MA, Westra J, Limburg PC, van Riel PL, van Rijswijk MH. Clinical significance of interleukin-6 measurement in early rheumatoid arthritis: relation with laboratory and clinical variables and radiological progression in a three year prospective study. Ann Rheum Dis. 1995;54:674–7.
38. Rho YH, Solus J, Sokka T, Oeser A, Chung CP, Gebretsadik T, et al. Adipocytokines are associated with radiographic joint damage in rheumatoid arthritis. Arthritis Rheum. 2009;60:1906–14.
39. Hammer HB, Odegard S, Syversen SW, Landewe R, van der Heijde D, Uhlig T, et al. Calprotectin (a major S100 leucocyte protein) predicts 10-year radiographic progression in patients with rheumatoid arthritis. Ann Rheum Dis. 2010;69:150–4.
40. Clavel G, Bessis N, Lemeiter D, Fardellone P, Mejjad O, Menard JF, et al. Angiogenesis markers (VEGF, soluble receptor of VEGF and angiopoietin-1) in very early arthritis and their association with inflammation and joint destruction. Clin Immunol. 2007;124:158–64.
41. Ballara S, Taylor PC, Reusch P, Marme D, Feldmann M, Maini RN, et al. Raised serum vascular endothelial growth factor levels are associated with destructive change in inflammatory arthritis. Arthritis Rheum. 2001;44:2055–64.
42. Garnero P, Landewe R, Boers M, Verhoeven A, Van Der Linden S, Christgau S, et al. Association of baseline levels of markers of bone and cartilage degradation with long-term progression of joint damage in patients with early rheumatoid arthritis: the COBRA study. Arthritis Rheum. 2002;46:2847–56.
43. van Tuyl LH, Voskuyl AE, Boers M, Geusens P, Landewe RB, Dijkmans BA, et al. Baseline RANKL:OPG ratio and markers of bone and cartilage degradation predict annual radiological progression over 11 years in rheumatoid arthritis. Ann Rheum Dis. 2010;69:1623–8.
44. Syversen SW, Haavardsholm EA, Boyesen P, Goll GL, Okkenhaug C, Gaarder PI, et al. Biomarkers in early rheumatoid arthritis: longitudinal associations with inflammation and joint destruction measured by magnetic resonance imaging and conventional radiographs. Ann Rheum Dis. 2010;69:845–50.
45. Bakker MF, Verstappen SM, Welsing PM, Jacobs JW, Jahangier ZN, van der Veen MJ, et al. The relation between cartilage biomarkers (C2C, C1,2C, CS846, and CPII) and the long-term outcome of rheumatoid arthritis patients within the CAMERA trial. Arthritis Res Ther. 2011;13:R70.
46. Verstappen SM, Poole AR, Ionescu M, King LE, Abrahamowicz M, Hofman DM, et al. Radiographic joint damage in rheumatoid arthritis is associated with differences in cartilage turnover and can be predicted by serum biomarkers: an evaluation from 1 to 4 years after diagnosis. Arthritis Res Ther. 2006;8:R31.
47. Andersson ML, Svensson B, Petersson IF, Hafstrom I, Albertsson K, Forslind K, et al. Early increase in serum-COMP is associated with joint damage progression over the first five years in patients with rheumatoid arthritis. BMC Musculoskelet Disord. 2013;14:229.
48. Posthumus MD, Limburg PC, Westra J, Cats HA, Stewart RE, van Leeuwen MA, et al. Serum levels of matrix metalloproteinase-3 in relation to the development of radiological damage in patients with early rheumatoid arthritis. Rheumatology. 1999;38:1081–7.
49. Green MJ, Gough AK, Devlin J, Smith J, Astin P, Taylor D, et al. Serum MMP-3 and MMP-1 and progression of joint damage in early rheumatoid arthritis. Rheumatology. 2003;42:83–8.
50. Young-Min S, Cawston T, Marshall N, Coady D, Christgau S, Saxne T, et al. Biomarkers predict radiographic progression in early rheumatoid arthritis and perform well compared with traditional markers. Arthritis Rheum. 2007;56:3236–47.
51. Cunnane G, Fitzgerald O, Beeton C, Cawston TE, Bresnihan B. Early joint erosions and serum levels of matrix metalloproteinase 1, matrix metalloproteinase 3, and tissue inhibitor of metalloproteinases 1 in rheumatoid arthritis. Arthritis Rheum. 2001;44:2263–74.
52. Moran EM, Mullan R, McCormick J, Connolly M, Sullivan O, Fitzgerald O, et al. Human rheumatoid arthritis tissue production of IL-17A drives matrix and cartilage degradation: synergy with tumour necrosis factor-alpha. Oncostatin M and response to biologic therapies. Arthritis Res Ther. 2009;11:R113.
53. Punzi L, Bertazzolo N, Pianon M, Rizzi E, Rossini P, Gambari P. Value of synovial fluid interleukin-1 beta determination in predicting the outcome of psoriatic monoarthritis. Ann Rheum Dis. 1996;55:642–44.
54. Szodoray P, Alex P, Chappell-Woodward CM, Madland TM, Knowlton N, Dozmorov I, et al. Circulating cytokines in Norwegian patients with psoriatic arthritis determined by a multiplex cytokine array system. Rheumatology. 2007;46:417–25.
55. Kane D, Roth J, Frosch M, Vogl T, Bresnihan B, FitzGerald O. Increased perivascular synovial membrane expression of myeloid-related proteins in psoriatic arthritis. Arthritis Rheum. 2003;48:1676–85.
56. Aochi S, Tsuji K, Sakaguchi M, Huh N, Tsuda T, Yamanishi K, et al. Markedly elevated serum levels of calcium-binding S100A8/A9 proteins in psoriatic arthritis are due to activated monocytes/macrophages. J Am Acad Dermatol. 2011;64:879–87.
57. Fink AM, Cauza E, Hassfeld W, Dunky A, Bayer PM, Jurecka W, et al. Vascular endothelial growth factor in patients with psoriatic arthritis. Clin Exp Rheumatol. 2007;25:305–8.
58. Fearon U, Griosios K, Fraser A, Reece R, Emery P, Jones PF, et al. Angiopoietins, growth factors, and vascular morphology in early arthritis. J Rheumatol. 2003;30:260–8.
59. Dalbeth N, Pool B, Smith T, Callon KE, Lobo M, Taylor WJ, et al. Circulating mediators of bone remodeling in psoriatic arthritis: implications for disordered osteoclastogenesis and bone erosion. Arthritis Res Ther. 2010;12:R164.
60. Rifai NGM, Carr SA. Protein biomarker discovery and validation: the long and uncertain path to clinical utility. Nat Biotechnol. 2006;24:971–83.
61. Sahab ZJ, Semaan SM, Sang QX. Methodology and applications of disease biomarker identification in human serum. Biomarker Insights. 2007;2:21–43.
62. O'Leary PC, Penny SA, Dolan RT, Kelly CM, Madden SF, Rexhepaj E, et al. Systematic antibody generation and validation via tissue microarray technology leading to identification of a novel protein prognostic panel in breast cancer. BMC Cancer. 2013;13:175.

63. Gillette MA, Carr SA. Quantitative analysis of peptides and proteins in biomedicine by targeted mass spectrometry. Nat Methods. 2013;10:28–34.
64. Picotti P, Bodenmiller B, Aebersold R. Proteomics meets the scientific method. Nat Methods. 2013;10:24–7.
65. Staunton L, Clancy T, Torny C, Ademowo OS, Dharsee M, Hernandez B. Protein Quantification by MRM for Biomarker Validation. In: Eyers CE, Gaskell SJ, editors New developments in mass spectrometry. Quantitative proteomics. Cambridge: Royal Society of Chemistry; 2014. p. 279–315.
66. Chang CY, Picotti P, Huttenhain R, Heinzelmann-Schwarz V, Jovanovic M, Aebersold R, et al. Protein significance analysis in selected reaction monitoring (SRM) measurements. Mol Cell Proteomics. 2012;11:M111 014662.
67. Prassas I, Chrystoja CC, Makawita S, Diamandis EP. Bioinformatic identification of proteins with tissue-specific expression for biomarker discovery. BMC Med. 2012;10:39.
68. Valencia A, Hidalgo M. Getting personalized cancer genome analysis into the clinic: the challenges in bioinformatics. Genome Med. 2012;4:61.
69. Chen YT, Chen HW, Domanski D, Smith DS, Liang KH, Wu CC, et al. Multiplexed quantification of 63 proteins in human urine by multiple reaction monitoring-based mass spectrometry for discovery of potential bladder cancer biomarkers. J Proteomics. 2012;75:3529–45.
70. Domanski D, Percy AJ, Yang J, Chambers AG, Hill JS, Freue GV, et al. MRM-based multiplexed quantitation of 67 putative cardiovascular disease biomarkers in human plasma. Proteomics. 2012;12:1222–43.
71. Collins BC, Miller CA, Sposny A, Hewitt P, Wells M, Gallagher WM, et al. Development of a pharmaceutical hepatotoxicity biomarker panel using a discovery to targeted proteomics approach. Mol Cell Proteomics. 2012;11:394–410.
72. Li XJ, Hayward C, Fong PY, Dominguez M, Hunsucker SW, Lee LW, et al. A blood-based proteomic classifier for the molecular characterization of pulmonary nodules. Sci Transl Med. 2013;5:207ra142.
73. Morrissey B, O'Shea C, Armstrong J, Rooney C, Staunton L, Sheehan M, et al. Development of a label-free LC-MS/MS strategy to approach the identification of candidate protein biomarkers of disease recurrence in prostate cancer patients in a clinical trial of combined hormone and radiation therapy. Proteomics Clin Appl. 2013;7:316–26.
74. Kuhn E, Wu J, Karl J, Liao H, Zolg W, Guild B. Quantification of C-reactive protein in the serum of patients with rheumatoid arthritis using multiple reaction monitoring mass spectrometry and 13C-labeled peptide standards. Proteomics. 2004;4:1175–86.
75. Ademowo OS, Hernandez B, Collins E, Rooney C, Fearon U, van Kuijk AW, et al. Discovery and confirmation of a protein biomarker panel with potential to predict response to biological therapy in psoriatic arthritis. Ann Rheum Dis. 2014 doi: 10.1136/annrheumdis-2014-205417.
76. Chowdhury F, Williams A, Johnson P. Validation and comparison of two multiplex technologies, luminex and mesoscale discovery, for human cytokine profiling. J Immunol Methods. 2009;340:55–64.
77. Elshal MF, McCoy JP. Multiplex bead array assays: performance evaluation and comparison of sensitivity to ELISA. Methods. 2006;38:317–23.
78. Zhi W, Wang M, She JX. Selected reaction monitoring (SRM) mass spectrometry without isotope labeling can be used for rapid protein quantification. Rapid Commun Mass Spectrom. 2011;25:1583–8.
79. Li W, Haney DJ, Cavet G, Huzinga TW, Sasso EH, van der Helm-van Mil AHM. The multi-biomarker disease activity test (Vectra® DA) estimates risk of radiographic progression for patients with rheumatoid arthritis from the Leiden Early Arthritis Clinic [abstract]. Arthritis Rheum. 2013;65:1788.
80. Hambardzumyan K, Bolce R, Saevarsdottir S, Cruickshank SE, Sasso EH, Chernoff D, et al. Pretreatment multi-biomarker disease activity score and radiographic progression in early RA: results from the SWEFOT trial. Ann Rheum Dis. 2014 doi:10.1136/annrheumdis-2013-204986.
81. van der Helm-van Mil AH, Knevel R, Cavet G, Huizinga TW, Haney DJ. An evaluation of molecular and clinical remission in rheumatoid arthritis by assessing radiographic progression. Rheumatology. 2013;52:839–46.
82. Finzel S, Englbrecht M, Engelke K, Stach C, Schett G. A comparative study of periarticular bone lesions in rheumatoid arthritis and psoriatic arthritis. Ann Rheum Dis. 2011;70:122–7.
83. Albrecht A, Finzel S, Englbrecht M, Rech J, Hueber A, Schlechtweg P, et al. The structural basis of MRI bone erosions: an assessment by microCT. Ann Rheum Dis. 2013;72:1351–7.
84. Wiell C, Szkudlarek M, Hasselquist M, Moller JM, Vestergaard A, Norregaard J, et al. Ultrasonography, magnetic resonance imaging, radiography, and clinical assessment of inflammatory and destructive changes in fingers and toes of patients with psoriatic arthritis. Arthritis Res Ther. 2007;9:R119.
85. Frediani B, Falsetti P, Storri L, Allegri A, Bisogno S, Baldi F, et al. Ultrasound and clinical evaluation of quadricipital tendon enthesitis in patients with psoriatic arthritis and rheumatoid arthritis. Clin Rheumatol. 2002;21:294–8.
86. Healy PJ, Helliwell PS. Measuring dactylitis in clinical trials: which is the best instrument to use? J Rheumatol. 2007;34:1302–6.
87. Marsal S, Armadans-Gil L, Martinez M, Gallardo D, Ribera A, Lience E. Clinical, radiographic and HLA associations as markers for different patterns of psoriatic arthritis. Rheumatology. 1999;38:332–7.

13

Pathogenic roles of CXCL10 signaling through CXCR3 and TLR4 in macrophages and T cells: relevance for arthritis

Jong-Ho Lee[2†], Bongjun Kim[1†], Won Jong Jin[1], Hong-Hee Kim[1], Hyunil Ha[3*] and Zang Hee Lee[1*]

Abstract

Background: Rheumatoid arthritis (RA) is a chronic autoimmune disease characterized by uncontrolled joint inflammation and destruction of bone and cartilage. We previously reported that C-X-C motif chemokine 10 (CXCL10; also called IP-10) has important roles in joint inflammation and bone destruction in arthritis. However, the specific mechanisms by which CXCL10 regulates the recruitment of inflammatory cells and the production of osteoclastogenic cytokines in RA progression are not fully understood.

Methods: Bone marrow-derived macrophages and $CD4^+$ T cells were isolated from wild-type (WT), *Cxcl10*$^{-/-}$, and *Cxcr3*$^{-/-}$ mice. CXCL10-induced migration was performed using a Boyden chamber, and CXCL10-stimulated production of osteoclastogenic cytokines was measured by quantitative real-time PCR and ELISA. Collagen antibody-induced arthritis (CAIA) was induced by administration of collagen type II antibodies and lipopolysaccharide to the mice. Clinical scores were analyzed and hind paws were collected for high-resolution micro-CT, and histomorphometry. Serum was used to assess bone turnover and levels of osteoclastogenic cytokines.

Results: CXCL10 increased the migration of inflammatory cells through C-X-C chemokine receptor 3 (CXCR3)-mediated, but not toll-like receptor 4 (TLR4)-mediated, ERK activation. Interestingly, both receptors CXCR3 and TLR4 were simultaneously required for CXCL10-stimulated production of osteoclastogenic cytokines in $CD4^+$ T cells. Furthermore, calcineurin-dependent NFATc1 activation was essential for CXCL10-induced RANKL expression. In vivo, F4/80$^+$ macrophages and $CD4^+$ T cells robustly infiltrated into synovium of WT mice with CAIA but were significantly reduced in both *Cxcl10*$^{-/-}$ and *Cxcr3*$^{-/-}$ mice. Serum concentrations of osteoclastogenic cytokines and bone destruction were also reduced in the knockout mice, leading to attenuated progression of arthritis.

Conclusion: These findings highlight the importance of CXCL10 signaling in the pathogenesis of RA and provide previously unidentified details of the mechanisms by which CXCL10 promotes the development of arthritis.

Keywords: CXCL10, CXCR3, TLR4, RANKL, Rheumatoid arthritis, Collagen antibody-induced arthritis

Background

Osteoclasts, multinucleated bone-resorbing cells, are essential mediators of inflammatory bone erosion and are derived from monocyte/macrophage lineage precursor cells through the action of RANKL, a key factor for osteoclastogenesis [1]. Increased bone resorption by activated osteoclasts can be caused by systemic alterations such as the upregulation of osteotropic or osteoclastogenic cytokines, including RANKL, TNFα, and IL-6, which in turn cause bone-destructive diseases, including rheumatoid arthritis (RA) [2].

RA is a common, chronic inflammatory and systemic autoimmune disease characterized by progressive infiltration of lymphocytes and macrophages into synovium, leading to persistent synovial inflammation and destruction of bone and cartilage [3]. Abnormal activation of T cells, one of the most abundant cell populations in the

* Correspondence: hyunil74@kiom.re.kr; zang1959@snu.ac.kr
†Equal contributors
[3]Clinical Research Division, Korean Medicine-Based Herbal Drug Development Group, Korea Institute of Oriental Medicine, 483 Expo-Ro, Yuseong-Gu, Daejeon 305-811, Republic of Korea
[1]Department of Cell and Developmental Biology, Dental Research Institute, School of Dentistry, Seoul National University, 28 Yeongon-dong, Jongno-gu, Seoul 110-749, Republic of Korea
Full list of author information is available at the end of the article

RA synovium, drives chronic inflammation and joint destruction [4]. The T cells interact with other immune and resident cells including macrophages by secreting cytokines and chemokines or by direct cell-to-cell contact, leading to a boost in production of proinflammatory cytokines and chemokines [5, 6]. The increased cytokines and chemokines in turn alter the activation or differentiation state of one or both of the cell types [4]. In particular, elevated proinflammatory cytokines and chemokines increase the expression of osteoclastogenic cytokines including RANKL, TNFα, and IL-6 from $CD4^+$ T cells of RA patients [7–9].

Synovitis, inflammation of a synovial membrane, is initiated by infiltration of inflammatory cells into the synovial compartment, followed by synovial hyperplasia, also called pannus, in RA synovial tissue [3, 10]. The hyperplastic synovial pannus in RA produces proinflammatory cytokines, chemokines, and proteases and subsequently invades and destroys bone and cartilage [10, 11]. Particularly, macrophages and fibroblast-like synoviocytes are central effectors of synovitis and synovial pannus formation, respectively [3, 10]. Thus, infiltration of inflammatory cells into the synovium is an essential step for the progression of RA.

C-X-C motif chemokine 10 (CXCL10), also known as interferon-gamma-inducible protein 10 (IP-10), was initially identified as a chemokine secreted by several cell types including macrophages, endothelial cells, and fibroblasts in response to interferon gamma (IFN-γ) [12]. CXCL10 binds to its receptor CXCR3 and regulates immune responses through recruitment of leukocytes, including T cells and monocytes/macrophages [12]. In addition to its binding to CXCR3, CXCL10 has been shown to bind with and activate toll-like receptor 4 (TLR4) [13]. The crucial role of CXCL10 has been well characterized in chronic Th1 inflammatory diseases. In inflamed tissues, CXCL10 recruits Th1 cells via CXCR3 where IFN-γ is secreted, which in turn stimulates CXCL10 expression in various cell types, resulting in positive feedback to amplify CXCL10 and Th1 responses [14]. It has been shown that CXCL10 levels in synovial fluid and serum are elevated in human RA patients and in mice with collagen-induced arthritis (CIA) [6, 15, 16]. Blockade of the CXCL10–CXCR3 axis has been shown to inhibit the infiltration of inflammatory cells, including T cells and macrophages, into inflamed joints and to decrease the severity of arthritis and bone and cartilage destruction in animal models of RA [6, 17]. In addition to its chemotactic effect, CXCL10 has been shown to increase RANKL expression in $CD4^+$ T cells [6, 18]. However, the exact mechanisms by which CXCL10 regulates inflammatory cell infiltration and osteoclastogenic cytokine production in RA are not fully understood.

In general, the CIA model is widely used in animal studies and shares many pathological and histological similarities with RA, which is known to be both T-cell and B-cell dependent. The model is commonly used to evaluate both the antigen-recognition phase and the inflammatory phase of arthritis [19]. However, the susceptibility for CIA is poor in mice of the C57BL/6 background, the strain widely used for knockout models. By contrast, collagen antibody-induced arthritis (CAIA) is induced by infiltration of neutrophils and macrophages into the inflamed joints [20, 21]. Many of the pathological symptoms that are typical of RA can be seen in the joints of animals with CAIA, such as synovitis, pannus formation, and destruction of cartilage and bone [22, 23]. In addition, the CAIA model not only is a suitable model for studies of arthritis-induced osteoporosis [24] but also can be used in genetically modified C57BL/6 mice, such as transgenics and knockouts [22].

In this study, we investigated the functional roles and specific mechanisms of CXCL10 signaling in RA progression using *Cxcl10*$^{-/-}$, *Cxcr3*$^{-/-}$, and *Tlr4*$^{-/-}$ knockout mice.

Methods

Animals

Wild-type (WT), *Cxcl10*$^{-/-}$, and *Cxcr3*$^{-/-}$ mice (C57BL/6 background) were obtained from The Jackson Laboratory (Bar Harbor, ME, USA). *Tlr4*$^{-/-}$ mice were kindly provided by Dr Sung Joong Lee (Seoul National University, Seoul, Korea). All animal procedures were reviewed and approved by the animal care committee of the Institute of Laboratory Animal Resources of Seoul National University.

Induction and evaluation of CAIA

Male 8-week-old mice were injected intravenously with a five-clone cocktail of collagen type II antibodies (5 mg/mouse; Chondrex, Redmond, WA, USA) to induce arthritis (CAIA group). Nonarthritic control mice received phosphate-buffered saline (control group). Three days after antibody administration, 100 μg lipopolysaccharide (LPS) was injected intraperitoneally in both CAIA and control mice.

The severity of arthritis was assessed according to paw swelling and was scored on a scale of 0–3 (where 0 = normal, 1 = swelling of the toes, 2 = swelling of the sole of the foot or increased swelling, and 3 = severe swelling or swelling of the entire paw). The arthritic score for each mouse was expressed as the sum of the scores of the four limbs. Mice were sacrificed on day 12, and serum and paws were collected. Paws were fixed in 4% paraformaldehyde overnight and were then washed with PBS. Three-dimensional images of posterior paws were obtained by microfocal computed tomography (micro-CT) scanning (SMX-90CT; Shimadzu, Japan). An eroded bone surface per total bone surface was determined using TRI 3D-BON software (RATOC System Engineering Co., Kyoto, Japan). For histological analysis, posterior paws were decalcified in 12% EDTA and then embedded in paraffin.

Histological evaluation

Paraffin-embedded sections of decalcified posterior paws were prepared as described previously [25]. The sections were stained with Harris hematoxylin and eosin (H&E), Safranin O and methyl green staining, and tartrate-resistant acid phosphatase (TRAP; Sigma-Aldrich, St Louis, MO, USA) and then scored as described previously [26, 27].

The H&E-stained sections were scored for inflammation and pannus formation. Inflammation was scored according to the following criteria: 0 = normal, 1 = minimal infiltration, 2 = mild infiltration, 3 = moderate infiltration, 4 = marked infiltration, and 5 = severe infiltration. Pannus formation was scored according to the following criteria: 0 = no pannus formation, 1 = minimal pannus formation, 2 = mild pannus formation, 3 = moderate pannus formation, 4 = marked pannus formation, and 5 = severe pannus formation.

The Safranin O-stained sections were scored for cartilage damage. Cartilage damage was scored according to the following criteria: 0 = no damage, 1 = minimal loss of cartilage, 2 = mild loss of cartilage, 3 = moderate loss of cartilage, 4 = marked loss of cartilage, and 5 = severe diffuse loss of cartilage.

The TRAP-stained sections were scored for osteoclast activity. Osteoclast activity was scored according to the following criteria: 0 = no staining, 1 = rare positive cells, 2 = scattered staining, 3 = multiple foci of positive cells, 4 = clusters of positive cells, and 5 = diffuse staining.

Immunohistochemistry

Immunohistochemical analysis was performed on decalcified paraffin-embedded tissue sections as described previously [28]. The anti-F4/80 antibody clone CI:A3-1 (Abcam, Cambridge, MA, USA) that recognizes the mouse F4/80 antigen, a cell surface glycoprotein expressed at high levels on various murine macrophages, was used to detect macrophages in arthritic joints. Detection of the primary antibody was performed using the VECTASTAIN® Elite ABC kit (Vector Laboratories, Burlingame, CA, USA), followed by 3,3-diaminobenzidine (Vector Laboratories) incubation and nuclear staining with hematoxylin. Six randomly chosen fields per slide were analyzed and averaged.

Immunohistofluorescence

The deparaffinized sections were treated with a citrate buffer (pH 6.0) for antigen retrieval in a microwave oven for 30 min. After washing, tissue sections were blocked for nonspecific binding with 5% horse serum/0.3% Tween-20/TBS and incubated with FITC-labeled rat anti-mouse CD4 (clone GK1.5, 1:100; eBioscience, San Diego, CA, USA) antibody at 4 °C overnight. The FITC-labeled rat igG2b K isotype control (clone eB149/10H5, 1:100; eBioscience) was used to control staining specificity. After a final washing, cover slips were mounted onto slides with fluoroshield mounting medium with DAPI (four slips were mounted on indole; Abcam). These sections were examined using an LSM 700 confocal laser-scanning microscope (Zeiss, Oberkochen, Germany).

Isolation of bone marrow-derived macrophages and activated CD4$^+$ T cells and gene transduction

Bone marrow-derived macrophages (BMMs) were prepared as described previously [25]. In brief, mouse bone marrow cells were obtained from femurs and tibias and incubated in α-MEM complete media containing 10% fetal bovine serum, 100 units/ml penicillin, and 100 μg/ml streptomycin on 10-cm culture dishes in the presence of M-CSF (10 ng/ml) overnight. Nonadherent cells were transferred to 10-cm bacterial culture dishes and were further cultured in the presence of M-CSF (30 ng/ml) for 3 days. Adherent cells were used as BMMs after the nonadherent cells were washed out.

CD4$^+$ T cells were isolated from mouse spleens as described previously [6]. Briefly, spleens were mashed in Hanks' balanced salt solution containing 3× antibiotics. Cells were harvested, and red blood cells were removed by ammonium–chloride–potassium (ACK) lysing buffer. The remaining cells were collected and separated with a Ficoll-Histopaque (Sigma-Aldrich) discontinuous gradient. The interface containing the cells was washed with PBS, resuspended in RPMI 1640 (Welgene, Daegu, Korea) containing 10% FBS, and then cultured for 1 day. Nonadherent cells were then cultured for 3 days in the presence of 50 ng/ml IL-2 (PeproTech, London, UK). Activated CD4$^+$ T cells were purified by negative selection using CD4$^+$ T-cell isolation kits (Miltenyi Biotec, Bergisch Gladbach, Germany) according to the manufacturer's instructions.

CD4$^+$ T cells were transduced with the retroviral vectors pMX-IRES-EGFP (control) or pMX-CA-NFATc1-IRES-EGFP encoding a constitutively active (CA) form of NFATc1 as described previously [25]. BMMs were transduced with the adenoviral vectors Ax1w1 (control) or AxMEK^{CA} carrying CA-MEK1 (Ser 218 and Ser222 to Glu) as described previously [29].

Migration assay

Amounts of 1×10^5 BMMs in 200 μl of serum-free α-MEM were seeded in the upper well of a Boyden chamber with polycarbonate filters containing 8-μm pore membranes (Corning Costar, Cambridge, MA, USA). The lower well was loaded with 600 μl of serum-free α-MEM with or without recombinant mouse CXCL10 (PeproTech). After 12 hours of incubation, cells attached on the lower surface of the membrane were fixed with 100% methanol for 10 min and then stained with Harris H&E. Migrated cells were quantified using an image analysis system (Image J; National Institutes of Health, Bethesda, MD, USA).

Amounts of 5×10^5 $CD4^+$ T cells in 200 μl serum-free RPMI 1640 medium were seeded in the upper well of the Boyden chamber with polycarbonate filters containing 5-μm pore membranes. The lower well was loaded with 600 μl serum-free RPMI 1640 medium with or without recombinant mouse CXCL10 and the cells were allowed to migrate for 12 hours. The migrated cells recovered from each bottom well were counted as follows: 100 μl of culture media containing migrated cells was collected from each bottom chamber and counted as migrated cells.

ELISA

The amount of CXCL10, RANKL, TNFα, IL-6, and C-terminal telopeptides of type I collagen (CTX) in serum was determined using the corresponding ELISA kits (R&D Systems, Minneapolis, MN, USA) according to the manufacturer's instructions. In some experiments, protein amounts of RANKL and TNFα in $CD4^+$ T-cell culture supernatants were determined using the same ELISA kits mentioned earlier.

Immunoblotting

Immunoblot analysis was performed as described previously [25]. Specific antibodies against NFATc1 (Santa Cruz Biotechnology, Santa Cruz, CA, USA), phospho-ERK1/2 (Thr202/Tyr204) and ERK (Cell Signaling Technology, Danvers, MA, USA), MEK1 (Millipore, Boston, MA, USA), and β-actin (Sigma-Aldrich) were used.

Reverse transcription and real-time PCR analysis

Total RNA was prepared from cells or spleens using an RNeasy Mini kit (Qiagen, Valencia, CA, USA) according to the manufacturer's instructions, and cDNA was synthesized from 2 μg of total RNA by reverse transcriptase (Superscript II Preamplification System; Gibco-BRL, Gaithersburg, MD, USA). Real-time PCR was performed on an ABI Prism 7500 sequence detection system using a SYBR® Green PCR Master Mix (Applied Biosystems, Foster City, CA, USA) and following the manufacturer's protocols. The ABI 7500 sequence detector was programmed with the following PCR conditions: 40 cycles of 15-s denaturation at 95 °C and 1-minute amplification at 60 °C. All reactions were run in triplicate and normalized to the housekeeping gene β-actin. The evaluation of relative differences of PCR results was calculated using the comparative cycle threshold (C_T) method. The following primer sets were used: mouse RANKL forward, 5′-TGGAAGGCTCATGGTTGGAT-3′ and reverse, 5′-CATTGATGGTGAGGTGTGCA-3′; mouse TNFα forward, 5′-GACCCTCACACTCAGATCATCTTCT-3′ and reverse, 5′-CCTCCACTTGGTGGTTTGCT-3′; mouse IL-6 forward, 5′-GTCCTTCCTACCCCAATTTCC A-3′ and reverse, 5′-GGATGGTCTTGGTCCTTAGCC-3′; mouse CXCR3 forward, 5′-CAGCCTGAACTTTGACAGAACC T-3′ and reverse, 5′-GCAGCCCCAGCAAGAAGA-3′; mouse TLR4 forward, 5′-AATCCTCTGGGGAGGCAC AT-3′ and reverse, 5′-CAGGTCCAAGTTGCCGTTTC-3′; and mouse β-actin forward, 5′-ATGTGGATCAGC AAGCAGGA-3′ and reverse, 5′-AAGGGTGTAAAACGC AGCTC-3′.

Statistical analysis

Data are presented as the mean ± SD (in-vitro data) or the mean ± SEM (in-vivo data). Statistical analysis was performed by either unpaired, two-tailed Student's t test, one-way ANOVA followed by Dunnett's test, or two-way repeated-measures ANOVA followed by Bonferroni's test using GraphPad Prism 5.0 (GraphPad Software, San Diego, CA, USA). Values of $P < 0.05$ were considered significant.

Results

CXCL10 induces migration of inflammatory cells through CXCR3-mediated ERK activation but not TLR4

Because CXCL10 has been reported to bind to TLR4 as well as to CXCR3 [13], we first investigated whether TLR4 is involved in CXCL10-induced cell migration. We isolated BMMs and $CD4^+$ T cells from WT, *Tlr4*$^{-/-}$, and *Cxcr3*$^{-/-}$ mice. In our experimental condition, $CD4^+$ T cells from the WT, *Tlr4*$^{-/-}$, and *Cxcr3*$^{-/-}$ spleens were enriched to about 94% purity by magnetic bead separation (Additional file 1: Figure S1a), and IL-2 treatment successfully increased CXCR3 and IL-2 mRNA expression with similar maintained viability of all $CD4^+$ T cells from WT, *Tlr4*$^{-/-}$, and *Cxcr3*$^{-/-}$ mice (Additional file 1: Figure S1b, c). We next carried out chemotactic assay experiments. As expected, the CXCL10-induced migration of BMMs (Fig. 1a and Additional file 1: Figure S2) and $CD4^+$ T cells (Fig. 1b and Additional file 1: Figure S3) was blocked in *Cxcr3*$^{-/-}$ or si-CXCR3 cells compared with WT or si-Control cells. TLR4 knockout, however, did not affect CXCL10-induced migration (Fig. 1a, b).

CXCL10 stimulates ERK [6], which positively regulates cell migration [30]. Therefore, we checked whether CXCL10 induces cell migration through the CXCR3–ERK axis. ERK inhibition by PD98059, a specific MEK inhibitor, greatly reduced CXCL10-induced migration of

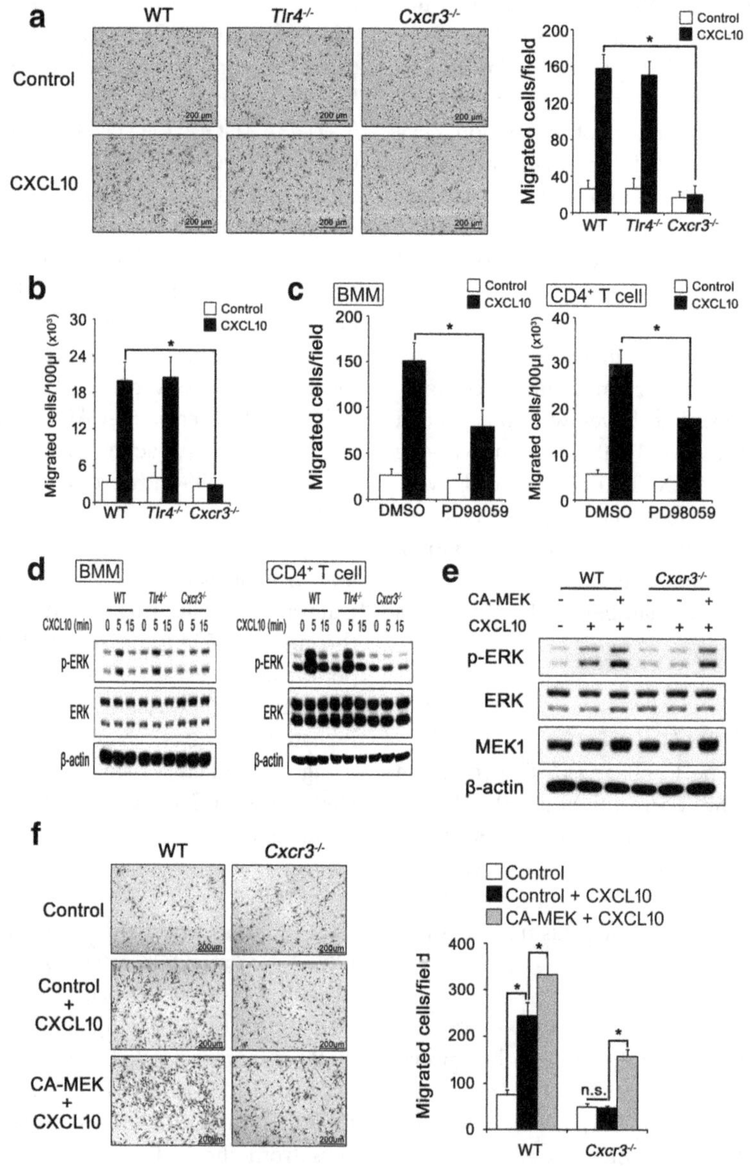

Fig. 1 CXCL10 induces migration of BMMs and CD4$^+$ T cells through CXCR3 but not TLR4. **a**, **b** BMMs and CD4$^+$ T cells were isolated from wild-type (*WT*), *Tlr4*$^{-/-}$, and *Cxcr3*$^{-/-}$ mice and then the cells were serum starved. Cell migration in response to CXCL10 (100 ng/ml) was assessed in transwell chambers for 12 hours. Representative images of migrated BMMs. (**a**, *left panel*; *scale bar*, 200 μm). Number of migrated BMMs (**a**, *right panel*) and CD4$^+$ T cells (**b**). **c** Serum-starved BMMs (*left panel*) and CD4$^+$ T cells (*right panel*) were preincubated with DMSO or 10 μM PD98059 for 1 hour, and migration was measured in the absence or presence of CXCL10 (100 ng/ml) after 12 hours. **d** Serum-starved BMMs (*left panel*) and CD4$^+$ T cells (*right panel*) were stimulated with CXCL10 (100 ng/ml) for the indicated times. Total cell lysates were immunoblotted with the indicated antibodies. **e**, **f** WT or *Cxcr3*$^{-/-}$ BMMs were infected with adenovirus carrying empty vector (Ax1w1) or CA-MEK1 (AxMEK^{CA}). After 24 hours, the infected cells were serum starved and stimulated with PBS (vehicle) or CXCL10 (100 ng/ml) for 5 min. Total cell lysates were immunoblotted with the indicated antibodies (**e**). Migration of the infected cells in response to CXCL10 (100 ng/ml) was assessed in transwell chambers for 12 hours. Representative images of migrated BMMs (**f**, *left panel*; *scale bar*, 200 μm) and the number of migrated BMMs (**f**, *right panel*). Results shown are representative of three independent experiments ($n = 3$), and values are expressed as mean ± SD. *$P < 0.001$ by one-way ANOVA followed by Dunnett's test. *CXCL10* C-X-C motif chemokine 10, *Tlr4* toll-like receptor 4, *Cxcr3* CXC chemokine receptor 3, *n.s.* nonsignificant, *BMM* bone marrow-derived macrophage

BMMs and CD4$^+$ T cells (Fig. 1c and Additional file 1: Figure S4). In addition, CXCR3 deficiency resulted in failed CXCL10-induced ERK phosphorylation in both BMMs and CD4$^+$ T cells, whereas TLR4 deficiency did not (Fig. 1d). The inhibition of CXCL10-induced ERK phosphorylation and migration was largely rescued by overexpression of a constitutively active MEK1 in *Cxcr3*$^{-/-}$ cells (Fig. 1e, f). These results suggest that CXCR3-mediated ERK activation is crucial for the CXCL10-induced cell migration.

CXCL10 induces the production of osteoclastogenic cytokines in CD4$^+$ T cells through both TLR4 and CXCR3

Beyond its chemotactic effect, CXCL10 has been shown to induce osteoclastogenic cytokines [6, 18]. Therefore, we next investigated the functional role of CXCR3 and TLR4 in response to CXCL10 in the expression of osteoclastogenic cytokines. Consistent with our previous report [6], CXCL10 significantly induced RANKL, TNFα, and IL-6 mRNA in CD4$^+$ T cells isolated from WT mice, but not in *Cxcr3*$^{-/-}$ CD4$^+$ T cells (Fig. 2a). In line with these results, the CXCL10-induced upregulation of RANKL, TNFα, and IL-6 mRNA was greatly inhibited in CXCR3-depleted CD4$^+$ T cells (Additional file 1: Figure S3). Interestingly, the inhibition was also found in CD4$^+$ T cells isolated from *Tlr4*$^{-/-}$ mice (Fig. 2a). To confirm this result, we measured the amount of RANKL, TNFα, and IL-6 secreted into the culture medium by ELISA, and the results were consistent with the mRNA expression (Fig. 2b). To exclude the possibility that the inhibitory effect was a side effect of a genetic disorder, we treated the CD4$^+$ T cells with PMA/ionomycin to induce RANKL expression [31]. As shown in Fig. 2c, PMA/ionomycin-induced expression of both mRNA and protein for RANKL was not significantly different between the cells. Altogether, these results suggest that both CXCR3 and TLR4 are specifically required for CXCL10-stimulated production of osteoclastogenic cytokines.

NFAT-binding sites exist in the RANKL promoter to induce RANKL expression in CD4$^+$ T cells, which is regulated by the calcineurin signaling pathway [31, 32]. Moreover, autoamplification of NFATc1 expression is mediated by activated calcineurin-dependent NFATc1 activation [33, 34]. We reported previously that CXCL10 induces NFATc1 expression in CD4$^+$ T cells [6], which was abolished in both *Cxcr3*$^{-/-}$ and *Tlr4*$^{-/-}$ CD4$^+$ T cells (Fig. 2d). To investigate whether calcineurin signaling plays a critical role in CXCL10-induced RANKL and NFATc1 expression, we performed real-time PCR and western blot analysis on samples prepared in the absence or presence of cyclosporin A (CsA, an inhibitor of calcineurin activity). Compared with the control, CsA pretreatment greatly inhibited CXCL10-induced RANKL (Fig. 2e) and NFATc1 expression (Fig. 2f). Furthermore, overexpression of CA-NFATc1 fully rescued the failed RANKL expression in both *Cxcr3*$^{-/-}$ and *Tlr4*$^{-/-}$ CD4$^+$ T cells (Fig. 2g, h). These data indicate that the calcineurin/NFATc1 pathway is essential for CXCL10-induced RANKL expression as well as NFATc1 expression in T cells.

CAIA progression is ameliorated in *Cxcl10*$^{-/-}$ and *Cxcr3*$^{-/-}$ mice

To determine the role of CXCL10 signaling in the development of arthritis, we used the CAIA model in mice lacking *Cxcl10*$^{-/-}$ and *Cxcr3*$^{-/-}$. As shown in Fig. 3a, LPS was used as a booster after injection of collagen type II antibodies to induce severe arthritis in the CAIA model. Because LPS is a specific ligand for TLR4, we excluded *Tlr4*$^{-/-}$ mice in this study. In C57BL/6 WT mice, clinical signs of arthritis were first observed 6 days after injection of collagen type II antibodies and reached a maximum on days 9–10. *Cxcl10*$^{-/-}$ and *Cxcr3*$^{-/-}$ mice developed less severe arthritis than WT mice (Fig. 3b, c). Consistent with the results of clinical scores, both *Cxcl10*$^{-/-}$ and *Cxcr3*$^{-/-}$ mice had attenuated paw swelling compared with WT mice (Fig. 3d). Next, we performed three-dimensional reconstruction and analysis of paws by micro-CT to check bone erosion status. Micro-CT scans revealed erosive bone lesions and an increase in eroded surface per total bone surface following CAIA, which were significantly decreased in *Cxcl10*$^{-/-}$ and *Cxcr3*$^{-/-}$ mice compared with WT mice (Fig. 3e, f).

To accurately evaluate the degree of inflammation, pannus formation, and cartilage destruction, joint tissue sections were examined using a histopathologic scoring system [26, 27]. Histopathologic studies also revealed milder inflammation, pannus formation, and cartilage degeneration following CAIA in *Cxcl10*$^{-/-}$ and *Cxcr3*$^{-/-}$ mice than in WT mice (Fig. 4a–d). In order to detect osteoclasts, we performed TRAP staining. In line with the results of micro-CT analysis, lower osteoclast activity was observed in *Cxcl10*$^{-/-}$ and *Cxcr3*$^{-/-}$ mice than in WT mice (Fig. 4a–d).

Taken together, these results demonstrate that the clinically observed amelioration of arthritis in *Cxcl10*$^{-/-}$ and *Cxcr3*$^{-/-}$ mice was reflected by suppression of joint inflammation and destruction of bone and cartilage.

Cxcl10$^{-/-}$ and *Cxcr3*$^{-/-}$ mice with CAIA have decreased F4/80$^+$ macrophages and CD4$^+$ T-cell accumulation in arthritic joints and serum concentrations of osteoclastogenic cytokines

Next, we carried out immunohistochemistry with an anti-F4/80 antibody and immunohistofluorescence with an anti-CD4-FITC antibody to check the extent of F4/80$^+$ macrophages and CD4$^+$ T-cell infiltration into the synovium, respectively. A significant reduction in both F4/80$^+$ macrophages and CD4$^+$ T-cell infiltration was observed in *Cxcl10*$^{-/-}$ and *Cxcr3*$^{-/-}$ mice compared with WT mice under the CAIA condition (Fig. 5a–d).

We have shown previously that CXCL10 levels are markedly increased in the inflamed joints and serum of CIA mice and that neutralization of CXCL10 by antibodies decreases CIA-induced elevation of RANKL and TNFα levels in serum [6]. Similar to the previous findings, C57BL/6 WT mice with CAIA exhibited a significant elevation of CXCL10, RANKL, TNFα, and IL-6 levels in serum compared with control mice. However,

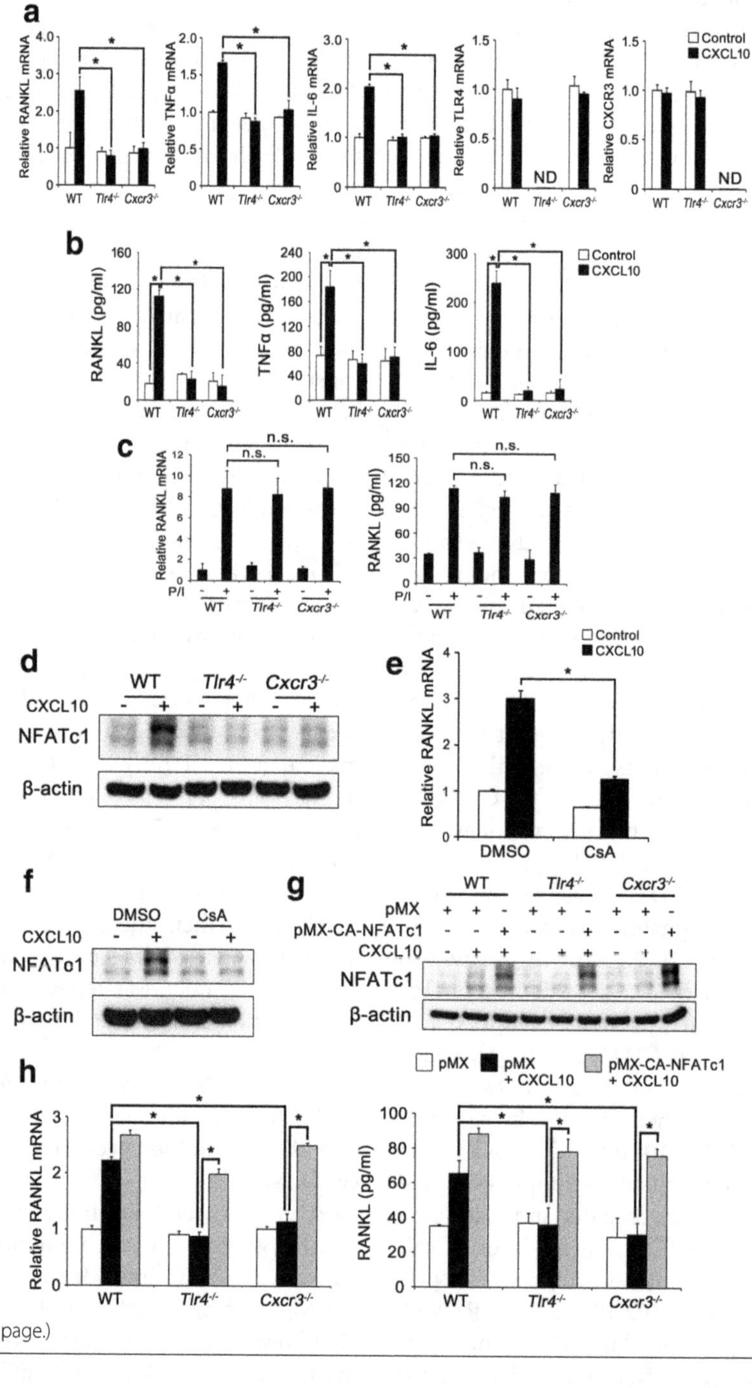

Fig. 2 (See legend on next page.)

(See figure on previous page.)
Fig. 2 CXCL10 stimulates production of osteoclastogenic cytokines in CD4$^+$ T cells through TLR4 and CXCR3. **a**, **b** CD4$^+$ T cells were isolated from WT, *Tlr4*$^{-/-}$, and *Cxcr3*$^{-/-}$ mice, and serum-starved CD4$^+$ T cells were cultured with or without CXCL10 (100 ng/ml) for 24 hours. RANKL, TNFα, IL-6, CXCR3, and TLR4 mRNA levels were analyzed by real-time PCR (**a**). RANKL, TNFα, and IL-6 protein levels in culture media were quantified by ELISA (**b**). **c** CD4$^+$ T cells from WT, *Tlr4*$^{-/-}$, and *Cxcr3*$^{-/-}$ mice were serum starved and treated with or without 500 ng/ml ionomycin and 20 ng/ml PMA (P/I) for 6 hours. RANKL mRNA levels and RANKL protein levels in culture media were measured by real-time PCR (*left panel*) and ELISA (*right panel*), respectively. **d** CD4$^+$ T cells were serum starved and treated with or without CXCL10 (100 ng/ml) for 24 hours. Total cell lysates were immunoblotted with the indicated antibodies. **e**, **f** Serum-starved WT CD4$^+$ T cells were preincubated with DMSO or 10 nM CsA and then stimulated with or without CXCL10 (100 ng/ml) for 24 hours. RANKL mRNA levels were analyzed by real-time PCR (**e**). NFATc1 protein levels were measured by western blotting (**f**). **g**, **h** CD4$^+$ T cells from the indicated mice were transduced with the retroviral vectors pMX-IRES-EGFP (*pMX*) or pMX-CA-NFATc1-IRES-EGFP (*pMX-CA-NFATc1*). The cells were serum starved and cultured with or without CXCL10 (100 ng/ml) for 24 hours. Total cell lysates were immunoblotted with the indicated antibodies (**g**). RANKL mRNA levels (**h**, *left panel*) and RANKL protein levels in culture media (**h**, *right panel*) were measured. Results shown are representative of three independent experiments ($n = 3$), and values are expressed as mean ± SD. *$P < 0.001$ by one-way ANOVA followed by Dunnett's test. *CXCL10* C-X-C motif chemokine 10, *RANKL* receptor activator of nuclear factor kappa-B ligand, *TNFα* tumor necrosis factor alpha, *IL-6* interleukin 6, *Tlr4* toll-like receptor 4, *Cxcr3* CXC chemokine receptor 3, *WT* wild-type, *NFATc1* nuclear factor of activated T cells, cytoplasmic 1, *DMSO* dimethyl sulfoxide, *CsA* cyclosporin A, *ND* not detected, *n.s.* nonsignificant

the CAIA-induced protein levels of RANKL, TNFα, and IL-6 in serum were markedly suppressed in *Cxcl10*$^{-/-}$ and *Cxcr3*$^{-/-}$ mice compared with their WT counterparts (Fig. 6a, b). In addition, CAIA greatly induced the mRNA expression of CXCL10, RANKL, TNFα, and IL-6 in spleens from WT mice, but not in spleens from *Cxcl10*$^{-/-}$ and *Cxcr3*$^{-/-}$ mice (Fig. 6c, d). Interestingly, we also found that the elevated protein or mRNA expression of CXCL10 in serum or spleen from WT mice with CAIA is abrogated in *Cxcr3*$^{-/-}$ mice (Fig. 6b, d), suggesting that CXCR3 signaling may involve an amplification of its ligand CXCL10 in the CAIA model.

Because CAIA-induced osteoclast activity was significantly decreased in *Cxcl10*$^{-/-}$ and *Cxcr3*$^{-/-}$ mice (Fig. 4), we measured serum CTX levels, a marker of bone resorption. As shown in Fig. 6a, b, serum CTX levels were increased by CAIA in WT mice, which was greatly inhibited in *Cxcl10*$^{-/-}$ and *Cxcr3*$^{-/-}$ mice.

Discussion

CXCL10 has been found to be highly expressed in the serum and synovial fluid of RA patients [15, 16]. Furthermore, previous studies have shown that pharmacologic blockade of CXCL10 signaling inhibits arthritis progression in animal models, mainly via inhibition of T-cell migration into the joint [6, 17, 35]. In the present study with *Cxcl10*$^{-/-}$ and *Cxcr3*$^{-/-}$ mice, we showed that the CXCL10–CXCR3 axis plays important roles in local and systemic inflammation in a CAIA model.

Infiltration of inflammatory cells into synovium is a crucial step in the progression of RA. The accumulation of inflammatory cells in the synovium mainly reflects migration rather than local proliferation [3]. CAIA is reported to be induced by infiltration of neutrophils and macrophages, which are the main effector cells in CAIA, into the inflamed joints [20, 21, 36]. Al-Banna et al. [37] showed that the accumulation of T cells in inflamed lymph nodes is highly CXCR3 dependent and that CXCR3 deficiency reduces the development of arthritis in a CIA model. In addition, Mohan and Issekutz [17] showed that blockade of CXCR3 inhibits T-cell and neutrophil recruitment to inflamed joints and decreases the severity of adjuvant arthritis. In the present study, we found that CXCL10 stimulates migration of BMMs and CD4$^+$ T cells through CXCR3-mediated ERK activation (Fig. 1). We also found that *Cxcl10*$^{-/-}$ and *Cxcr3*$^{-/-}$ mice showed less joint inflammation (Figs. 3 and 4) with reduced accumulation of F4/80$^+$ macrophages and CD4$^+$ T cells in the synovium (Fig. 5) compared with WT mice. Taken together, these results suggest that the CXCL10–CXCR3–ERK pathway may play a role in the accumulation of inflammatory cells during the development of arthritis.

It has been shown that inflammatory cytokine-expressing CD4$^+$ T cells in the spleen and RANKL-expressing CD4$^+$ T cells in blood are increased in the CAIA model [38]. In addition, inflammatory cytokine levels are systemically elevated in blood in CAIA mice [39]. Consistent with these reports, the protein and mRNA levels of RANKL, TNFα, IL-6, and CXCL10 in serum or spleens were elevated in WT mice with CAIA; however, elevation of these cytokines was abrogated in *Cxcl10*$^{-/-}$ and *Cxcr3*$^{-/-}$ mice (Fig. 6). We also found that CXCL10 stimulated the expression of RANKL, TNFα, and IL-6 in CD4$^+$ T cells in a CXCR3-dependent and TLR4-dependent manner (Fig. 2a, b). Enhanced levels of RANKL and TNFα play an essential role in inflammation and mediate cartilage and bone destruction in RA [2, 40, 41]. CD4$^+$ T cells are considered one of the major sources of inflammatory cytokines, especially of soluble RANKL, in arthritis. In fact, activated CD4$^+$ T cells expressing soluble RANKL have been shown to cause severe joint inflammation and bone and cartilage destruction in adjuvant arthritis [42]. It is thus likely that CXCL10 signaling contributes to CAIA-induced RANKL production at least in part through CD4$^+$ T cells in vivo. Recently, Grahnemo et al. [24] showed that CAIA is associated with an increased number of osteoclasts and

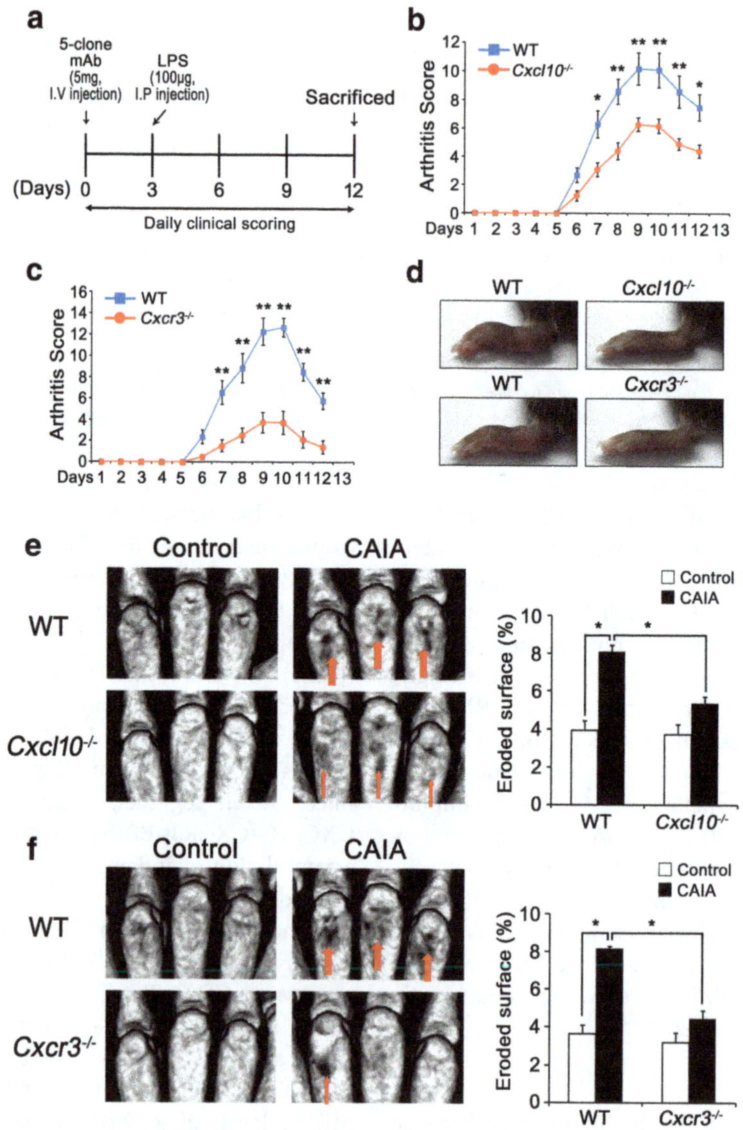

Fig. 3 Amelioration of CAIA development in *Cxcl10*$^{-/-}$ and *Cxcr3*$^{-/-}$ mice. **a** Experimental design of CAIA. WT, *Cxcl10*$^{-/-}$, and *Cxcr3*$^{-/-}$ mice were subjected to collagen type II antibodies + LPS (CAIA) or LPS injection (control). **b–d** Development of CAIA was monitored for 12 days, and arthritic scores were assessed by the degree of swelling in each paw (scored 0–3). Arthritic scores in WT and *Cxcl10*$^{-/-}$ mice (**b**, $n = 5$ each) and WT and *Cxcr3*$^{-/-}$ mice (**c**, $n = 5$ each) subjected to CAIA. Data represent mean ± SEM. *$P < 0.01$; **$P < 0.001$ vs WT at each time point by two-way repeated-measures ANOVA followed by Bonferroni's test. Representative photographs of CAIA-induced paw swelling on day 9 (**d**). **e**, **f** Representative micro-CT images and quantification of bone surface erosion in the hind paws from WT and *Cxcl10*$^{-/-}$ mice (**e**; $n = 5$ each group) and WT and *Cxcr3*$^{-/-}$ mice (**f**, $n = 5$ each group) on day 12. *Arrows* indicate bone erosions. Data represent mean ± SEM. *$P < 0.001$ by one-way ANOVA followed by Dunnett's test. *LPS* lipopolysaccharide, *WT* wild-type, *CXCL10* C-X-C motif chemokine 10, *Cxcr3* CXC chemokine receptor 3, *CAIA* collagen antibody-induced arthritis

trabecular bone loss. In the present study, CAIA-induced destruction of bone and cartilage in inflamed joints (Figs. 3 and 4) and elevation of CTX levels in serum (Fig. 6a, b) were significantly reduced in *Cxcl10*$^{-/-}$ and *Cxcr3*$^{-/-}$ mice. Collectively, these findings suggest that the elevation of CXCL10 signaling increases the production of cytokines including RANKL, TNFα, and IL-6, leading to destruction of bone and cartilage during the development of CAIA.

The RANKL gene promoter region in CD4^{+} T cells contains several recognition sequences for transcription factors, including NFAT, c-Fos, and NF-κB [31]. Wang et al. [32] have shown that intracellular calcineurin signaling downstream of T-cell receptor activation is critical for RANKL expression, which suggests that calcineurin-dependent NFAT activation may be involved in RANKL expression in CD4^{+} T cells. Activated calcineurin signaling can induce autoamplification of NFATc1

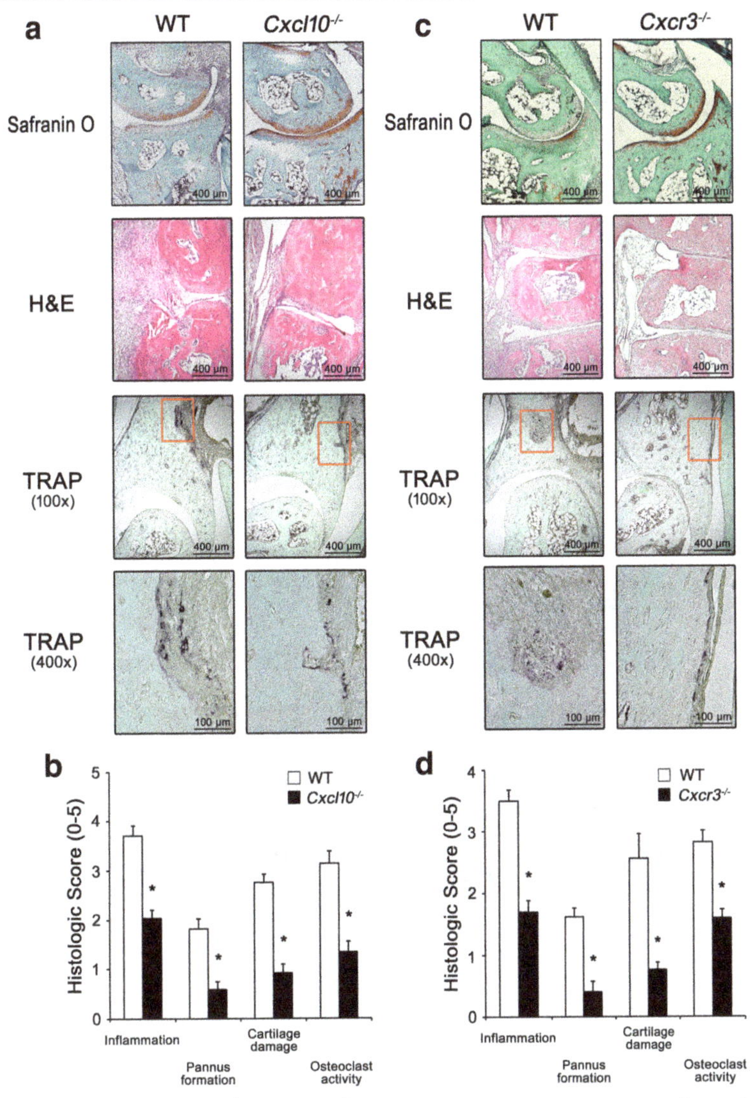

Fig. 4 Histological analysis of arthritic lesions in *Cxcl10*$^{-/-}$ and *Cxcr3*$^{-/-}$ mice with CAIA. Tissue sections were obtained from paw joints of the same mice as in Fig. 3 on day 12 after arthritic induction. Representative images of Safranin O, H&E, and TRAP staining (**a**, **c**) and quantification of histological analysis (**b**, **d**) of joint tissue sections from WT and *Cxcl10*$^{-/-}$ mice (**a**, **b**) and WT and *Cxcr3*$^{-/-}$ mice (**c**, **d**) with CAIA. *Fourth panel* (**a**, **c**) is a higher magnification image of the boxed area in the *third panel*. *Scale bar*, 400 μm (*first–third panels*) and 100 μm (*fourth panel*). Data represent mean ± SEM of results in five samples of staining ($n = 5$). *$P < 0.001$ vs WT mice by unpaired Student's *t* test. *WT* wild-type, *CXCL10* C-X-C motif chemokine 10, *Cxcr3* CXC chemokine receptor 3, *H&E* hematoxylin and eosin, *TRAP* tartrate-resistant acid phosphatase (Color figure online)

through NFATc1-dependent NFATc1 gene transcription [33]. In the present study, we found that CXCL10 increases NFATc1 and RANKL expression in CD4^{+} T cells in a CXCR3-dependent and TLR4-dependent manner (Fig. 2). Treatment of CD4^{+} T cells with CsA, an inhibitor of calcineurin activity, suppressed CXCL10-induced NFATc1 and RANKL expression. Moreover, the impairment of CXCL10-induced RANKL expression in *Cxcr3*$^{-/-}$ and *Tlr4*$^{-/-}$ CD4^{+} T cells was greatly rescued by overexpression of CA-NFATc1 (Fig. 2g, h). Therefore, our results indicate that CXCL10 induces RANKL expression in CD4^{+} T cells via the activation of NFATc1 in a CXCR3-dependent and TLR4-dependent manner. Although it has been shown that TLR4 is involved in the pathophysiology of RA in CIA and K/BxN serum transfer animal models [43, 44], the functional role of TLR4 in CXCL10-mediated production of cytokines contributing to destruction of bone and cartilage during the development of RA remains to be elucidated.

It is well known that CXCR3 is the main receptor for CXCL10. In line with this fact, CXCL10-induced cell migration and cytokine production were completely abolished in BMMs and CD4^{+} T cells from *Cxcr3*$^{-/-}$ cells (Figs. 1 and 2). Interestingly, however, we found that CXCL10-induced cytokine production was also abolished in *Tlr4*$^{-/-}$ CD4^{+} T cells even though the CXCR3 expression

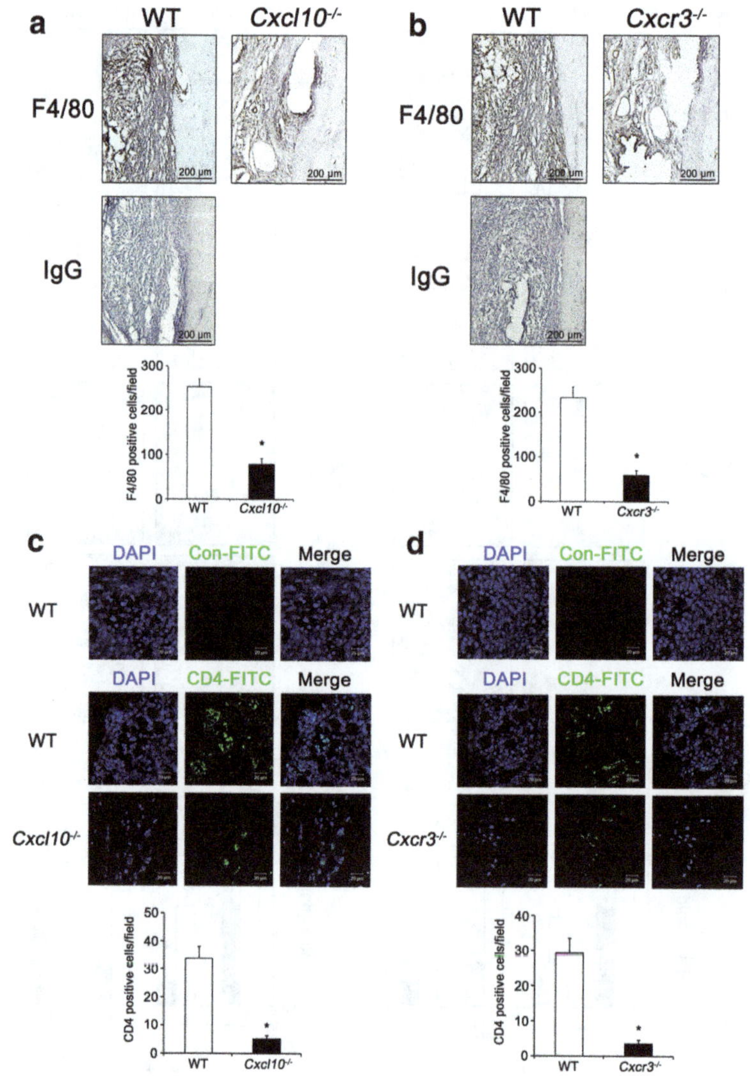

Fig. 5 Reduction of macrophages and $CD4^+$ T cells accumulation in arthritic joints of *Cxcl10*$^{-/-}$ and *Cxcr3*$^{-/-}$ mice with CAIA. **a**, **b** Joint tissue sections from WT, *Cxcl10*$^{-/-}$ (**a**), and *Cxcr3*$^{-/-}$ (**b**) mice with CAIA used in Fig. 4 were stained with an IgG or an anti-F4/80 antibody. Representative images of F4/80 staining of joint tissue sections from each group (*top panel*) and quantification of F4/80-positive cells (*bottom panel*). IgG, negative control. *Scale bar*, 200 μm. Data represent mean ± SEM of results in five samples ($n = 5$). $^*P < 0.001$ vs WT mice by unpaired Student's *t* test. **c**, **d** Joint tissue sections from WT, *Cxcl10*$^{-/-}$ (**c**), and *Cxcr3*$^{-/-}$ (**d**) mice with CAIA used in Fig. 4 were stained with a control-FITC or an anti-CD4-FITC antibody. Representative images of CD4-FITC staining of joint tissue sections from each group (*second and third topmost panels*) and quantification of CD4-positive cells (*bottom panel*). Con-FITC, negative control. *Scale bar*, 20 μm. Data represent mean ± SEM of results in five samples ($n = 5$). $^*P < 0.001$ vs WT mice by unpaired Student's *t* test. *WT* wild-type, *CXCL10* C-X-C motif chemokine 10, *Cxcr3* CXC chemokine receptor 3, *IgG* immunoglobulin G, *DAPI* 4′,6-diamidino-2-phenylindole, *FITC* fluorescein isothiocyanate

was intact in these cells (Fig. 2). These results suggest that TLR4 is specifically required for CXCR3 signaling in CXCL10-induced cytokine production, but not in CXCL10-induced cell migration. It has been reported that TLR4 activation induces an upregulation of chemokine expression including CXCL10 [45]. Recently, we have reported that CXCL10 induces CXCL10 expression through CXCR3 [46]. The TLR4 activation-induced or CXCR3-mediated CXCL10 upregulation can exert important roles in arthritis progression through TLR4 and CXCR3, suggesting that it could form a positive feedback loop between CXCL10 and its receptors TLR4 and/or CXCR3. In addition, several studies have shown crosstalk between TLRs and GPCR signaling. Eskan et al. [47] showed that TLR4 and S1P receptors coordinate to enhance inflammatory cytokine production in epithelial cells. GPCR agonist has been shown to transactivate TLRs via mammalian neuraminidase-1 sialidase and matrix metalloproteinase-9 crosstalk [48]. Moreover, TLR signaling has been reported to regulate GPCR signals by altering

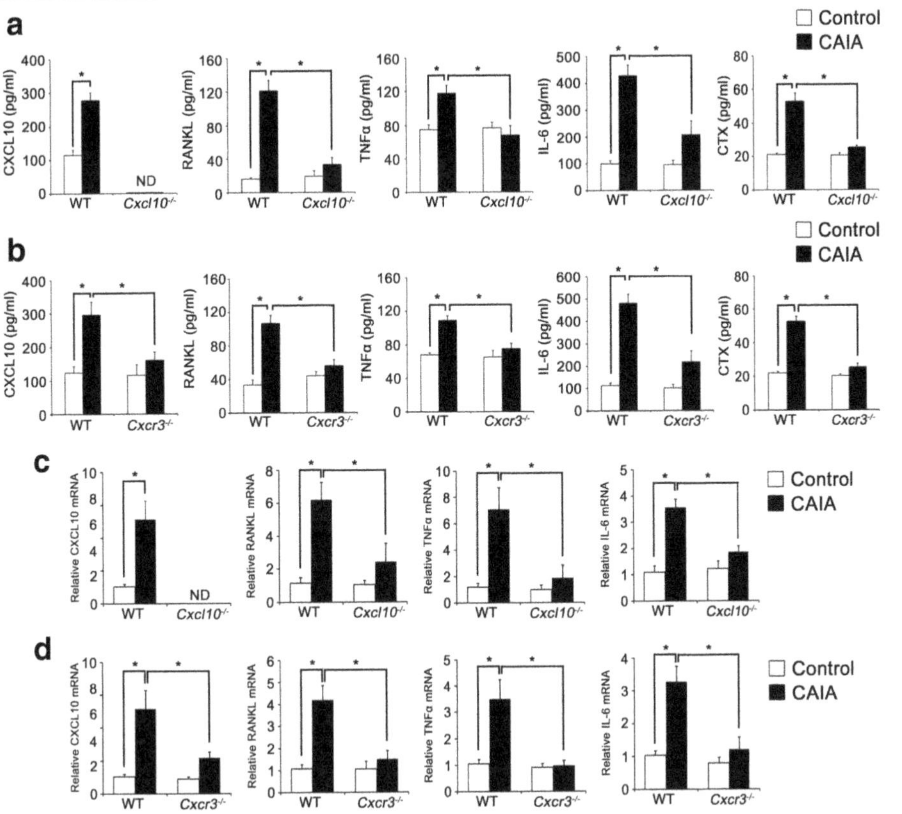

Fig. 6 Reduction of osteoclastogenic cytokine levels in serum and spleen of *Cxcl10*$^{-/-}$ and *Cxcr3*$^{-/-}$ mice with CAIA. **a**, **b** Serum was collected from the same WT, *Cxcl10*$^{-/-}$ (**a**), and *Cxcr3*$^{-/-}$ (**b**) mice as in Fig. 3 on day 12. Serum levels of CXCL10, RANKL, TNFα, IL-6, and CTX were measured by ELISA. Data represent mean ± SEM. *$P < 0.001$ by one-way ANOVA followed by Dunnett's test. **c**, **d** Spleens were collected from the same WT, *Cxcl10*$^{-/-}$ (**c**), and *Cxcr3*$^{-/-}$ (**d**) mice as in Fig. 3 on day 12. RANKL, TNFα, IL-6, and CXCL10 mRNA levels were analyzed by real-time PCR. Data represent mean ± SEM of results in five samples ($n = 5$). *$P < 0.001$ vs WT mice by unpaired Student's *t* test. *WT* wild-type, *CXCL10* C-X-C motif chemokine 10, *Cxcr3* CXC chemokine receptor 3, *CAIA* collagen antibody-induced arthritis, *RANKL* receptor activator of nuclear factor kappa-B ligand, *TNFα* tumor necrosis factor α, *IL-6* interleukin 6, *CTX* C-terminal telopeptide, *ND* not detected

the expression of regulator of G protein signaling proteins in inflammatory cells [49, 50]. However, analysis of how TLR4 cooperates with CXCR3 in CXCL10-induced cytokine production remains to be elucidated.

As mentioned earlier, several cells including macrophages, T cells, neutrophils, and fibroblast-like synoviocytes have been considered relevant components of RA progression. These cells in the inflamed joint or other organs have roles in secretion of proinflammatory cytokines/chemokines, synovitis, and synovial pannus formation, leading to chronic inflammation and joint destruction [3]. In the present study, we used global *Cxcl10*$^{-/-}$ and *Cxcr3*$^{-/-}$ mice to investigate the pathogenic roles of CXCL10 signaling in a CAIA model and obtained less inflammation, accumulation of F4/80$^+$ macrophages and CD4$^+$ T cells, cytokine production, cartilage degeneration, and bone destruction in those mice. Accumulating evidence has shown that neutrophil recruitment in the joints is reduced by blockade of CXCR3 [17] and that CXCL10/CXCR3 signaling regulates invasion of fibroblast-like synoviocytes [51]. Given these reports, we cannot rule out that defective CXCL10 signaling in those cells including neutrophil and fibroblast-like synoviocytes might contribute to the inhibitory results of arthritis progression seen in *Cxcl10*$^{-/-}$ and *Cxcr3*$^{-/-}$ mice in our study. Furthermore, it has been reported that the accumulation of T cells in inflamed lymph nodes is highly CXCR3 dependent, but not CCR4 dependent [37]. Thus, we speculated that decreased recruitment of T cells in other organs including inflamed lymph nodes, not only in the synovium, would be observed in *Cxcl10*$^{-/-}$ and *Cxcr3*$^{-/-}$ mice; however, this hypothesis remains to be elucidated.

Collectively, our study provides data on the functional roles and molecular mechanisms of CXCL10 signaling in local and systemic inflammatory processes in RA. A study from human phase II clinical trials using anti-CXCL10 monoclonal antibody (MDX-1100) in RA patients has shown an improved response rate on day 58 [52]. In the present study, reducing the clinical severity of CAIA was more effective in *Cxcr3*$^{-/-}$ mice than in

Cxcl10$^{-/-}$ mice (Fig. 3b, c). This might be due to the presence of other CXCR3 ligands including CXCL9 and CXCL11. Indeed, CXCL9 has been shown to be increased in the serum of RA patients [16]. In addition, CAIA-induced elevation of CXCL10 levels was abrogated in *Cxcr3*$^{-/-}$ mice (Fig. 6b, d). Thus, these findings suggest that CXCR3 would be a more attractive therapeutic target for RA than CXCL10.

Conclusions

CXCL10 increased cell migration via CXCR3, not TLR4. However, both the CXCR3 and TLR4 receptors were required for CXCL10 to stimulate cytokine production in CD4$^+$ T cells. The activated calcineurin-dependent NFATc1 pathway was essential for CXCL10-induced RANKL expression in CD4$^+$ T cells. Arthritic *Cxcl10*$^{-/-}$ and *Cxcr3*$^{-/-}$ mice showed milder bone destruction, serum cytokines, and cell infiltration into synovium. These results indicate that CXCL10 may exert pathogenic roles through CXCR3 or TLR4 during arthritis progression.

Abbreviations

ACK: Ammonium–chloride–potassium; BMM: Bone marrow-derived macrophage; CAIA: Collagen antibody-induced arthritis; CIA: Collagen-induced arthritis; CsA: Cyclosporin A; CTX: C-terminal telopeptide; CXCL10: C-X-C motif chemokine 10; CXCR3: Chemokine receptor 3; DAPI: 4',6-Diamidino-2-phenylindole; EDTA: Ethylenediaminetetraacetic acid; ELISA: Enzyme-linked immunosorbent assay; FITC: Fluorescein isothiocyanate; H&E: Hematoxylin and eosin; IFN-γ: Interferon gamma; IL: Interleukin; LPS: Lipopolysaccharide; NFATc1: Nuclear factor of activated T cells, cytoplasmic 1; PBS: Phosphate-buffered saline; RA: Rheumatoid arthritis; RANKL: Receptor activator of nuclear factor kappa-B; TLR4: Toll-like receptor 4; TNFα: Tumor necrosis factor alpha; TRAP: Tartrate-resistant acid phosphatase; WT: Wild-type

Acknowledgements
Not applicable.

Funding
This study was supported by the Basic Science Research Program through the National Research Foundation of Korea funded by the Ministry of Science, ICT & Future Planning (NRF-2014R1A2A2A01002531).

Authors' contributions

J-HL and BK designated almost studies together. J-HL participated in the molecular studies of CD4$^+$ T cells and BMMs, carried out the CAIA experiment, drafted the manuscript and revised the manuscript. BK carried out the molecular studies of CD4$^+$ T cells and BMMs, participated in the CAIA experiment, drafted the manuscript and revised the manuscript. J-HL and BK cooperated in the study with each other. WJJ participated in design of the CAIA experiment and acquired the data of the CAIA experiments. H-HK provided insightful guidance, participated in design of experiments, and analyzed the data of the BMM assay. ZHL provided insightful guidance, critical appraisal of the manuscript and the revised manuscript, participated in its design, and performed statistical analyses. HH provided critical appraisal of the manuscript and performed statistical analyses. All other experiments were done by J-HL and BK. All authors read and approved the final manuscript.

Competing interests

The authors declare that they have no competing interests.

Author details
[1]Department of Cell and Developmental Biology, Dental Research Institute, School of Dentistry, Seoul National University, 28 Yeongon-dong, Jongno-gu, Seoul 110-749, Republic of Korea. [2]Brain Tumor Center and Department of Neuro-Oncology, The University of Texas MD Anderson Cancer Center, Houston, TX 77030, USA. [3]Clinical Research Division, Korean Medicine-Based Herbal Drug Development Group, Korea Institute of Oriental Medicine, 483 Expo-Ro, Yuseong-Gu, Daejeon 305-811, Republic of Korea.

References

1. Boyle WJ, Simonet WS, Lacey DL. Osteoclast differentiation and activation. Nature. 2003;423(6937):337–42.
2. Walsh NC, Crotti TN, Goldring SR, Gravallese EM. Rheumatic diseases: the effects of inflammation on bone. Immunol Rev. 2005;208:228–51.
3. McInnes IB, Schett G. The pathogenesis of rheumatoid arthritis. N Engl J Med. 2011;365(23):2205–19.
4. Tran CN, Lundy SK, Fox DA. Synovial biology and T cells in rheumatoid arthritis. Pathophysiology. 2005;12(3):183–9.
5. Beech JT, Andreakos E, Ciesielski CJ, Green P, Foxwell BM, Brennan FM. T-cell contact-dependent regulation of CC and CXC chemokine production in monocytes through differential involvement of NFkappaB: implications for rheumatoid arthritis. Arthritis Res Ther. 2006;8(6):R168.
6. Kwak HB, Ha H, Kim HN, Lee JH, Kim HS, Lee S, Kim HM, Kim JY, Kim HH, Song YW, et al. Reciprocal cross-talk between RANKL and interferon-gamma-inducible protein 10 is responsible for bone-erosive experimental arthritis. Arthritis Rheum. 2008;58(5):1332–42.
7. Schett G, Hayer S, Zwerina J, Redlich K, Smolen JS. Mechanisms of disease: the link between RANKL and arthritic bone disease. Nat Clin Pract Rheumatol. 2005;1(1):47–54.
8. Gravallese EM, Manning C, Tsay A, Naito A, Pan C, Amento E, Goldring SR. Synovial tissue in rheumatoid arthritis is a source of osteoclast differentiation factor. Arthritis Rheum. 2000;43(2):250–8.
9. Kotake S, Udagawa N, Hakoda M, Mogi M, Yano K, Tsuda E, Takahashi K, Furuya T, Ishiyama S, Kim KJ, et al. Activated human T cells directly induce osteoclastogenesis from human monocytes: possible role of T cells in bone destruction in rheumatoid arthritis patients. Arthritis Rheum. 2001;44(5):1003–12.
10. Bartok B, Firestein GS. Fibroblast-like synoviocytes: key effector cells in rheumatoid arthritis. Immunol Rev. 2010;233(1):233–55.
11. Muller-Ladner U, Kriegsmann J, Franklin BN, Matsumoto S, Geiler T, Gay RE, Gay S. Synovial fibroblasts of patients with rheumatoid arthritis attach to and invade normal human cartilage when engrafted into SCID mice. Am J Pathol. 1996;149(5):1607–15.
12. Lee EY, Lee ZH, Song YW. CXCL10 and autoimmune diseases. Autoimmun Rev. 2009;8(5):379–83.
13. Schulthess FT, Paroni F, Sauter NS, Shu L, Ribaux P, Haataja L, Strieter RM, Oberholzer J, King CC, Maedler K. CXCL10 impairs beta cell function and viability in diabetes through TLR4 signaling. Cell Metab. 2009;9(2):125–39.
14. Rotondi M, Chiovato L, Romagnani S, Serio M, Romagnani P. Role of chemokines in endocrine autoimmune diseases. Endocr Rev. 2007;28(5):492–520.
15. Hanaoka R, Kasama T, Muramatsu M, Yajima N, Shiozawa F, Miwa Y, Negishi M, Ide H, Miyaoka H, Uchida H, et al. A novel mechanism for the regulation of IFN-gamma inducible protein-10 expression in rheumatoid arthritis. Arthritis Res Ther. 2003;5(2):R74–81.
16. Kuan WP, Tam LS, Wong CK, Ko FW, Li T, Zhu T, Li EK. CXCL 9 and CXCL 10 as Sensitive markers of disease activity in patients with rheumatoid arthritis. J Rheumatol. 2010;37(2):257–64.
17. Mohan K, Issekutz TB. Blockade of chemokine receptor CXCR3 inhibits T cell recruitment to inflamed joints and decreases the severity of adjuvant arthritis. J Immunol. 2007;179(12):8463–9.
18. Lee EY, Seo M, Juhnn YS, Kim JY, Hong YJ, Lee YJ, Lee EB, Song YW. Potential role and mechanism of IFN-gamma inducible protein-10 on receptor activator of nuclear factor kappa-B ligand (RANKL) expression in rheumatoid arthritis. Arthritis Res Ther. 2011;13(3):R104.

19. Cho YG, Cho ML, Min SY, Kim HY. Type II collagen autoimmunity in a mouse model of human rheumatoid arthritis. Autoimmun Rev. 2007;7(1):65–70.
20. Nandakumar KS, Svensson L, Holmdahl R. Collagen type II-specific monoclonal antibody-induced arthritis in mice: description of the disease and the influence of age, sex, and genes. Am J Pathol. 2003;163(5):1827–37.
21. Tanaka D, Kagari T, Doi H, Shimozato T. Essential role of neutrophils in anti-type II collagen antibody and lipopolysaccharide-induced arthritis. Immunology. 2006;119(2):195–202.
22. Khachigian LM. Collagen antibody-induced arthritis. Nat Protoc. 2006; 1(5):2512–6.
23. Wang J, Fathman JW, Lugo-Villarino G, Scimone L, von Andrian U, Dorfman DM, Glimcher LH. Transcription factor T-bet regulates inflammatory arthritis through its function in dendritic cells. J Clin Invest. 2006;116(2):414–21.
24. Grahnemo L, Andersson A, Nurkkala-Karlsson M, Stubelius A, Lagerquist MK, Svensson MN, Ohlsson C, Carlsten H, Islander U. Trabecular bone loss in collagen antibody-induced arthritis. Arthritis Res Ther. 2015;17:189.
25. Lee JH, Kim HN, Yang D, Jung K, Kim HM, Kim HH, Ha H, Lee ZH. Trolox prevents osteoclastogenesis by suppressing RANKL expression and signaling. J Biol Chem. 2009;284(20):13725–34.
26. Bendele A, McAbee T, Sennello G, Frazier J, Chlipala E, McCabe D. Efficacy of sustained blood levels of interleukin-1 receptor antagonist in animal models of arthritis: comparison of efficacy in animal models with human clinical data. Arthritis Rheum. 1999;42(3):498–506.
27. Pettit AR, Ji H, von Stechow D, Muller R, Goldring SR, Choi Y, Benoist C, Gravallese EM. TRANCE/RANKL knockout mice are protected from bone erosion in a serum transfer model of arthritis. Am J Pathol. 2001;159(5):1689–99.
28. Lee JH, Kim HN, Kim KO, Jin WJ, Lee S, Kim HH, Ha H, Lee ZH. CXCL10 promotes osteolytic bone metastasis by enhancing cancer outgrowth and osteoclastogenesis. Cancer Res. 2012;72(13):3175–86.
29. Kwak HB, Sun HM, Ha H, Lee JH, Kim HN, Lee ZH. AG490, a Jak2-specific inhibitor, induces osteoclast survival by activating the Akt and ERK signaling pathways. Mol Cells. 2008;26(5):436–42.
30. Bonacchi A, Romagnani P, Romanelli RG, Efsen E, Annunziato F, Lasagni L, Francalanci M, Serio M, Laffi G, Pinzani M, et al. Signal transduction by the chemokine receptor CXCR3: activation of Ras/ERK, Src, and phosphatidylinositol 3-kinase/Akt controls cell migration and proliferation in human vascular pericytes. J Biol Chem. 2001;276(13):9945–54.
31. Bishop KA, Coy HM, Nerenz RD, Meyer MB, Pike JW. Mouse Rankl expression is regulated in T cells by c-Fos through a cluster of distal regulatory enhancers designated the T cell control region. J Biol Chem. 2011;286(23):20880–91.
32. Wang R, Zhang L, Zhang X, Moreno J, Celluzzi C, Tondravi M, Shi Y. Regulation of activation-induced receptor activator of NF-kappaB ligand (RANKL) expression in T cells. Eur J Immunol. 2002;32(4):1090–8.
33. Takayanagi H, Kim S, Koga T, Nishina H, Isshiki M, Yoshida H, Saiura A, Isobe M, Yokochi T, Inoue J, et al. Induction and activation of the transcription factor NFATc1 (NFAT2) integrate RANKL signaling in terminal differentiation of osteoclasts. Dev Cell. 2002;3(6):889–901.
34. Kiani A, Rao A, Aramburu J. Manipulating immune responses with immunosuppressive agents that target NFAT. Immunity. 2000;12(4):359–72.
35. O'Boyle G, Fox CR, Walden HR, Willet JD, Mavin ER, Hine DW, Palmer JM, Barker CE, Lamb CA, Ali S, et al. Chemokine receptor CXCR3 agonist prevents human T-cell migration in a humanized model of arthritic inflammation. Proc Natl Acad Sci U S A. 2012;109(12):4598–603.
36. Murata K, Inami M, Hasegawa A, Kubo S, Kimura M, Yamashita M, Hosokawa H, Nagao T, Suzuki K, Hashimoto K, et al. CD69-null mice protected from arthritis induced with anti-type II collagen antibodies. Int Immunol. 2003; 15(8):987–92.
37. Al-Banna NA, Vaci M, Slauenwhite D, Johnston B, Issekutz TB. CCR4 and CXCR3 play different roles in the migration of T cells to inflammation in skin, arthritic joints, and lymph nodes. Eur J Immunol. 2014;44(6):1633–43.
38. Dimitrova P, Ivanovska N, Belenska L, Milanova V, Schwaeble W, Stover C. Abrogated RANKL expression in properdin-deficient mice is associated with better outcome from collagen-antibody-induced arthritis. Arthritis Res Ther. 2012;14(4):R173.
39. Park MH, Yoon DY, Ban JO, Kim DH, Lee DH, Song S, Kim Y, Han SB, Lee HP, Hong JT. Decreased severity of collagen antibody and lipopolysaccharide-induced arthritis in human IL-32beta overexpressed transgenic mice. Oncotarget. 2015;6(36):38566–77.
40. Ehrenstein MR, Evans JG, Singh A, Moore S, Warnes G, Isenberg DA, Mauri C. Compromised function of regulatory T cells in rheumatoid arthritis and reversal by anti-TNFalpha therapy. J Exp Med. 2004;200(3):277–85.
41. Saidenberg-Kermanac'h N, Corrado A, Lemeiter D, deVernejoul MC, Boissier MC, Cohen-Solal ME. TNF-alpha antibodies and osteoprotegerin decrease systemic bone loss associated with inflammation through distinct mechanisms in collagen-induced arthritis. Bone. 2004;35(5):1200–7.
42. Kong YY, Feige U, Sarosi I, Bolon B, Tafuri A, Morony S, Capparelli C, Li J, Elliott R, McCabe S, et al. Activated T cells regulate bone loss and joint destruction in adjuvant arthritis through osteoprotegerin ligand. Nature. 1999;402(6759):304–9.
43. Pierer M, Wagner U, Rossol M, Ibrahim S. Toll-like receptor 4 is involved in inflammatory and joint destructive pathways in collagen-induced arthritis in DBA1J mice. PLoS One. 2011;6(8):e23539.
44. Kim HS, Chung DH. TLR4-mediated IL-12 production enhances IFN-gamma and IL-1beta production, which inhibits TGF-beta production and promotes antibody-induced joint inflammation. Arthritis Res Ther. 2012;14(5):R210.
45. Kawai T, Takeuchi O, Fujita T, Inoue J, Muhlradt PF, Sato S, Hoshino K, Akira S. Lipopolysaccharide stimulates the MyD88-independent pathway and results in activation of IFN-regulatory factor 3 and the expression of a subset of lipopolysaccharide-inducible genes. J Immunol. 2001;167(10):5887–94.
46. Jin WJ, Kim B, Kim D, Park Choo HY, Kim HH, Ha H, Lee ZH. NF-kappaB signaling regulates cell-autonomous regulation of CXCL10 in breast cancer 4 T1 cells. Exp Mol Med. 2017;49(2):e295.
47. Eskan MA, Rose BG, Benakanakere MR, Zeng Q, Fujioka D, Martin MH, Lee MJ, Kinane DF. TLR4 and S1P receptors cooperate to enhance inflammatory cytokine production in human gingival epithelial cells. Eur J Immunol. 2008; 38(4):1138–47.
48. Abdulkhalek S, Szewczuk MR. Neu1 sialidase and matrix metalloproteinase-9 cross-talk regulates nucleic acid-induced endosomal TOLL-like receptor-7 and -9 activation, cellular signaling and pro-inflammatory responses. Cell Signal. 2013;25(11):2093–105.
49. Loniewski K, Shi Y, Pestka J, Parameswaran N. Toll-like receptors differentially regulate GPCR kinases and arrestins in primary macrophages. Mol Immunol. 2008;45(8):2312–22.
50. Shi GX, Harrison K, Han SB, Moratz C, Kehrl JH. Toll-like receptor signaling alters the expression of regulator of G protein signaling proteins in dendritic cells: implications for G protein-coupled receptor signaling. J Immunol. 2004;172(9):5175–84.
51. Laragione T, Brenner M, Sherry B, Gulko PS. CXCL10 and its receptor CXCR3 regulate synovial fibroblast invasion in rheumatoid arthritis. Arthritis Rheum. 2011;63(11):3274–83.
52. Yellin M, Paliienko I, Balanescu A, Ter-Vartanian S, Tseluyko V, Xu LA, Tao X, Cardarelli PM, Leblanc H, Nichol G, et al. A phase II, randomized, double-blind, placebo-controlled study evaluating the efficacy and safety of MDX-1100, a fully human anti-CXCL10 monoclonal antibody, in combination with methotrexate in patients with rheumatoid arthritis. Arthritis Rheum. 2012; 64(6):1730–9.

14

Lymphatic delivery of etanercept via nanotopography improves response to collagen-induced arthritis

Melissa B. Aldrich[1], Fred C. Velasquez[1], Sunkuk Kwon[1], Ali Azhdarinia[1], Kenneth Pinkston[1], Barrett R. Harvey[1], Wenyaw Chan[2], John C. Rasmussen[1], Russell F. Ross[3], Caroline E. Fife[4] and E. M. Sevick-Muraca[1*]

Abstract

Background: Evidence suggests lymphatic function mediates local rheumatoid arthritis (RA) flares. Yet biologics that target the immune system are dosed systemically via the subcutaneous (SC) administration route, thereby inefficiently reaching local lymphatic compartments. Nanotopography has previously been shown to disrupt tight cellular junctions, potentially enhancing local lymphatic delivery and potentially improving overall therapeutic efficacy.

Method: We first characterized nanotopography (SOFUSA™) delivery of an anti-TNF drug, etanercept, by comparing pharmacokinetic profiles to those obtained by conventional SC, intravenous (IV), and intradermal (ID) routes of administration, and assessed uptake of radiolabeled etanercept in draining lymph nodes (LNs) in single dosing studies. We then compared etanercept efficacy in a progressive rat model of collagen-induced arthritis (CIA), administered systemically via SC route of administration; via the regional lymphatics through ID delivery; or through a nanotopography (SOFUSA™) device at 10, 12, and 14 days post CIA induction. Measurements of hind limb swelling and near-infrared fluorescence (NIRF) imaging of afferent lymph pumping function and reflux were conducted on days 11, 13, and 18 post CIA induction and compared to untreated CIA animals. Univariate and multivariate analysis of variance were used to compare the group differences for percentage swelling and lymphatic contractile activity.

Results: Even though all three modes of administration delivered an equal amount of etanercept, SOFUSA™ delivery resulted in increased lymphatic pumping and significantly reduced swelling as compared to untreated, ID, and SC groups. Pharmacokinetic profiles in serum and LN uptake studies showed that using the nanotopography device resulted in the greatest uptake and retention in draining LNs.

Conclusions: Locoregional lymphatic delivery of biologics that target the immune system may have more favorable pharmacodynamics than SC or IV administration. Nanotopography may provide a more efficient method for delivery of anti-TNF drugs to reverse impairment of lymphatic function and reduce swelling associated with RA flares.

Keywords: Lymphatic pumping function, Nanotopography, Delivery systems, Route of administration, Etanercept, Near-infrared fluorescence lymphatic imaging

* Correspondence: Eva.Sevick@uth.tmc.edu
[1]The Center for Molecular Imaging, The Brown Foundation Institute of Molecular Medicine, The University of Texas Health Science Center, Houston, TX 77030, USA
Full list of author information is available at the end of the article

Background

Rheumatoid arthritis (RA) is a chronic inflammatory joint disease and one of several immune-mediated inflammatory disorders with etiology that is not well-understood. RA is characterized by inflammation in the synovial membrane, cartilage, and bone, where accumulation of immune cells is observed. Patients experience severe pain, swelling, and erosion of the joints that leads to joint deformity and disability. In patients who are unresponsive to non-steroidal anti-inflammatory drugs or disease modifying anti-rheumatic drugs, a number of biologic agents (antibodies or recombinant proteins) that block activity of inflammatory mediators or signaling molecules provide another line of defense [1]. Examples include biologics that: (1) deplete B-cells that produce autoantibodies characteristic of RA or (2) block co-stimulatory signals needed to activate T-cells within the lymph nodes (LNs). In the latter case, biologic targets are pro-inflammatory cytokines such as anti-tumor necrosis factor (TNF), interleukin-6 (IL-6), and interleukin-1 (IL-1) that are secreted by macrophages and play important roles in T-cell activation. Interestingly, while the sites of action of these cytokine and signaling molecules may be in regional LNs and lymphatic vasculature, biologics that target the immune system are provided through intravenous (IV) or subcutaneous (SC) routes that may not efficiently reach the lymphatics.

The lymphatic vasculature is a unidirectional highway for the transit of immune cells, activation of T cells and B cells, and return of activated immune cells, cellular waste, and excess fluid to the blood vasculature [2]. The lymphatic vasculature starts with initial lymphatic capillaries beneath the epidermis that surround most organs and the synovium. These capillaries are composed of single layers of lymphatic endothelial cells with no basement membrane. Immune cells, waste products, and fluid enter between specialized button-like, lymphatic endothelial cell junctions [3] and are propelled through mature conducting lymphatic vessel segments called lymphangions, which are bounded by valves that open and close in concert with lymphatic smooth muscle contraction to efficiently pump lymph proximally and through regional LNs, before emptying into the blood stream. Entrance of exogenous agents into the lymphatic vasculature can occur via an intradermal (ID) injection into space occupied by the initial lymphatics under the epidermis, or to a lesser extent, into the high endothelial venules of LNs following IV injection. SC administration may enable indirect entry into both venous and lymphatic vasculatures, but is limited from efficient uptake from the interstitium into blood vessels due to the intact tight endothelial junctions and glycocalyx that severely regulates the flow of high molecular-weight molecules across the blood vessel wall [4]. SC administration thus misses the ID space beneath the epidermis containing the initial lymphatics that efficiently take up macromolecules. As a consequence, SC administration is associated with reduced bioavailability and impaired systemic and lymphatic delivery.

As reviewed elsewhere [5, 6], several recent clinical and experimental observations implicate the lymphatic vasculature in the pathogenesis of RA. Lymphedema and RA are known comorbidities [7], and lymphangiography studies show that RA patients have abnormal lymphatic vasculature with extensive dermal reflux, consistent with lymphedema [8]. In addition, enlarged and greater numbers of popliteal LNs, and increased synovial fluid volumes in the knees of RA patients, have been reported along with elevated pro-inflammatory cytokine levels in lymph-draining synovial joints, as compared to levels found in serum [9]. In animal studies, elevated levels of the pro-inflammatory and pro-lymphangiogenic cytokine vascular endothelial growth factor C (VEGF-C) have been found in the joints of tumor necrosis factor transgenic (TNF-Tg) animals, which mimic human RA pathogenesis [10]. TNF-Tg animals experience B-cell expansion in draining LNs with concomitant collapse and loss of afferent lymph vessel pumping, as measured by non-invasive near-infrared fluorescence (NIRF) lymphatic imaging [11], and proinflammatory cytokines TNF-α and IL-1β cause lymphatic vessel dilation and arrest of the lymphatic pump that can be rescued by ID-administered inducible nitric oxide (iNOS) inhibitors [12]. Because the draining lymphatic vasculature and LNs have been shown to mediate adaptive immune responses [13] and may mediate RA flares, [14] delivery of therapeutic agents through the lymphatic compartment could be expected to mediate a systemic response with an enhanced effect on local disease manifestation.

While systemic anti-TNF therapy is considered successful in the treatment of RA, a substantial percentage of patients (~30 – 40%) fail to respond, exposing them to unnecessary adverse events while disease progresses [15, 16]. Similar failure rates are reported for other biologics administered for RA, and efforts to identify biomarkers that could predict response rates have failed [17].

Given the importance of the draining lymphatics in RA, we sought to determine whether nanotopography-directed lymphatic delivery of an anti-TNF drug, etanercept, could result in improvement of lymphatic pumping function and reduced swelling in the collagen-induced arthritis (CIA) model of RA progression. We first characterized the pharmacokinetic (PK) profiles and measured the accumulation of etanercept in draining LNs using nanotopography, ID, and SC local administration, and using systemic IV administration. Because CIA animals have varying disease severity that could impact measurements, we performed these measurements in normal animals. Then in CIA animals, we monitored hind limb swelling and lymphatic pumping function using NIRF lymphatic imaging [18] before, during, and following a course of etanercept administered SC, ID, or with a nanotopographic device that infused drug directly into the intradermal space containing the initial lymphatics. We show that lymphatic delivery of etanercept predominated with nanotopography (SOFUSA™) and resulted in improved pumping function of afferent lymphatic vessels and reduced hind limb swelling in CIA animals when compared to animals treated with SC-administered or ID-administered etanercept.

Methods

General procedures and reagents

Animals and housing

Male Lewis rats, each weighing approximately 350 g, were obtained from Charles River (Wilmington, MA, USA) and housed in an Association for Assessment and Accreditation of Laboratory Animal Care-approved facility, according to institutional guidelines. All animal protocols were reviewed and approved by the Institutional Animal Care and Use Committee at the University of Texas Health Science Center-Houston. Animals used for CIA induction, PK, and LN uptake studies were ear-tagged prior to handling.

Reagents

All reagents were analytical grade and used without further purification unless otherwise stated. Etanercept (Enbrel, Amgen, CA, USA) was received in 50 mg/ml dosage form and diluted to 10 mg/ml for dosing.

Radiolabeled etanercept

Radiolabeled ^{64}Cu-NODAGA-etanercept was used to validate the amount of drug delivered by SOFUSA™ and the amount of etanercept in LNs following the different routes of administration. To synthesize NODAGA-etanercept, a 10-mg aliquot of etanercept was buffer-exchanged into 0.1 M sodium phosphate buffer (pH 8.3) and reacted with a 20-fold molar excess of NODAGA-NHS (Chematech, Dijon, France) for 4 h at room temperature, then kept in a fridge at 4 °C overnight. The reaction was purified with Zeba desalting spin columns (Thermo Scientific, Rockford, IL, USA) and collected in PBS for radiolabeling and immunoreactivity studies. The average number of NODAGA molecules per protein was quantified by isotopic dilution as previously described [19] and was 1.4. Solution concentration was determined by ND-1000 spectrophotometer (NanoDrop, Wilmington, DE, USA). Retention of TNF-α binding affinity of NODAGA-etanercept bioconjugate was validated by comparing ELISA binding of naïve etanercept with NODAGA-etanercept. For final radiolabeling prior to administration, 1 mg of NODAGA-Enbrel was then buffer-exchanged into 0.1 M NaOAc (pH 6) and reacted with 50 μl of ^{64}Cu in buffer. $^{64}CuCl_2$ was produced by Washington University School of Medicine (St. Louis, MO, USA). After incubation at room temperature for 1 h, 3 μL of 10 mmol EDTA was added, and samples were incubated for an additional 15 minutes. The samples were Zeba-purified and collected with 80.7 ± 8.3% radiochemical yield and >99% radiochemical purity, as determined by high-performance liquid chromatography (HPLC) analysis. For radiolabeled etanercept dosing, we added a 9:1 stoichiometric ratio of naïve, unlabeled etanercept to radiolabeled etanercept, yielding a 10-mg/mL solution for dosing. The radioactivity of the dosing solution was measured using CRC-25R dose calibrator (Capintec, Inc., Florham Park, NJ, USA).

Nanotopographic device for drug delivery (SOFUSA™)

SOFUSA™ is a microneedle drug delivery device with a nanotopographical imprinted polyether, ether, ketone film heat-formed over each microneedle on the array (Fig. 1a). The nanotopographical film-microneedle combination has been found to increase permeability through the skin epidermis layer by remodeling tight junction proteins initiated via integrin binding to the nanotopography [20]. The increased permeability enables SOFUSA™ to deliver therapeutic drug levels and control targeting to the lymphatic system based on the delivery occurring between the stratum corneum and initial lymphatic capillaries, and the ability to change the number of microneedles and the microneedle flowrate.

Twenty-four hours prior to SOFUSA™ administration, rats were anesthetized with isofluorane and the dorsal region was shaved and covered with depilatory cream (Nair Sensitive) for 8 minutes. The cream was then wiped off with warm, wet paper towels, followed by alcohol wipes. SOFUSA™ was then applied to the dorsal region using a plastic shell with a skin adhesive (Fig. 1b). A hand-held applicator was then placed over the plastic shell to insert the microneedles into the skin. The operation of the device was as follows. The applicator strikes the microneedles with a post traveling at a velocity of 6 m/s. There are a total of 100 microneedles over the applicator area of 66 mm^2. With the microneedles inserted in the skin, the syringe pump is started to deliver the agent. In these studies, the syringe pump was set at a constant rate of 100 μL/h and was run for 1 h to deliver the 1 mg etanercept. The etanercept dosing was 10 mg/mL.

Characterization of etanercept delivery via SOFUSA™, IV, SC, and ID routes of administration

PK profiles

In order to characterize differences in etanercept delivery by the different routes of administration, we used normal rats

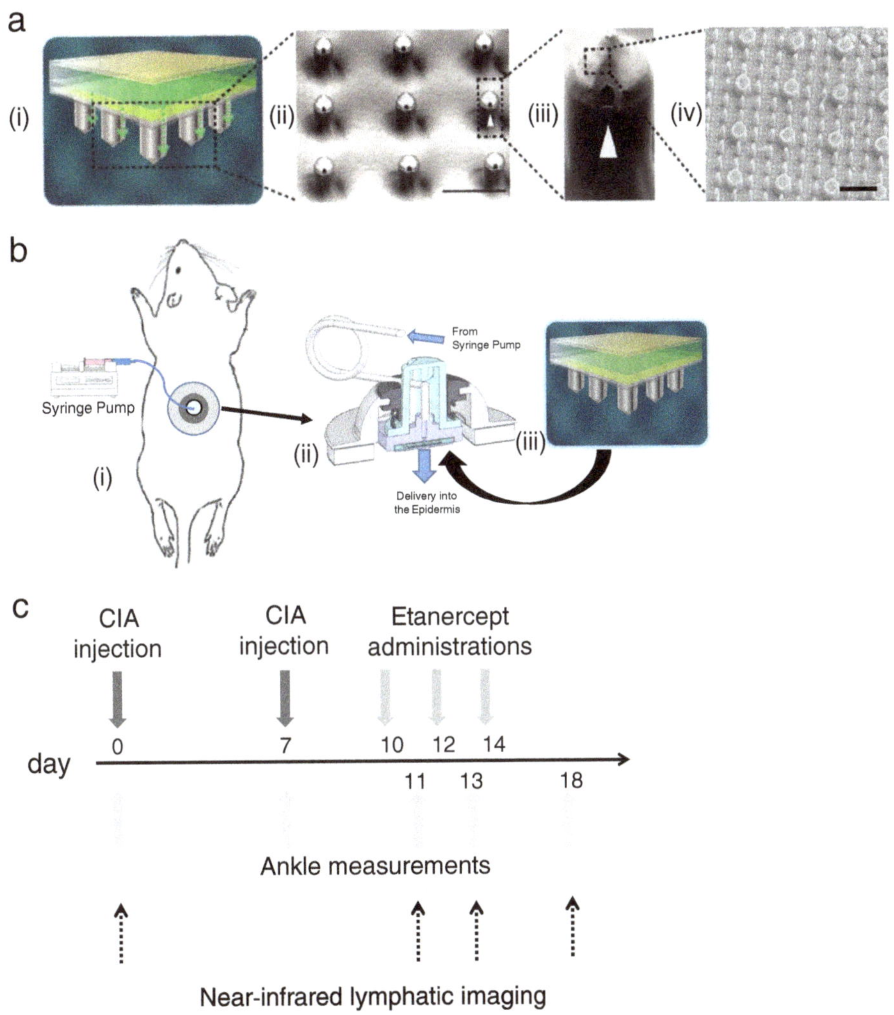

Fig. 1 a The SOFUSA™ nanotopographical device. (*i*) Microfluidic fluid block with a perforated attachment adhesive (*tan*), microfluidic distributor (*green*), perforated attachment adhesive (*yellow*), and silicon microneedle array (*gray*). Each microneedle is 350 μm long and 110 μm wide, with a 30-μm hole located off-center, through which the drug flows out of a total of 100 microneedles (*ii*) Scanning electron microscopy (SEM) image of nanotopographic film heat formed over the silicon microneedles (*scale bar* represents 300 μm); (*iii*) SEM of individual microneedle, and (*iv*) SEM image of the nanostructures on each microneedle (*scale bar* represents 3 μm). **b** Administration procedure for the SOFUSA™ nanotopographical device. (*i*) Location of SOFUSA™ on the rat dorsal region during drug delivery experiments; (*ii*) cross-sectional illustration of the complete SOFUSA™ device, and (*iii*) microfluidic fluid block as defined in panel **a**. **c** Timeline for induction, measurements, and treatments of animals with collagen-induced arthritis

to determine the PK profiles following a single dose of 1 mg etanercept in 100 uL delivered via SOFUSA™ ($n = 6$), conventional IV (in the tail vein, $n = 6$), SC (dorsolateral injection at the same site as the SOFUSA™ application, $n = 4$), or ID injections (symmetrical dorsolateral injections 2 × 50 uL for a total dose of 1 mg etanercept, $n = 6$). Other than the SOFUSA™ delivery, all administration was conducted using a 31-gauge needle. At 2, 4, 8, 12, 24, and 36 h after administration, animals were anesthetized under isoflurane, and 200 μL of blood was drawn from the jugular vein. The etanercept concentration in serum was quantified using the Etanercept ELISA Kit (ABIN: 1540251) (Matriks Biotechnology Co., LTD., Ankara, Turkey). Optical density was measured at 450 nm using Thermo Scientific Multiskan EX (Thermo Fisher Scientific, Waltham, MA, USA).

Measurement of LN uptake of etanercept via different routes of administration in normal rats

In order to determine the etanercept delivered to the LNs, we administrated the radiolabeled etanercept solution via SOFUSA™ (1 mg etanercept in 100 uL), IV (1 mg etanercept in the tail vein in 100 uL), SC (1 mg etanercept in the dorsolateral side at the same site as the SOFUSA™ application, 100 uL), and ID (1 mg total etanercept in two 50-μL injections). Animals were harvested at 12 and 36 h after administration, and the left/

right axillary and inguinal LNs were collected, weighed, and counted for radioactivity using a 2480 Wizard^2 automatic gamma counter (PerkinElmer, Waltham, MA, USA). The time-corrected radioactivity was then used to compute the μg/mL of tissue etanercept concentration from the specific radioactivity of the dosing solution with animals that were euthanized at 12 h ($n = 4$, SOFUSA™; $n = 6$, IV; $n = 6$, ID; and $n = 6$, SC) and at 36 h ($n = 6$, SOFUSA™; $n = 6$, IV; $n = 6$, ID; and $n = 6$, SC).

Quantification of etanercept delivered

In order to validate the amount of etanercept delivered, we measured the radioactivity in the SOFUSA™ device and tubing before and after the 1-h infusion. Measurement was conducted using the dose calibrator. We computed the amount of etanercept as the difference in the time-corrected radioactivity before and after administration,. We similarly computed the amount of etanercept delivered via conventional syringes using the same method, with the expectation that the amount delivered matched that determined from radioactivity balance.

To directly visualize SOFUSA™ delivery, 100 μL of 645 μM indocyanine green (ICG) (Akorn, Inc.) in sterile saline was delivered over 1 h using a syringe pump (model NE-300, SyringePump.com) connected to the SOFUSA™, which was applied to the dorsal surface on the right side of the rat. NIRF imaging was conducted as described subsequently.

Treatment of CIA animals with etanercept administered by SOFUSA™, SC, and ID routes of administration

CIA induction, hind limb measurement, and measurements

Type II porcine collagen (Chondrex, Inc. catalog #20031), solubilized in 0.05 N of acetic acid in sterile water at a concentration of 2 mg/mL was emulsified with an equal volume of incomplete Freud's adjuvant (Chondrex, Inc. catalog #7002) using homogenization at 35,000 rpm (Omni International homogenizer TH, homogenizer probe #32750): 100 μL emulsion was injected subcutaneously at the base of the tails on both sides for initial administration (day 0, 200 μL of emulsion total), and then again, 7 days later, on the right side only, for booster administration (day 7, 100 μL of emulsion total). Hind limb swelling usually became evident at day 14. Hind limb swelling was assessed by caliper measurements of the rear ankle cross (side-to-side) and oblique (front-to-back) dimensions. The two measurements for each hind limb were multiplied together for assessment of swelling as done in other studies [21] and percent change from baseline was computed. These measurements and lymphatic imaging (as described subsequently) were performed on days 0, 7, 11, 13, and 18, in *the* early stages of CIA before the onset of joint destruction [22]. Four groups of animals were studied: (1) untreated ($n = 20$), (2) treated with etanercept given by SC administration ($n = 20$, 1 mg in 100 μL), (3) treated with etanercept given by ID administration ($n = 20$, two administrations of 0.5 mg in 50 μL), and (4) treated with etanercept given via SOFUSA™ ($n = 18$, one administration of 1 mg in 100 μL delivered). Figure 1c shows the timeline for induction, measurement, and treatment of CIA animals. *We* did not include IV treatment of CIA animals *b*ecause etanercept is not administered IV in RA patients, and because repetitive IV administration in animals is invasive.

Imaging of lymphatic pumping function

Rats were anesthetized with isoflurane and shaved before imaging: 10 μL of 625 μM ICG was then injected ID with a 31-gauge needle/syringe (BD #328438, Fisher Scientific) at the base of the tail and on the dorsal side of the paw on both the right and left sides of the rats to perform NIRF imaging of the lymphatics. NIRF images were collected with a custom-built system that employed illumination of tissue surfaces with 785-nm light from a laser diode (85 mA and 80 mW, DL7140-201, Sanyo) that was diffused to cover a circular area approximately 8 cm in diameter [23]. Fluorescent light generated from the ICG within the lymphatic vasculature was collected with an electron-multiplying charge-coupled device (EMCCD) (model 7827-0001, Princeton Instruments). Filter sets were used to reject backscattered and reflected excitation light. Images were acquired with V++ software (Total Turnkey Solutions, Sydney, Australia). The integration time for fluorescence images was 200 ms: 300–900 images were collected per lateral side per rat for lymph propulsive frequency measurements. Images were collected at or before day zero (when the first CIA injection was administered) and at days 11, 13, and 18 following CIA induction.

Data analysis

NIRF images were loaded into ImageJ software (NIH), and fluorescence intensity values were quantified and imported into Microsoft Excel for computation of lymphatic pumping function as previously described [24]. Briefly, the number of forward lymphatic pulses minus those observed traveling in the distal direction in the hind limbs over a period of 5 minutes was computed and reported as a measure of lymphatic pumping function. The lymphatic vessels afferent to the popliteal LNs were interrogated. Quantification was done blinded. Statistical significance for comparison of the amount of etanercept delivered and LN uptake on the basis of μg/mL for the administration groups was determined from univariate and multivariate analysis of variance (ANOVA and MANOVA). Pairwise comparisons using contrast and the ANOVA model were used to compare the group differences for percent swelling and lymphatic pumping function, among the SOFUSA™, untreated, SC, and ID groups. These comparisons were performed separately for data collected at days 11, 13, and 18 post-CIA and the results can be used for examining influence of disease progression/regression upon measurements of swelling and lymphatic pumping function.

Results

PK and quantification studies show lymphatic delivery of etanercept via SOFUSA™

Figure 2 shows the early time course of normalized mean plus or minus the standard deviation of etanercept serum concentration normalized to peak concentration following 1 mg of etanercept delivery via SOFUSA™ and IV, SC, and ID administration. Table 1 shows the actual values at peak times, and the values at the 36-h time point. Consistent with past PK modeling studies of varying routes of antibody administration, the profile following IV administration shows initially high serum concentrations with moderately rapid clearance from the blood vasculature. In contrast, the PK profile associated with SC administration demonstrates a comparatively slower uptake into the blood vasculature with substantially lower serum values and reduced bioavailability [25] than found following the IV administration. In contrast to SC administration, the ID and SOFUSA™ PK profiles show rapid uptake from the intradermal space into the lymphatic plexus beneath the epidermis, and through the lymphatics, which empty into the blood vasculature. The SOFUSA™ PK profile shows more rapid uptake than the ID profile, due possibly to the larger area of administration (infusion area of 66 mm^2 as compared to two ID injection sites of < 1 mm^2) and enhanced update mechanisms that may be attributed to nanotopography. Due to the potential variability of the injection depth beneath the epidermis, ID administrations may penetrate too deeply, miss the initial lymphatics, and in part may mimic an SC injection, with loss of bioavailability.

Despite the differences in serum PK profiles and values, Table 2 shows that the amount of etanercept delivered to the body was statistically identical with SOFUSA™, IV, SC, and ID administration, as determined through radioactive balance. These results suggest that the delayed and attenuated PK profiles from SC, ID, and SOFUSA™ administration at early time points arise from delayed input into the blood vascular compartment from the intradermal (from SOFUSA™ and ID administrations) and interstitial (from SC administration) tissue compartments.

SOFUSA™ delivers material directly into the intradermal space drained by initial lymphatics

Two approaches were utilized to track delivery via SOFUSA™. Figure 3 shows that the SOFUSA™ device delivers ICG directly into the intradermal space drained by the initial lymphatics for efficient uptake into the lymphatic vasculature, as shown by the highlighted lymphatic vessels, and the lymphatic pumping to draining LNs, shown in Additional file 1: Video 1 and Additional file 2: Video 2. Because SOFUSA™ administration provides local intradermal delivery that feeds into draining LN basins that vary widely between animals (see Additional file 3: Figure S1), we observed a large variation between

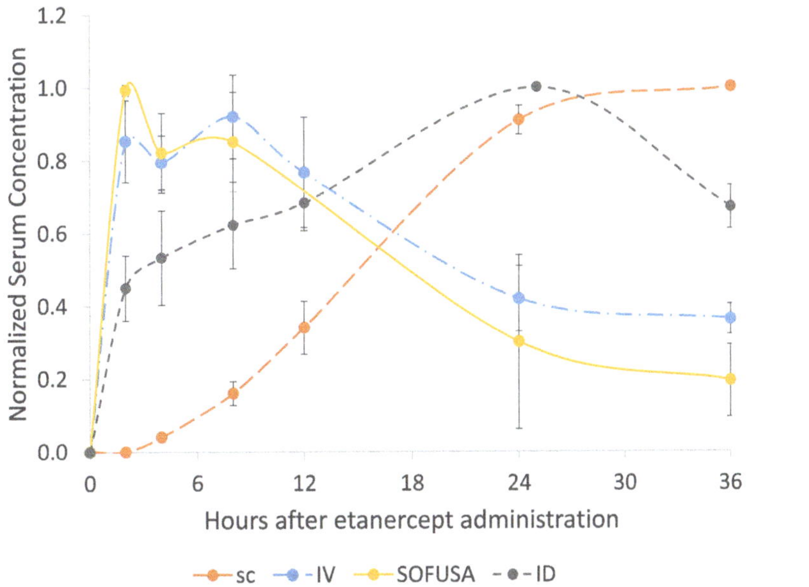

Fig. 2 Normalized mean serum concentration of etanercept plus or minus standard deviation as a function of time following subcutaneous (*SC*), intradermal (*ID*), intravenous (*IV*), and SOFUSA™ administration of 1 mg of drug

Table 1 Mean plus or minus the SD of etanercept serum concentration (μg/mL) at the time of maximum concentration (in parentheses) and 36 h after administration

Route of administration	Mean ± SD maximum serum concentration of etanercept, μg/mL (time of maximum concentration)	Mean ± SD serum concentration of etanercept, μg/mL after 36 h administration
SOFUSA™ ($n = 6$)	18.28 ± 6.95 (2 h)	4.91 ± 3.76
IV ($n = 6$)	110.84 ± 15.03 (2 h)	47.06 ± 4.81
	119.62 ± 16.73 (8 h)	
ID ($n = 6$)	31.08 ± 5.68 (25 h)	20.65 ± 2.94
SC ($n = 4$)	13.50 ± 3.21 (24 h)	13.50 ± 3.21

IV intravenous, *ID* intradermal, *SC* subcutaneous

radiolabeled etanercept delivery to right, left axillary/brachial and right, left inguinal LNs, often seeing one, but not all LNs, as radioactive. Likewise, variation in the levels of radiolabeled etanercept in regional draining LNs was also seen in SC and ID administration, but not in systemic IV administration, with which there were uniform but low tissue-concentrations of etanercept. To account for the different locoregional lymph drainage patterns between different animals, we compared etanercept concentration in the single LN with the highest radioactivity after administering radiolabeled etanercept via SOFUSA™ and the SC and ID route. Due to the more uniform systemic delivery to LNs following IV administration, we reported the mean radioactivity across all LNs at 12 and 36 h after administration. Figure 4 shows that SC and IV administration resulted in lower etanercept concentration in the LNs after 12 h as compared to SOFUSA™ and ID administration. In addition, the tissue concentration of etanercept in the LNs after 36 h was significantly greater ($p < 0.05$) when administered via SOFUSA™ than via the ID or SC routes, despite the potentially large variation in drainage routes, or via IV administration. The SOFUSA™ group variation was likely due to the larger area for infusion as compared to the SC and ID injection sites and to the drainage to one or more lymphatic basins.

Table 2 Amount of etanercept administered (mg) as determined from radioactivity balance

Route of administration	Dose ± SD of etanercept from radioactivity balance, mg
SOFUSA™ ($n = 10$)	1.07 ± 0.031
IV ($n = 12$)	0.96 ± 0.004
ID ($n = 12$)	1.00 ± 0.007
SC ($n = 12$)	0.91 ± 0.031

IV intravenous, *ID* intradermal, *SC* subcutaneous

This finding may be consistent with the PK results (Fig. 2, Table 1), showing that etanercept is predominantly located in the lymphatic vasculature following SOFUSA™ administration, with the smallest amount of drug in the systemic circulation at 36 h after administration when compared to IV, ID, and SC administration. Due to radioactivity half-life considerations, we were unable to determine the time at which clearance from draining LNs occurred.

Nonetheless, when taken together our results showing reduced blood serum concentration and increased concentration in draining LNs suggests there may be a mechanism by which etanercept administered by SOFUSA™ is retained within the lymphatic vasculature. Blood circulation times for therapeutic antibodies can be prolonged by enhanced neonatal Fc receptor (FcRN) binding, cellular uptake, and non-destructive recycling that occurs in epithelial and endothelial cells. FcRN expression has been identified in blood vascular endothelium [26] and elevated by pro-inflammatory cytokines TNF-α and IL-1β [27], but has not previously been identified in lymphatic endothelial cells. Using flow cytometry, we demonstrated FcRN expression in immortalized lymphatic endothelial cells (data not shown for brevity), further suggesting that FcRN-mediated retention may occur in the lymphatics as it does in the blood vasculature. It remains unknown whether FcRN expression in the lymphatics changes with inflammation and whether it may alter retention of etanercept.

Etanercept administration into the lymphatics via SOFUSA™ delivery improves lymphatic pumping

Additional file 4: Video 3 and Additional file 5: Video 4 show examples of the sluggish flow and reflux in the lymphatic vessels afferent to the popliteal LNs in untreated rats that consistently occurred 18 days after CIA induction. Impaired lymphatic pumping function has also been visualized in the arms and legs of humans with peripheral vascular disease and lymphedema [28]. In contrast to Additional file 4: Video 3 and Additional file 5: Video 4, Additional file 6: Video 5 shows an example of lymphatic pumping of the lymphatic vessels afferent to popliteal LNs in animals treated by SOFUSA™ 18 days after CIA induction. It is noteworthy that we observed no differences between the groups in the lymphatic pump function in the large vessel efferent to the inguinal LN and afferent to the axillary LN. In addition, we found no significant correlation between percent swelling and the lymphatic pumping function of vessels afferent to the popliteal LNs measured at days 11, 13, and 18 in untreated animals, although these results do not rule out the expected relationship between lymphatic pump efficiency and onset of swelling.

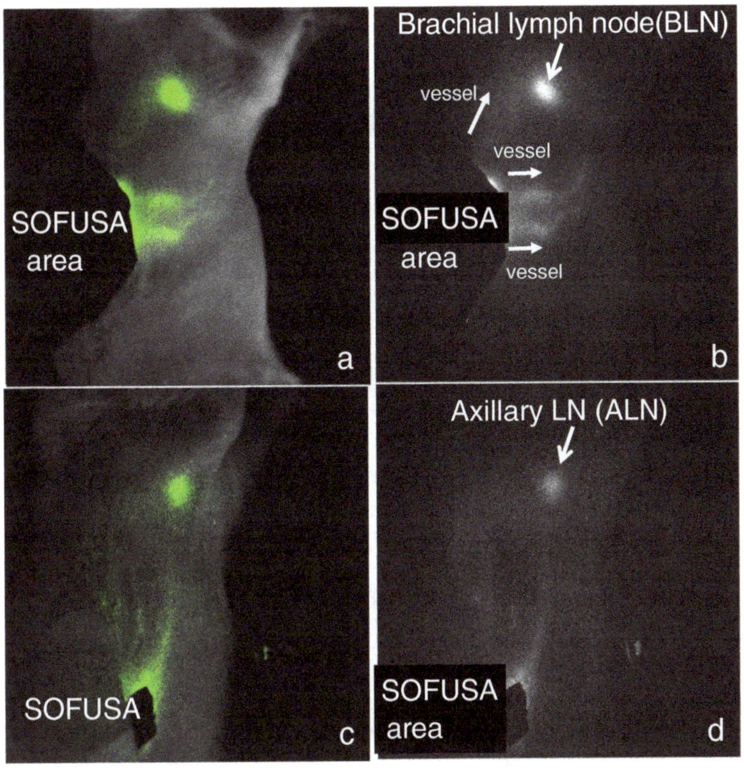

Fig. 3 Near-infrared fluorescence lymphatic imaging of indocyanine green (ICG) delivered via SOFUSA™ in normal rats showing different drainage patterns. **a** Fluorescence image shows drainage to brachial lymph nodes (BLNs) overlaid onto a white light image. **b** Fluorescence image alone (see Additional file 1: Video 1 showing lymphatic pumping of ICG delivered via SOFUSA™ to the BLN). **c** Fluorescence image shows drainage to axillary lymph nodes overlaid onto a white light image. **d** Fluorescence image alone (see Additional file 2: Video 2 showing lymphatic pumping of ICG delivered via SOFUSA™ to the BLN)

Figures 5a and b shows the histogram of the lymphatic pumping function and percent swelling in both hind limbs of each animal 11, 13, and 18 days after CIA induction in the untreated groups, and in those treated with etanercept administered by the ID and SC route and by SOFUSA™. No animals were excluded from the analysis, even those that had minimal swelling. At days 13 and 18 post CIA induction, univariate analyses showed: (1) statistically significant greater lymphatic pumping in the hind limbs of animals treated with SOFUSA™ and SC administrations than in untreated animals and (2) significant reduction in swelling of the hind limbs of all treated groups when compared to untreated animals. In addition, animals treated by SOFUSA™ had significantly reduced hind limb swelling at days 13 and 18 when compared to SC-treated animals.

Paired group comparisons using contrast in the ANOVA model showed that the lymphatic pumping function was significantly decreased with progression of disease in untreated animals and swelling was significantly increased with progression of disease in untreated animals and animals treated by SC and ID administration. No statistically significant increase in swelling was observed in animals treated by SOFUSA™ administration.

Simultaneous comparison of both metrics of swelling and lymphatic pumping function were performed using Wilk's lambda test, with the level of significance determined ($p = 0.008$ after Bonferroni adjustment). Multivariate analyses (Table 3) showed that there were no significant differences between the SOFUSA™ and all other treated groups based upon the combination of percent swelling and pumping function comparisons at day 11. However on day 13 and 18, all treated groups were statistically different compared to untreated animals.

Discussion

In this work we showed that the function of afferent lymphatic vessels in the hind limbs of rats with CIA-induced arthritis declined with disease progression, but may be reversed through SOFUSA™ administration of etanercept to draining inguinal and axillary LNs, consistent with the hypothesis that the lymphatic system mediates inflammatory-erosive arthritis [5, 6]. Furthermore, we showed reduced swelling with etanercept administration to the lymphatics, via the nanotopography device (SOFUSA™) compared to administration via the clinically used SC route.

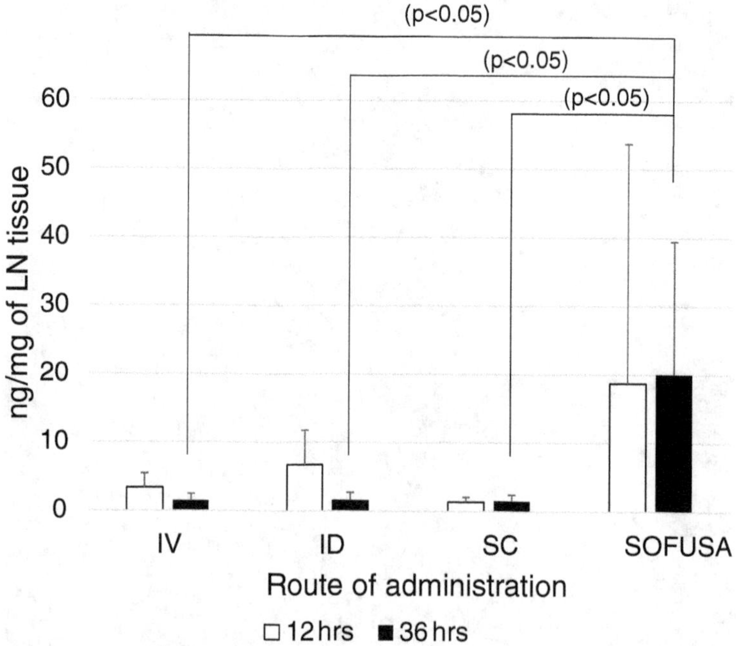

Fig. 4 Mean ± SD ng/mg of etanercept in lymph nodes (*LNs*) with the greatest radioactivity in animals 12 and 36 h following etanercept administration via intravenous (*IV*), intradermal (*ID*), subcutaneous (*SC*), and SOFUSA™ administration. Values of etanercept concentration following systemic IV administration represent the mean ± standard deviation of all LNs harvested. Values of etanercept concentration following ID, SC and SOFUSA™ administration represent the mean ± standard deviation of the most radioactive LN harvested from each animal. Two-tailed *p* values denote significant differences between etanercept LN concentrations at 36 h following administration via the SOFUSA™, IV, ID, and SC routes

It is noteworthy that prior studies have employed IV and SC administration of etanercept to effect changes in swelling in CIA animals [29]. Systemic intraperitoneal (IP) administration of anti-CD20 (depletion of B cells) has also been used to effect decreased knee synovium volume, enhanced afferent lymphatic pumping function, and macrophage egress from inflamed joints in TNF-Tg mice, presumably by "unclogging" the draining LN through removal of B cells [11]. Because our work shows improvement in afferent lymphatic function and reduced swelling with SOFUSA™ delivery over that of SC administration of etanercept, one could speculate that direct lymphatic administration of anti-CD20 therapy to reach B cells in draining LNs could result in improved response with lower dose, reduced systemic exposure, and lower incidence of adverse events. Another mechanism that may be responsible for impairment of afferent lymph drainage could be the well-known neutrophil recruitment to subcapsules of draining LNs in inflamed peripheral tissues [30]. Recently it has been shown that RA patients have elevated numbers of neutrophils that participate in the process of NETosis induced by pro-inflammatory cytokines, including TNF-α. NETosis occurs when neutrophils spew DNA nets that display autoantigens [31] and can intravascularly trap cells and cellular debris to play a critical role in hemovascular thrombi formation [32].

Whether NETosis can impair afferent lymph draining in the synovial fluid of RA patients and whether TNF-α antagonists delivered into the lymphatics can restrict NETosis or other immune processes that impact drainage, remains to be answered. Other biologics that target the immune system could be delivered into the lymphatics for regional treatment of localized autoimmune skin diseases through direct targeting of the immune system. In addition, stimulation of the immune system using systemic IV administration of biologics to block checkpoint inhibition may be less effective when compared to SOFUSA™ or ID-directed lymphatic delivery, which can directly access LNs at the sites where immune cell activation is induced [33]. The presence of FcRN receptor expression on the lymphatic endothelium may prolong the presence of therapeutic biologics in the lymphatic vasculature that feeds draining LNs. It is also noteworthy that SOFUSA™ resulted in unilateral delivery to draining inguinal and axillary LNs, not direct delivery to the bilateral popliteal LNs draining the inflamed hind limbs. Future work is needed to understand the interaction of biologics with the lymphatic endothelium and LN stroma and whether the "abscopal" effect, i.e., the well-known distant immune responses observed away from the site of cancer treatment [34], may play a role in RA treatments. The hypothesis that delivery of anti-TNF to inguinal or axillary LNs can efficiently suppress the

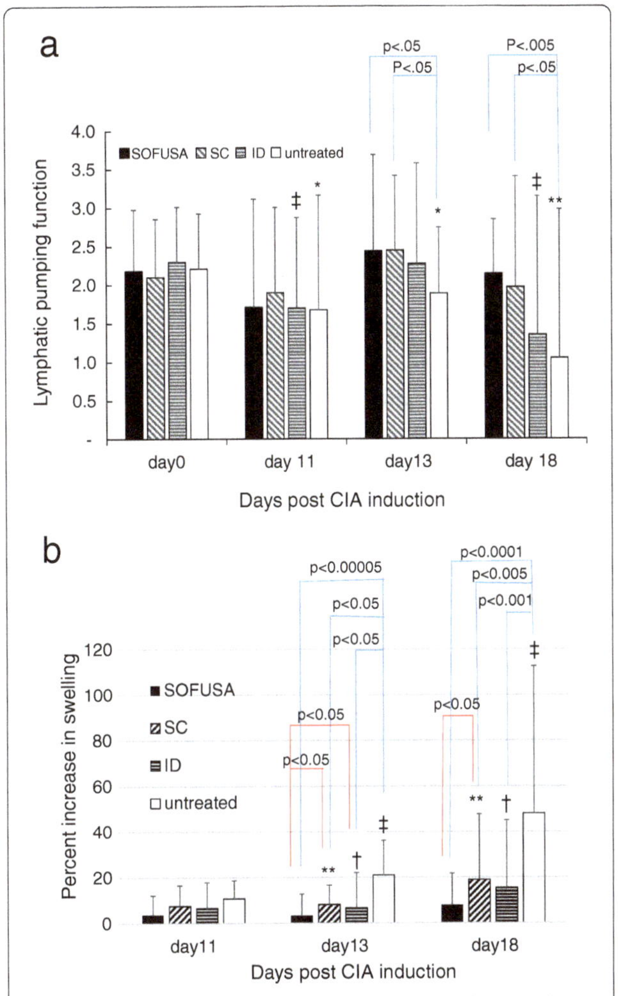

Fig. 5 a Mean ± SD of lymphatic pumping function as a function of time after induction of collagen-induced arthritis (*CIA*) in the four groups: untreated (*white bars*), treated by SOFUSA™ (*solid bars*) and treated by the subcutaneous (*SC*) (*diagonal lined bars*), and intradermal (*ID*) (*horizontal lined bars*) routes. Two-tailed, pairwise test *p* values in the framework of the analysis of variance (ANOVA) model at days 13 and 18 after CIA induction (*bars* connecting the different groups) show significant reduction in lymphatic pumping function in the untreated groups compared to SOFUSA™ and SC administration groups: significant decrease ($^*p < 0.005$, $^{**}p < 0.05$, paired Student's *t* test, one-tailed) in lymphatic pumping in untreated animals at 11, 13, and 18 days after CIA induction compared to baseline (day 0); significant decrease ($^‡p < 0.005$, paired Student's *t* test, one-tailed) in lymphatic pumping at 11 and 18 days after CIA induction in animals treated with ID administration of etanercept as compared to baseline (day 0). **b** Mean ± SD of percent increase in swelling as a function of time after CIA induction in the four groups: untreated (*white bars*), and treated by SOFUSA (*solid bars*) and by the SC (*diagonal lined bars*), and ID (*horizontal lined bars*) routes. Pairwise *F* test *p* values using contrast in the ANOVA model at days 13 and 18 after CIA induction (*bars* connecting the different groups) denote significant reduction in swelling in the SOFUSA™ and SC administration groups when compared to the untreated group: $^{**}p < 0.005$ for significant increase in swelling at day 18 compared to day 13 in animals treated with SC administration; $^†p < 0.05$ for significant increase in swelling at day 18 compared to day 13 in animals treated with ID administration; $^‡p < 0.005$ for significant increase in swelling at day 18 compared to day 13 in untreated animals

Table 3 Multivariate *p* values to assess the differences in swelling and lymphatic pumping function at days 11, 13, and 18 in animals with etanercept administered by SOFUSA™ and the SC and ID routes and in untreated animals

	ID	SC	Untreated
Day 11 (overall, $p = 0.62$)			
SOFUSA™	0.17	0.43	0.84
ID		0.70	0.35
SC			0.76
Day 13 (overall, $p = 0.0002$)			
SOFUSA™	0.07	0.39	<0.0001
ID		0.69	0.0017
SC			0.0015
Day 18 (overall, $p < 0.0001$)			
SOFUSA™	0.48	0.10	<0.0001
ID		0.13	0.0006
SC			0.004

ID intradermal, SC subcutaneous. $P < 0.008$ is statistically significant due to application of the Bonferroni adjustment for multiple comparisons

progression of systemic disease, thus reducing joint swelling and preserving lymphatic pumping in other anatomical locations, needs to be further explored.

However, it also important to note that while ID or SOFUSA™ administration affords delivery through draining LNs, the lymphatics *do* empty into the blood vasculature, enabling systemic delivery, as evidenced by the early PK data presented herein. While SC, IP, and IV routes of administration provide systemic delivery into the blood circulation by which biologics could enter the lymphatics via high endothelial venules in LNs, administration into the intradermal space via ID or SOFUSA™ delivery may enable systemic delivery through regional lymphatics with maximal exposure to draining LNs.

In the clinic, ID injection may be irrelevant because: (1) the intradermal space is too small to receive therapeutic drug volumes and (2) advanced skill is required for successful ID injection. However, it is relevant to compare ID injection with SOFUSA™ infusion, because the device may mimic drug placement in the intradermal space of a successful ID injection and could potentially infuse a therapeutic dose into the intradermal space in humans. Indeed, it may be surprising in this animal study that ID administration did not impact the lymphatic pumping function and swelling as well as the nanotopography device did. This observation could arise from accidental penetration of conventional needles beyond the initial lymphatics, where lymphatic uptake is most efficient. Indeed, in our NIRF imaging studies conducted in humans (for review see [18]), we often observed operator error in performing the intradermal injections: if the Mantoux procedure is not accurate and a weal is not formed on the skin, there is considerable delay (10–60 minutes) until the partial lymphatic uptake of ICG enabling lymphatic imaging. Another reason for the improved performance of nanotopography infusion over ID administration may be the enhanced area of SOFUSA™ microneedle coverage and the enhanced disruption of tight junctions through mechanotransduction mechanisms [20] that could facilitate lymphatic uptake. Compared to SOFUSA™ administration, the delayed PK profile and reduced radiolabeled etanercept uptake into draining LNs (Figs. 2 and 4) after ID administration are consistent with improved lymphatic uptake with nanotopographic delivery.

There have been several academic and commercial efforts to develop microneedle-based delivery systems [35–37], but this is the first to demonstrate improved pharmacodynamics over conventional Mantoux procedures. It is noteworthy that, unlike other studies that demonstrate efficacy in animals with at least a 50% increase in swelling in one hind limb [29], we conservatively included all animals in our study, including those with minimal swelling. While there are several rodent models of RA, the CIA model is a commonly used to mimic both the innate and adaptive immune responses that are important in RA progression. When used in combination with adjuvant-induced arthritis, and genetic models (such as TNF-Tg mice), the CIA rat model provides an efficient means for predicting therapeutic efficacy in humans [38]. Since completing our work, another study in TNF-Tg animals has shown that systemic IP administration of anti-TNF drugs increase the lymphatic pump [14], in agreement with our data on early CIA progression in rats treated with etanercept versus untreated CIA rats. Extension of this work to adjuvant-induced arthritis, genetic models of RA, and human RA patients remains to be shown.

Finally, there are limitations to the study presented herein. First, we are unaware of a commercially available isotype control protein that is identical to etanercept but with abrogated TNF binding. It is possible that the Fc portion of etanercept could itself evoke an immune response within the lymphatics, necessitating further study of the interaction with biologics within the lymphatic vasculature. Another limitation for quantifying lymphatic pumping function using our approach should be noted. Because we quantified the pumping function as the number of proximally propelled minus the number of distally propelled lymph "packets" imaged by NIRF, our metric may not discriminate between: (1) the arrest of lymphatic pumping and (2) a strong lymphatic pump that pumped and refluxed lymph equally in both proximal and distal directions. A more suitable metric of lymphatic efficiency from NIRF imaging needs to be developed that might better predict swelling and response to therapy. Nonetheless, these preclinical studies demonstrate modification of the lymphatic pump function in a CIA animal model and suggest that future work to therapeutically mediate lymphatic function through nanotopography delivery of immune targets could result in more effective treatments for RA.

Conclusion

Administration of etanercept into the draining lymphatics of inflamed joints significantly reduced swelling and improved lymphatic pumping when administered using nanotopography (SOFUSA™). This work suggests that alternative routes of locoregional administration could provide more effective delivery than SC or IV administration.

Additional files

Additional file 1: Video 1. Lymphatic pumping of ICG delivered via SOFUSA™ to the brachial lymph node shown in Fig. 3. (AVI 9656.32 kb)

Additional file 2: Video 2. Lymphatic pumping of ICG delivered via SOFUSA™ to the axillary lymph node shown in Fig. 3. (AVI 9861.12 kb)

Additional file 3: Figure S1. Variation of lymphatic pathways draining to inguinal lymph nodes (*ILN*) following ICG injection (*yellow dotted arrow*) with conventional needle on the dorsal surface of the rat. (PDF 146 kb)

Additional file 4: Video 3. Example of sluggish lymphatic pump function in the hind limb of an untreated rat 18 days post CIA induction. (AVI 2242.56 kb)

Additional file 5: Video 4. Example of forward and retrograde lymphatic pump function in the hind limb of an untreated rat 18 days post CIA induction. (AVI 1843.2 kb)

Additional file 6: Video 5. Example of lymphatic pumping function in the hind limb of a SOFUSA™-treated rat 18 days post CIA induction. (AVI 2027.52 kb)

Abbreviations

ANOVA: Analysis of variance; CIA: Collagen induced arthritis; ELISA: Enzyme-linked immunosorbent assay; FcRN: Neonatal Fc receptor; ICG: indocyanine green; ID: Intradermal; IL-1: Interleukin-1; IL-6: Interleukin-6; iNOS: Inducible nitric oxide synthase; IP: Intraperitoneal; IV: Intravenous; LN: Lymph node; NIRF: Near-infrared fluorescence; PBS: Phosphate-buffered saline; PK: Pharmacokinetic; RA: Rheumatoid arthritis; SC: Subcutaneous; TNF: Tumor necrosis factor; TNF-Tg: Tumor necrosis factor transgenic

Acknowledgements

We acknowledge the assistance of Holly Robinson, Julie Voss, and Randy Hickman for animal handling; Ken Pinkston for assisting in ELISA of labeled etanercept; and Nathaniel Wilganowski for serum ELISA testing.

Funding

This work was supported by an industrial grant from Kimberly-Clark Corporation and clinical studies were funded in part by NIH R01 HL092923 (EMS).

Authors' contributions

MBA designed and conducted CIA animal studies, performed imaging, analyzed data, and wrote the manuscript; FCV performed radiolabeling and all data analysis; SK conducted near-infrared lymphatic imaging of animals; BRH and KP designed analyses of labeled and unlabeled etanercept; WC conducted statistical analyses; AA designed the radiolabeling of etanercept; RFR conducted SOFUSA™ delivery studies and designed studies; EMS-M, JCR, CEF, and MBA designed the study and wrote the manuscript; All authors have read and approved the manuscript.

Authors' information

Eva M Sevick, Melissa Aldrich, Barrett Harvey, Ali Azhdarinia, Sunkuk Kwon, and Fred Christian Velasquez are with the Center for Molecular Imaging, The Brown Foundation Institute of Molecular Medicine, The University of Texas Health Science Center. Wenyaw Chan is with the Department of Biostatistics, The School of Public Health, The University of Texas Health Science Center. Russell F. Ross is with the Kimberly Clark Corporation.

Competing interests

RFR is employed by the Kimberly Clark Corporation, which manufacturers the SOFUSA™ device. EMS-M receives research funding from the Kimberly Clark Corporation. EMS-M, CEF, and JCR have royalty and financial interests in NIRF Imaging, Inc. a University of Texas Health Science Center Portfolio Company, which is commercializing clinical NIRF imaging. The remaining authors declare that they have no competing interests.

Declarations

All figures and video files in this publication are original to this article.

Author details

[1]The Center for Molecular Imaging, The Brown Foundation Institute of Molecular Medicine, The University of Texas Health Science Center, Houston, TX 77030, USA. [2]Department of Biostatistics, The School of Public Health, The University of Texas Health Science Center, Houston, TX 77030, USA. [3]Kimberly Clark Corporation, Atlanta, GA, USA. [4]The Wound Care Clinic, CHI St. Luke's Health, The Woodlands Hospital, The Woodlands, TX 77382, USA.

References

1. Emery P. Treatment of rheumatoid arthritis. BMJ. 2006;332(7534):152–5. doi:10.1136/bmj.332.7534.152. PubMed PMID: 16424492; PubMed Central PMCID: PMCPMC1336767.
2. Alitalo K. The lymphatic vasculature in disease. Nat Med. 2011;17(11):1371–80. doi:10.1038/nm.2545.
3. Baluk P, Fuxe J, Hashizume H, Romano T, Lashnits E, Butz S, et al. Functionally specialized junctions between endothelial cells of lymphatic vessels. J Exp Med. 2007;204(10):2349–62. doi:10.1084/jem.2006259. PubMed PMID: 17846148; PubMed Central PMCID: PMCPMC2118470.
4. Levick JR, Michel CC. Microvascular fluid exchange and the revised Starling principle. Cardiovasc Res. 2010;87(2):198–210. doi:10.1093/cvr/cvq062.
5. Bouta EM, Li J, Ju Y, Brown EB, Ritchlin CT, Xing L, et al. The role of the lymphatic system in inflammatory-erosive arthritis. Semin Cell Dev Biol. 2015;38:90–7. doi:10.1016/j.semcdb.2015.01.001. PubMed PMID: 25598390; PubMed Central PMCID: PMCPMC4397133.
6. Benaglio F, Vitolo B, Scarabelli M, Binda E, Bugatti S, Caporali R, et al. The draining lymph node in rheumatoid arthritis: current concepts and research perspectives. Biomed Res Int. 2015;2015:420251. doi:10.1155/2015/420251. PubMed PMID: 25793195; PubMed Central PMCID: PMCPMC4352497.
7. Joos E, Bourgeois P, Famaey JP. Lymphatic disorders in rheumatoid arthritis. Semin Arthritis Rheum. 1993;22(6):392–8.
8. Grillet B, Dequeker J. Rheumatoid lymphedema. J Rheumatol. 1987;14(6):1095–7.
9. Olszewski WL, Pazdur J, Kubasiewicz E, Zaleska M, Cooke CJ, Miller NE. Lymph draining from foot joints in rheumatoid arthritis provides insight into local cytokine and chemokine production and transport to lymph nodes. Arthritis Rheum. 2001;44(3):541–9. doi:10.1002/1529-0131(200103)44:3<541::AID-ANR102>3.0.CO;2-6.
10. Polzer K, Baeten D, Soleiman A, Distler J, Gerlag DM, Tak PP, et al. Tumour necrosis factor blockade increases lymphangiogenesis in murine and human arthritic joints. Ann Rheum Dis. 2008;67(11):1610–6. doi:10.1136/ard.2007.083394.
11. Li J, Ju Y, Bouta EM, Xing L, Wood RW, Kuzin I, et al. Efficacy of B cell depletion therapy for murine joint arthritis flare is associated with increased lymphatic flow. Arthritis Rheum. 2013;65(1):130–8. doi:10.1002/art.37709. PubMed PMID: 23002006; PubMed Central PMCID: PMCPMC3535508.
12. Aldrich MB, Sevick-Muraca EM. Cytokines are systemic effectors of lymphatic function in acute inflammation. Cytokine. 2013;64(1):362–9. doi:10.1016/j.cyto.2013.05.015. PubMed PMID: 23764549; PubMed Central PMCID: PMCPMC3771384.
13. Swartz MA. Immunomodulatory roles of lymphatic vessels in cancer progression. Cancer Immunol Res. 2014;2(8):701–7. doi:10.1158/2326-6066.CIR-14-0115.
14. Bouta EM, Kuzin I, de Mesy BK, Wood RW, Rahimi H, Ji RC, et al. Treatment of TNF-Tg mice with anti-TNF restores lymphatic contraction, repairs lymphatic vessels, and may increase monocyte/macrophage egress. Arthritis Rheumatol. 2017. doi:10.1002/art.40047.
15. Maini RN, Feldmann M. How does infliximab work in rheumatoid arthritis? Arthritis Res. 2002;4 Suppl 2:S22–8. doi:10.1186/ar549. PubMed PMID: 12110154; PubMed Central PMCID: PMCPMC3238217.
16. Prajapati R, Plant D, Barton A. Genetic and genomic predictors of anti-TNF response. Pharmacogenomics. 2011;12(11):1571–85. doi:10.2217/pgs.11.114.
17. Thomson TM, Lescarbeau RM, Drubin DA, Laifenfeld D, de Graaf D, Fryburg DA, et al. Blood-based identification of non-responders to anti-TNF therapy in rheumatoid arthritis. BMC Med Genet. 2015;8:26. doi:10.1186/s12920-015-0100-6. PubMed PMID: 26036272; PubMed Central PMCID: PMCPMC4455917.
18. Sevick-Muraca EM, Kwon S, Rasmussen JC. Emerging lymphatic imaging technologies for mouse and man. J Clin Invest. 2014;124(3):905–14. doi:10.1172/JCI71612. PubMed PMID: 24590275; PubMed Central PMCID: PMCPMC3938259.
19. Ghosh SC, Pinkston KL, Robinson H, Harvey BR, Wilganowski N, Gore K, et al. Comparison of DOTA and NODAGA as chelators for (64)Cu-labeled immunoconjugates. Nucl Med Biol. 2015;42(2):177–83. doi:10.1016/j.nucmedbio.2014.09.009.
20. Walsh L, Ryu J, Bock S, Koval M, Mauro T, Ross R, et al. Nanotopography facilitates in vivo transdermal delivery of high molecular weight therapeutics through an integrin-dependent mechanism. Nano Lett. 2015;15(4):2434–41. doi:10.1021/nl504829f. PubMed PMID: 25790174; PubMed Central PMCID: PMCPMC4478088.
21. Earp JC, Dubois DC, Almon RR, Jusko WJ. Quantitative dynamic models of arthritis progression in the rat. Pharm Res. 2009;26(1):196–203. doi:10.1007/s11095-008-9711-3. PubMed PMID: 18758921; PubMed Central PMCID: PMCPMC3725549.
22. Yamashita A, Yonemitsu Y, Okano S, Nakagawa K, Nakashima Y, Irisa T, et al. Fibroblast growth factor-2 determines severity of joint disease in adjuvant-induced arthritis in rats. J Immunol. 2002;168(1):450–7.
23. Kwon S, Sevick-Muraca EM. Noninvasive quantitative imaging of lymph function in mice. Lymphat Res Biol. 2007;5(4):219–31. doi:10.1089/lrb.2007.1013.
24. Tan IC, Maus EA, Rasmussen JC, Marshall MV, Adams KE, Fife CE, et al. Assessment of lymphatic contractile function after manual lymphatic drainage using near-infrared fluorescence imaging. Arch Phys Med Rehabil. 2011;92(5):756–64 e1. doi:10.1016/j.apmr.2010.12.027. PubMed PMID: 21530723; PubMed Central PMCID: PMCPMC3109491.
25. Kagan L. Pharmacokinetic modeling of the subcutaneous absorption of therapeutic proteins. Drug Metab Dispos. 2014;42(11):1890–905. doi:10.1124/dmd.114.059121.
26. Roopenian DC, Akilesh S. FcRn: the neonatal Fc receptor comes of age. Nat Rev Immunol. 2007;7(9):715–25. doi:10.1038/nri2155.
27. Liu X, Ye L, Christianson GJ, Yang JQ, Roopenian DC, Zhu X. NF-kappaB signaling regulates functional expression of the MHC class I-related neonatal Fc receptor for IgG via intronic binding sequences. J Immunol. 2007;179(5):2999–3011. PubMed PMID: 17709515; PubMed Central PMCID: PMCPMC2667116.
28. Rasmussen JC, Aldrich MB, Tan IC, Darne C, Zhu B, O'Donnell Jr TF, et al. Lymphatic transport in patients with chronic venous insufficiency and venous leg ulcers following sequential pneumatic compression. J Vasc Surg Venous Lymphat Disord. 2016;4(1):9–17. doi:10.1016/j.jvsv.2015.06.001. PubMed PMID: 26946890; PubMed Central PMCID: PMCPMC4782606.
29. Lon HK, Liu D, Zhang Q, DuBois DC, Almon RR, Jusko WJ. Pharmacokinetic-pharmacodynamic disease progression model for effect of etanercept in Lewis rats with collagen-induced arthritis. Pharm Res. 2011;28(7):1622–30. doi:10.1007/s11095-011-0396-7. PubMed PMID: 21360252; PubMed Central PMCID: PMCPMC3726066.
30. Hampton HR, Chtanova T. The lymph node neutrophil. Semin Immunol. 2016;28(2):129–36. doi:10.1016/j.smim.2016.03.008.
31. Khandpur R, Carmona-Rivera C, Vivekanandan-Giri A, Gizinski A, Yalavarthi S, Knight JS, et al. NETs are a source of citrullinated autoantigens and stimulate inflammatory responses in rheumatoid arthritis. Sci Transl Med. 2013;5(178):178ra40. doi:10.1126/scitranslmed.3005580. PubMed PMID: 23536012; PubMed Central PMCID: PMCPMC3727661.

32. Martinod K, Wagner DD. Thrombosis: tangled up in NETs. Blood. 2014; 123(18):2768–76. doi:10.1182/blood-2013-10-463646. PubMed PMID: 24366358; PubMed Central PMCID: PMCPMC4007606.
33. Fransen MF, Arens R, Melief CJ. Local targets for immune therapy to cancer: tumor draining lymph nodes and tumor microenvironment. Int J Cancer. 2013;132(9):1971–6. doi:10.1002/ijc.27755.
34. Kaminski JM, Shinohara E, Summers JB, Niermann KJ, Morimoto A, Brousal J. The controversial abscopal effect. Cancer Treat Rev. 2005;31(3):159–72. doi:10.1016/j.ctrv.2005.03.004.
35. Harvey AJ, Kaestner SA, Sutter DE, Harvey NG, Mikszta JA, Pettis RJ. Microneedle-based intradermal delivery enables rapid lymphatic uptake and distribution of protein drugs. Pharm Res. 2011;28(1):107–16. doi:10.1007/s11095-010-0123-9.
36. Norman JJ, Choi SO, Tong NT, Aiyar AR, Patel SR, Prausnitz MR, et al. Hollow microneedles for intradermal injection fabricated by sacrificial micromolding and selective electrodeposition. Biomed Microdevices. 2013;15(2):203–10. doi:10.1007/s10544-012-9717-9. PubMed PMID: 23053452; PubMed Central PMCID: PMCPMC3572334.
37. Korkmaz E, Friedrich EE, Ramadan MH, Erdos G, Mathers AR, Ozdoganlar OB, et al. Tip-loaded dissolvable microneedle arrays effectively deliver polymer-conjugated antibody inhibitors of tumor-necrosis-factor-alpha into human skin. J Pharm Sci. 2016;105(11):3453–7. doi:10.1016/j.xphs.2016.07.008.
38. Asquith DL, Miller AM, McInnes IB, Liew FY. Animal models of rheumatoid arthritis. Eur J Immunol. 2009;39(8):2040–4. doi:10.1002/eji.200939578.

15

Differences in serum and synovial CD4+ T cells and cytokine profiles to stratify patients with inflammatory osteoarthritis and rheumatoid arthritis

Alessandra Penatti[1,3*†], Federica Facciotti[2*†], Roberta De Matteis[5], Paola Larghi[2,6], Moira Paroni[2], Antonella Murgo[3], Orazio De Lucia[3], Massimiliano Pagani[2], Luca Pierannunzii[3], Marcello Truzzi[3], Andreea Ioan-Facsinay[4], Sergio Abrignani[1,2], Jens Geginat[2†] and Pier Luigi Meroni[1,3,5†]

Abstract

Background: The aim was to investigate CD4+T-cell subsets, immune cells and their cytokine profiles in blood and synovial compartments in rheumatoid arthritis (RA) and inflammatory osteoarthritis (OA) to define specific immune signatures.

Methods: Peripheral blood, synovial fluid (SF) and synovial membranes (SM) of RA and OA patients were analyzed. CD4+T-cell subset frequencies were determined by flow cytometry, and cytokine concentrations in serum and SF were measured by ELISA.

Results: In peripheral blood, OA patients had altered frequencies of regulatory T-cell subsets, and higher frequencies of Th17 and of Th1/17 cells than RA patients. In the synovial compartment of OA patients, conventional Th17 cells were largely excluded, while Th1/17 cells were enriched and more frequent than in RA patients. Conversely, in the synovial compartment of RA patients, regulatory T cells and Tfh cells were enriched and more frequent then in OA patients. IL-17 and Blys were increased both in serum and SF of RA patients, and correlated with autoantibodies and disease activity. Notably, Blys levels were already significantly elevated in RA patients with low disease activity score in 28 joints (DAS28) and without autoantibody positivity.

Conclusions: Although patients with inflammatory OA have immune activation in the synovial compartment, they display different T-cell subset frequencies and cytokine profiles. Soluble mediators such as Blys might help to discriminate mild clinical forms of RA from inflammatory OA particularly at the onset of the disease.

Keywords: Rheumatoid arthritis, Inflammatory osteoarthritis, T helper subsets, Cytokines, Blys

Background

Rheumatoid arthritis (RA) and osteoarthritis (OA) represent two manifestations of inflammatory arthritides. Although the etiopathology of these diseases is different, they both involve synovial inflammation [1]. While RA is an autoimmune disease characterized by chronic relapsing-remitting inflammation of the peripheral joints [2], OA is induced by multifactorial mechanisms established primarily by biomechanical stress [3]. Thus, for a long time it has been believed that only patients with RA may have immune cells in the synovial infiltrate. However, recent reports showed that patients with OA also have inflammatory synovial infiltrates that, particularly in the most severe forms, are characterized by high-grade inflammation and could lead to abrupt onset, marked clinical symptoms and structural damage [4]. Those patients with inflammatory OA have inflammatory features that in some

* Correspondence: alessandra.penatti@gmail.com; Federica.facciotti@ieo.it; federica.facciotti@ieo.ie
†Equal contributors
[1]DISCCO-Department of Clinical Science and Community Health Università degli Studi di Milano, 20122 Milan, Italy
[2]INGM-National Institute of Molecular Genetics "Romeo ed Enrica Invernizzi", 20122 Milan, Italy
Full list of author information is available at the end of the article

instances resemble those of RA. $CD4^{+}$T-cells are key to the initiation and progression of synovitis [2, 5] in patients with RA, and cytokines released into the synovial fluid (SF) by the inflamed tissue likely reflect the composition of effector and regulatory T cells infiltrating the synovia [6]. Relatively little is known about the characteristics of synovial immune cells in patients with inflammatory OA, although recent studies suggest that CD4 + T cells might contribute to the pathophysiology of OA and correlated symptoms, such as pain [7, 8].

Here, we further evaluated the role of $CD4^{+}$ T cells by in-depth analysis of subset composition and the cytokine milieu in peripheral blood and SF during effusion episodes in patients with RA and OA, and of the synovial membrane in patients who also underwent joint biopsy or surgery. We tested correlation between the disease activity parameters and the immunologic alterations in order to determine whether different synovial profiles of immune cells or cytokines could be specifically associated with different types of arthropathy. We report that patients with inflammatory OA display synovial immune activation that presents different signatures in comparison to RA.

Methods

Human samples and patients

Buffy-coat blood from 25 healthy age-matched and sex-matched donors (mean age 42 years; age range 26–58 years; male/female ratio 10/15) were obtained from the IRCCS Policlinico Ospedale Maggiore, Milan, Italy. There were 25 patients with RA (mean age 56 years; age range 40–72 years; male/female ratio 12/13) and 18 patients with inflammatory OA (mean age 69 years; age range 57–86 years; male/female ratio 8/10), who were attending the Rheumatology Department of the ASST-Gaetano Pini/CTO Orthopedic and Traumatology Specialist Center of Milan, enrolled in this study. All patients with RA fulfilled the European League Against Rheumatism/American College of Rheumatologists (EULAR/ACR) 2010 classification criteria and their disease activity were assessed using the disease activity score in 28 joints (DAS28) based on the erythrocyte sedimentation rate (ESR) [9]. The median duration of RA was 4.3 ± 3.9 years. We included symptomatic patients with radiographic evidence of mild knee OA (Kellgren and Lawrence grade 2) with an active inflammatory phenotype characterized by the presence of knee effusion synovitis and synovial thickening detected by ultrasound (US) [10]. Clinical, biochemical and cellular data on the enrolled patients with RA and OA are summarized in Table 1.

Peripheral blood (PB) was obtained and collected in heparinized tubes. SF samples from the knee joints of patients with RA and OA were collected during therapeutic needle aspiration into heparinized tubes. SM samples were taken from two patients with RA who also underwent knee

Table 1 Summary of clinical, biochemical and cellular data on patients with RA and OA

Characteristic	Rheumatoid arthritis			Osteoarthritis		
	PB[a]	SF[b]	SM[c]	PB[a]	SF[b]	SM[c]
Number	25	9	4	11	10	9
RF (*n*)[d]	17	9	4			
ACPA (*n*)[e]	17	9	4	-	-	-
DAS28[f] index, low (0–3) mean 2.42	10/25	0/9	3/4	-	-	-
DAS28[f] index, medium (3–5) mean 4.26	12/25	6/9	1/4	-	-	-
DAS28[f] index, high (>5) mean 5.55	3/25	3/9	0/4	-	-	-
ESR[g] (mm/h)	56.3 (5–87)			10.3 (1–25)		
CRP[h] (mg/dl)	4.3 (0.4–7.5)			0.27 (0–0.6)		
NSAID[i] (+/−)	8/25			14/18		
Corticosteroids (+/−)	14/25			0/18		
DMARDs[j] (+/−)	25/25			0/18		
PBMCs[k] (10^6/ml)	1.8 (1.4–2.3)			1.6 (1.3–1.9)		
SFMCs[l]	6.2 (3.6–11.3) *10^5/ml			9.2 (4.6–18.2) *10^4/ml		
SMMCs[m]	3.2 *10^6			1.3 *10^6		

[a]*PB* peripheral blood, [b]*SF* synovial fluid, [c]*SM* synovial membrane, [d]*RF* rheumatoid factor, [e]*ACPA* anti-citrullinated protein antibody, [f]*DAS28* disease activity score based on 28 joint counts, [g]*ESR* erythrocyte sedimentation rate, [h]*CRP* C-reactive protein (CRP), [i]*NSAIDs* non-steroidal anti-inflammatory drugs, [j]*DMARDs* disease-modifying anti-rheumatic drugs, [k]*PBMCs* peripheral blood mononuclear cells, [l]*SFMCs* synovial fluid mononuclear cells, [m]*SMMCs* synovial membrane mononuclear cells. *Mean, (values range). [d]RF nephelometry assay, cutoff value >15 UI/ml. All patients with RA had high positive [d]RF levels (more than three times the ULN for the laboratory and assay): 264 ± 190. [e]ACPA: QUANTA Lite® CCP3.1 IgG/IgA ELISA (INOVA Diagnostics), cutoff value >20 UI/ml. All patients with RA had high positive [e]ACPA levels (more than three times the ULN for the laboratory and assay):125 ± 64. [h]CRP cutoff value 1 mg/dl.

joint biopsy and from nine patients with OA and two patients with RA who additionally had knee replacement surgery.

The majority of patients with RA had medium/low disease activity (as summarized in Table 1), and were on medium/low doses of disease modifying anti-rheumatic drugs (DMARDs) (hydroxychloroquine, methotrexate or leflunomide). Thirteen out of twenty-four patients were on low-dose corticosteroid therapy (<8 mg/day). No patient was treated with biological therapy. See Table 1 for details.

Cell isolation

PB, SF and SM were collected. Peripheral blood mononuclear cells (PBMCs) and synovial fluid mononuclear cells (SFMCs) were directly isolated by Ficoll-Hypaque gradient (Sigma-Aldrich). Synovial membrane mononuclear cells (SMMCs) were isolated by Ficoll-Hypaque gradient (Sigma-Aldrich) after digestion of the tissue with Collagenase Type II (1 ml solution per 40 mg tissue; Sigma-Aldrich) for a variable length of time ranging from 1 h up to 6 h according to the size of the tissue sample.

Flow cytometry

Single-cell suspension of cells was stained with the following antibodies: CD3 (UCHT1), CD4 (RPA-T4; VIT4), CD8 (RPA-T8; OKT8), CD19 (HIB19), CD56 (B159,), CD127 (eBioRDR5), CD25 (M-A251 BD; BC96), ICOS (ISA-3), CXCR5 (51505), CCR6 (11A9) and CCR5 (27D/CCR5), obtained from BD Bioscience (Becton, Dickinson and Company, NJ, USA), eBioscience (eBioscience Inc, CA, USA), Miltenyi (Miltenyi Biotec GmbH, DE) or R&D (R&D Systems, MN, USA). Samples were passed on a FACSCanto flow cytometer. $CD4^+$ T-cell subsets were gated according to well-established phenotypic markers [11]. Thus, Tfh-cells were gated as $CD4^+CXCR5^+ICOS^+$ [12], Th1 cells as $CD4^+CD127^{hi}CD25^-CXCR3^+CCR6^-$, Th17 cells as $CD4^+CD127^{hi}CD25^-CXCR3^-CCR6^+$ [13] and Th1/17-cells as $CD4^+CD127^{hi}CD25^-CXCR3^+CCR6^+$ [14]. T regulatory cells (Tregs) were gated as $CD4^+CD127^{lo}CD25^+$ and Tr1 cells as $CD4^+CD127^-CD25^-CCR5^+CCR6^-$ [15]. Data were analyzed using FlowJo software (Tristar, Palo Alto, CA, USA).

ELISA

Cytokines in serum and SF were assessed by ELISA. IL-10 was measured with antibody pairs from BD, IL-17-A and IL-21 with antibody pairs from eBioscience (eBioscience Inc, CA, USA). Blys/B cell activating factor (BAFF) was measured using an ELISA kit from Biosupply (BioSupply Ltd, UK).

Statistics

Statistical significance was calculated using the two-tailed Student *t* test in the case of a Gaussian distribution (determined by the use of SPSS software, IBM); otherwise, the Mann-Whitney test was used for unmatched groups and the Wilcoxon test was used for paired groups. *P* values <0.05 were regarded as statistically significant and are denoted as $^*p < 0.05$, $^{**}p < 0.005$ and $^{***}p < 0.0005$.

Results

Patients with inflammatory OA manifest qualitative and quantitative differences in immune cell infiltrates in the synovial compartment compared to patients with RA

To evaluate whether the immune cell compartments in Patients with RA or OA differed from those in healthy donors (HD), we first compared the frequencies and performed statistical analysis of major circulating immune cell subsets, i.e. B cells, $CD4^+$ and $CD8^+$ T cells, monocytes and natural killer (NK) cells in PB. B cells were more frequent in patients with OA and in those with RA, whereas $CD14^+$monocytes were selectively reduced in patients with OA (Fig. 1a and b). Interestingly, although total T-cell frequencies were largely unchanged, patients with RA and those with OA had an increased CD4:CD8 ratio (Fig. 1a, b).

We then analyzed infiltrating immune cells in the SF (Fig. 1c, d) and in the SM (Additional file 1: Figure S1). Immune cells were present in the SF and in the SM of patients with RA and those with OA, as expected [7], and the immune infiltrate was composed mostly of T cells in both cases (Fig. 1c, d and Additional file 1: Figure S1). However, the number of immune cells per milliliter in SF from patients with OA was significantly lower than that in patients with RA (10^4 vs 10^5/ml) (Table 1). Moreover, patients with RA had a higher CD4:CD8 ratio in SF (Fig. 1d).

$CD4^+$ T cell subset frequencies in PB and in the synovial compartment distinguish patients with RA from patients with inflammatory OA

Next, we compared the frequencies of relevant $CD4^+$ T helper and regulatory subsets in PB and in SF from patients with RA and OA, identified according to well-established phenotypic markers [11] (Fig. 2 and Additional file 2: Figure S2).

Patients with RA had lower frequencies of circulating $CCR6^+CXCR3^-$Th17, $CCR6^+CXCR3^+$Th1/17 [12] and of $CXCR5^+ICOS^+$Tfh cells [13] as compared to patients with OA (Fig. 2a), and the reduction in Th1/17 and Th17 cells was statistically significant. Interestingly, patients with OA had significantly increased frequencies of circulating Tr1 cells [15] as compared to both patients with RA and HD, while frequencies of conventional $CD25^+$ Tregs were significantly reduced (Fig. 2b).

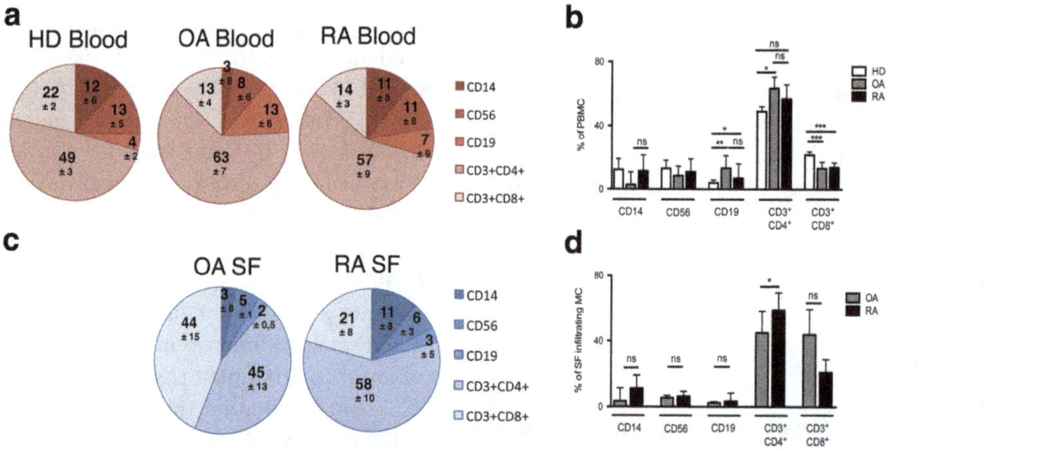

Fig. 1 Patients with osteoarthritis (*OA*) manifest qualitative and quantitative differences in the immune cell infiltrates in the synovial compartment as compared to patients with rheumatoid arthritis (*RA*). Frequencies (**a**) and cumulative statistical analysis (**b**) of immune cell populations (monocytes, $CD14^+$, B cells $CD19^+$, natural killer cells, $CD56^+$, $CD3^+$ $CD4^+$ T cells and $CD3^+$ $CD8^+$ T cells) in peripheral blood (**a**, **b**) from healthy donors (*HD*, $n = 25$) patients with OA ($n = 11$) and patients with RA ($n = 24$). Frequencies (**c**) and cumulative statistical analysis (**d**) of immune cell populations in synovial fluid (*SF*) from patients with OA ($n = 6$) and patients with RA ($n = 8$): $^*p \leq 0.05$, $^{**}p \leq 0.005$, $^{***}p \leq 0.0005$, Mann-Whitney unpaired two-tailed *t* test. Mean value ± SEM are reported. *ns* not significant, *PBMC* peripheral blood mononuclear cells, *MC* mononuclear cells

Consistent with previous studies, we observed an immune infiltrate of T helper cells in the synovial environment of patients with inflammatory OA [16] (Fig. 2c, d). In the SF, patients with OA and patients with RA both had high frequencies of Th1 cells and surprisingly, also of Th1/17 cells, which are thought to play a prominent pathogenic role in autoimmune arthritis [17] (Fig. 2c). Conversely, patients with RA had higher frequencies of Th17 [18, 19] and of Tfh cells than patients with OA (Fig. 2c). However, the frequencies of Th17 cells were low in a fraction of patients with RA, and therefore these differences were not statistically significant ($p = 0.0625$). Patients with RA had also higher frequencies of regulatory T-cell subsets, and the increased frequency of conventional $CD25^+$ Treg cells was highly significant (Fig. 2d). Notably, we observed very similar differences in the

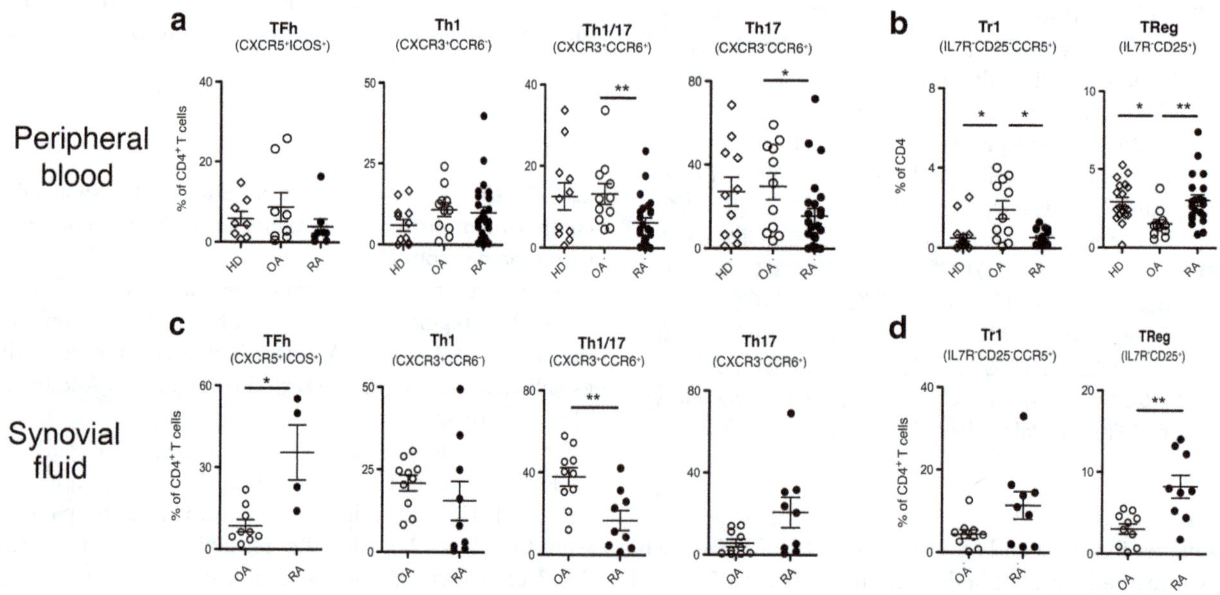

Fig. 2 $CD4^+$ T cell subset frequencies in blood and synovial fluid distinguish patients with rheumatoid arthritis (*RA*) from patients with osteoarthritis (*OA*). Frequency of $CD4^+$ T helper subsets (**a**, **c**) and T regulatory subsets (**b**, **d**) identified according to phenotypic markers in blood and synovial fluid from healthy donors (*HD*) (*open diamonds*), patients with OA (*open circles*) and patients with RA (*closed circles*): $^*p \leq 0.05$, $^{**}p \leq 0.005$, Mann-Whitney unpaired two-tailed *t* test. Mean value ± SEM are reported. *Treg* T regulatory cells, *Th* T helper cells

synovial membranes (SM) collected from the subgroup of patients who also underwent joint needle biopsy or surgery for joint replacement (Additional file 3: Figure S3A/B).

We then performed analysis of correlation between T helper and regulatory subset frequencies in paired blood and SF samples (Fig. 3). Interestingly, while no differences were observed in Th1 cells (Fig. 3a), in patients with OA there was significant and strong enrichment of Th1/17 cells in the SF (Fig. 3b), while conventional Th17 cells were largely excluded (Fig. 3c). Conversely, patients with RA did not have significant differences in the frequencies of helper T-cell subsets in PB and SF, with the notable exception of Tfh cells (Fig. 3a-d). Finally, we compared the distribution of T regulatory subsets in blood and SF from patients with RA and OA (Fig. 3e, f). Patients with RA had significantly increased frequencies of both Tr1 (Fig. 3e) and Treg (Fig. 3f) subsets in SF as compared to PB, whereas only Tr1 cells were significantly enriched in SF from patients with OA (Fig. 3d). Notably, there were no significant differences between SF and SM, consistent with the view that T-cell subset distribution in the two synovial compartments is similar (Additional file 3: Figure S3C/D).

Cytokine levels in serum and SF differ in patients with inflammatory OA and patients with RA, and correlate with disease activity and ACPA positivity

Different T-cell subsets preferentially infiltrate the synovium of patients with OA and RA. We asked if their characteristic cytokine products in serum or SF might be useful biomarkers to distinguish patients with RA from patients with OA. We therefore analyzed the prototypical cytokines that are produced by Th17 cells (IL-17, IL-21), Tfh cells (Blys, IL-21) and by regulatory T-cell subsets (IL-10). Notably, however, IL-10 was produced by both IL-7R- and IL-7R$^+$ T-cell subsets (Additional file 4: Figure S4), which contain respectively mainly regulatory and helper T cells [11, 15], suggesting that IL-10 is not exclusively derived from regulatory T cells in patients with OA and patients with RA, in particular in the synovial compartment. IL-17A (Fig. 4a), IL-10 (Fig. 4b) and Blys (Fig. 4c) serum levels were significantly elevated in patients with RA but not OA, as compared to HD. Moreover, IL-17A and in particular Blys were also abundant in SF from patients with RA (Fig. 4a and c) [20], but were hardly detectable in patients with OA. In marked contrast, similar amounts of IL-10 were present in SF from patients with RA and patients with OA (Fig. 4b). Interestingly, IL-21 was present in serum from both patients with OA and those with RA, but was completely absent in SF (Fig. 4d).

As cytokine levels in serum and SF differed between patients with RA and OA, we asked if cytokine levels could be useful also to distinguish patients with mild RA from patients with inflammatory OA. Thus, we tested correlation between the levels of cytokines in serum and SF from patients with RA, and the DAS28 and anti-citrullinated protein antibody (ACPA) positivity in these patients and compared them to the levels measured in serum and SF from patients with OA (Fig. 5).

Blys, a cytokine that induces differentiation and proliferation of B cells and promotes the production of

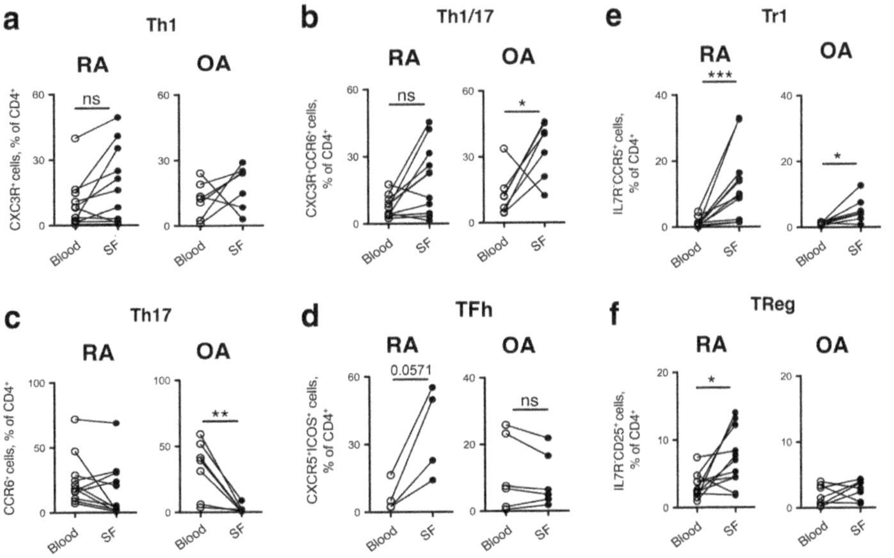

Fig. 3 Tissue distribution of T-helper (*Th*) and T-regulatory (*Treg*) subsets in patients with rheumatoid arthritis (*RA*) and patients with osteoarthritis (*OA*). Correlation between Th1 (**a**), Th1/17 (**b**), Th17 (**c**), Tfh (**d**), Tr1 (**e**) and Treg (**f**) subsets in paired samples of blood and synovial fluid (*SF*) isolated from the same patients with OA and the same patients with RA on the same day (values from the same patients are connected by *lines*): *$p \leq 0.05$, **$p \leq 0.005$, ***$p \leq 0.0005$, Wilcoxon paired two-tailed *t* test

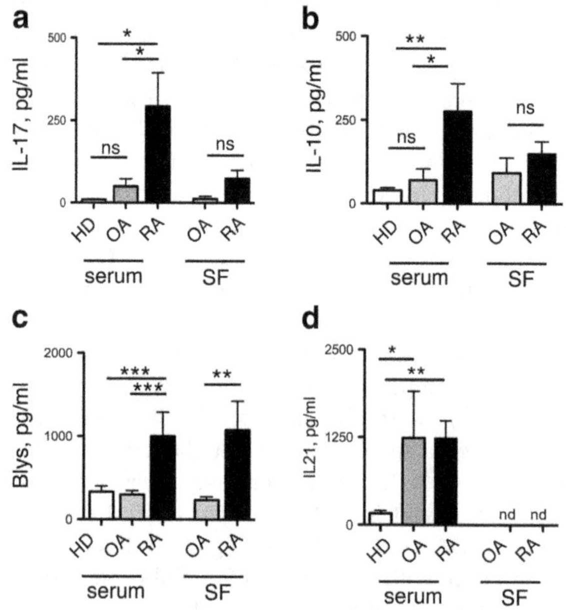

Fig. 4 Cytokine levels in serum and synovial fluid discriminate between patients with osteoarthritis (*OA*) and rheumatoid arthritis (*RA*). Blys (**a**), IL-10 (**b**), IL-17A (**c**) and IL-21 (**d**) levels in serum from healthy donors (*HD*) ($n = 25$), patients with OA ($n = 11$) and patients with RA ($n = 24$) and in synovial fluid (*SF*) from patients with OA ($n = 10$) and patients with RA ($n = 8$) patients: $^{*}p \leq 0.05$, $^{**}p \leq 0.005$, $^{***}p \leq 0.0005$, Mann-Whitney unpaired two-tailed *t* test. Mean value ± SEM are reported. *ns* not significant

autoantibodies [21], was elevated in patients with RA who had a low DAS28, and, surprisingly, independent of ACPA positivity, both in serum and in SF (Fig. 5a, b). In marked contrast, serum IL-10 and IL17A was selectively increased in patients with RA with ACPA (Fig. 5c, e), and/or with an increased DAS28 (Fig. 5 d,f), and there was no significant association between the levels of these cytokines and ACPA positivity or the DAS28 in the SF. A statistically non-significant tendency was observed for increased serum IL-21, ACPA positivity and DAS28 (Additional file 5: Figure S5). Of note, all patients positive for ACPA were also positive for rheumatoid factor (RF) and there were no patients positive for RF only.

As expected, patients with OA had a higher mean age than patients with RA, but on analysis of correlation none of the analyzed parameters were significantly associated with age in the two patient groups (Additional file 6: Figure S6 and Additional file 7: Figure S7). Moreover, we also analyzed a possible impact of corticosteroid therapy, but again found no significant association (Additional file 8: Figure S8).

We concluded that levels of serum cytokine and Blys in the SF could help to distinguish patients with RA from those with OA. Most important, the levels of Blys both in the serum and in the SF might distinguish patients with mild RA from patients with inflammatory OA, whereas elevated serum IL-17A is a more selective feature of severe and/or ACPA-positive patients with RA.

Discussion

Tissue-specific compartmentalization of immune cells is a distinct pathogenic mechanism that accounts for the selective accumulation of immune mediators in the synovium of both patients with RA and patients with OA. The striking differences in T-cell subset frequencies that we observed in the analyzed patients underline the pathogenic and clinical relevance of the analysis of tissues from the affected joint during active effusion. Indeed, SF samples directly reflect the inflammatory changes in the synovial membrane, and are more easily accessible for research and diagnostic purposes than needle biopsies.

To the best of our knowledge, this study is the first to perform a comprehensive and simultaneous analysis of both helper and regulatory T-cell subsets and their functional products in PB and in the affected tissues of patients with RA or OA. Consistent with previous studies, we observed an immune infiltrate in the synovium of patients with inflammatory OA that contained many Th1 cells [16]. Surprisingly, we also observed strong enrichment of Th1/17 cells, which are thought to play a prominent pathogenic role in autoimmune arthritis [18] and also other organ-specific autoimmune diseases [14]. However, the total cellularity in the SF was lower than in patients with RA, and regulatory T cells were quite frequent.

Consistent with the view that IL-10-producing Treg and/or Tr1 cells control potentially pathogenic IL-17-producing Th1/17 cells in the synovium of patients with OA, IL-10 was quite abundant in SF, whereas IL-17A was hardly detectable. Moreover, $CD4^{+}IL\text{-}7R^{-}$ T cells, which contain both Tr1 cells and Tregs [11, 15], produced IL-10 in the synovium of patients with OA following polyclonal stimulation. Surprisingly however, we also observed an increase in IL-10-producing $IL\text{-}7R^{+}CD4^{+}$ T cells, in particular in the synovial compartment and in patients with RA. Interestingly, as compared to patients with OA, there are higher numbers of $CCR6^{+}IL\text{-}7R^{+}$TH17-cells [18, 19] and $CXCR5^{+}ICOS^{+}$Tfh-cells in SF among many but not all patients with RA. Importantly, both subsets can produce IL-10, but provide help to B cells in the production of IgG, and could play a pathogenic role in autoantibody-driven autoimmune disease [22].

Of note, $CD25^{+}$ Tregs and Tr1 cells were highly enriched in SF and in the SM in patients with RA, but were insufficient to control the local production of IL-17A and Blys. We recently demonstrated that both $CD25^{+}$ Treg cells and Tr1 cells can regulate B-cell and T-cell responses, and that Tr1-mediated suppression of T-cell-dependent IgG production is selectively impaired in patients with systemic lupus erythematosus

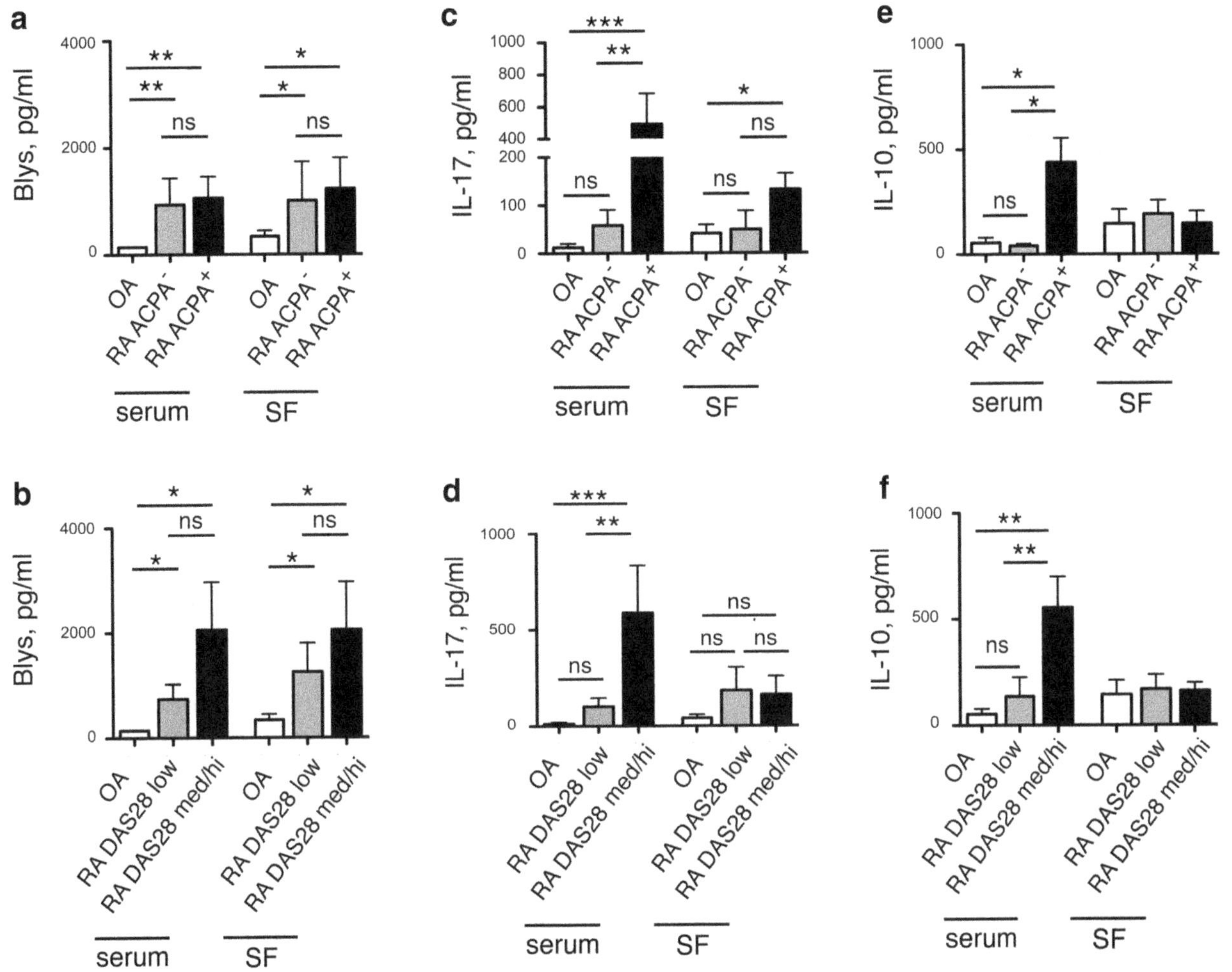

Fig. 5 Cytokine levels in serum and synovial fluid (*SF*) correlate with disease activity and anti-citrullinated protein antibody (*ACPA*) positivity. Correlation between serum and synovial fluid levels of Blys (**a**, **b**), IL-17 (**c**, **d**) and IL-10 (**e**, **f**) in patients with rheumatoid arthritis (*RA*) stratified according to ACPA positivity (**a**, **c**, **e**) or to the disease activity score in 28 joints (*DAS28*) (**b**, **d**, **f**), and cytokine levels in serum and synovial fluid from patients with osteoarthritis (*OA*). Cytokine concentrations were determined by ELISA: $*p \leq 0.05$, $**p \leq 0.005$, $***p \leq 0.0005$, two-tailed *t* test. Mean value ± SEM are reported. *ns* not significant

[15]. It seems likely therefore that Tregs and/or Tr1 cells are also functionally impaired in the synovium of patients with RA [23, 24]. In addition, we detected a cytokine storm in serum from patients with RA who had an elevated DAS28, suggesting that the function of regulatory T cells in patients with severe RA is also systemically compromised. Notably, however, while cytokines such as IL-21 and IL-17 are predominantly or exclusively produced by T cells, other cytokines such as IL-10 and Blys are also secreted by myeloid cells or B cells. Indeed, preliminary data suggests that B cells in SF in patients with RA could spontaneously secrete IL-10, indicating that B cells represent a relevant source (data not shown). Blys induces differentiation and proliferation of B cells and promotes the production of autoantibodies [21]. We observed significant increased levels of Blys both in serum and in SF from patients with RA, and virtual absence of Blys in patients with OA. Most important, although Blys serum and SF levels increased with disease activity in patients with RA, Blys was also significantly increased in patients with RA who had a low DAS28, and the levels of Blys were surprisingly independent of the presence of ACPA or RF (data not shown). These findings, generated by the analysis in a cohort of patients with relatively rare inflammatory OA, indicate that Blys might be a useful biomarker to discriminate between mild RA and inflammatory OA at the onset. These findings might help to support the stratification of patients in the future, and provide an additional tool to monitor disease activity at diagnosis and upon subsequent therapeutic interventions.

Conclusions

Although patients with inflammatory OA have immune activation in the synovial compartment, they display a specific immune signature, which is distinct from that in patients with RA, and this is characterized by different T-cell subset frequencies and cytokine profiles. In addition, soluble mediators such as Blys might serve as biomarkers to discriminate mild clinical forms of RA from inflammatory OA at onset and during acute episodes.

Additional files

Additional file 1: Figure S1. Frequencies of immune cell populations (monocytes CD14$^+$, B cells CD19$^+$, NK cells CD56$^+$, CD3$^+$ CD4$^+$ T cells and CD3$^+$ CD8$^+$ T cells) in the synovial membrane (*SM*) of patients with OA (n = 9) and patients with RA (n = 4): $*p \leq 0.05$, unpaired two-tailed Student *t* test. Mean value ± SEM are reported. (TIF 200 kb)

Additional file 2: Figure S2. Gating strategy to identify CD4$^+$ T helper and regulatory subsets. **a** Forward and side scatter indicating living lymphocytes; **b** gate to identify CD4$^+$ T cells; **c** CD127/CD25 gate to identify memory (CD127$^+$CD25$^-$), effector (CD127$^-$CD25$^-$) and Treg cells (CD127$^-$CD25$^+$); **d** among memory cells (CD127$^+$CD25$^-$), gates to identify Th1 cells (CXCR3$^+$CCR6$^-$), Th1/17 cells (CXCR3$^+$CCR6$^+$) and Th17 cells (CXCR3$^-$CCR6$^+$); **e** among memory cells (CD127$^+$CD25$^-$), gate to identify Tfh cells (CXCR5$^+$ICOS$^+$); **f** Among effector cells (CD127$^-$CD25$^-$), gate to identify Tr1 cells (CCR5$^+$CCR6$^-$). (TIF 5405 kb)

Additional file 3: Figure S3. Frequencies and statistical analysis of CD4 + helper (**a**) and regulatory T cell subsets (**b**) among CD4$^+$ lymphocytes in the synovial membrane (*SM*) of patients with OA (n = 9) and patients with RA (n = 4): $*p \leq 0.05$, unpaired two-tailed Student *t* test. Mean value ± SEM are reported. **c, d** Comparison of the frequencies of helper and regulatory T-cell subsets in synovial fluid and membranes in paired samples of the same patients with OA (*lower panels*) or RA (*upper panels*) (values from the same patients are connected by *lines*). (TIF 2769 kb)

Additional file 4: Figure S4. Intracellular IL-10 staining among IL-7R$^-$ (**a**) and IL7R$^+$ (**b**) CD4$^+$ T cells in the peripheral blood of healthy donors (*HD*), in the peripheral blood of patients with OA or RA (*OA Blood, RA Blood*), in the synovial fluid of patients with OA or RA (*OA SF, RA SF*) and in the synovial membrane of patients with OA or RA (*OA SM, RA SM*) following brief polyclonal activation with phorbole ester and calcium ionophore. (TIF 443 kb)

Additional file 5: Figure S5. Correlation of serum levels of IL-21 between patients with RA stratified according to positivity for autoantibodies (*ACPA*) or to the DAS28 disease activity index compared to cytokines serum levels in patients with OA. Cytokine concentrations were determined by ELISA. Unpaired two-tailed Mann-Whitney test. Mean value ± SEM are reported. (TIF 766 kb)

Additional file 6: Figure S6. Correlation between frequencies of CD4$^+$ subsets significantly different between patients with RA and patients with OA, and age of patients with RA. Frequency variations in Th17, Th1/17 and TFh CD4$^+$ T helper subsets (**a**, **b**) and of Tr1 and CD25$^+$ Treg regulatory subsets (**c**, **d**) in peripheral blood (**a**, **c**) and synovial fluid (**b**, **d**) in patients with RA and patients with OA are largely independent of patient age. Pearson's correlation coefficient: $p > 0.05$ for all. (TIF 439 kb)

Additional file 7: Figure S7. Serum (**a**) and synovial fluid (**b**) levels of IL-10 (*blue graphs*), IL-17 (*light blue graphs*) and Blys (*red graphs*) in patients with RA and patients with OA are largely independent of patient age. Pearson's correlation coefficient: $p > 0.05$ for all. (TIF 642 kb)

Additional file 8: Figure S8. Distribution of T helper (**a**, **c**) and T regulatory (**b**, **d**) subsets in peripheral blood (*upper panels*) and synovial fluid (*lower panels*) of significantly different subsets in patients with RA according to CS therapy: statistical analysis by Mann-Whitney test, $p > 0.05$. Peripheral blood: (**a**) Th1/17, Th17; (**b**) Tr1 and TReg subsets. Synovial fluid: (**c**) Th1/17; (**d**) TReg subsets. (TIF 607 kb)

Abbreviations

ACPA: Anti-citrullinated protein antibody; DAS29: disease activity score in 28 joints; DMARDs: Disease-modifying anti-rheumatic drugs; ELISA: Enzyme-linked immunosorbent assay; ESR: erythrocyte sedimentation rate; HD: Healthy donors; IL: interleukin; NK: Natural killer; NSAIDs: non-steroidal anti-inflammatory drugs; OA: Osteoarthritis; PB: Peripheral blood; PBMCs: Peripheral blood mononuclear cells; RA: Rheumatoid arthritis; RF: Rheumatoid factor; SF: Synovial fluid; SFMCs: Synovial fluid mononuclear cells; SM: Synovial membranes; SMMCs: Synovial membrane mononuclear cells; Th: T helper; Tregs: T regulatory cells; US: Ultrasound

Acknowledgements

Not applicable.

Funding

This work was supported by the Cariplo foundation, by the Romeo ed Enrica Invernizzi foundation and by Ricerca Corrente 2015–16 IRCCS Istituto Auxologico Italiano.

Authors' contributions

AP participated in the study design, obtained data, participated in the statistical analysis and drafted the manuscript; FF participated in the study design and coordination, obtained data, participated in the statistical analysis and wrote the manuscript; RDM and PL performed experiments; MP participated in the analysis of the data and in the drafting of the manuscript; AM and ODL recruited patients with OA and RA and obtained biological samples; LP and MT obtained biological samples; SA, MP and AIF participated in the design of the study, in the interpretation of the data and in the drafting of the manuscript; JG and PLM conceived the study, participated in its design and coordination, in analysis and interpretation of data and in the drafting of the manuscript. All authors read and approved the final manuscript.

Competing interests

The authors declare that they have no competing interests.

Source of support

None declared.

Author details

[1]DISCCO-Department of Clinical Science and Community Health Università degli Studi di Milano, 20122 Milan, Italy. [2]INGM-National Institute of Molecular Genetics "Romeo ed Enrica Invernizzi", 20122 Milan, Italy. [3]ASST-Gaetano Pini/CTO Orthopedic and Traumatology Specialist Center, Rheumatology and Orthopedic Department, 20122 Milan, Italy. [4]Department of Rheumatology, Leiden University Medical Center, 2300 Leiden, The Netherlands. [5]Laboratory of immuno-rheumatological researches, IRCCS Istituto Auxologico Italiano, 20149 Milan, Italy. [6]Department of Pathophysiology and Transplantation, Università degli Studi di Milano, 20122 Milan, Italy.

References

1. Beaten D, et al. Comparative study of the synovial histology in rheumatoid arthritis, spondyloarthropathy, and osteoarthritis: influence of disease duration and activity. Ann Rheum Dis. 2000;59:945–53.
2. McInnes IB, Schett G. The pathogenesis of rheumatoid arthritis. NEJM. 2011; 365:2205–19.
3. Hunter DJ. Osteoarthritis. Best Pract Res Clin Rheumatol. 2011;25:801–14.
4. Sellam J, Berenbaum F. The role of synovitis in pathophysiology and clinical symptoms of osteoarthritis. Nat Rev Rheumatol. 2010;6:625–35.
5. Mellado M, et al. T cell migration in rheumatoid arthritis. Front Immunol. 2015;6:384.

6. McInnes IB, Schett G. Cytokines in the pathogenesis of rheumatoid arthritis. Nat Rev Immunol. 2007;7:429–42.
7. Lange-Brokaar BJE, et al. Synovial inflammation, immune cells and their cytokines in osteoarthritis: a review. Osteoarthritis Cartilage. 2012;20:1484–99.
8. Klein-Wieringa IR, et al. Inflammatory cells in patients with endstage knee osteoarthritis: a comparison between the synovium and the infrapatellar fat pad. J Rheumatol. 2016;43(4):771–8.
9. Aletaha D, et al. Rheumatoid arthritis classification criteria: an American College of Rheumatology/European League Against Rheumatism collaborative initiative. Arthritis Rheum. 2010;62:2569–81.
10. Hart DJ, Spector TD. The classification and assessment of osteoarthritis. Baillieres Clin Rheumatol. 1995;9(2):407–32.
11. Geginat J, Paroni M, Facciotti F, Gruarin P, Kastirr I, Caprioli F, Pagani M, Abrignani S. The CD4-centered universe of human T cell subsets. Semin Immunol. 2013;25(4):252–62. Epub 2013 Nov 1.
12. Morita R, et al. Human blood CXCR5(+)CD4(+) T cells are counterparts of T follicular cells and contain specific subsets that differentially support antibody secretion. Immunity. 2011;34:108–21.
13. Acosta-Rodriguez EV, Rivino L, Geginat J, et al. Surface phenotype and antigenic specificity of human interleukin 17-producing T helper memory cells. Nat Immunol. 2007;8:639–46.
14. Paroni M, Maltese V, De Simone M, Ranzani V, Larghi P, et al. Recognition of viral and self-antigens by Th1 and Th1/Th17 central memory cells in patients with multiple sclerosis reveals distinct roles in immune surveillance and relapses. J Allergy Clin Immunol. 2017 [Epub ahead of print].
15. Facciotti F, Gagliani N, Häringer B, Alfen JS, Penatti A, et al. IL-10-producing forkhead box protein 3-negative regulatory T cells inhibit B-cell responses and are involved in systemic lupus erythematosus. J Allergy Clin Immunol. 2016;137(1):318–21.
16. Yamada H, et al. Preferential accumulation of activated Th1 cells not only in rheumatoid arthritis but also in osteoarthritis joints. J Rheumatol. 2011;38:1569–75.
17. Nistala K, et al. Th17 plasticity in human autoimmune arthritis is driven by the inflammatory environment. Proc Natl Acad Sci USA. 2010;107:14751–6.
18. Paulissen SMJ, et al. The role and modulation of CCR6+ Th17 cell populations in rheumatoid arthritis. Cytokine. 2015;74:43–53.
19. Paulissen SMJ, et al. CCR6+ Th cell populations distinguish ACPA positive from ACPA negative rheumatoid arthritis. Arthritis Res Ther. 2015;17:344.
20. Cheema GS, et al. Elevated serum B Lymphocyte stimulator levels in patients with systemic immune-based rheumatic diseases. Arthritis Rheum. 2001;44(6):1313–9.
21. Wei F, et al. The role of BAFF in the progression of rheumatoid arthritis. Cytokine. 2015;76:537–44.
22. Geginat J, et al. The light and the dark sides of Interleukin-10 in immune-mediated diseases and cancer. Cytokine Growth Factor Rev. 2016;30:87–93.
23. Moradi B, et al. CD4 + CD25 + hiCd127lw regulatory T cells are enriched in rheumatoid arthritis and ostheoarthritis joints-analysis of frequency and phenotype in synovial membrane, synovial fluid and peripheral blood. Arthritis Res Ther. 2014;16:R97.
24. Appel H, et al. An elevated level of IL-10- and TGF β-secreting T cells, B cells and macrophages in the synovial membrane of patients with reactive arthritis compared to rheumatoid arthritis. Clin Rheumatol. 2004;23:435–40.

16

Multicenter inception cohort of enthesitis-related arthritis: variation in disease characteristics and treatment approaches

Sabrina Gmuca[1], Rui Xiao[2], Timothy G. Brandon[1], Ilaria Pagnini[3], Tracey B. Wright[4], Timothy Beukelman[5], Esi M. Morgan[6] and Pamela F. Weiss[7,8*]

Abstract

Background: Enthesitis-related arthritis (ERA) is a specific subtype of juvenile idiopathic arthritis (JIA) defined according to the International League of Associations for Rheumatology (ILAR) criteria. We aimed to characterize the clinical features and treatment regimens in an inception cohort of children with ERA.

Methods: We performed a retrospective, cross-sectional, multicenter cohort study including subjects diagnosed with ERA between 1989 and 2012. Patients all fulfilled the ILAR criteria for ERA within 3 months of initial presentation to the rheumatology clinic. Differences in the prevalence of clinical criteria across study sites and by human leukocyte antigen (HLA)-B27 status were assessed using the Wilcoxon rank-sum or chi-square test, as appropriate.

Results: Two hundred thirty-four children met the inclusion criteria. Their median age at diagnosis was 11.6 years, and 59% were HLA-B27-positive. Sixty-nine percent had enthesitis and arthritis at the time of diagnosis. Seventy-eight percent had a pauciarticular onset. The prevalence of all ILAR criteria at diagnosis, except arthritis and acute anterior uveitis, differed significantly across sites (all $p < 0.01$). Medication use varied significantly across sites for children with peripheral arthritis ($p < 0.001$), but not for sacroiliitis or enthesitis only. Nonsteroidal anti-inflammatory drugs and disease-modifying antirheumatic drugs were the most commonly prescribed treatments, with anti-TNF agents primarily being initiation for sacroiliitis. HLA-B27 positivity was associated with male sex, higher active joint count, sacroiliitis, and higher disease activity at disease onset.

Conclusions: The majority of children had a pauciarticular onset, and several statistically significant clinical differences based on HLA-B27 status were identified. The observed heterogeneity in clinical presentation across sites reflects either true differences in patient populations or differences in how the ILAR criteria are being applied.

Keywords: Enthesitis-related arthritis, Juvenile idiopathic arthritis, HLA-B27, Classification criteria

Background

Juvenile idiopathic arthritis (JIA) is the most common pediatric rheumatic disease [1] and includes a number of heterogeneous arthritides. JIA is classified into seven mutually exclusive categories by the International League of Associations of Rheumatology (ILAR) classification [2]. Enthesitis-related arthritis (ERA) accounts for approximately 10% to 20% of JIA cases [3, 4] and, as alluded to by its name, is distinguished mainly by involvement of the entheses (where tendons and ligaments insert into bone). A significant proportion of current knowledge regarding ERA is based on data from adults with ankylosing spondylitis and spondyloarthritis (SpA), with a paucity of studies specifically focused on the ERA population. Additionally, application of adult data to children with ERA is not ideal, as evidenced by recognized clinical differences between the two populations, including less severe spinal involvement and more pronounced enthesitis and peripheral arthritis in children [5, 6]. Therefore, there is a

* Correspondence: weisspa@email.chop.edu
[7]University of Pennsylvania Perelman School of Medicine and Children's Hospital of Philadelphia, Philadelphia, PA, USA
[8]Department of Pediatric Rheumatology, The Children's Hospital of Philadelphia, 34th Street and Civic Center Boulevard, Wood Building, Fourth Floor, Philadelphia, PA 19104, USA
Full list of author information is available at the end of the article

critical need for research focused specifically on the ERA population.

The majority of research conducted in children with ERA has been in the context of juvenile SpA, which includes other conditions such as inflammatory bowel disease and psoriatic arthritis. Epidemiologic studies focused on children with ERA as a distinct cohort are scarce. The largest study to date included 312 ERA subjects from a single center in northern India [7]. In this study, the mean age was 11.3 years, there was a male predominance (9:1), and 87% were human leukocyte antigen (HLA)-B27-positive. The high HLA-B27 positivity and single-center nature of the study make its applicability to other populations uncertain. Other studies focused on this JIA category have limited sample sizes ranging from 19 to 84 subjects [8–12]. Additionally, few studies have examined treatment practices for this group of children. Treatment recommendations have been published by the American College of Rheumatology (ACR) and are based primarily on the number of active joints and the presence of sacroiliitis [13]. It is unknown whether routine practice reflects these recommendations.

The significance of HLA-B27 positivity in this population has also not been well characterized. In children classified as having ERA on the basis of ILAR criteria, the proportion of HLA-B27 positivity ranges from 45% to 88% in published studies [6, 7, 9, 10, 12]. HLA-B27 positivity in this group of children also seems to vary by geographic location. Cohorts from India and Mexico have higher reported prevalence of HLA-B27 positivity than North American and European cohorts [7, 14]. The importance, or lack thereof, of HLA-B27 in shaping the clinical phenotype and course of these patients remains unclear. Both acute anterior uveitis (AAU) and sacroiliitis have been reported to have an association with HLA-B27 [15, 16]. Researchers in prior studies have also reported HLA-B27 as an indicator of a poor prognosis among all categories of JIA, with HLA-B27-positive patients having more inflammatory back pain [17], greater disease activity [18], and decreased likelihood of remission after 8 years of disease [19] than children with JIA who are HLA-B27-negative.

We performed a retrospective, cross-sectional, multicenter cohort study that included subjects from five pediatric rheumatology centers (in North America and Europe) to evaluate the clinical presentation and treatment regimens of children with ERA. We also aimed to test whether children classified as having ERA are phenotypically distinct based on HLA-B27 positivity, which might have implications for the assessment or management of these two subgroups of ERA.

Methods

The protocol for this study was reviewed and approved by each institution's committee for the protection of human subjects.

Study site and participants

We performed a retrospective cross-sectional study using a multicenter database of children with ERA from five pediatric rheumatology centers. The study sites were Children's Hospital of Philadelphia (Philadelphia, PA, USA), Children's of Alabama (Birmingham, AL, USA), Cincinnati Children's Hospital Medical Center (Cincinnati, OH, USA), Texas Scottish Rite Hospital for Children (Dallas, TX, USA), and Meyer Children's Hospital (Florence, Italy). All subjects met the following inclusion criteria: (1) diagnosis of ERA according to the ILAR criteria (Table 1) within 3 months of initial presentation to rheumatology clinic with signs or symptoms of juvenile arthritis, (2) aged ≤16 years at symptom onset, and (3) evaluated at one of the study sites during the study period (1989–2012). Chart reviewers independently applied the ILAR criteria to all study subjects to establish the diagnosis of ERA, given that this nomenclature did not exist for the years prior to 1995. Eligibility criteria were verified by the coordinating center (Children's Hospital of Philadelphia); 85 children were excluded after this process.

Clinical characteristics

The baseline visit was defined as the first rheumatology appointment at which the patient exhibited clinical signs or symptoms of JIA (enthesitis, arthritis, AAU, or inflammatory back pain), regardless of whether the child was classified as having ERA at that time. Patient data were abstracted from the medical charts and included the following: demographics, family history, clinical features, patient-reported outcomes, and medications

Table 1 International League of Associations for Rheumatology criteria for enthesitis-related arthritis

Inclusion criteria	Exclusion criteria
Arthritis and enthesitis	• Psoriasis or a history of psoriasis in the patient or a first degree relative
or	• Presence of IgM RF on at least two occasions at least 3 months apart
Arthritis *or* enthesitis with at least two of the following: • Sacroiliac joint tenderness and/or inflammatory spinal pain • Presence of HLA-B27 • Onset of arthritis in a male over 6 years of age • Family history in at least one first degree relative of ankylosing spondylitis, ERA, sacroiliitis with IBD, reactive arthritis or acute anterior uveitis • Acute anterior uveitis	• Systemic JIA in the patient

Abbreviations: ERA Enthesitis-related arthritis, *HLA* Human leukocyte antigen, *IBD* Inflammatory bowel disease, *IgM* Immunoglobulin M, *RF* Rheumatoid factor, *JIA* Juvenile idiopathic arthritis

prescribed. Peripheral arthritis was defined as joint swelling or, in the absence of swelling, limited range of motion plus tenderness [20, 21]. Enthesitis was defined as tenderness to palpation according to the ILAR criteria [2]. Because there is no standardized pediatric examination of the entheses, the sites routinely examined at each study site varied. The entheses insertion sites routinely examined included interosseous ligaments of the sacroiliac joint (all sites), hip flexors at the greater trochanter (four sites), quadriceps at the patella (all sites), infrapatellar tendon at the patella (all sites), infrapatellar tendon at the tibial tubercle (four sites), Achilles tendon (all sites), and plantar fascia at calcaneus (all sites). Sacroiliitis was defined as evidence of inflammation (e.g., bone marrow edema, joint space enhancement, or erosions/sclerosis) visualized by magnetic resonance imaging (MRI) [22, 23]. Ascertained laboratory values included the C-reactive protein (CRP), erythrocyte sedimentation rate (ESR), antinuclear antibody (ANA), and HLA-B27.

Patient-reported outcomes included patient-reported pain over the past week using a visual analogue scale (range 0–10); the Childhood Health Assessment Questionnaire (CHAQ), which is 30-item questionnaire that assesses 8 domains of physical function with scores ranging from 0 to 3 [24, 25]; and patient global assessment of disease activity using a visual analogue scale (range 0–10). CHAQ scores of 0.13, 0.63, and 1.75 represent mild, mild to moderate, and moderate impairment, respectively [26]. Physician global assessment of disease activity (physician global) was also abstracted (range 0–10) [27, 28]. Two composite disease activity scores were calculated: the clinical Juvenile Arthritis Disease Activity Score (cJADAS) (comprised of the active joint count, physician global evaluation, and parent global evaluation) and the Juvenile Spondyloarthritis Disease Activity Index (JSpADA). The cJADAS was developed for use in all categories of JIA, with a score ranging from 0 to 30, where higher scores indicate more active disease [29]. Cutoffs for minimal and high disease activity using the cJADAS are <1.5 and >4, respectively, in oligoarticular disease and <2.5 and >8.5, respectively, in polyarticular disease [30]. The JSpADA was developed specifically for use in juvenile SpA and consists of eight items (arthritis, enthesitis, patient pain assessment, inflammatory markers, morning stiffness, clinical sacroiliitis, AAU, and back mobility). Scores range from 0 to 8, with higher scores being indicative of more active disease [31].

Because this study involved retrospective data collection, there were missing data. Missing data for laboratory values (ANA, HLA-B27, ESR, or CRP) did not exceed 13%. Patient-reported outcomes were missing for approximately 50% of visits; missing values were not imputed. Age, sex, and active joint count did not significantly differ between those visits with and without missing patient-reported outcomes (all $p > 0.05$) or between those with and without calculable cJADAS and JSpADA scores ($p > 0.05$).

For evaluation of treatments, children were considered to belong to one of the following three mutually exclusive phenotypes with the following hierarchy: (1) sacroiliitis (MRI-defined), (2) peripheral arthritis, and (3) enthesitis only. Treatments evaluated included nonsteroidal anti-inflammatory drugs (NSAIDs), intra-articular (IA) glucocorticoid injections, disease-modifying antirheumatic drugs (DMARDs: methotrexate, leflunomide, sulfasalazine), and biologic therapy with tumor necrosis factor (TNF)-α blockade (adalimumab, etanercept, infliximab). For comparison of clinical features between children based on HLA-B27 status, the cohort was restricted to those who had both arthritis and enthesitis. We reasoned that if we were to compare those who were HLA-B27-positive with those who were HLA-B27-negative without restricting the analyses to those with both arthritis and enthesitis, we might be detecting differences based on the classification criteria met rather than true differences between these groups based on HLA-B27 status.

Analysis

Subject characteristics were summarized by median and interquartile range (IQR) for continuous variables and frequency and percentage for categorical variables. Differences in the prevalence of clinical criteria and medication use for clinical phenotypes across study sites were assessed by the chi-square test. Differences in clinical characteristics by HLA-B27 status were assessed using the Wilcoxon rank-sum or chi-square test, as appropriate. *P* values less than 0.05 were considered statistically significant. All analyses were performed using Stata release 14.2 statistical software (StataCorp, College Station, TX, USA).

Results

Clinical characteristics

Two hundred thirty-four children and adolescents met the study inclusion criteria. Table 2 shows the demographic and clinical characteristics of this cohort at diagnosis. Children and adolescents with ERA were predominantly male (72.2%) and Caucasian (82.9%). The median age at diagnosis was 11.6 years (IQR 9.8–13.7). One hundred thirty-five (59.2%) children were HLA-B27-positive. The median number of active joints was 2 (IQR 1–4), and the median number of tender entheses was 2 (IQR 1–4). The most commonly affected joints were the knee (107 patients with at least one affected knee [45.7%]), ankle (n = 84 patients [35.9%]), wrist (n = 46 [19.7%]), and hip (n = 45 [19.2%]). Seventy-eight percent of children had a

Table 2 Patient characteristics at time of enthesitis-related arthritis classification

	All subjects ($n = 234$)
Demographics, median (IQR) or n (%)	
Age in years	11.6 (9.8–13.7)
Sex, male	169 (72.2)
Race, Caucasian	194 (82.9)
Family history of HLA-B27-associated disease	36 (15.4)
Clinical characteristics, median (IQR) or n (%)	
HLA-B27 positivity	135 (59.2)
Active joint count	2 (1–4)
Tender entheses count	2 (1–4)
MRI-defined sacroiliitis ($n = 45$ with imaging)	25 (55.6)
Polyarticular onset	52 (22.2)
ANA-positive	49 (23.4)
CRP, abnormal/elevated	39 (26.9)
ESR, abnormal/elevated	93 (45.8)
Patient-/physician-reported outcomes, median (IQR)	
Physician global disease activity assessment (0–10)	2.5 (2–4)
Juvenile Spondyloarthritis Disease Activity Index (JSpADA) (0–8)	3 (2.5–4)
Juvenile Arthritis Disease Activity Score (cJADAS), excluding ESR (0–30)	9 (5–14)
Patient/parent global disease activity assessment (0–10)	4 (2–6)
Function (CHAQ) (0–3)	0.563 (0–1)
Patient/parent pain assessment (0–10)	4 (2–7)

Abbreviations: IQR Interquartile range, *HLA* Human leukocyte antigen, *MRI* Magnetic resonance imaging, *ANA* Antinuclear antibody, *CRP* C-reactive protein, *ESR* Erythrocyte sedimentation rate, *CHAQ* Childhood Health Assessment Questionnaire

Denominators for clinical characteristics varied because of missing data: HLA-B27 status ($n = 228$), magnetic resonance imaging-defined sacroiliitis ($n = 45$), ANA ($n = 209$), CRP ($n = 145$), ESR ($n = 203$), physician global disease activity assessment ($n = 126$), JSpADA ($n = 116$), patient/parent global disease activity assessment ($n = 102$), CHAQ ($n = 120$), patient/parent pain assessment ($n = 129$), cJADAS (JADAS3–10) ($n = 86$)

pauciarticular onset (fewer than five joints). The most frequently tender entheses were the insertions of the infrapatellar tendon on the patella ($n = 103$ patients [44%]), Achilles tendon ($n = 77$ [32.9%]), and the interosseous ligaments of the sacroiliac joint ($n = 71$ [30.3%]).

Figure 1 shows the percentage of children who met each of the ILAR ERA criteria. The majority of patients met the ILAR criteria for a diagnosis of ERA at the first rheumatology visit ($n = 214$ [91.5%]), with 18 subjects (7.7%) meeting the criteria at the second visit and 2 subjects (0.9%) meeting the criteria by the third visit. One hundred sixty-two (69.2%) children had arthritis *and* enthesitis, and 72 (30.8%) children had arthritis *or* enthesitis plus at least two additional ILAR criteria. Of the 72 children presenting with arthritis or enthesitis plus at least two additional ILAR criteria, 55 had arthritis only and 17 had enthesitis only. Because arthritis (91.5%) and enthesitis (75.2%) are requirements under the ILAR criteria for ERA, it was not surprising that they were the two most common disease manifestations followed by the presence of arthritis in a male over the age of 6 years (62.8%). Sacroiliac tenderness was present in 25.6% ($n = 60$) of patients, and AAU was present in only 5.6% ($n = 13$) of patients. Although more than half (59.2%) of all patients were HLA-B27-positive, this proportion varied significantly across sites, ranging from 35% to 89% ($p < 0.001$) (Fig. 1). The prevalence of arthritis and AAU did not differ significantly across sites. The prevalence of each of the remaining ILAR criteria, however, was also significantly different across sites (Fig. 1) (all $p < 0.01$): enthesitis (range: 57% to 91%), sacroiliac tenderness or inflammatory lumbosacral pain (range: 12% to 43%), onset of arthritis in a male over 6 years (range: 46% to 79%), and history of HLA-B27-associated disease in a first-degree relative (range: 6% to 43%).

Table 2 lists patient- and physician-reported disease activity assessments. Disease activity at diagnosis was moderate as assessed globally by patients/parents (median 4, IQR 2–6) and physicians (median 2.5, IQR 2–4). Patients also had moderate disease activity as evaluated by composite disease activity measures (JSpADA median 3, IQR 2.5–4; cJADAS median 9, IQR 5–14). Patients reported moderate pain (median score of 4, IQR 2–7) and between mild and mild to moderate disability as assessed by the CHAQ (median score of 0.563, IQR 0–1). Twenty-seven percent ($n = 39$) had systemic inflammation as evidenced by an elevated CRP level, and 45.8% ($n = 93$) had an elevated ESR (Table 2).

Medication use

Figure 2 demonstrates unadjusted medication use at diagnosis based on clinical phenotype. Overall, NSAIDs were the most commonly prescribed medication class ($n = 189$ [80.8%]), followed by DMARDs ($n = 75$ [32.1%]). Oral glucocorticoids (14.6%), IA glucocorticoid injections (15.0%), and biologic agents (15.4%) were less commonly used. Medication use varied significantly among sites for children with peripheral arthritis ($p < 0.001$) but not for those with sacroiliitis or enthesitis only. NSAIDs-only was the most prevalent treatment across every disease phenotype. Children presenting with MRI-defined sacroiliitis were prescribed NSAIDs only (40%), biologic monotherapy (32%), or a combination of a biologic and a DMARD (4%). Children with arthritis at diagnosis were most commonly prescribed NSAIDs only (43%) or DMARD monotherapy (27%). Subjects with only enthesitis at diagnosis were treated primarily with NSAIDs (82%). IA glucocorticoid injections were

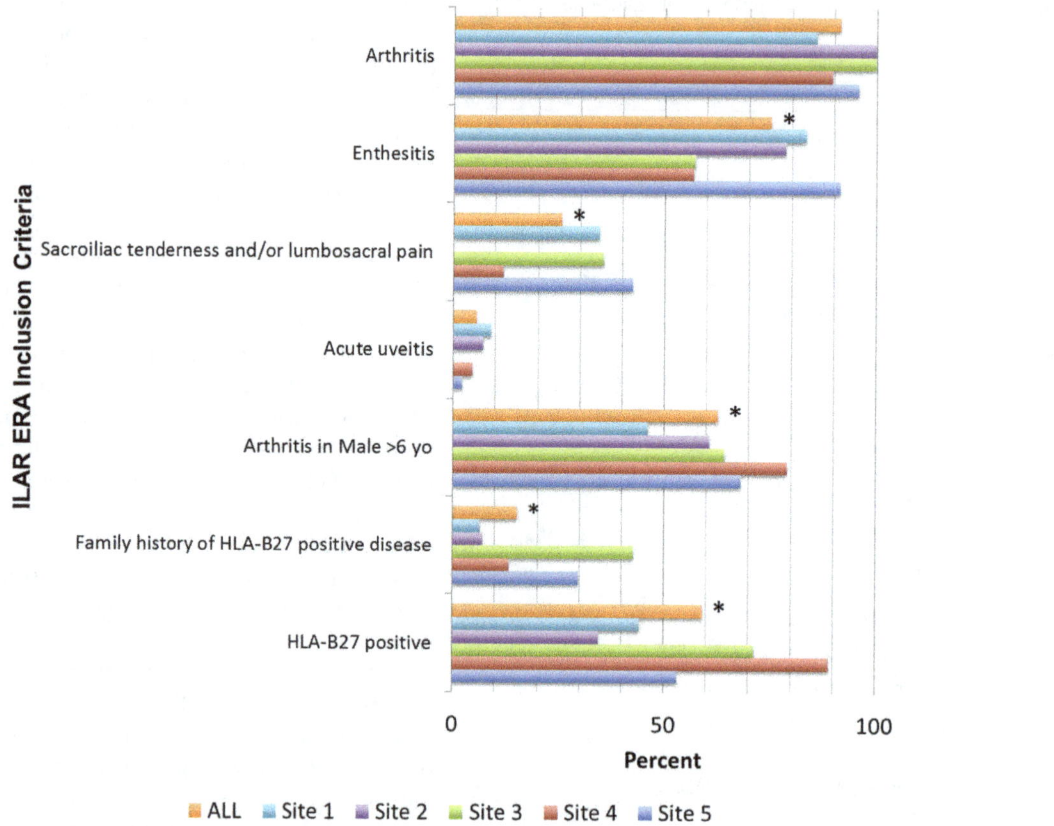

Fig. 1 International League of Associations for Rheumatology (ILAR) enthesitis-related arthritis (ERA) inclusion criteria by enrollment site. * $p < 0.05$ for between-group comparisons. *HLA* Human leukocyte antigen

reserved for children with peripheral arthritis (11.3%). Oral corticosteroids were prescribed for those with sacroiliitis (4.0%) and peripheral arthritis (5.9%).

HLA-B27 status and clinical phenotype

In order to determine whether patient demographics, clinical characteristics, or ILAR criteria fulfillment differed on the basis of HLA-B27 status, we restricted our analyses to patients who met ILAR criteria by having both arthritis *and* enthesitis ($n = 156$). Clinical characteristics of HLA-B27-positive versus HLA-B27-negative children are presented in Table 3. Among this restricted cohort, 44% ($n = 69$) were HLA-B27-positive. As in the primary analysis, male sex and Caucasian racial predominance persisted.

There was an older median age of onset in the HLA-B27-positive children (12.3 versus 11.0 years; $p = 0.01$). In comparison with HLA-B27-negative children, HLA-B27-positive children had a higher active joint count ($p < 0.01$) and were more likely to have sacroiliitis ($p < 0.01$). A greater proportion of HLA-B27-positive children had an elevated ESR (54.8% versus 31.1%; $p < 0.01$). The JSpADA was significantly higher in those who were HLA-B27-positive than in those who were HLA-B27-negative ($p = 0.04$), whereas there was no significant difference in the cJADAS or physician global disease activity assessment. Those who were HLA-B27-positive were more likely to develop arthritis after the age of 6 years ($p < 0.01$). There were no other differences in the ILAR criteria based on HLA-B27 status.

Discussion

To our knowledge, this study comprises the largest multicenter international inception cohort of children with ERA to date. Children with ERA were predominantly male, Caucasian, and HLA-B27-positive; these findings are in accordance with previously published cohorts [9, 32]. An overwhelming majority of patients (91.5%) met the ILAR criteria for a diagnosis of ERA at their first visit to a pediatric rheumatologist. The majority of subjects had both arthritis and enthesitis at the time of diagnosis. Most children had a pauciarticular onset of disease, and the most commonly affected joints were the knees, ankles, wrists, and hips. Enthesitis was most common at the attachments of the infrapatellar tendon on the inferior pole of the patella, the interosseous ligaments of the sacroiliac joints, and the Achilles tendon. These findings highlight the importance of carefully assessing for arthritis

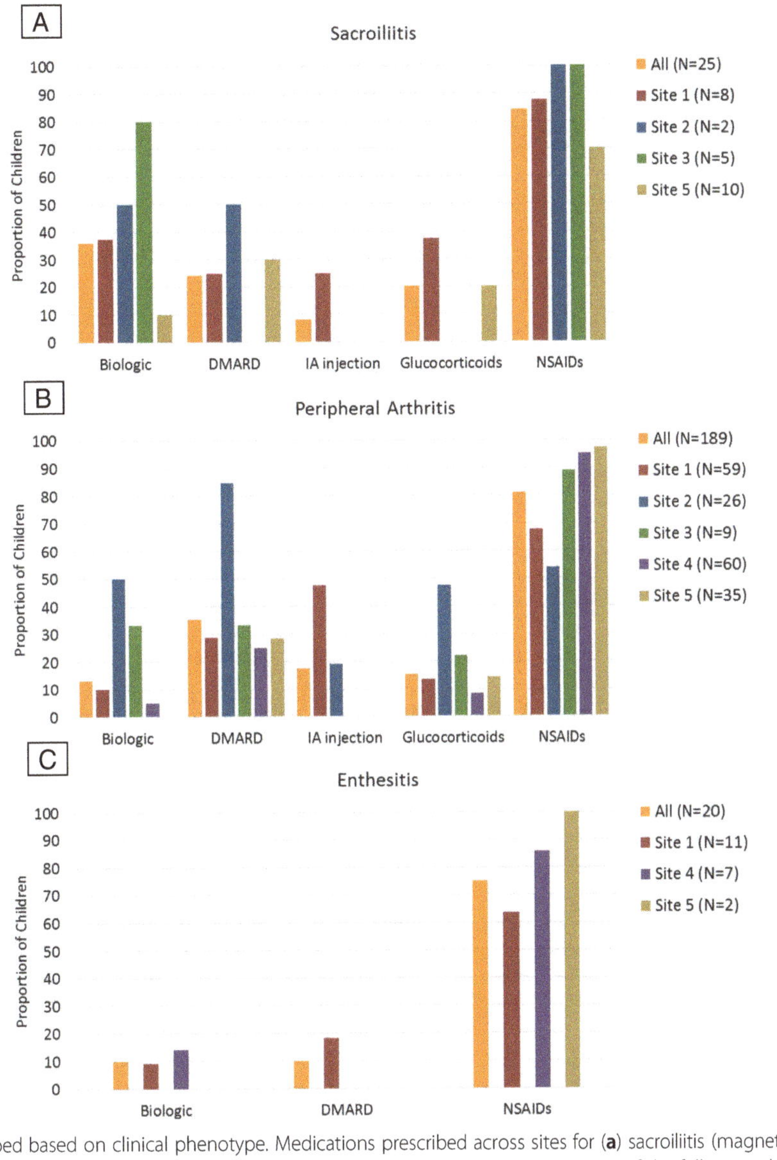

Fig. 2 Medications prescribed based on clinical phenotype. Medications prescribed across sites for (**a**) sacroiliitis (magnetic resonance imaging [MRI]-defined), (**b**) peripheral arthritis, and (**c**) enthesitis only. Children were considered as having one of the following three mutually exclusive phenotypes with the following hierarchy: (1) sacroiliitis (MRI-defined), (2) peripheral arthritis, and (3) enthesitis. Biologic medications included tumor necrosis factor-α inhibitors (adalimumab, etanercept, infliximab). Sacroiliitis data were not available for site 4. No children from site 2 or 3 were diagnosed with isolated enthesitis, and of those with enthesitis, none were prescribed IA injections or glucocorticoids. *DMARD* Disease-modifying antirheumatic drug, *Glucocorticoids* Oral glucocorticoids, *IA* Intra-articular glucocorticoid injection, NSAIDs Nonsteroidal anti-inflammatory drugs

and enthesitis in all possible locations when examining a new patient presenting with concern for JIA. Perhaps special attention should be paid to the aforementioned anatomical sites when considering a diagnosis of ERA. NSAIDs and DMARDs were the most often prescribed first-line therapies. There was increased use of biologic agents, however, for the treatment of children with sacroiliitis. Systemic glucocorticoids were reserved for children with arthritis or sacroiliitis. Children who were HLA-B27-positive tended to be older and male, with a higher active joint count, more sacroiliitis, and higher disease activity.

Several findings warrant additional discussion. First, we found significant variability in the presenting features and initial treatment strategies between sites. The variation in presenting features may reflect either true differences by geographic location or differences between sites in the assessment of particular features. There are no standardized definitions for what constitutes positive enthesitis. The entheses examined and thresholds for declaring positive findings varied not only between sites but also between physicians at each site. Variation in family history could reflect recall bias, differences in

Table 3 Clinical features by human leukocyte antigen B27 status

	All[a] ($n = 156$)	HLA-B27 positive ($n = 69$)	HLA-B27 negative ($n = 87$)	p Value
Demographics and clinical findings, n (%) or median (IQR)				
Age in years	11.5 (9.6, 13.6)	12.3 (10.3, 14.1)	11.0 (8.8,13.2)	*<0.01*
Sex, male	100 (64.1)	50 (72.5)	50 (57.5)	0.05
Race, Caucasian	129 (82.7)	59 (85.5)	70 (80.5)	0.66
Active joint count	2 (1–4)	3 (2–5)	2 (1–4)	*<0.01*
Tender entheses count	2 (2–4)	2 (1–3)	2 (2–5)	*0.01*
MRI-defined sacroiliitis	22 (57.9)	15 (83.3)	7 (35.0)	*<0.01*
Polyarticular onset	36 (23.1)	20 (29.0)	16 (18.4)	0.15
ANA-positive	31 (21.4)	10 (15.6)	21 (25.9)	0.13
CRP, abnormal/elevated	31 (28.4)	13 (31.0)	18 (26.9)	0.65
ESR, abnormal/elevated	57 (41.9)	34 (54.8)	23 (31.1)	*<0.01*
Outcome measures, median (IQR)				
Physician disease activity (0–10)	2.4 (2–3)	2 (2–3)	2.6 (2–4)	0.07
Juvenile Spondyloarthritis Disease Activity Index (JSpADA) (0–8)	3 (2.5–4)	3.5 (2.5–4)	3 (2.5–3.5)	*0.04*
Patient/parent disease activity (0–10)	4 (2–6)	4 (2–5)	4 (2–6)	0.63
Function (CHAQ) (0–3)	0.625 (0–1)	0.375 (0–1)	0.625 (0–1)	0.85
Patient/parent pain (0–10)	4 (2–7)	4 (3–7)	4 (2–7)	0.71
Juvenile Arthritis Disease Activity Score, excluding ESR (cJADAS) (0–30)	9 (5–13)	9 (5–13)	9 (5–14)	0.98
ILAR criteria, n (%)				
Acute, symptomatic uveitis	7 (4.5)	4 (5.8)	3 (3.5)	0.48
Arthritis in a male over 6 years of age	93 (59.6)	50 (72.5)	43 (49.4)	*<0.01*
Family history of HLA-B27-associated disease	18 (11.5)	7 (10.1)	11 (12.6)	0.63
Sacroiliac tenderness or lumbosacral pain	46 (29.5)	20 (29.0)	26 (29.9)	0.9

Abbreviations: HLA-B27 Human leukocyte antigen B27, *MRI* Magnetic resonance imaging, *ANA* Antinuclear antibody, *CRP* C-reactive protein, *ESR* Erythrocyte sedimentation rate, *IQR* Interquartile range, *CHAQ* Childhood Health Assessment Questionnaire

Analyses restricted to patients who had both arthritis and enthesitis at the time of diagnosis. Denominators varied due to missing data: MRI-defined sacroiliitis ($n = 38$); ANA ($n = 145$); CRP ($n = 109$); ESR ($n = 136$); Physician disease activity ($n = 97$); JSpADA ($n = 92$); Patient/parent disease activity ($n = 79$); CHAQ ($n = 92$); Patient/parent pain ($n = 100$); cJADAS (JADAS3-10) ($n = 69$)

[a] Six subjects who had arthritis and enthesitis at diagnosis were excluded because they were missing HLA-B27 status. *P*-values less than 0.05 are in italics and considered clinically significant

how family history was recorded at each site, or true variation. In terms of the initial treatment of ERA, we found that NSAIDs and DMARDs were most often prescribed. We did note, however, that there was increased use of biologic agents for the treatment of children with sacroiliitis, and IA glucocorticoids were reserved for cases of peripheral arthritis. Despite the intersite variation in treatments, our findings suggest that pediatric rheumatologists are generally adhering to ACR-recommended treatment guidelines [13, 33, 34] to initiate a TNF-α blocker for axial disease, especially early in the disease course [35]; however, barriers imposed by insurance companies may account for the fact that only 15% of patients received biologic agents in the first 3 months of disease. Because many insurance companies require that patients first fail methotrexate before they will provide coverage for a biologic agent, this logistical issue may be driving our findings. These differences highlight the need for standardized assessments for ERA as well as comparative effectiveness studies of the different treatment options.

Second, this study demonstrates a few statistically significant clinical differences based on HLA-B27 status. Children who were HLA-B27-positive tended to be older and male, with a higher active joint count and more sacroiliitis. We restricted our analyses of HLA-B27-positive versus HLA-B27-negative patients to children with both arthritis and enthesitis because of a concern for selection bias owing to the inherent nature of the minor inclusion classification criteria. Doing so strengthened our findings by removing any reliance on criteria selecting for HLA-B27 status, sex, and age. HLA-B27-positive children also had a higher disease activity as assessed by the JSpADA. Surprisingly, in contrast to adult studies, we did not find an association between HLA-B27 status and the presence of AAU [15, 36]. However, in a recent study of patients with ERA in which researchers enrolled subjects prospectively over a 3-year period an overall prevalence of AAU of 15.4% was found with no statistically significant difference based on HLA-B27 status [7]. This suggests that there may be additional phenotypic differences between child- and adult-onset diseases. Alternatively, one might theorize that AAU manifests later in the disease course of ERA and is not a frequent symptom at the time of initial presentation. Because this was a cross-sectional study at the time of diagnosis, it is possible that a larger proportion of patients eventually developed AAU. Additionally, we did not find any statistically significant difference in HLA-B27-positive and HLA-B27-negative children with regard to a family history of HLA-B27-associated disease, which challenges current understanding of the genetic susceptibility of patients to ERA. One possibility is that adult-onset SpA is more greatly affected by one's genetic milieu and therefore is more common among related family members. Perhaps the development of ERA is influenced less by genetics but more so by environmental factors. Alternatively, given that family history was based on patients' individual reports, it could be that patients' knowledge of HLA-B27-associated diseases in their own family history may be limited. Longitudinal studies should further assess the significance of HLA-B27 as a prognostic marker over the natural history of ERA and whether enthesitis follows a different pattern in HLA-B27-negative versus HLA-B27-positive patients.

Our findings should be interpreted in light of several limitations. First, this was a retrospective study spanning several decades from the earliest to the most recent patient. As such, there was not uniform collection of data at the time of initial evaluation, and clinical examinations may have varied between providers and sites. We suspect that treatment practices did vary over time with likely increasing use of TNF-α blockade, but this type of time-series analysis would be best suited as its own separate study. Second, imaging was done at the discretion of the caregiver; there was no uniform screening for hip arthritis or sacroiliitis with imaging. Several reports have shown that sacroiliitis (with sclerotic changes and erosions) is frequently present in children who do not complain of back pain [16, 37, 38]. Therefore, the prevalence of MRI-confirmed sacroiliitis in both groups in this cohort was likely underreported, and our results are likely biased toward the null.

To our knowledge, this study is the largest multicenter international study of children with ERA to date. Both the presenting clinical features and treatment algorithms used for various phenotypes of ERA significantly differed across sites. This heterogeneity in clinical presentation reflects either true differences in patient populations or differences in how the ILAR criteria are being applied. The variation in treatment algorithms emphasizes the need for efficacy and effectiveness studies to help establish evidence-based treatment guidelines tailored to the various clinical phenotypes in this understudied population.

Conclusions

To our knowledge, this study comprises the largest multicenter international inception cohort of children with ERA to date. Both the presenting clinical features and treatment algorithms used for the various phenotypes of ERA differed significantly across clinical sites. NSAIDs and DMARDs were prescribed as first-line treatments for newly diagnosed ERA, with biologic agents used primarily for sacroiliitis. In comparison with children who were HLA-B27-negative, children who were HLA-B27-positive tended to be older and male and had a higher active joint count, more sacroiliitis, and greater disease activity.

Abbreviations

AAU: Acute anterior uveitis; ACR: American College of Rheumatology; ANA: Antinuclear antibody; CHAQ: Childhood Health Assessment Questionnaire; cJADAS: clinical Juvenile Arthritis Disease Activity Score; CRP: C-reactive protein; DMARD: Disease-modifying antirheumatic drug; ERA: Enthesitis-related arthritis; ESR: Erythrocyte sedimentation rate; HLA: Human leukocyte antigen; IA: Intra-articular; IBD: Inflammatory bowel disease; IgM: Immunoglobulin M; ILAR: International League of Associations for Rheumatology; IQR: Interquartile range; JIA: Juvenile idiopathic arthritis; JSpADA: Juvenile Spondyloarthritis Disease Activity Index; MRI: Magnetic resonance imaging; NSAID: Nonsteroidal anti-inflammatory drug; RF: Rheumatoid factor; SpA: Spondyloarthritis; TNF-α: Tumor necrosis factor-α

Acknowledgements

The authors thank Colden Broderick, Andrew Klink, Keshia Maughn, Christy Reed, Davide Moretti, Roxanna Sabghi, and Carla Upperman for their assistance in review of the medical charts and data entry.

Funding

Research reported in this publication was supported by the National Institute of Arthritis and Musculoskeletal and Skin Diseases of the National Institutes of Health under award numbers T32-AR007442 (to SG) and K23-AR059749 (to PFW). The content is solely the responsibility of the authors and does not necessarily represent the official views of the National Institutes of Health.

Authors' contributions

PFW was responsible for study conception and design. EMM, IP, TB, TBW, TGB, and PFW were responsible for acquisition of the data. PFW, RX, SG, and TGB participated in interpretation and analysis of the data. PFW, RX, SG, and TGB drafted and wrote the manuscript. EMM, IP, TB, and TBW were involved in critically revising the manuscript for important intellectual content. All authors read and approved the final manuscript and take accountability for the accuracy and integrity of the final version.

Competing interests

The authors declare that they have no competing interests.

Author details
[1]Division of Rheumatology, Department of Pediatrics, The Children's Hospital of Philadelphia, Philadelphia, PA, USA. [2]Department of Biostatistics and Epidemiology, Perelman School of Medicine, University of Pennsylvania, Philadelphia, PA, USA. [3]University of Florence and Anna Meyer Children's Hospital, Florence, Italy. [4]University of Texas Southwestern Medical Center and Texas Scottish Rite Hospital of Children, Dallas, TX, USA. [5]University of Alabama at Birmingham, Birmingham, AL, USA. [6]Cincinnati Children's Hospital, Cincinnati, OH, USA. [7]University of Pennsylvania Perelman School of Medicine and Children's Hospital of Philadelphia, Philadelphia, PA, USA. [8]Department of Pediatric Rheumatology, The Children's Hospital of Philadelphia, 34th Street and Civic Center Boulevard, Wood Building, Fourth Floor, Philadelphia, PA 19104, USA.

References

1. Ravelli A, Martini A. Juvenile idiopathic arthritis. Lancet. 2007;369:767–78.
2. Petty RE, Southwood TR, Manners P, Baum J, Glass DN, Goldenberg J, et al. International League of Associations for Rheumatology classification of juvenile idiopathic arthritis: second revision, Edmonton, 2001. J Rheumatol. 2004;31:390–2.
3. Flato B, Hoffmann-Vold AM, Reiff A, Forre O, Lien G, Vinje O. Long-term outcome and prognostic factors in enthesitis-related arthritis: a case-control study. Arthritis Rheum. 2006;54:3573–82.
4. Bryan AR, Rabinovich CE. Enthesitis-related arthritis: time to re-define? Curr Rheumatol Rep. 2014;16:466.
5. Hofer M. Spondylarthropathies in children—are they different from those in adults? Best Pract Res Clin Rheumatol. 2006;20:315–28.
6. Adrovic A, Barut K, Sahin S, Kasapcopur O. Juvenile spondyloarthropathies. Curr Rheumatol Rep. 2016;18:55.
7. Srivastava R, Phatak S, Yadav A, Bajpai P, Aggarwal A. HLA B27 typing in 511 children with juvenile idiopathic arthritis from India. Rheumatol Int. 2016;36: 1407–11.
8. Weiss PF, Klink AJ, Behrens EM, Sherry DD, Finkel TH, Feudtner C, et al. Enthesitis in an inception cohort of enthesitis-related arthritis. Arthritis Care Res (Hoboken). 2011;63:1307–12.
9. Nordal E, Zak M, Aalto K, Berntson L, Fasth A, Herlin T, et al. Ongoing disease activity and changing categories in a long-term Nordic cohort study of juvenile idiopathic arthritis. Arthritis Rheum. 2011;63:2809–18.
10. Thomson W, Barrett JH, Donn R, Pepper L, Kennedy LJ, Ollier WE, et al. Juvenile idiopathic arthritis classified by the ILAR criteria: HLA associations in UK patients. Rheumatology (Oxford). 2002;41:1183–9.
11. Di Paola M, Cavalieri D, Albanese D, Sordo M, Pindo M, Donati C, et al. Alteration of fecal microbiota profiles in juvenile idiopathic arthritis: associations with HLA-B27 allele and disease status. Front Microbiol. 2016;7:1703.
12. Kunjir V, Venugopalan A, Chopra A. Profile of Indian patients with juvenile onset chronic inflammatory joint disease using the ILAR classification criteria for JIA: a community-based cohort study. J Rheumatol. 2010;37: 1756–62.
13. Beukelman T, Patkar NM, Saag KG, Tolleson-Rinehart S, Cron RQ, DeWitt EM, et al. 2011 American College of Rheumatology recommendations for the treatment of juvenile idiopathic arthritis: initiation and safety monitoring of therapeutic agents for the treatment of arthritis and systemic features. Arthritis Care Res (Hoboken). 2011;63:465–82.
14. Silva-Ramirez B, Vargas-Alarcon G, Granados J, Burgos-Vargas R. HLA antigens and juvenile onset spondyloarthritides: negative association with non-B27 alleles. Clin Exp Rheumatol. 2005;23:721–3.
15. Khan MA, Kushner I, Braun WE. Comparison of clinical features in HLA-B27 positive and negative patients with ankylosing spondylitis. Arthritis Rheum. 1977;20:909–12.
16. Weiss PF, Xiao R, Biko DM, Chauvin NA. Assessment of sacroiliitis at diagnosis of juvenile spondyloarthritis by radiography, magnetic resonance imaging, and clinical examination. Arthritis Care Res (Hoboken). 2016;68: 187–94.
17. Berntson L, Damgard M, Andersson-Gare B, Herlin T, Nielsen S, Nordal E, et al. HLA-B27 predicts a more extended disease with increasing age at onset in boys with juvenile idiopathic arthritis. J Rheumatol. 2008;35: 2055–61.
18. Gare BA, Fasth A. The natural history of juvenile chronic arthritis: a population based cohort study. I. Onset and disease process. J Rheumatol. 1995;22:295–307.
19. Berntson L, Nordal E, Aalto K, Peltoniemi S, Herlin T, Zak M, et al. HLA-B27 predicts a more chronic disease course in an 8-year followup cohort of patients with juvenile idiopathic arthritis. J Rheumatol. 2013;40:725–31.
20. Giannini EH, Ruperto N, Ravelli A, Lovell DJ, Felson DT, Martini A. Preliminary definition of improvement in juvenile arthritis. Arthritis Rheum. 1997;40: 1202–9.
21. Brewer Jr EJ, Bass J, Baum J, Cassidy JT, Fink C, Jacobs J, et al. JRA Criteria Subcommittee of the Diagnostic and Therapeutic Criteria Committee of the American Rheumatism Section of The Arthritis Foundation. Current proposed revision of JRA criteria. Arthritis Rheum. 1977;20(2 Suppl):195–9.
22. Weiss PF, Xiao R, Biko DM, Johnson AM, Chauvin NA. Detection of inflammatory sacroiliitis in children with magnetic resonance imaging: is gadolinium contrast enhancement necessary? Arthritis Rheumatol. 2015;67: 2250–6.
23. Sieper J, Rudwaleit M, Baraliakos X, Brandt J, Braun J, Burgos-Vargas R, et al. The Assessment of SpondyloArthritis international Society (ASAS) handbook: a guide to assess spondyloarthritis. Ann Rheum Dis. 2009;68 Suppl 2:ii1–44.
24. Tennant A, Kearns S, Turner F, Wyatt S, Haigh R, Chamberlain MA. Measuring the function of children with juvenile arthritis. Rheumatology (Oxford). 2001;40:1274–8.
25. Lam C, Young N, Marwaha J, McLimont M, Feldman BM. Revised versions of the Childhood Health Assessment Questionnaire (CHAQ) are more sensitive and suffer less from a ceiling effect. Arthritis Rheum. 2004;51:881–9.
26. Dempster H, Porepa M, Young N, Feldman BM. The clinical meaning of functional outcome scores in children with juvenile arthritis. Arthritis Rheum. 2001;44:1768–74.
27. Consolaro A, Ruperto N, Bazso A, Pistorio A, Magni-Manzoni S, Filocamo G, et al. Development and validation of a composite disease activity score for juvenile idiopathic arthritis. Arthritis Rheum. 2009;61:658–66.
28. Consolaro A, Giancane G, Schiappapietra B, Davì S, Calandra S, Lanni S, et al. Clinical outcome measures in juvenile idiopathic arthritis. Pediatr Rheumatol Online J. 2016;14:23.
29. McErlane F, Beresford MW, Baildam EM, Chieng SE, Davidson JE, Foster HE, et al. Validity of a three-variable Juvenile Arthritis Disease Activity Score in children with new-onset juvenile idiopathic arthritis. Ann Rheum Dis. 2013; 72:1983–8.
30. Consolaro A, Negro G, Chiara Gallo M, Bracciolini G, Ferrari C, Schiappapietra B, et al. Defining criteria for disease activity states in nonsystemic juvenile idiopathic arthritis based on a three-variable juvenile arthritis disease activity score. Arthritis Care Res (Hoboken). 2014;66:1703–9.
31. Weiss PF, Colbert RA, Xiao R, Feudtner C, Beukelman T, DeWitt EM, et al. Development and retrospective validation of the Juvenile Spondyloarthritis Disease Activity Index. Arthritis Care Res (Hoboken). 2014;66:1775–82.
32. Burgos-Vargas R. The juvenile-onset spondyloarthritides. Rheum Dis Clin North Am. 2002;28:531–60.
33. Katsicas MM, Russo R. Biologic agents in juvenile spondyloarthropathies. Pediatr Rheumatol Online J. 2016;14:17.
34. Horneff G, Burgos-Vargas R. TNF-α antagonists for the treatment of juvenile-onset spondyloarthritides. Clin Exp Rheumatol. 2002;20(6 Suppl 28): S137–42.
35. Tse S, Burgos-Vargas R, Colbert RA. Juvenile spondyloarthritis treatment recommendations. Am J Med Sci. 2012;343:367–70.
36. Zeboulon N, Dougados M, Gossec L. Prevalence and characteristics of uveitis in the spondyloarthropathies: a systematic literature review. Ann Rheum Dis. 2008;67:955–9.
37. Stoll ML, Bhore R, Dempsey-Robertson M, Punaro M. Spondyloarthritis in a pediatric population: risk factors for sacroiliitis. J Rheumatol. 2010;37: 2402–8.
38. Bollow M, Biedermann T, Kannenberg J, Paris S, Schauer-Petrowski C, Minden K, et al. Use of dynamic magnetic resonance imaging to detect sacroiliitis in HLA-B27 positive and negative children with juvenile arthritides. J Rheumatol. 1998;25:556–64.

Prolactin blocks the expression of receptor activator of nuclear factor κB ligand and reduces osteoclastogenesis and bone loss in murine inflammatory arthritis

Maria G. Ledesma-Colunga, Norma Adán, Georgina Ortiz, Mariana Solís-Gutiérrez, Fernando López-Barrera, Gonzalo Martínez de la Escalera and Carmen Clapp*

Abstract

Background: Prolactin (PRL) reduces joint inflammation, pannus formation, and bone destruction in rats with polyarticular adjuvant-induced arthritis (AIA). Here, we investigate the mechanism of PRL protection against bone loss in AIA and in monoarticular AIA (MAIA).

Methods: Joint inflammation, trabecular bone loss, and osteoclastogenesis were evaluated in rats with AIA treated with PRL (via osmotic minipumps) and in mice with MAIA that were null (*Prlr-/-*) or not (*Prlr+/+*) for the PRL receptor. To help define target cells, synovial fibroblasts from *Prlr+/+* mice were treated or not with proinflammatory cytokines ((Cyt), including TNFα, IL-1β, and interferon (IFN)γ) with or without PRL, and these synovial cells were co-cultured or not with bone marrow osteoclast progenitors from *Prlr+/+* or *Prlr-/-* mice.

Results: In AIA, PRL treatment reduced joint swelling, increased trabecular bone area, lowered osteoclast density, and reduced mRNA levels of osteoclast-associated genes (tartrate-resistant acid phosphatase (*Trap*)), cathepsin K (*Ctsk*), matrix metalloproteinase 9 (*Mmp9*), and receptor activator of nuclear factor κB or RANK (*Tnfrsf11a*)), of genes encoding cytokines with osteoclastogenic activity (*Tnfa, Il1b, Il6,* and receptor activator of nuclear factor κB ligand or RANKL (*Tnfrsf11*)), and of genes encoding for transcription factors and cytokines related to T helper (Th)17 cells (*Rora, Rorc, Il17a, Il21, Il22*) and to regulatory T cells (*Foxp3, Ebi3, Il12a, Tgfb1, Il10*). *Prlr-/-* mice with MAIA showed enhanced joint swelling, reduced trabecular bone area, increased osteoclast density, and elevated expression of *Tnfa, Il1b, Il6, Trap, Tnfrsf11a, Tnfrsf11, Il17a, Il21, Il22, 1 l23, Foxp3,* and *Il10.* The expression of the long PRL receptor form increased in arthritic joints, and in synovial membranes and cultured synovial fibroblasts treated with Cyt. PRL induced the phosphorylation/activation of signal transducer and activator of transcription-3 (STAT3) and inhibited the Cyt-induced expression of *Il1b, Il6,* and *Tnfrsf11* in synovial fibroblast cultures. The STAT3 inhibitor S31-201 blocked inhibition of *Tnfrsf11* by PRL. Finally, PRL acted on both synovial fibroblasts and osteoclast precursor cells to downregulate Cyt-induced osteoclast differentiation.

Conclusion: PRL protects against osteoclastogenesis and bone loss in inflammatory arthritis by inhibiting cytokine-induced expression of RANKL in joints and synovial fibroblasts via its canonical STAT3 signaling pathway.

Keywords: Hormones, Bone, Inflammation, Experimental arthritis, Osteoclasts, Synovial fibroblasts, Prolactin receptor, RANKL, RANK

* Correspondence: clapp@unam.mx
Instituto de Neurobiología, Universidad Nacional Autónoma de México (UNAM), Campus UNAM-Juriquilla, 76230 Querétaro, México

Background

Rheumatoid arthritis (RA) is an immune-mediated type of inflammatory arthritis that causes massive bone destruction by increasing osteoclast development (osteoclastogenesis) and activity. Receptor activator of nuclear factor κB ligand (RANKL), its cellular receptor, receptor activator of nuclear factor κB (RANK), and the decoy soluble RANKL receptor osteoprotegerin (OPG) are key regulators of osteoclastogenesis in RA [1–3]. RANKL is produced by osteoblastic lineage cells, activated T cells, synovial fibroblasts, and other stromal cells, and it binds to RANK on osteoclast precursors to stimulate their differentiation, activity, and survival [4–8]. The effects of RANKL are neutralized by OPG which, by binding to RANKL, prevents it from activating RANK. RANKL and OPG are pivotal downstream signals upon which many cytokines, growth factors, and steroid and peptide hormones converge to regulate bone homeostasis [7, 8]. Shifting the RANKL-to-OPG ratio in favor of bone protection is a promising therapeutic strategy against joint destruction in RA. Prolactin (PRL), the hormone essential for mammary gland development and milk production, may have this protective effect.

The female preponderance and the influence of reproductive states in RA, together with PRL immune-enhancing actions, have long linked this disease to a detrimental effect of PRL [9–11]. However, accumulating evidence has challenged this view by showing that PRL is also immunosuppressive [12–14], and that hyperprolactinemia occurring during pregnancy and lactation [15, 16] or induced pharmacologically by the dopamine D2 receptor antagonist haloperidol [17], is associated with a reduction in the severity and risk of RA. Moreover, increasing prolactinemia by PRL infusion or treatment with haloperidol ameliorates inflammation and joint destruction in AIA as revealed by reduced joint swelling, lower local expression of proinflammatory cytokines TNFα, IL-1β, IFNγ, and IL-6, and inhibition of chondrocyte apoptosis, pannus formation, and bone erosion [18].

PRL protection against bone loss in inflammatory arthritis is not unexpected. PRL-receptor-null mice are osteopenic [19] and PRL treatment increases bone formation during growth by decreasing the RANKL/OPG ratio in osteoblasts [20]. Moreover, PRL stimulates the proliferation of pancreatic β cells by promoting OPG-mediated inhibition of RANKL [21], and RANKL is under the control of PRL to promote mammary gland lobulo-alveolar development during pregnancy [22].

Here, we investigated whether PRL, either by its exogenous administration or by the genetic deletion of the its receptor, reduces trabecular bone loss and osteoclastogenesis by modifying proinflammatory cytokine-induced upregulation of the RANKL/RANK/OPG system in rodent polyarticular AIA and monoarticular AIA (MAIA), and whether these actions involve a direct effect of PRL on synovial fibroblasts and osteoclast progenitor cells.

Methods

Animals

Male Sprague-Dawley rats (200–250 g) and female C57BL6 mice, wild type (*Prlr+/+)* or null for the PRL receptor (*Prlr-/-)* (8 weeks old, 20–25 g), were housed under standard laboratory conditions (22 °C; 12-hour/12-hour light/dark cycle; free access to food and water).

Induction of AIA

AIA was induced in rats as described [18], by a single intradermal injection at the base of the tail of 0.2 ml complete Freund's adjuvant (CFA, Difco Laboratories, Detroit, MI, USA; 10 mg heat-killed *Mycobacterium tuberculosis* per 1 ml of Freund's adjuvant). Three days before CFA injection some rats were rendered hyperprolactinemic by the subcutaneous implantation of a 28-day osmotic minipump (Alza, Palo Alto, CA, USA) containing 1.6 mg of ovine PRL (Sigma Aldrich, St. Louis, MO, USA). Ankle swelling, monitored as described [18], indicated that the onset of arthritis appeared on day 12 after CFA injection and was maximal by day 21, when the animals were euthanized, serum samples collected for PRL and cytokine determinations, and ankle joints processed for histological examination, quantitative (q)PCR, and western blot.

Induction of MAIA

Monoarticular AIA was induced and assessed in mice as described [23]. Briefly, mice were injected into the articular space of the right knee joint with CFA (5 μg in 10 μl) once every 7 days for 18 days. The diameter across the knee joint (left and right) was measured twice a week with a micro-caliper. Mice were euthanized 18 days after the initial CFA injection, and knee joints were removed and processed as above.

Intra-articular injection of TNFα, IL-1β, and IFNγ (Cyt)

Mice were injected in the articular space of the knee joints with Cyt in a final volume of 20 μl (62.5 ng TNFα, 25 ng IL-1β, and 25 ng IFNγ; R&D Systems, Minneapolis, MN,USA) or with endotoxin-free water as vehicle. Forty-eight hours after Cyt or vehicle injection, mice were euthanized and synovial membranes were extracted and processed for quantitative real-time (qRT)-PCR evaluation.

Serum measurements

Infused ovine PRL was measured in serum by the Nb2 cell bioassay, a standard procedure based on the proliferative response of the Nb2 lymphoma cells to PRL, carried out as described [18]. The serum levels of C-reactive protein and TNFα were quantified using ELISA kits from BD Biosciences (San Jose, CA, USA) and R&D systems (Minneapolis, MN, USA), respectively.

Histological examination and image analysis

Ankle and knee joints were fixed, decalcified, and dehydrated for paraffin embedding. Four 7-μm-thick sections spaced 380 μm or 126 μm apart, per each rat tibia/tarsal joint or mouse femur/tibia joint, respectively, were stained with Harris's hematoxylin-eosin solution for measurement of trabecular bone area and with tartrate-resistant acid phosphatase (TRAP) for evaluation of osteoclast number. For the latter, deparaffinized sections were washed, and incubated for 3 hours at 37 °C in TRAP activity staining mix (Fast Red Violet LB Salt (80 mg; Sigma Aldrich), Naphtol AS-MX (40 mg; Sigma Aldrich), formamide (4 ml; Invitrogen, Carlsbad, CA, USA), 0.04 M sodium acetate (0.656 g), 0.2 M disodium tartrate dihydrate (9.2 g), and distilled water (200 ml)). The pH was adjusted to 5.0 and pre-incubated to 37 °C before use. After incubation, sections were rinsed with distilled water, counterstained with Mayer's hematoxilin (Sigma Aldrich), and coverslipped with mounting medium (Entellan, Merck Millipore Corporation, Billerica, MA, USA). Hematoxylin-eosin-stained and TRAP-stained tissue sections were visualized by light microscopy (Olympus BX60F5, Olympus Tokyo, Japan). Trabecular bone surface and number of TRAP-stained purple spots (osteoclasts) were quantified (Image-Pro Plus analysis software; Media Cybernetics, Silver Spring, MD, USA) and divided by total bone area to obtain trabecular bone area and osteoclast density. Two independent observers, blind to the experiments, performed the measurements.

qRT-PCR

Frozen whole ankle and knee joints were pulverized in liquid nitrogen using a mortar and pestle. Total RNA was isolated using TRIzol reagent (Invitrogen, Carlsbad, CA, USA) and reverse transcribed using the High-Capacity cDNA Reverse Transcription Kit (Applied Biosystems, Foster City, CA, USA). PCR products were detected and quantified using Maxima SYBR Green qPCR Master Mix (Thermo Fisher Scientific, Waltham, MA, USA) in a final reaction of 10 μl containing template and 0.5 μM of each of the primer pairs for different genes (see Additional file 1: Table S1). Amplification performed in the CFX96 real-time PCR detection system (Bio-Rad, Richmond, CA, USA) included a 10-minute denaturation step at 95 ° C, followed by 35 cycles of amplification (10 sec at 95 °C, 30 sec at the primer pair-specific annealing temperature, and 30 sec at 72 °C). The PCR data were analyzed by the $2^{-\Delta\Delta CT}$ method, and cycle thresholds (CT) normalized to the housekeeping gene hypoxanthine-guanine phosphoribosyltransferase (*Hprt*) were used to calculate the mRNA levels of interest.

Isolation and culture of synovial fibroblasts

Synovial fibroblasts were isolated from the hind limbs of wild-type mice separated at the femur/fibula/tibia junctions, as previously described [24]. Briefly, limbs were washed in Hanks' balanced salt solution (HBSS), and dissected while immersed in high glucose DMEM (Invitrogen, Carlsbad, CA, USA) supplemented with 20% heat-inactivated fetal bovine serum (FBS; Gibco, Grand Island, NY, USA) and antibiotics (50 U/ml of penicillin and 50 μg/ml of streptomycin; Invitrogen) to remove all soft tissues from bones. The joint space was opened with a scalpel to expose the synovial tissues and incubated in culture medium containing 1 mg/ml collagenase type IV (Difco Laboratories) and 0.1 mg/ml of deoxyribonuclease I (Sigma Aldrich) in a shaking bath for 3 hours at 37 °C. Tissues were then vortexed vigorously to release cells. The supernatant was passed through an 80-μm filter and centrifuged; cells were re-suspended in fresh culture media and grown to confluency. Cells were used for experiments after 2–4 passages, when the cultures showed >98% synovial fibroblast phenotype (CD90.2+, VCAM1+, and ICAM-1+) as described [24].

Synovial fibroblasts were seeded at 10^6 cells/well in 6-well plates and incubated in 2 ml of culture medium for 16 hours with or without PRL (100 nM, recombinant human PRL provided by Michael E. Hodsdon, Yale University, New Haven, CT, USA). Cyt (0.25 ng/ml TNFα, 0.05 ng/ml IL-1β, and 0.05 ng/ml IFNγ) were then added or not to the culture for an additional period of 24 hours. Other cell cultures were pre-incubated for 2 hours with or without the STAT inhibitor, S31-201 at 50 nM (Santa Cruz Biotechnology, Santa Cruz, CA, USA), and then incubated or not with 100 nM PRL for 16 hours, followed by the treatment with or without Cyt for 24 hours. To evaluate PRL effects on phosphorylation/activation of STAT3, synovial fibroblasts were seeded in complete medium for 24 hours, cultured in serum-free medium for another 24 hours, and then pre-treated for 6 hours with the Cyt followed by a 30-minute incubation in the presence or absence of Cyt with or without 100 nM PRL.

Co-culture of synovial fibroblasts and osteoclast progenitors

Synovial fibroblasts (passage 4) were seeded at 5×10^5 cells in 48-well plates and after 12 hours the cells were treated or not with PRL for 16 hours. Cyt were then added or not to the culture, and after 24 hours, bone marrow cells (2×10^6) containing osteoclast progenitors, harvested from the tibias and femurs of 8-week-old C57BL/6 mice, wild type (*Prlr+/+*) or null for the PRL receptor (*Prlr-/-*), were delivered in culture medium with 1, 25 dihydroxy-vitamin D3 (10^{-8} M, Sigma-Aldrich). Co-cultures were incubated for 10 days changing for new medium (containing 1, 25 dihydroxy-vitamin D3, +/- Cyt, +/- PRL) every 2 days. Co-cultures were fixed with 3.7% formaldehyde for 10 minutes at room temperature, washed twice with PBS, air-dried, and incubated for 20 minutes at 37 °C with TRAP activity staining mix. Osteoclastogenesis was assessed by counting the number of enlarged TRAP-positive (TRAP+) cells.

Isolation of chondrocytes, osteoblasts, and osteoclast-like cells

To identify other joint cells expressing the PRL receptor, chondrocytes, osteoblasts, and osteoclast-like cells were obtained from *Prlr+/+* and *Prlr-/-* mice. Synovial fibroblasts obtained from both mouse groups served as positive controls. Articular chondrocytes were isolated from femoral epiphyseal cartilage as described previously [25]. Murine bone marrow stromal cells were obtained by flushing the bone marrow from femur and tibia with PBS. Cells were maintained in DMEM with 20% FBS and antibiotics until 70% confluence, when they were differentiated into osteoblasts by treatment with 100 μM ascorbate phosphate and 5 mM β-glycerol phosphate for 10 days and medium replacement every 2 days [26]. Other bone marrow cells were differentiated into osteoclasts by their culture in α-MEM (Sigma-Aldrich) supplemented with 10% FBS and antibiotics, 25 ng/ml recombinant macrophage colony stimulating factor and 50 ng/ml RANKL (PreproTech, Rocky Hill, NJ, USA) for 10 days and medium replacement every 2 days [27]. All cells were processed for PCR.

The purity of the different cell types has been documented [27–29] and was confirmed by the mRNA expression of specific markers: collagen type II (chondrocytes), runt related transcription factor 2, alkaline phosphatase, and osteocalcin (osteoblasts), and RANK, calcitonin receptor, and TRAP (osteoclast-like cells). Total RNA was isolated, reverse transcribed, and used for the PCR amplification of a 139-bp fragment from exon 5 of the PRL receptor gene (exon 5 is deleted in *Prlr-/-* mice) in a final reaction mixture (10 μl) containing template, 0.02 U/μl of Phusion DNA Polymerase (Thermo Fisher, Waltham, MA, USA), 2 μl of 5X Phusion Buffer HF (Thermo Fisher), 0.4 mM of deoxyribonucleotide triphosphates (dNTPs) and 0.5 μM of each of the primer pairs for *PRLr* (forward 5′-CAC ATA AAG TGG ATC CGA GGT A-3′; reverse 5′-TGA ATG TCC AGA CTA CAA AAC CA -3′), using *Hprt* as loading control (Additional file 1: Table S1). The amplification in the Eppendorf Mastercycler ep Gradient S equipment (Eppendorf, Hamburg, Germany) included denaturation for 2 minutes at 95 °C, followed by 36 cycles of 15 sec at 95 °C, 15 sec at 56 °C, and 30 sec at 72 °C, followed by one cycle of 5 minutes at 72 °C. PCR products were resolved on a 1.2% agarose gel. The specificity of the reaction was confirmed by the lack of amplification products in samples from *Prlr-/-* mice.

Western blot

Pulverized ankle joints or synovial fibroblasts were resuspended in lysis buffer (0.1 M Tris-HCl, 0.2 M EGTA, 0.2 M EDTA, 100 mM sodium orthovanadate, 50 mM sodium fluoride, 100 mM sodium acid pyrophosphate, 250 mM sucrose, pH 7.5) and total protein (60 μg), subjected to SDS/PAGE, blotted, and probed overnight with 1:1000 anti-PRL receptor (sc-300; Santa Cruz Biotechnology, Santa Cruz, CA, USA), 1:250 anti-phospho-STAT3 (Tyrosine 705) (9131; Cell Signaling, Beverly, MA, USA), 1:250 anti STAT3 (sc-483; Santa Cruz Biotechnology), or 1:1000 anti-β tubulin (ab6046; Abcam, Cambridge, MA, USA) primary antibodies. Blots were washed in Tris-buffered saline/Tween-20 and detection was performed using goat anti-rabbit conjugated to alkaline phosphatase (1:5000) or to horseradish peroxidase (1:10,000) as secondary antibodies (both from Jackson ImmunoResearch Laboratories Inc., West Grove, PA, USA). Protein densities were quantified with Quantity One software (Bio-Rad, Richmond, CA, USA).

Statistical analysis

The Sigma Stat 7.0 software (Systat Software, San Jose, CA, USA) was used. Data distribution and equality of variances were determined by the D'Agostino-Pearson test. When the distribution was normal and variances were equal, the t test was used to evaluate differences between two groups and one-way analysis of variance (ANOVA) followed by Tukey's post-hoc test was used to compare differences between more than three groups. In the case of data with a non-parametric distribution, statistical differences between two groups and more than three groups were determined by the Mann-Whitney U test and Kruskal-Wallis test followed by Dunn's post-hoc correction, respectively. The threshold for significance was set at $P < 0.05$.

Results

The long PRL receptor isoform increases in the joints and PRL reduces the systemic levels of C-reactive protein and TNFα and the expression of transcription factors and cytokines related to Th17 cells and regulatory T cells in the joints of rats subjected to AIA

Confirming our previous findings [18], osmotic minipumps delivering PRL, implanted 3 days before the injection of CFA, elevated serum PRL fivefold (Fig. 1a), reduced ankle joint swelling (ankle circumference, Fig. 1b), and lowered joint expression of the proinflammatory cytokine genes, *Tnfa, Il1b, Il6, and Ifng* (Fig. 1c) at day 21 after inducing AIA with CFA in rats. At this

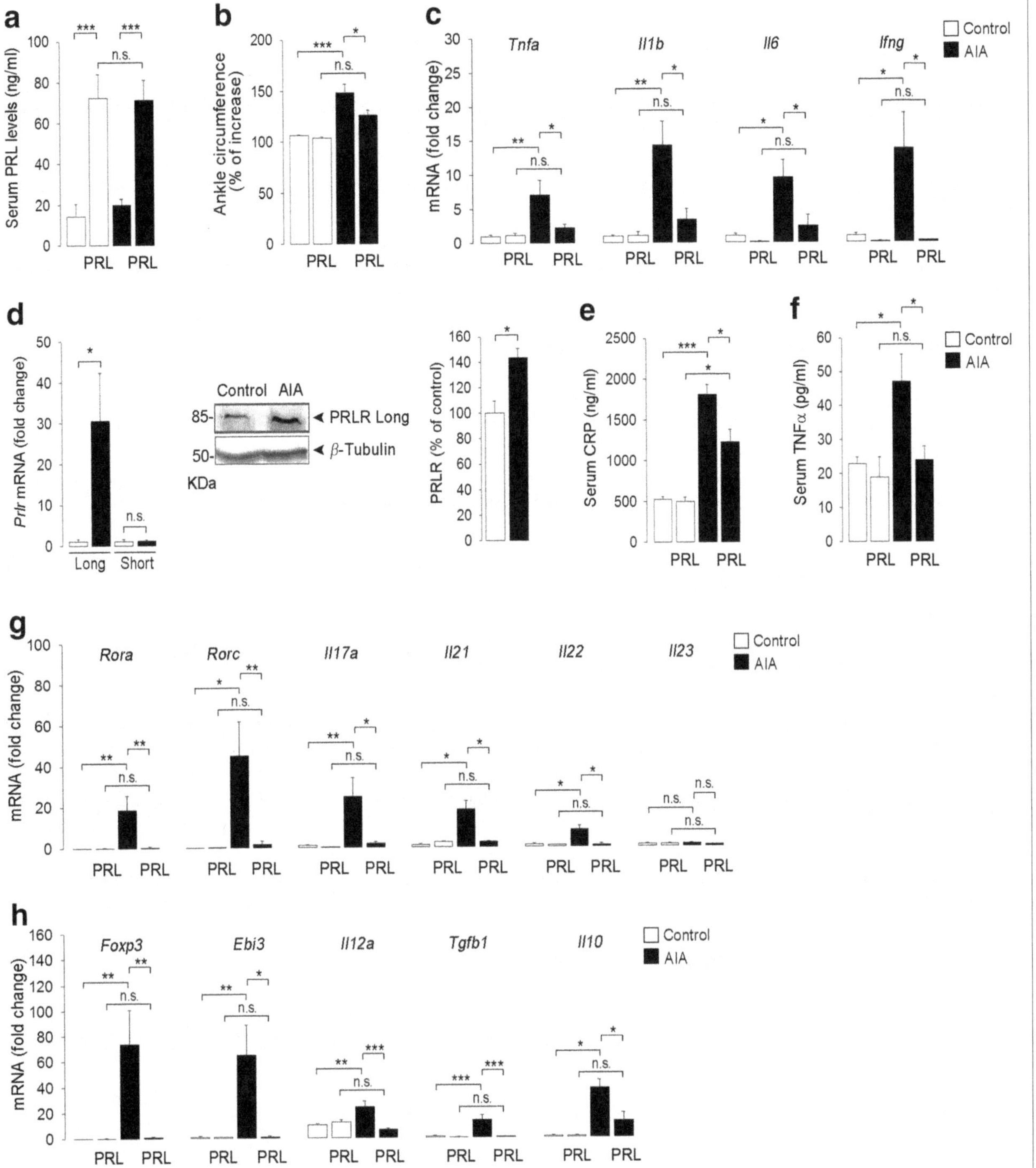

Fig. 1 The long prolactin (*PRL*) receptor isoform increases in the joints and PRL reduces the systemic levels of C-reactive protein and TNFα and the expression of transcription factors and cytokines related to T helper 17 (*Th17*) cells and regulatory T cells in the joints of rats subjected to polyarticular adjuvant-induced arthritis (*AIA*). Osmotic minipumps delivering PRL were positioned (or not positioned) 3 days before the intradermal injection of complete Freund's adjuvant (*CFA*) to induce AIA in rats. All evaluations were performed 21 days after injection of CFA. **a** Serum PRL levels, **b** ankle circumference, and **c** quantitative real-time PCR (qRT-PCR) quantification of *Tnfa*, *Il1b*, *Il6*, and *Ifng* mRNA levels in ankle joints. **d** qRT-PCR and western blot evaluation of PRL receptor (*Prlr*) long (*Long*) and short (*Short*) isoform mRNA and long PRL receptor protein (*PRLR Long*), respectively. *Bars* show the quantification of PRLR Long/β-Tubulin by densitometry (n = 3). **e** C-reactive protein (*CRP*) and **f** TNFα levels in serum. **g** qRT-PCR quantification of the mRNA levels of the Th17-cell-related transcription factors, *Rora* and *Rorc*, and cytokine genes *Il17a*, *Il21*, *Il22*, and *Il23* in the ankle joints. **h** qRT-PCR quantification of the mRNA levels of the regulatory-T-cell-related transcription factor *Foxp3* and cytokine genes *Ebi3*, *Il12a*, *Tgfb1*, *Il10* in the ankle joints. Values are means ± SEM (n = 5–12). *$P < 0.05$, **$P < 0.01$, ***$P < 0.001$, *n.s.* non-significant

time, the levels of the long form of the PRL receptor mRNA and protein increased in the AIA joints, whereas no changes in the transcript of the short PRL receptor isoform were detected (Fig. 1d). PRL infusion in AIA was associated with reduced serum levels of C-reactive protein (CRP, Fig. 1e) and TNFα (Fig. 1f), two biomarkers of systemic inflammation in arthritis. Moreover, the imbalance between Th17 and T-regulatory lymphocytes influences inflammation and osteoclastogenesis in arthritis [30], and PRL blocked the AIA-induced increase in the joint expression of the genes *Rorc* and *Rora* encoding for retinoic acid orphan nuclear receptors RORγt and RORα, respectively, which are transcription factors specific for Th17 cells, and the expression of the Th17 cell cytokine genes, *Il17a*, *Il21*, and *Il22* (Fig. 1g). Also, PRL inhibited the AIA-induced expression of the gene encoding for fork-head box protein 3 (*Foxp3*), a transcription factor specific for regulatory T cells, and the AIA-induced expression of the regulatory-T-cell-related genes encoding for the cytokines IL-35 (a heterodimer composed of IL12a and Ebi3 subunits), TGFβ-1, and IL-10 (Fig. 1h). PRL had no effects in non-arthritic, control animals (Fig. 1a-c and e-g).

PRL reduces loss of trabecular bone and osteoclast density in AIA

Because systemic and local CRP, TNFα, IL-1β, IL-6, and IL-17A trigger osteoclastogenesis by upregulating RANKL in the arthritic joint [2, 31, 32], we evaluated the effect of PRL infusion on trabecular bone loss and osteoclastogenesis in rats with AIA. PRL reduced the loss of trabecular bone area (Fig. 2a) and blocked the increase in osteoclast density in arthritic joints (Fig. 2b). Moreover, PRL decreased osteoclastogenesis as revealed by the reduction in the mRNA levels of the osteoclast-associated genes: *Trap, Mmp9, Ctsk*, and the gene encoding for RANK *(Tnfrsf11a)* (Fig. 2c). Also, PRL blocked the AIA-induced increase in the mRNA levels of the gene encoding for RANKL (*Tnfrsf11)* (Fig. 2d). The expression of the gene encoding for OPG (*Tnfrsf11b*) was not modified by AIA or by PRL, but this hormone reduced the *Tnfrsf11/Tnfrsf11b* mRNA ratio in the arthritic joint (Fig. 2d). PRL had no effects on trabecular bone area and osteoclastogenesis in the joints of control rats.

MAIA-induced joint inflammation and expression of proinflammatory cytokines and that of transcription factors and cytokines related to Th17 cells and regulatory T cells are enhanced in PRL-receptor-null mice

To further explore the protective effect of PRL against inflammation and osteoclastogenesis in arthritis, mice null (*Prlr-/-*) or not (*Prlr+/+)* for the PRL receptor were subjected to MAIA, as this is a highly efficient model for inducing unilateral joint inflammation and bone erosion in the genetic background (C57BL6) of these mice [23]. Inflammation was greater (Fig. 3a) and the expression of the proinflammatory cytokine genes, *Tnfa, Il1b, Il6, Infg* (Fig. 3b), the Th17 cell-related genes, *Il17a, Il21, Il22, Il23* (Fig. 3c); and the regulatory-T-cell-associated genes, *Foxp3* and *Il10,* were significantly elevated (Fig. 3d) in the arthritic knee-joint of *Prlr-/-* mice compared to *Prlr+/+* mice. The expression of *Il12a* was increased in MAIA joints but that of *Rora, Rorc,* and *Tgfb1* was not, and these four genes remained unchanged in the absence of PRL receptors (Fig. 3c and d).

Trabecular bone area is reduced and osteoclast density is increased in PRL receptor-null mice subjected to MAIA

Confirming that PRL-receptor-null mice are osteopenic [19], the loss of trabecular bone area was greater in control non-arthritic *Prlr-/-* mice relative to *Prlr+/+* mice (Fig. 4a). Moreover, the trabecular bone area was reduced (Fig. 4a), whereas the density of osteoclasts (Fig. 4b) and the mRNA levels of *Trap* and *Tnfrsf11* (Fig. 4c, d) were higher in the arthritic joints of *Prlr-/-* mice compared to wild-type mice. There were no differences in the expression levels of *Mmp9, Ctsk, Tnfrsf11a*, and *Tnfrsf11b* between *Prlr-/-* and *Prlr+/+* mice, but the *Tnfrsf11/Tnfrsf11b* ratio was higher in *Prlr-/-* mice. Non-arthritic, control *Prlr-/-* mice showed elevated, albeit non-significant, osteoclastogenesis parameters relative to non-arthritic, control *Prlr+/+* mice (Fig. 4b, c, d). These findings indicate that bone loss and osteoclast development are potentiated in arthritic joints in the absence of PRL signaling and that this hormone influences the maintenance of bone mass under normal conditions.

TNFα, IL-1β, and IFNγ induce the expression of the long PRL receptor in synovial membranes and synovial fibroblasts

To further investigate the role of PRL receptor signaling in the arthritic joint, a combination of proinflammatory cytokines (Cyt: TNFα, IL-1β, and IFNγ) was injected into the intra-articular space of knee joints of mice in an attempt to mimic the AIA inflammatory condition. The intra-articular Cyt injection elevated the levels of the long form of the PRL receptor mRNA in whole synovial membranes 48 hours after injection (Fig. 5a). Likewise, Cyt treatment for 24 hours stimulated the expression of the long PRL receptor mRNA and protein in primary cultures of mouse synovial fibroblasts (Fig. 5b), implying that these cells become relevant targets of PRL under inflammatory conditions.

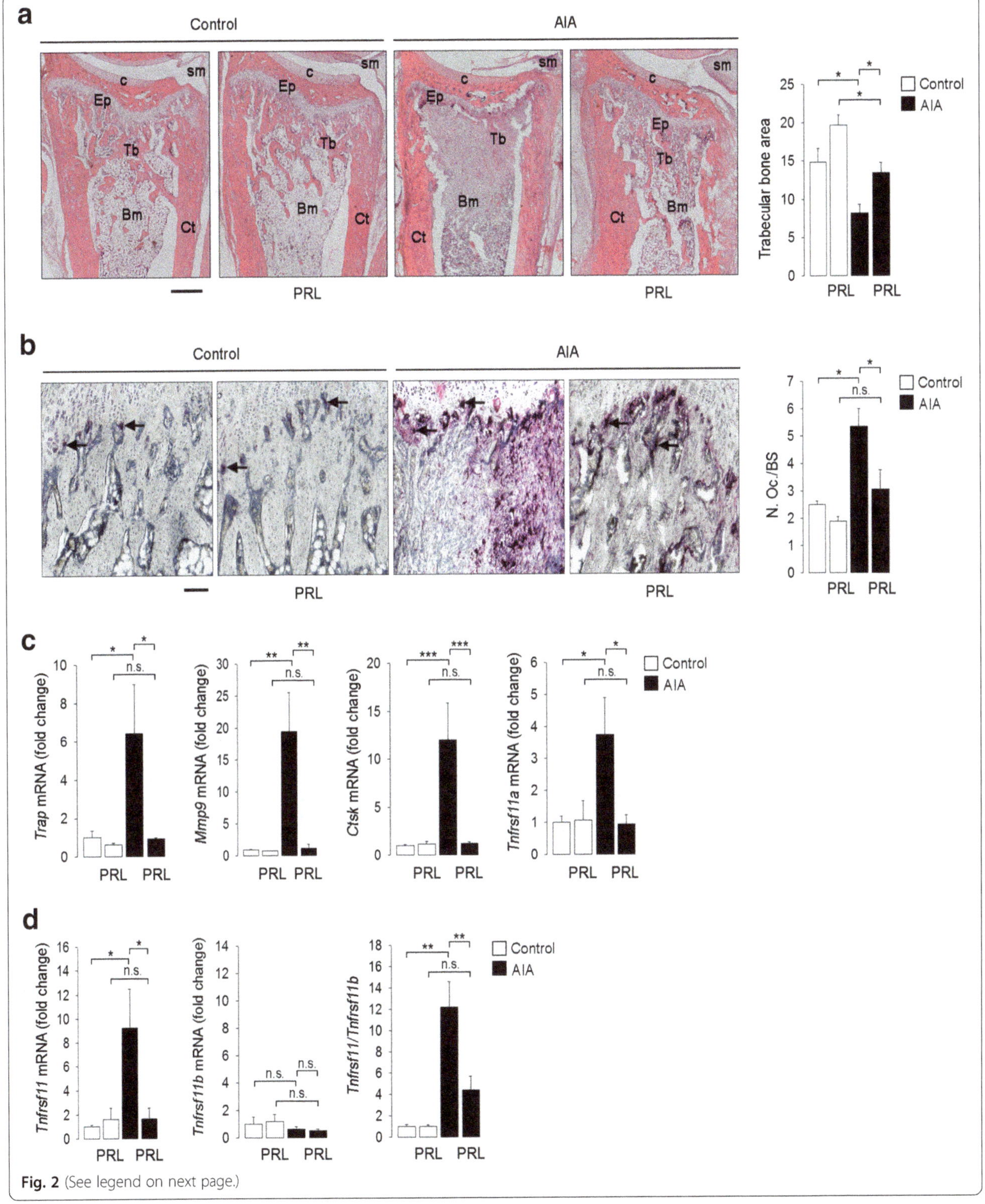

Fig. 2 (See legend on next page.)

(See figure on previous page.)

Fig. 2 Prolactin (*PRL*) reduces loss of trabecular bone area and osteoclastogenesis in polyarticular adjuvant-induced arthritis (*AIA*). Osmotic minipumps delivering PRL were positioned (or were not positioned) 3 days before the intradermal injection of complete Freund's adjuvant (*CFA*) to induce AIA in rats. The experiments ended on day 21 after injection of CFA, when all evaluations were performed. **a** Representative images of hematoxylin-eosin-stained tibiotarsal joint sections. *Scale bar* 500 μm. *Ep* epiphyseal plate, *Bm* bone marrow, *Ct* cortical bone, *Tb* trabecular bone, *c* cartilage, *sm* synovial membrane. Graph indicates the values of trabecular bone area (trabecular surface area divided by the total bone area). **b** Representative images of tartrate-resistant alkaline phosphatase (*TRAP*)-stained tibiotarsal joint sections where TRAP-positive *purple spots* (multinucleated cells (osteoclasts)) below the growth plate are indicated (*arrows*). *Scale bar* 200 μm. *Graph* shows the number of osteoclasts per bone surface (*N.Oc/BS*). **c** Quantification by quantitative real-time PCR (qRT-PCR) of the mRNA levels of the osteoclast gene markers: *Trap*, *Mmp9*, *Ctsk*, and *Tnfrsf11a* in the ankle joints. **d** qRT-PCR quantification of the mRNA levels of *Tnfrsf11* and *Tnfrsf11b* and of the *Tnfrsf11/Tnfrsf11b* mRNA ratio in the ankle joints. Values are means ± SEM (n = 5–8). *$P < 0.05$, **$P < 0.01$, ***$P < 0.001$, *n.s.* non-significant

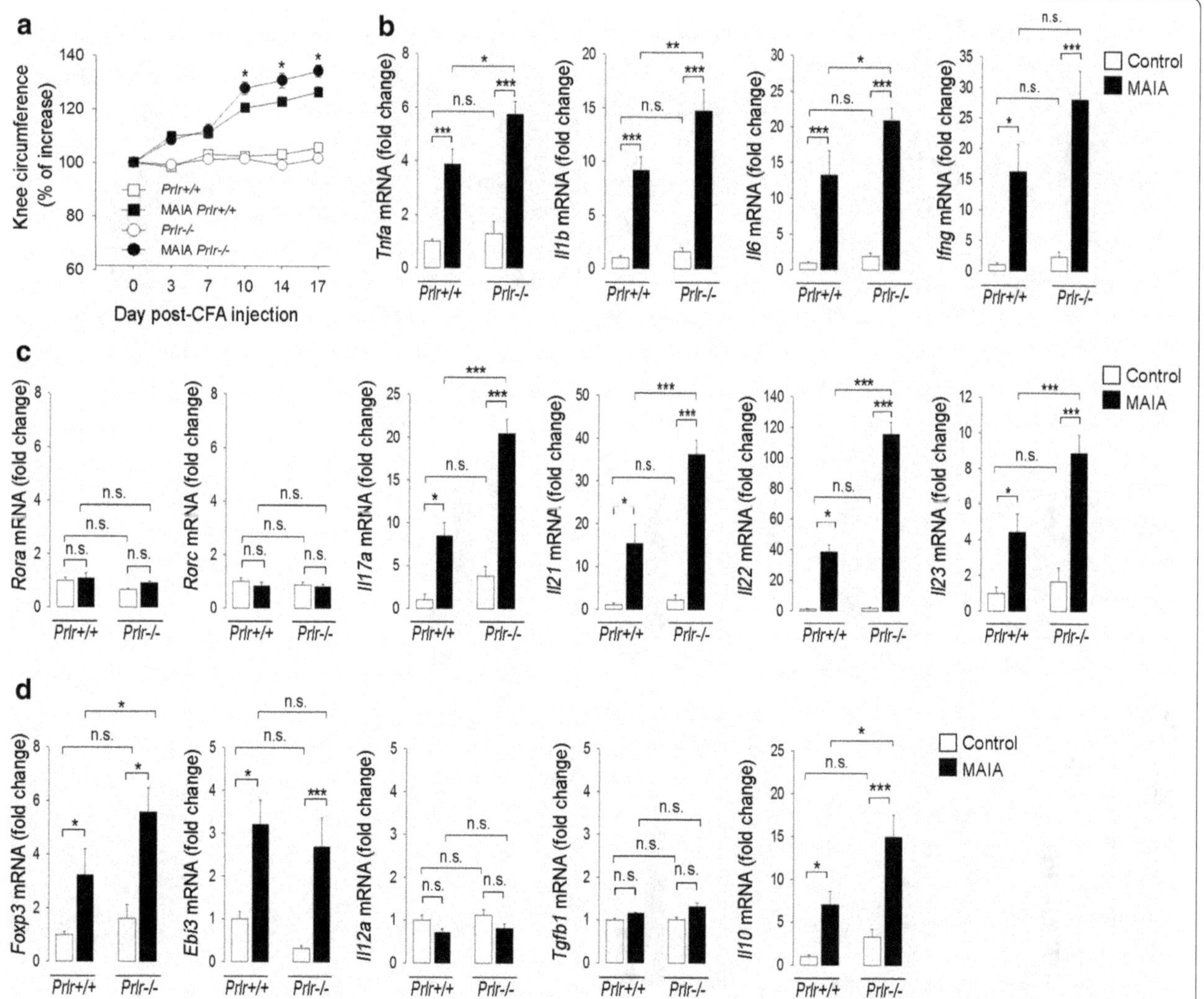

Fig. 3 Joint inflammation and expression of proinflammatory cytokines and of transcription factors and cytokines related to T helper 17 (*Th17*) cells and regulatory T cells are enhanced in prolactin (*PRL*)-receptor-null mice with monoarticular adjuvant-induced arthritis (*MAIA*). Mice null (*Prlr-/-*) or not (*Prlr+/+*) for PRL receptors were injected with complete Freund's adjuvant (*CFA*) into the right knee joint once every 7 days to induce MAIA. The experiments ended on day 18 after the initial CFA injection, when all evaluations were performed. **a** Time course of knee circumference in control and MAIA groups. **b** Quantification by quantitative real-time PCR (*qRT-PCR*) of *Tnfa*, *Il1b*, *Il6*, and *Ifng* mRNA levels in the knee joints. **c** qRT-PCR quantification of the mRNA levels of the Th17-cell-related transcription factors, *Rora* and *Rorc*, and cytokine genes *Il17a*, *Il21*, *Il22*, and *Il23* in the knee joints. **d** qRT-PCR quantification of the mRNA levels of the regulatory-T-cell-related transcription factor *Foxp3* and cytokine genes *Ebi3*, *Il12a*, *Tgfb1*, *Il10* in the knee joints. Values are means ± SEM (n = 8–12). *$P < 0.05$, **$P < 0.01$, ***$P < 0.001$, *n.s.* non-significant

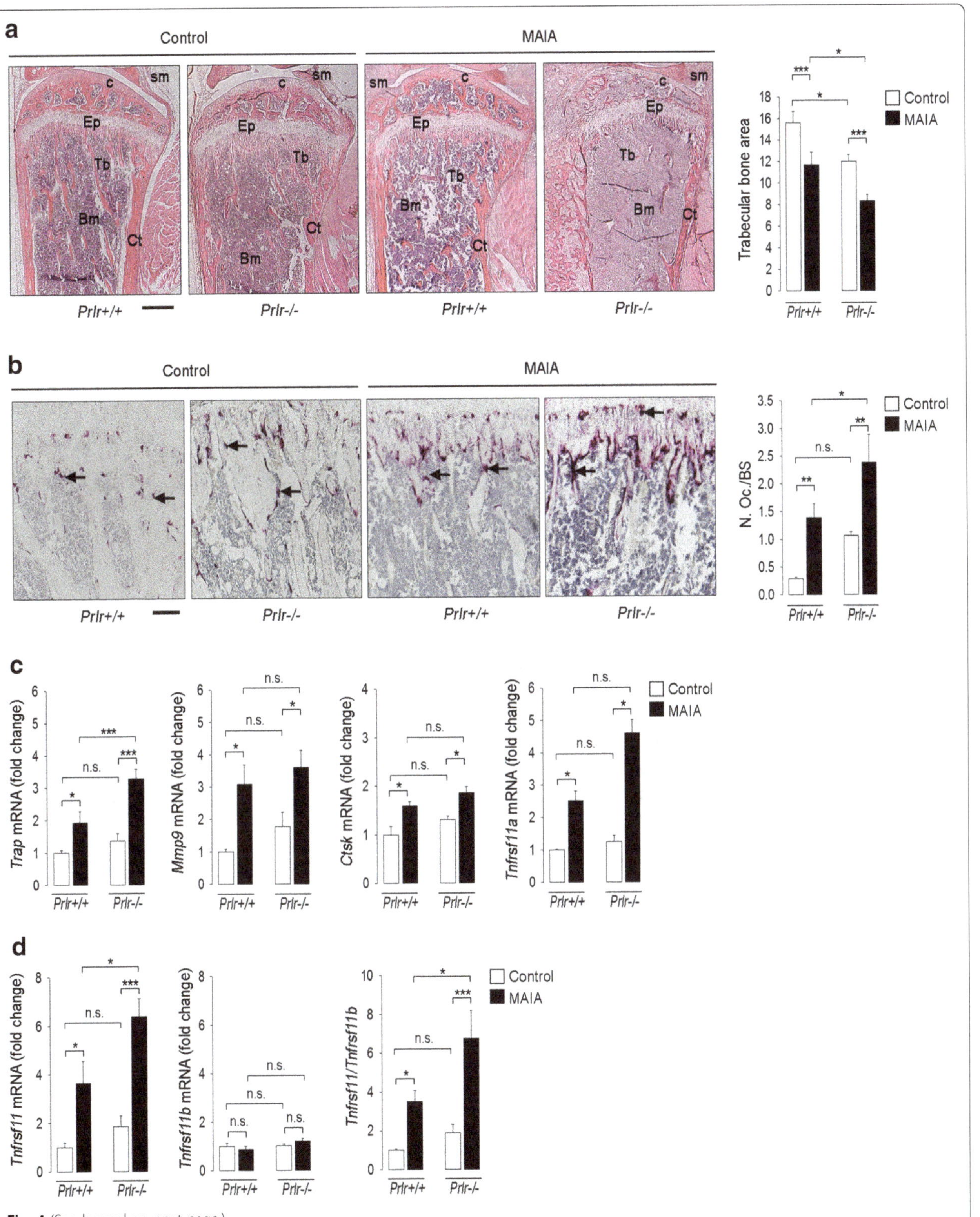

Fig. 4 (See legend on next page.)

(See figure on previous page.)

Fig. 4 Trabecular bone area is reduced and osteoclastogenesis is enhanced in prolactin (*PRL*)-receptor-null mice subjected to monoarticular adjuvant-induced arthritis (*MAIA*). Mice null (*Prlr-/-*) or not (*Prlr+/+*) for the PRL receptor were injected with complete Freund's adjuvant (*CFA*) into the right knee joint once every 7 days to induce MAIA. The experiments ended on day 18 after the initial CFA injection, when all evaluations were performed. **a** Representative images of hematoxylin-eosin-stained tibiofemoral joint sections. *Scale bar* 500 μm. *Ep* epiphyseal plate, *Bm* bone marrow, *Ct* cortical bone, *Tb* trabecular bone, *c* cartilage, *sm* synovial membrane. *Graph* indicates the values of trabecular bone area (trabecular surface area divided by the total bone area). **b** Representative images of tartrate-resistance alkaline phosphatase (*TRAP*)-stained tibiofemoral joint sections where TRAP-positive *purple spots* (multinucleated cells (osteoclasts)) below the growth plate are indicated (*arrows*). *Scale bar* 200 μm. *Graph* shows the number of osteoclast per bone surface (*N.Oc/BS*). **c** Quantification by quantitative real-time PCR (*qRT-PCR*) of the mRNA levels of the osteoclast gene markers: *Trap*, *Mmp9*, *Ctsk*, and *Tnfrsf11a* in the knee joints. **d** qRT-PCR-based quantification of the mRNA levels of *Tnfrsf11* and *Tnfrsf11b* and of the *Tnfrsf11/Tnfrsf11b* mRNA ratio in the knee joints. Values are means ± SEM (n = 5–12). *$P < 0.05$, **$P < 0.01$, ***$P < 0.001$, *n.s.* non-significant

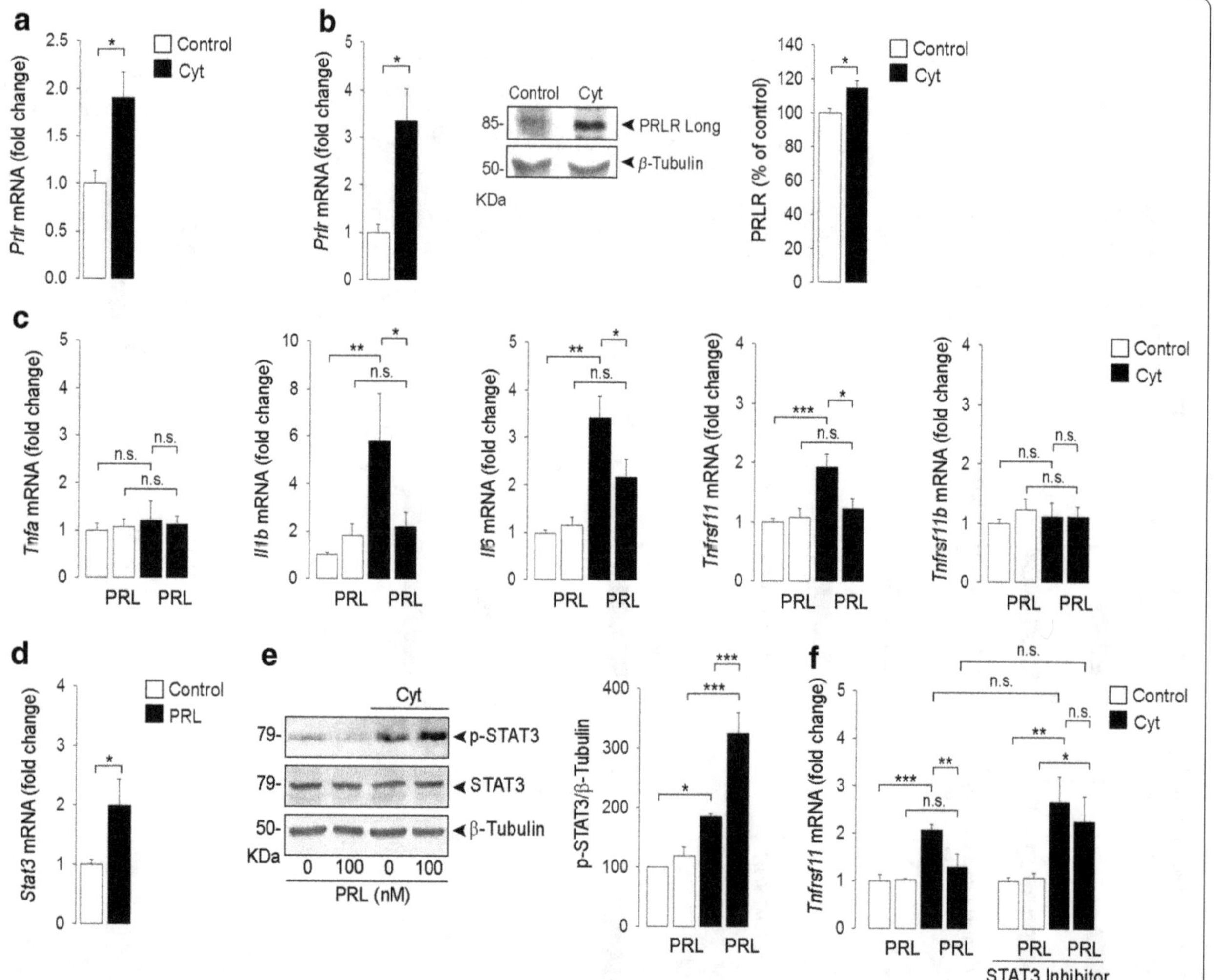

Fig. 5 TNFα, IL-1β, and IFNγ (*Cyt*) induce the expression of the long prolactin (*PRL*) receptor (*Prlr*) in synovial membrane and synovial fibroblasts and PRL blocks Cyt-induced *Tnfrsf11* expression in synovial fibroblasts by a STAT3-dependent pathway. **a** Quantification by quantitative real-time PCR (*qRT-PCR*) of PRL receptor long isoform mRNA levels in synovial membrane from mouse knees injected with or without Cyt. **b** qRT-PCR and western blot evaluation of PRL receptor long isoform mRNA and protein in primary cultures of synovial fibroblasts incubated with or without Cyt. *Bars* show the quantification of PRLR Long/β-Tubulin by densitometry. **c** qRT-PCR quantification of *Tnfa*, *Il1b*, *Il6*, *Tnfrsf11*, and *Tnfrsf11b* mRNA levels in primary cultures of synovial fibroblasts incubated or not with Cyt in the absence or presence of 100 nM PRL. **d** qRT-PCR and **e** western blot evaluation of *Stat3* mRNA levels and phosphorylated STAT3 (*p-STAT3*), respectively, in primary cultures of synovial fibroblasts incubated with or without Cyt and with or without 100 nM PRL. *Bars* show the quantification of pSTAT3/β-Tubulin by densitometry. **f** qRT-PCR quantification of *Tnfrsf11* mRNA levels in primary cultures of synovial fibroblasts incubated with or without Cyt and with or without 100 nM PRL in the absence or presence of 50 μM of the STAT3 inhibitor S31-201. Values are means ± SEM of three independent experiments. *$P < 0.05$, **$P < 0.01$, ***$P < 0.001$, *n.s.* non-significant

PRL blocks Cyt-induced Tnfrsf11 expression in synovial fibroblasts by a STAT3-dependent pathway

We next studied the contribution of synovial fibroblasts to the anti-osteoclastogenic effects of PRL by culturing synovial fibroblasts with Cyt in the absence or presence of PRL. Cyt induced the expression of the osteoclastogenesis-inducing cytokine genes *Il1b, Il6,* and *Tnfrsf11,* and this effect was blocked by PRL (Fig. 5c). Cyt and PRL did not alter the expression of *Tnfa* or *Tbfrsf11b* (Fig. 5c). Because PRL signals through STAT3 to promote chondrocyte survival [18] and STAT3 inhibits osteoclastogenesis [33], we examined whether PRL signals through STAT3 in synovial fibroblasts. PRL stimulated the expression of *Stat3* mRNA in synovial fibroblasts in culture (Fig. 5d) and promoted the phosphorylation/activation of STAT3 when the cells were cultured in the presence of Cyt (Fig. 5e). Moreover, incubation of synovial fibroblasts with the STAT3 inhibitor S31-201 [34] blocked PRL inhibition of Cyt-induced *Tnfrsf11* expression (Fig. 5f), thereby suggesting that PRL signals through STAT3 to inhibit osteoclastogenesis in joints under inflammatory conditions.

PRL reduces Cyt-induced osteoclast formation in co-cultures of synovial fibroblasts and osteoclast progenitor cells

To investigate synovial fibroblasts and osteoclast progenitor cells as targets of PRL inhibition of osteoclastogenesis, we evaluated the effect of PRL on synovial fibroblasts co-cultured with bone-marrow-derived osteoclast progenitors in the presence of Cyt, which act on synovial fibroblasts to induce the secretion of RANKL necessary for osteoclast differentiation [6] (Fig. 6a). The time course of the co-culture was as follows: 12 hours after being seeded, synovial fibroblasts were treated or not with PRL for 16 hours. Cyt were then added or not to the culture and after 24 hours osteoclast progenitors were delivered in medium containing 1, 25-dihydroxy-vitamin D3. Co-cultures were incubated for 10 days, replacing with new medium (containing +/- Cyt, +/- PRL, and 1, 25-dihydroxy-vitamin D3) every 2 days. Cyt treatment promoted the differentiation of osteoclast precursors into TRAP+, enlarged, multinucleated cells (mature osteoclasts), and this effect was significantly reduced by PRL (Fig. 6a). PRL can act on synovial fibroblasts to inhibit osteoclastogenesis (Fig. 5). To investigate osteoclast progenitors as PRL targets, synovial fibroblasts derived from *Prlr* +/+ mice were co-cultured with osteoclast progenitors from either *Prlr+/+* mice or *Prlr-/-* mice. PRL had no significant effect on the number of mature osteoclasts when osteoclast precursors were derived from *Prlr-/-* mice. However, the number of mature osteoclasts was similar between the co-cultures treated with Cyt and PRL, whether or not osteoclast progenitors were derived from PRL-receptor-null mice (Fig. 6b). These findings support a direct effect of PRL on both synovial fibroblasts and osteoclast progenitors to reduce osteoclastogenesis.

Expression of PRL receptor transcripts in chondrocytes, osteoblasts, and osteoclast-like cells

In addition to synovial fibroblasts, other cells in joint tissues express PRL receptors. RT-PCR performed on chondrocytes, osteoblasts, osteoclast-like cells, and synovial fibroblasts (positive controls) from *Prlr+/+* mice revealed a single band of 139 bp, the size of which corresponded to the region amplified from exon 5 of the *Prlr* gene (Fig. 6c). Specificity of the reaction was confirmed by the absence of such a transcript in cells obtained from *Prlr-/-* mice. In these knockout mice, exon 5 of the PRL receptor has been deleted, which results in a very short peptide unable to bind to PRL.

Discussion

Articular bone loss and increased fracture risk in arthritis are indicative of an imbalance between bone resorption and formation. Bone resorption depends on the development of bone resorbing osteoclasts (osteoclastogenesis) in response to systemic and local signals that converge to regulate the RANKL/RANK/OPG system [2, 3, 7, 8]. Here, we showed that PRL reduces the systemic levels and the joint production of cytokines with osteoclastogenic activity, lowers the joint expression of the genes encoding for RANKL and RANK, decreases osteoclast density, and reduces trabecular bone area in two murine models of inflammatory arthritis. Moreover, synovial fibroblasts are an important source for RANKL-induced bone loss in arthritis [6], and we showed that PRL downregulates cytokine-induced expression of the RANKL gene in cultured synovial fibroblasts via a STAT3-dependent pathway, and that this hormone reduces osteoclastogenesis in co-cultures of synovial fibroblasts and osteoclast progenitor cells.

Chronic inflammation determines local and systemic bone loss in RA [2, 3] and may be attenuated by PRL. PRL treatment reduces joint swelling, proinflammatory cytokine expression (TNFα, IL-1β, IL-6, and IFNγ), pannus formation, and the destruction of bone trabeculae in rats with AIA [18], a model of inflammatory arthritis. Here, we have extended these findings by showing that increasing serum PRL to levels similar to those (40 ng/ml) found in the circulation of some patients with RA [35] reduced systemic levels of CRP and TNFα, two osteoclastogenic cytokines [2, 3, 31]. The serum levels of CRP and TNFα in RA patients correlate with their levels in the

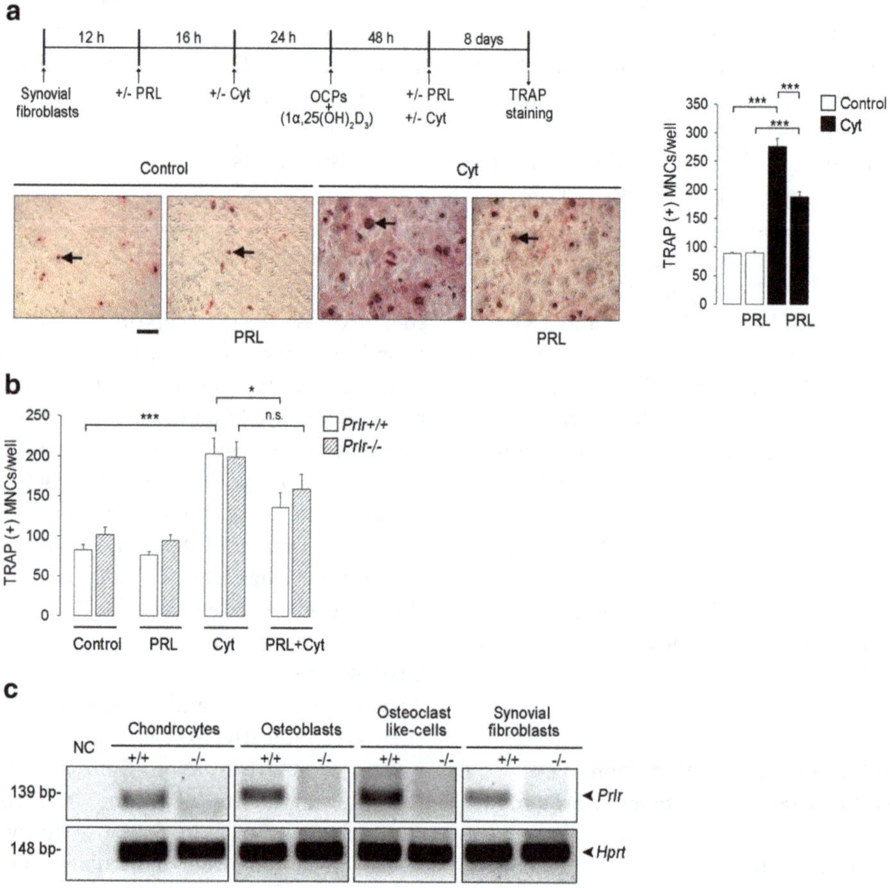

Fig. 6 Prolactin (*PRL*) reduces TNFα, IL-1β, and IFNγ (*Cyt*)-induced osteoclast formation in co-cultures of synovial fibroblast and osteoclast progenitor cells. **a** Time course of the co-culture: 12 hours after being seeded, synovial fibroblasts were treated or not with PRL for 16 hours. Cyt were then added or not to the culture and after 24 hours, osteoclast progenitors were delivered in medium containing 1, 25-dihydroxy-vitamin D3. Co-cultures were incubated for 10 days, replacing with new medium (containing +/- Cyt, +/- PRL, and 1, 25-dihydroxy-vitamin D3) every 2 days. Both synovial fibroblasts and osteoclast progenitors were from wild-type (*Prlr+/+*) mice. Osteclastogenesis, was assessed by the number of tartrate-resistant alkaline phosphatase (*TRAP*)-positive, multinucleated (≥3 nuclei) cells (*TRAP(+) MNCs*) (*arrows*). *Scale bar* 120 μm. **b** Number of TRAP(+) MNCs in co-cultures of synovial fibroblasts from *Prlr+/+* mice and osteoclast progenitors from *Prlr+/+* mice or from mice null for the PRL receptor (*Prlr-/-*). Co-cultures were carried out under the same conditions as in **a** Values are means ± SEM (n = 5). *$P < 0.05$, ***$P < 0.001$. **c** Real-time PCR amplification of the PRL receptor in joint cells obtained from *Prlr+/+* and *Prlr-/-* mice. mRNA levels of *Hprt* were amplified as internal control. *NC* without RNA negative control

synovial fluid and reflect systemic and joint inflammatory responses [31, 36]. Moreover, PRL treatment reduced the expression of transcription factors and cytokines associated with Th17 and T regulatory cells in arthritic joints. Th17 cells promote inflammation, osteoclastogenesis, and bone erosion in arthritis [32, 37], whereas T regulatory cells suppress immune responses [38], and the imbalance of the two T lymphocyte subpopulations has been identified as a key event in the pathogenesis of rheumatoid arthritis [30]. It remains to be determined how PRL actions, particularly the downregulation of T regulatory cells, would contribute to PRL protection against inflammation and osteoclastogenesis in arthritis. The matter is complex as the differentiation and function of Th17 and T regulatory cells are closely related and vary in the presence of strong inflammatory conditions [39, 40]. Both T cell populations require transforming growth factor (TGF)β for differentiation [41], and in vivo studies have identified a subset of T cells that dually express elements of both the T regulatory and Th17 phenotypes [40, 42] with potent inflammatory and osteoclastogenic effects in autoimmune arthritis [43].

In support of PRL acting locally on inflamed joint tissues, we show that the long PRL receptor isoform is upregulated in the joints of rats with AIA and in the synovial membranes and synovial fibroblasts of mice treated with the proinflammatory cytokines, TNFα, IL-1β, and IFNγ, which contribute to AIA inflammatory lesions [44]. PRL receptors exist in various molecular forms that differ primarily in the sequence and length of their cytoplasmic domain and are classified as long, intermediate, and short [45]. The long PRL receptor is considered the major isoform signaling all PRL actions, the intermediate isoform transmits cell proliferation and survival signals, and the short PRL receptor exerts dominant-negative effects on signals by the long form [46]. The long form of the PRL receptor appears to predominate in osteoblasts [19] and chondrocytes [25], where PRL promotes bone development and cartilage survival. Also, fibroblasts and T cells in the synovium of patients with RA express PRL receptors [47], and proinflammatory cytokines induce the expression of the long form of the PRL receptor in lung fibroblasts to mediate anti-inflammatory effects of PRL in the airways [48]. Therefore, these findings could imply that the long form of the PRL receptor mediates the protective effects of PRL in arthritis.

Supporting the anti-inflammatory role of PRL in arthritis, PRL-receptor-null mice exhibited increased joint swelling and higher joint expression of the genes encoding for TNFα, IL-1β, IL-6, IFNγ, IL-17A, IL-21, IL-22, IL-23, and IL-10 when subjected to monoarticular AIA (MAIA). These findings are consistent with PRL treatment inhibiting the expression of the same cytokines in the joints of rats with AIA [18] and with previous reports showing that targeted disruption of PRL [13] and of PRL receptors [49] enhances immune responses and mortality under stress-related conditions. Besides their crucial effects on joint inflammation, TNFα, IL-1β, IL-6, and IL-17A also drive bone loss. They promote osteoclastic bone resorption largely by stimulating the expression and function of RANKL and RANK [2, 32]. Accordingly, we next investigated whether PRL downregulates osteoclast development and bone loss in AIA and MAIA.

Increasing systemic PRL levels in rats with AIA and blocking PRL receptor signaling in *Prlr-/-* mice with MAIA reduced and increased, respectively, the loss of trabecular bone area, osteoclast density, the accumulation of phenotypic markers identifying osteoclasts (the gene for RANKL cognate receptor RANK and the genes encoding for acid (TRAP and cathepsin K) and neutral (MMP-9) proteases used by osteoclasts to degrade the organic matrix of bone [3]). Moreover, PRL and lack of PRL signaling reduced and increased, respectively, the expression of RANKL gene (*Tnfrsf11*) in the arthritic joint, which resulted in a lower and higher *Tnfrsf11/Tnfrsf11b* mRNA ratio for each condition, respectively. *Tnfrsf11b* encodes for OPG, a soluble decoy receptor that neutralizes RANKL and prevents bone erosion in AIA [4]. A high RANKL/OPG ratio occurs in patients with RA and is associated with increased bone resorption [50].

Our findings indicate that inhibition of RANKL-induced osteoclast development is a component of PRL protection against bone loss in inflammatory arthritis. It is unclear whether PRL signals directly on osteoclasts or indirectly through other cell types responsible for bone loss. Arguing against osteoclasts being direct targets of PRL is the finding that bone marrow cells differentiated into osteoclasts are devoid of the PRL receptor [19]. On the other hand, chondrocytes, osteoblasts, and synovial fibroblasts express PRL receptors and are major sources of osteoclastogenic cytokines including RANKL [2, 5, 6, 51]. Here, we support direct effects of PRL on chondrocytes, synovial fibroblasts, and osteoblasts, but also in osteoclasts by showing the PCR-mediated amplification of a PRL receptor transcript in the various cell types obtained from *Prlr+/+* mice but not in those obtained from *Prlr-/-* mice. While differences in osteoclast differentiation protocols may contribute to our contrasting finding [19], the presence of the PRL receptor in osteoclasts reinforces the role of PRL on bone remodeling.

Consistent with synovial fibroblasts being cellular targets of PRL-induced anti-osteoclastogenesis, the incubation of primary cultures of synovial fibroblasts with TNFα, IL-1β, and IFNγ (Cyt) elevated the expression of the PRL receptor, and treatment of these cells with PRL inhibited Cyt-induced expression of *Il1b*, *Il6*, and *Tnfrsf11*. PRL receptors signal through Janus kinase-2 (JAK-2)-STATs 1, 5, and 3 as their canonical pathway [52]. STATs, and in particular STAT3, are emerging as important regulators of bone homeostasis [33]. STAT3 mutations correlate with increased osteoclast number and bone resorption in the clinic [53, 54] and mice with an osteoblast-specific deletion of *Stat3* have an osteopenic phenotype [33]. Here, we demonstrate that PRL stimulates the expression of *Stat3* and enhances Cyt-induced phosphorylation/activation of STAT3 in synovial fibroblasts. The Cyt-induced STAT3 activation may be due to the production of IL-6 in response to the Cyt, as IL-6 activates STAT3 in synovial fibroblasts [55]. However, IL-6-mediated STAT3 activation may lead to either bone resorption [56] or bone formation [57]. In support of STAT3 being anti-osteoclastogenic when activated by PRL, pharmacological blockage of STAT3 prevented PRL inhibition of Cyt-induced *Tnfrsf11* expression. These findings suggest that PRL may signal through STAT3 in synovial fibroblasts to inhibit RANKL-induced osteoclastogenesis. Consistent with this notion, we found that PRL acts on co-cultures of synovial fibroblasts and osteoclast precursor cells to downregulate Cyt-induced osteoclast differentiation. The fact that such PRL inhibition was reduced when osteoclast precursors were derived from *Prlr-/-* mice implies that PRL receptors in osteoclast progenitor cells contribute to PRL protection against osteoclastogenesis. This is in agreement with the presence of PRL receptors in osteoclast-like cells and with the PRL downregulation of RANK in arthritic joints. Reduction of RANK levels may contribute to PRL inhibitory effects on osteoclastogenesis and bone loss at the level of osteoclast progenitors and mature osteoclasts.

PRL regulation of the RANKL/RANK/OPG system for physiological bone remodeling during growth and reproduction is well-substantiated [58]. PRL decreases the RANKL/OPG ratio by downregulating RANKL and upregulating OPG in osteoblasts to promote bone formation early in life [20], whereas in pregnancy and lactation, PRL accelerates bone turnover by raising the RANKL/OPG ratio in osteoblasts [59, 60] in order to supply calcium for fetal growth and milk production. The opposing effects of PRL on bone remodeling indicate that the outcome of its action depends on complex age-related and hormone-related interactions.

In experimental inflammatory arthritis, PRL appears to be beneficial; however, the role of PRL in RA is controversial (as reviewed [58]). PRL increases in the circulation of some patients with RA, but it is not clear whether systemic PRL levels correlate with disease severity. Confounding factors include the contribution of PRL synthesized locally by joint tissues like chondrocytes [61], endothelial cells [62], synoviocytes and immune cells [47]; and the ability of PRL to exert immunostimulatory or immunosuppressive effects, depending on its level and that of other cytokines and hormones [58]. Hyperprolactinemia in the context of reproduction [59] and non-inflammatory pathology (prolactinoma) [63] promotes bone loss, whereas high circulating PRL levels can be anti-inflammatory and reduce bone loss under inflammatory conditions [18, 64] (and present findings). The mechanisms governing the effects of PRL on bone remodeling are challenging but a better understanding of them could lead to the use of hyperprolactinemia-inducing drugs as therapeutic agents in the clinic.

Conclusion

We demonstrated in this study that PRL protects against bone loss and osteoclastogenesis in inflammatory arthritis by inhibiting cytokine-induced activation of RANKL in joints and synovial fibroblasts via its canonical STAT3 signaling pathway.

Abbreviations

AIA: Adjuvant-induced arthritis; bp: Base pairs; CD90.2: Cluster of differentiation 90; CFA: Complete Freund's adjuvant; CRP: C-reactive protein; *Ctsk*: Cathepsin K gene; Cyt: Combination of the proinflammatory cytokines TNFα, IL-1β, and interferon-γ; DMEM: Dulbecco's modified Eagle's medium; *Ebi3*: Gene encoding for Epstein-Barr virus induced 3; ELISA: Enzyme-linked immunosorbent assay; FBS: Fetal bovine serum; *Foxp3*: Gene encoding for forkhead box protein 3; Hprt: Hypoxanthine-guanine phosphoribosyltransferase; ICAM-1: Intercellular adhesion molecule 1; IFNγ: Interferon γ; IL: Interleukin; *Il10*: Gene encoding for interleukin 10; *Il12a*: Gene encoding for interleukin 12A; JAK-2: Janus kinase-2; MAIA: Monoarticular adjuvant-induced arthritis; Mmp9: Matrix metalloproteinase 9; OPG: Osteoprotegerin; PBS: phosphate-buffered saline; PRL: Prolactin; PRLR: Prolactin receptor; qPCR: Quantitative polymerase chain reaction; qRT-PCR: Quantitative real-time polymerase chain reaction; RA: Rheumatoid arthritis; RANK: Receptor activator of nuclear factor κB; RANKL: Receptor activator of nuclear factor κB ligand; *Rora*: Gene encoding for retinoic acid orphan nuclear receptors RORα; *Rorc*: Gene encoding for retinoic acid orphan nuclear receptors RORγt; STAT3: Signal transducer and activator of transcription 3; *Tgfb1*: Gene encoding for transforming growth factor β 1; Th: T helper; *Tnfrsf11*: Gene encoding for RANKL; *Tnfrsf11a*: Gene encoding for RANK; *Tnfrsf11b*: Gene encoding for OPG; TNFα: Tumor necrosis factor alpha; TRAP: Tartrate-resistant acid phosphatase; VCAM1: Vascular cell adhesion molecule 1

Acknowledgements

We thank Gabriel Nava, Martín García, Alejandra Castilla, and Maarten Werdler for their technical assistance, and Dorothy D. Pless, for critically editing the manuscript.

Funding

UNAM Grant PAPIIT, IN201315 to C. Clapp supported the work. M. G. Ledesma-Colunga is a doctoral student from Programa de Doctorado en Ciencias Biomédicas, Universidad Nacional Autónoma de México (UNAM) and received fellowship 245828 from the National Council of Science and Technology of Mexico (CONACYT).

Authors' contributions

Conception and design: MGL-C, CC. Acquisition of data: NA, GO, MS-G, FL-B. Analysis or interpretation of data: MGL-C, GME, CC. Drafting of the manuscript: MGL-C, CC. All authors were involved in critical revision of the manuscript for important intellectual content, and all authors approved the final version of the manuscript and take responsibility for appropriate portions of the content, accuracy and integrity.

Competing interests

The authors declare that they have no competing interests.

References

1. Cohen SB, Dore RK, Lane NE, Ory PA, Peterfy CG, Sharp JT, van der Heijde D, Zhou L, Tsuji W, Newmark R, et al. Denosumab treatment effects on structural damage, bone mineral density, and bone turnover in rheumatoid arthritis: a twelve-month, multicenter, randomized, double-blind, placebo-controlled, phase II clinical trial. Arthritis Rheum. 2008;58(5):1299–309.
2. Braun T, Zwerina J. Positive regulators of osteoclastogenesis and bone resorption in rheumatoid arthritis. Arthritis Res Ther. 2011;13(4):235.
3. Schett G, Gravallese E. Bone erosion in rheumatoid arthritis: mechanisms, diagnosis and treatment. Nat Rev Rheumatol. 2012;8(11):656–64.
4. Kong YY, Feige U, Sarosi I, Bolon B, Tafuri A, Morony S, Capparelli C, Li J, Elliott R, McCabe S, et al. Activated T cells regulate bone loss and joint destruction in adjuvant arthritis through osteoprotegerin ligand. Nature. 1999;402(6759):304–9.
5. Gravallese EM, Manning C, Tsay A, Naito A, Pan C, Amento E, Goldring SR. Synovial tissue in rheumatoid arthritis is a source of osteoclast differentiation factor. Arthritis Rheum. 2000;43(2):250–8.
6. Tunyogi-Csapo M, Kis-Toth K, Radacs M, Farkas B, Jacobs JJ, Finnegan A, Mikecz K, Glant TT. Cytokine-controlled RANKL and osteoprotegerin expression by human and mouse synovial fibroblasts: fibroblast-mediated pathologic bone resorption. Arthritis Rheum. 2008;58(8):2397–408.
7. Hofbauer LC, Heufelder AE. Role of receptor activator of nuclear factor-kappaB ligand and osteoprotegerin in bone cell biology. J Mol Med (Berl). 2001;79(5-6):243–53.

8. Jones DH, Kong YY, Penninger JM. Role of RANKL and RANK in bone loss and arthritis. Ann Rheum Dis. 2002;61 Suppl 2:ii32–39.
9. Brennan P, Ollier B, Worthington J, Hajeer A, Silman A. Are both genetic and reproductive associations with rheumatoid arthritis linked to prolactin? Lancet. 1996;348(9020):106–9.
10. Neidhart M, Gay RE, Gay S. Prolactin and prolactin-like polypeptides in rheumatoid arthritis. Biomed Pharmacother. 1999;53(5-6):218–22.
11. Costanza M, Binart N, Steinman L, Pedotti R. Prolactin: a versatile regulator of inflammation and autoimmune pathology. Autoimmun Rev. 2015;14(3):223–30.
12. Matera L, Cesano A, Bellone G, Oberholtzer E. Modulatory effect of prolactin on the resting and mitogen-induced activity of T, B, and NK lymphocytes. Brain Behav Immun. 1992;6(4):409–17.
13. Dugan AL, Thellin O, Buckley DJ, Buckley AR, Ogle CK, Horseman ND. Effects of prolactin deficiency on myelopoiesis and splenic T lymphocyte proliferation in thermally injured mice. Endocrinology. 2002;143(10):4147–51.
14. Oberbeck R, Schmitz D, Wilsenack K, Schuler M, Biskup C, Schedlowski M, Nast-Kolb D, Exton MS. Prolactin modulates survival and cellular immune functions in septic mice. J Surg Res. 2003;113(2):248–56.
15. de Man YA, Dolhain RJ, van de Geijn FE, Willemsen SP, Hazes JM. Disease activity of rheumatoid arthritis during pregnancy: results from a nationwide prospective study. Arthritis Rheum. 2008;59(9):1241–8.
16. Pikwer M, Bergstrom U, Nilsson JA, Jacobsson L, Berglund G, Turesson C. Breast feeding, but not use of oral contraceptives, is associated with a reduced risk of rheumatoid arthritis. Ann Rheum Dis. 2009;68(4):526–30.
17. Grimaldi MG. Long-term low dose haloperidol treatment in rheumatoid patients: effects on serum sulphydryl levels, technetium index, ESR, and clinical response. Br J Clin Pharmacol. 1981;12(4):579–81.
18. Adan N, Guzman-Morales J, Ledesma-Colunga MG, Perales-Canales SI, Quintanar-Stephano A, Lopez-Barrera F, Mendez I, Moreno-Carranza B, Triebel J, Binart N, et al. Prolactin promotes cartilage survival and attenuates inflammation in inflammatory arthritis. J Clin Invest. 2013;123(9):3902–13.
19. Clement-Lacroix P, Ormandy C, Lepescheux L, Ammann P, Damotte D, Goffin V, Bouchard B, Amling M, Gaillard-Kelly M, Binart N, et al. Osteoblasts are a new target for prolactin: analysis of bone formation in prolactin receptor knockout mice. Endocrinology. 1999;140(1):96–105.
20. Seriwatanachai D, Charoenphandhu N, Suthiphongchai T, Krishnamra N. Prolactin decreases the expression ratio of receptor activator of nuclear factor kappaB ligand/osteoprotegerin in human fetal osteoblast cells. Cell Biol Int. 2008;32(9):1126–35.
21. Kondegowda NG, Fenutria R, Pollack IR, Orthofer M, Garcia-Ocana A, Penninger JM, Vasavada RC. Osteoprotegerin and denosumab stimulate human beta cell proliferation through inhibition of the receptor activator of NF-kappaB ligand pathway. Cell Metab. 2015;22(1):77–85.
22. Srivastava S, Matsuda M, Hou Z, Bailey JP, Kitazawa R, Herbst MP, Horseman ND. Receptor activator of NF-kappaB ligand induction via Jak2 and Stat5a in mammary epithelial cells. J Biol Chem. 2003;278(46):46171–8.
23. Gauldie SD, McQueen DS, Clarke CJ, Chessell IP. A robust model of adjuvant-induced chronic unilateral arthritis in two mouse strains. J Neurosci Methods. 2004;139(2):281–91.
24. Armaka M, Gkretsi V, Kontoyiannis D, Kollias G. A standardized protocol for the isolation and culture of normal and arthritogenic murine synovial fibroblasts. Protocol Exch. 2009. doi:10.1038/nprot.2009.1102.
25. Zermeno C, Guzman-Morales J, Macotela Y, Nava G, Lopez-Barrera F, Kouri JB, Lavalle C, de la Escalera GM, Clapp C. Prolactin inhibits the apoptosis of chondrocytes induced by serum starvation. J Endocrinol. 2006;189(2):R1–8.
26. Rauner M, Foger-Samwald U, Kurz MF, Brunner-Kubath C, Schamall D, Kapfenberger A, Varga P, Kudlacek S, Wutzl A, Hoger H, et al. Cathepsin S controls adipocytic and osteoblastic differentiation, bone turnover, and bone microarchitecture. Bone. 2014;64:281–7.
27. Marino S, Logan JG, Mellis D, Capulli M. Generation and culture of osteoclasts. Bonekey Rep. 2014;3:570.
28. Shakibaei M, De Souza P, Merker HJ. Integrin expression and collagen type II implicated in maintenance of chondrocyte shape in monolayer culture: an immunomorphological study. Cell Biol Int. 1997;21(2):115–25.
29. Rauner M, Winzer M, Stupphann D, Krenbek D, Pietschmann P. RANKL and OPG gene expression bone marrow stromal cells and calvarial osteoblasts in mouse and rat. Osteologie. 2007;16:19–28.
30. Alunno A, Manetti M, Caterbi S, Ibba-Manneschi L, Bistoni O, Bartoloni E, Valentini V, Terenzi R, Gerli R. Altered immunoregulation in rheumatoid arthritis: the role of regulatory T cells and proinflammatory Th17 cells and therapeutic implications. Mediat Inflamm. 2015;2015:751793.
31. Kim KW, Kim BM, Moon HW, Lee SH, Kim HR. Role of C-reactive protein in osteoclastogenesis in rheumatoid arthritis. Arthritis Res Ther. 2015;17:41.
32. Sato K, Suematsu A, Okamoto K, Yamaguchi A, Morishita Y, Kadono Y, Tanaka S, Kodama T, Akira S, Iwakura Y, et al. Th17 functions as an osteoclastogenic helper T cell subset that links T cell activation and bone destruction. J Exp Med. 2006;203(12):2673–82.
33. Li J. JAK-STAT and bone metabolism. Jak-Stat. 2013;2(3), e23930.
34. Siddiquee K, Zhang S, Guida WC, Blaskovich MA, Greedy B, Lawrence HR, Yip ML, Jove R, McLaughlin MM, Lawrence NJ, et al. Selective chemical probe inhibitor of Stat3, identified through structure-based virtual screening, induces antitumor activity. Proc Natl Acad Sci USA. 2007; 104(18):7391–6.
35. Ghule S, Dhotre A, Gupta M, Dharme P, Vaidya S. Serum prolactin levels in women with rheumatoid arthritis. Biomed Res. 2009;20(2):2009–5. 2009-2008.
36. Hamed EA, Hamed EA, Hamed SA, Gamal H-A. Synovial fluid and serum levels of sE-selectin, IL-1β and TNF-α in rheumatoid arthritis. JKAU Med Sci. 2007;14(1):19–34.
37. Lubberts E. Th17 cytokines and arthritis. Semin Immunopathol. 2010; 32(1):43–53.
38. Sakaguchi S, Miyara M, Costantino CM, Hafler DA. FOXP3+ regulatory T cells in the human immune system. Nat Rev Immunol. 2010;10(7):490–500.
39. Deknuydt F, Bioley G, Valmori D, Ayyoub M. IL-1beta and IL-2 convert human Treg into T(H)17 cells. Clin Immunol. 2009;131(2):298–307.
40. Diller ML, Kudchadkar RR, Delman KA, Lawson DH, Ford ML. Balancing inflammation: the link between Th17 and regulatory T cells. Mediat Inflamm. 2016;2016:6309219.
41. Zhou L, Lopes JE, Chong MM, Ivanov II, Min R, Victora GD, Shen Y, Du J, Rubtsov YP, Rudensky AY, et al. TGF-beta-induced Foxp3 inhibits T(H)17 cell differentiation by antagonizing RORgammat function. Nature. 2008; 453(7192):236–40.
42. Voo KS, Wang YH, Santori FR, Boggiano C, Wang YH, Arima K, Bover L, Hanabuchi S, Khalili J, Marinova E, et al. Identification of IL-17-producing FOXP3+ regulatory T cells in humans. Proc Natl Acad Sci USA. 2009;106(12): 4793–8.
43. Komatsu N, Okamoto K, Sawa S, Nakashima T, Oh-hora M, Kodama T, Tanaka S, Bluestone JA, Takayanagi H. Pathogenic conversion of Foxp3+ T cells into TH17 cells in autoimmune arthritis. Nat Med. 2014;20(1):62–8.
44. Panayi GS, Lanchbury JS, Kingsley GH. The importance of the T cell in initiating and maintaining the chronic synovitis of rheumatoid arthritis. Arthritis Rheum. 1992;35(7):729–35.
45. Bole-Feysot C, Goffin V, Edery M, Binart N, Kelly PA. Prolactin (PRL) and its receptor: actions, signal transduction pathways and phenotypes observed in PRL receptor knockout mice. Endocr Rev. 1998;19(3):225–68.
46. Ben-Jonathan N, LaPensee CR, LaPensee EW. What can we learn from rodents about prolactin in humans? Endocr Rev. 2008;29(1):1–41.
47. Nagafuchi H, Suzuki N, Kaneko A, Asai T, Sakane T. Prolactin locally produced by synovium infiltrating T lymphocytes induces excessive synovial cell functions in patients with rheumatoid arthritis. J Rheumatol. 1999;26(9):1890–900.
48. Corbacho AM, Macotela Y, Nava G, Eiserich JP, Cross CE, Martinez de la Escalera G, Clapp C. Cytokine induction of prolactin receptors mediates prolactin inhibition of nitric oxide synthesis in pulmonary fibroblasts. FEBS Lett. 2003;544(1-3):171–5.
49. Moreno-Carranza B, Goya-Arce M, Vega C, Adan N, Triebel J, Lopez-Barrera F, Quintanar-Stephano A, Binart N, Martinez de la Escalera G, Clapp C. Prolactin promotes normal liver growth, survival, and regeneration in rodents: effects on hepatic IL-6, suppressor of cytokine signaling-3, and angiogenesis. Am J Physiol Regul Integr Comp Physiol. 2013;305(7):R720–6.
50. Fadda S, Hamdy A, Abulkhair E, Mahmoud Elsify H, Mostafa A. Serum levels of osteoprotegerin and RANKL in patients with rheumatoid arthritis and their relation to bone mineral density and disease activity. Egyptian Rheumatologist. 2015;37:1–6.
51. Martinez-Calatrava MJ, Prieto-Potin I, Roman-Blas JA, Tardio L, Largo R, Herrero-Beaumont G. RANKL synthesized by articular chondrocytes contributes to juxta-articular bone loss in chronic arthritis. Arthritis Res Ther. 2012;14(3):R149.
52. DaSilva L, Rui H, Erwin RA, Howard OM, Kirken RA, Malabarba MG, Hackett RH, Larner AC, Farrar WL. Prolactin recruits STAT1, STAT3 and STAT5 independent of conserved receptor tyrosines TYR402, TYR479, TYR515 and TYR580. Mol Cell Endocrinol. 1996;117(2):131–40.

53. Holland SM, DeLeo FR, Elloumi HZ, Hsu AP, Uzel G, Brodsky N, Freeman AF, Demidowich A, Davis J, Turner ML, et al. STAT3 mutations in the hyper-IgE syndrome. N Engl J Med. 2007;357(16):1608–19.
54. Minegishi Y, Saito M, Tsuchiya S, Tsuge I, Takada H, Hara T, Kawamura N, Ariga T, Pasic S, Stojkovic O, et al. Dominant-negative mutations in the DNA-binding domain of STAT3 cause hyper-IgE syndrome. Nature. 2007; 448(7157):1058–62.
55. Hashizume M, Hayakawa N, Mihara M. IL-6 trans-signalling directly induces RANKL on fibroblast-like synovial cells and is involved in RANKL induction by TNF-alpha and IL-17. Rheumatology. 2008;47(11):1635–40.
56. O'Brien CA, Gubrij I, Lin SC, Saylors RL, Manolagas SC. STAT3 activation in stromal/osteoblastic cells is required for induction of the receptor activator of NF-kappaB ligand and stimulation of osteoclastogenesis by gp130-utilizing cytokines or interleukin-1 but not 1,25-dihydroxyvitamin D3 or parathyroid hormone. J Biol Chem. 1999;274(27):19301–8.
57. Shin HI, Divieti P, Sims NA, Kobayashi T, Miao D, Karaplis AC, Baron R, Bringhurst R, Kronenberg HM. Gp130-mediated signaling is necessary for normal osteoblastic function in vivo and in vitro. Endocrinology. 2004; 145(3):1376–85.
58. Clapp C, Adan N, Ledesma-Colunga MG, Solís-Gutiérrez M, Triebel J, Martinez de la Escalera G. The role of the prolactin/vasoinhibin axis in rheumatoid arthritis: an integrative overview. Cell Mol Life Sci. 2016;73(15): 2929–48.
59. Lotinun S, Limlomwongse LC, Sirikulchayanonta V, Krishnamra N. Bone calcium turnover, formation, and resorption in bromocriptine- and prolactin-treated lactating rats. Endocrine. 2003;20(1-2):163–70.
60. Seriwatanachai D, Thongchote K, Charoenphandhu N, Pandaranandaka J, Tudpor K, Teerapornpuntakit J, Suthiphongchai T, Krishnamra N. Prolactin directly enhances bone turnover by raising osteoblast-expressed receptor activator of nuclear factor kappaB ligand/osteoprotegerin ratio. Bone. 2008; 42(3):535–46.
61. Macotela Y, Aguilar MB, Guzman-Morales J, Rivera JC, Zermeno C, Lopez-Barrera F, Nava G, Lavalle C, Martinez de la Escalera G, Clapp C. Matrix metalloproteases from chondrocytes generate an antiangiogenic 16 kDa prolactin. J Cell Sci. 2006;119(Pt 9):1790–800.
62. Corbacho AM, Macotela Y, Nava G, Torner L, Duenas Z, Noris G, Morales MA, Martinez De La Escalera G, Clapp C. Human umbilical vein endothelial cells express multiple prolactin isoforms. J Endocrinol. 2000;166(1):53–62.
63. Mazziotti G, Porcelli T, Mormando M, De Menis E, Bianchi A, Mejia C, Mancini T, De Marinis L, Giustina A. Vertebral fractures in males with prolactinoma. Endocrine. 2011;39(3):288–93.
64. Jacobi AM, Rohde W, Volk HD, Dorner T, Burmester GR, Hiepe F. Prolactin enhances the in vitro production of IgG in peripheral blood mononuclear cells from patients with systemic lupus erythematosus but not from healthy controls. Ann Rheum Dis. 2001;60(3):242–7.

18

Lapachol, a compound targeting pyrimidine metabolism, ameliorates experimental autoimmune arthritis

Raphael S. Peres[1], Gabriela B. Santos[2], Nerry T. Cecilio[1], Valquíria A. P. Jabor[3], Michael Niehues[3], Bruna G. S. Torres[4], Gabriela Buqui[3], Carlos H. T. P. Silva[2], Teresa Dalla Costa[4], Norberto P. Lopes[3], Maria C. Nonato[3], Fernando S. Ramalho[5], Paulo Louzada-Júnior[6], Thiago M. Cunha[1], Fernando Q. Cunha[1], Flavio S. Emery[2*] and Jose C. Alves-Filho[1*]

Abstract

Background: The inhibition of pyrimidine biosynthesis by blocking the dihydroorotate dehydrogenase (DHODH) activity, the prime target of leflunomide (LEF), has been proven to be an effective strategy for rheumatoid arthritis (RA) treatment. However, a considerable proportion of RA patients are refractory to LEF. Here, we investigated lapachol (LAP), a natural naphthoquinone, as a potential DHODH inhibitor and addressed its immunosuppressive properties.

Methods: Molecular flexible docking studies and bioactivity assays were performed to determine the ability of LAP to interact and inhibit DHODH. In vitro studies were conducted to assess the antiproliferative effect of LAP using isolated lymphocytes. Finally, collagen-induced arthritis (CIA) and antigen-induced arthritis (AIA) models were employed to address the anti-arthritic effects of LAP.

Results: We found that LAP is a potent DHODH inhibitor which had a remarkable ability to inhibit both human and murine lymphocyte proliferation in vitro. Importantly, uridine supplementation abrogated the antiproliferative effect of LAP, supporting that the pyrimidine metabolic pathway is the target of LAP. In vivo, LAP treatment markedly reduced CIA and AIA progression as evidenced by the reduction in clinical score, articular tissue damage, and inflammation.

Conclusions: Our findings propose a binding model of interaction and support the ability of LAP to inhibit DHODH, decreasing lymphocyte proliferation and attenuating the severity of experimental autoimmune arthritis. Therefore, LAP could be considered as a potential immunosuppressive lead candidate with potential therapeutic implications for RA.

Keywords: Rheumatoid arthritis, Lapachol, Inflammation, Collagen-induced arthritis, Dihydroorotate dehydrogenase, DMARDs, Pyrimidine metabolism

Background

Rheumatoid arthritis (RA) is an autoimmune disease that is characterized by chronic articular inflammation with progressive joint destruction [1]. The current first-line therapy for RA patients includes the use of conventional disease-modifying antirheumatic drugs (DMARDs), such as methotrexate or leflunomide (LEF), in combination with short-term glucocorticoids. Moreover, the use of biological agents is employed as an alternative therapy in patients whose disease failed to respond to conventional DMARDs [2].

LEF is an isoxazole derivative with a potent immunosuppressive activity that was approved for the treatment of RA in 1998 [3]. LEF is a prodrug that is converted in vivo to its primary active metabolite A771726 (also known as teriflunomide). LEF blocks lymphocyte proliferation and hence the clonal expansion of autoreactive T cells in RA patients by inhibiting dihydroorotate dehydrogenase (DHODH), the mitochondrial rate-limiting

* Correspondence: flavioemery@fcfrp.usp.br; jcafilho@usp.br
[2]Department of Pharmaceutical Sciences, Faculty of Pharmaceutical Sciences of Ribeirão Preto, University of São Paulo, Avenida do Café s/n, Ribeirão Preto CEP: 14040-903, Brazil
[1]Department of Pharmacology, Ribeirão Preto Medical School, Center of Research in Inflammatory Diseases (CRID), University of São Paulo, Avenida Bandeirantes, 3900, Ribeirão Preto, São Paulo CEP: 14049-900, Brazil
Full list of author information is available at the end of the article

enzyme in the de novo synthesis of pyrimidine ribonucleotides [4, 5]. The use of LEF is normally reserved for RA patients whose disease failed to respond to first-line DMARDs, before the introduction of biological DMARDs [6]. Nevertheless, despite it having demonstrated safety and efficacy, a substantial proportion of patients (around 30–40%) do not have an appropriate response to LEF [7]. Therefore, it is highly desirable to discover novel DHODH inhibitors as lead compounds for the development of new DMARD candidates.

Lapachol (LAP; 2-hydroxy-3-(3methyl-2-butenyl)-1,4-naphthoquinone) is a nonpolar naturally occurring naphthoquinone found in some Brazilian medicinal plants [8]. LAP and others naphthoquinones have been described as having a range of biological actions, including microbicidal, anti-inflammatory and antiproliferative activities [9–15]. In fact, it was demonstrated that LAP has potent antitumoral activity which was characterized by its ability to inhibit DNA and RNA synthesis in neoplastic cells [16]. Moreover, it was reported that LAP can reduce proliferation of the human keratinocytes in vitro, suggesting that it has potential antipsoriatic effects [17]. Despite the molecular mechanisms associated with these effects remaining poorly elucidated, it has been described that LAP and other naphthoquinones derivatives, such as lawsone and atovaquone, can inhibit DHODH activity [9]. However, the biological relevance of this effect was poorly characterized. In the present study, we investigated the potential immunosuppressive properties of LAP.

Methods

Preparation of LAP sodium salt

To a solution of LAP (500 mg, 2.06 mmol) in ethanol (20 ml) was added NaOH (112 mg, 0.28 mmol) and the reaction mixture was stirred for 24 h. After consumption of LAP, the reaction mixture was concentrated under reduced pressure and the solid residue was washed with dichloromethane (4×) and petroleum ether (4×) to afford a purple solid of 518 mg, 95% yield (^{1}H NMR (300 MHz, D_2O_{d6}) δ7.66 (br s, 1H), 7.64 (br s, 1H), 7.53 (*br* t, $J = 9$ Hz, 1H), 7.41 (*br* t, $J = 9$Hz, 1H), 5.15 (*br* t, $J = 9$Hz, 1H), (3.06, d, $J = 6$Hz, 2H), 1.72 (s, 3H), 1.63 (s, 3H); ^{13}C NMR (101 MHz, $DMSO_{d6}$) δ 187.2, 178.4, 169.6, 136.0, 133.2, 131.3, 129.7, 127.5, 125.76 124.81, 124.4, 117.9, 25.59, 20.8, 14.1; HRMS-ESI m/z cald for: $[M + Na]^+ = 265.0835$; found = 265.0834).

Molecular modeling and docking procedures

We used nine human DHODH high-resolution crystal structures in complex with the following inhibitors: DHO1B0033 (PDB id: 4LS0); DSM338 (PDB id: 4OQV); O57 (PDB id: 4JS3); a brequinar analogue (PDB id: 4JTU); 221290 (PDB ID: 2WV8); amino-benzoic acid inhibitor 715 (PDB id: 3KVL); LEF derivative inhibitor 1 (PDB id: 3F1Q); another brequinar analogue (PDB id: 2B0M); and antiproliferative agent A771726 (PDB id: 1D3H). The crystal structure of hDHODH in complex with antiproliferative agent A771726 (PDB id: 1D3H) has been considered for flexible docking with A771726 and LAP, and the calculations were carried out using the GOLD (Genetic Optimisation for Ligand Docking) 5.2 software [18]. GOLD was comprehensively validated, reliably identifying the correct binding mode for a large range of test set cases, in a vast set of independent studies, with a rate of success in 70–80% of the PDB protein-ligand structures thus analyzed, such as reported in the literature [18, 19].

Here, a parameter set including a population of 100 conformers, 100,000 operations, 95 mutations, and 95 crossovers has been used. The simulations were then performed inside a selected region of the active site (sphere of 8.5 Å radius centered at $x = 49.65$, $y = 42.13$, $z = -1.54$), keeping the Leu46 side chain flexible (using a rotamers library). The number of docking simulations to be performed with each inhibitor was specified under 10 GA (genetic algorithm) runs, once each docking run can evolve to different ligand poses (pose = conformation + orientation). Thus, ten poses of highest score (top-ranked GOLD solutions) obtained for each compound were selected by using the CHEMPLP score function. In this case, a Piecewise Linear Potential (fPLP) is used to model the steric complementarity between protein and ligand, and for CHEMPLP the distance- and angle-dependent hydrogen and metal bonding terms from other fitness function also implemented in GOLD, so called ChemScore, are considered. CHEMPLP has been found to give the highest success rates for docking pose prediction as well as virtual screening experiments against diverse validation test sets and it was here chosen as the fitness function. Based on this CHEMPLP function, GOLD classifies the orientations of the molecules by a decreasing order of affinity (scores) with the binding site of the receptor [19].

Previous to the docking calculations and after the removal of the ligand as well as crystallographic waters of the hDHODH/A771726 complex structure, hydrogen atoms of the residues side chains were added and oriented in the active site region. Also, suitable 3D structures of the inhibitors A771726 and LAP were previously built and optimized with molecular mechanics (MMFF force field), followed by Hartree-Fock/Density Functional methods (full optimization at B3LYP/6-31G* level of calculation), using the Spartan'06 software.

Pharmacokinetics study design

For administration to Wistar rats, LAP was dissolved in DMSO:Tween 80:glucose 5% in a proportion of 15:5:80 (v/v/v), resulting in a solution of 1 mg/ml (for intravenous (i.v.) administration) and another of 5 mg/ml (for oral administration). LAP was administered to rats as an i.v. bolus dose at 2 mg/kg ($n = 7$) and at two oral doses of 10 ($n = 8$) and 25 mg/kg ($n = 6$). LAP salt was administered as i.v. (2 mg/kg, $n = 6$) and oral doses (30 mg/kg equivalent to 27.5 mg/kg of LAP, $n = 8$). The i.v. doses were injected into the lateral tail vein, and oral doses were given by gavage. The doses were chosen based on previous toxicological and pharmacodynamic studies [20]. At predetermined time points (30 min before dosing and at 0.08, 0.25, 0.5, 1, 2, 4, 6, 8, 12, and 24 h) after LAP i.v. administration, blood samples (200–250 µl) were withdrawn into heparinized tubes via puncture of the lateral tail vein, opposite to the vein used for drug dosing. The same procedure was carried out after oral administration of LAP, with blood sampling at 0.25, 0.5, 1, 1.5, 2, 3, 6, 12, 24, and 30 h. After LAP sodium salt i.v. and oral dosing, blood samples were harvested up to 10 and 12 h, respectively. Plasma was obtained by centrifugation of blood samples (6800 × g, at 4 °C for 10 min) and stored at −80 °C until analysis by UPLC-MS/MS.

Pharmacokinetic analysis

LAP and LAP sodium salt pharmacokinetic parameters after i.v. and oral administration were determined from individual plasma profiles by a noncompartmental approach (NCA). The peak plasma concentration (Cmax) and the time of maximum concentration (Tmax) were obtained by visual inspection of the data from the plasma concentration–time curve after oral dosing. Pharmacokinetic parameters such an elimination rate constant (λ), area under the curve (AUC0–∞), clearance (CLtot), half-life (t1/2), volume of distribution (Vdss), mean residence time (MRT), and bioavailability (Fabs) were determined using classical equations. The compartmental analyses were performed using SCIENTIST v.2.0.1 software (MicroMath®, USA). One- and two-compartment models with or without weighting schemes were evaluated. The best model to fit the data was chosen based on the random distribution of residuals, the correlation coefficient, and the model selection criterion (MSC) given by the software.

The individual plasma profiles of LAP and LAP sodium salt after i.v. administration were best described by a two-compartmental open model. Plasma profiles after oral administration with two different doses of LAP and one dose of LAP sodium salt were best described by the one-compartmental model.

Plasma analysis by UPLC-MS/MS

LAP concentration in plasma samples was determined by a validated (FDA, US Food and Drug Administration, 2001) UPLC-MS/MS method [21]. Analyses were run on an Acquity UPLC BEH (Waters Acquity™) C18 column (2.1 × 50 mm, 1.7 µm particle size), with a flow of 300 µl/min at 35 °C. A gradient constituted of water (A) and acetonitrile (B) acidified with 0.1% acetic acid was used as follows: 0 min (90% A), 1 min (75% A), 7 min (50% A), 8.5 min (0% A) and 9.5 min (100% A). For the triple quadrupole, MS parameters were set as follows: capillary voltage (2.20 kV); extractor (3.0 V) source temperature (150 °C), desolvation temperature (300 °C), cone gas flow (50 l/h), and desolvation gas flow (700 l/h). For quantification, a multiple reaction monitoring method (MRM) was applied. For LAP, the transition of m/z 243 > 187 using cone energy of 24 V and collision energy of 19 V was determined as most appropriate for quantification (Calibration curves between 1 and 20,000 ng/ml of LAP, $R > 0.99$, low quantification limit of 1 ng/ml, and detection limit of 0.1 ng/ml).

Sample preparation for pharmacokinetics studies

A total of 200 µl cold acetonitrile containing internal standard (2-methyl-amino-lapachol) at 5 µg/ml and 0.05% trifluoroacetic acid was added to 100 µl of plasma and vortexed for 20 s. Precipitated protein was removed by centrifugation (6800 × g at 4 °C for 10 min). A total of 200 µl of the supernatant was diluted with purified water 1:1 and filtered by a 0.22-µm membrane before analysis. To prepare the calibration curves, blank plasma samples were spiked with LAP and further processed as indicated. Animal samples with concentrations at the higher upper limit of the calibration curve were diluted with blank plasma before processing.

Enzymatic assay

hDHODH activity was assessed using a colorimetric continuous assay that monitors 2,6-dichloroindophenol (DCIP) reduction. Change in absorbance at 610 nm was monitored over a period of 60 s at 25 °C using a microplate reader (Molecular Devices, SpectraMax 384 Plus, California, USA). The enzymatic reaction was analyzed in a total volume of 195 µl containing 50 mmol/l Tris, pH 8.15, 150 mmol/l KCl, 0.1% Triton X-100, 1 mmol/l L-dihydroorotate, 100 µmol/l CoQ0, and 60 µmol/l DCIP. The assay was started with 5 µl of 0.8 µmol/l stock of enzyme prepared in 50 mmol/l HEPES, pH 7.7, 400 mmol/l NaCl, 10% glycerol, 0.05% Thesit, and 1 mmol/l EDTA in a final concentration of enzyme at 20 nmol/l. A reference measurement was obtained by preparing the same solution without enzyme.

LAP was analyzed in quadruplicate for each concentration used. LAP sodium salt was prepared as a 10 mmol/l stock in DMSO. From this solution, dilutions were prepared in the assay mixture to achieve the range of 100 µmol/l to 0.35 nmol/l. Control enzyme activity in the absence of inhibitor was taken as 100%. The percentage of activity versus log of LAP concentration graph was drawn. The half maximal inhibitory concentration (IC_{50}) values were calculated using a nonlinear fitting of the concentration–response data to the equation:

$$activity\ (\%) = Bottom + \left[\frac{Top{-}Bottom}{10^{\log[I]-\log[IC_{50}]}+1}\right]$$

Animals

Collagen-induced arthritis (CIA) and antigen-induced arthritis (AIA) models were carried out in male DBA1/J mice (10–12 weeks old) and male C57BL/6 mice (6 weeks old), respectively. The mice were bred and housed in the animal facility of the Ribeirão Preto Medical School (FMRP) at University of São Paulo. For the pharmacokinetic studies, male Wistar rats (200–300 g) were purchased from the State Foundation for the Research and Production in Health (FEPPS, Porto Alegre, Brazil). Animals received water and food ad libitum. All protocols were conducted in accordance with ethical guidelines and approved by the Animal Welfare Committee of FMRP and the Federal University of Rio Grande do Sul (Protocols: 53/2013 and 20244, respectively).

Isolation of CD4 T cells

Human CD4 T cells were purified from the whole blood of healthy volunteers. Briefly, peripheral blood mononuclear cells (PBMCs) were isolated by Percoll gradient (Sigma-Aldrich, St. Louis, MO, USA). CD4 T cells were isolated from PBMCs using Isolation Kit (Miltenyi Biotec, Bergisch Gladbach, Germany). For murine CD4 T cells, lymph nodes from naive C57BL/6 male mice were harvested, and CD4 T cells were purified using Isolation Kit (Miltenyi Biotec, Bergisch Gladbach, Germany) according to the manufacturer's recommendations.

Proliferation assay

A total of 1×10^5 CD4 T cells were labeled with 1 μM Dye Efluor® 670 (eBioscience, San Diego, CA, USA) for 15 min at 37 °C and cultured in RPMI-1640 10% FBS for 4 days in a 96-well U-bottom plate (Falcon, Franklin Lakes, New Jersey, USA) with the LAP salt diluted in RPMI-1640 (10, 30, and 100 μM), LEF diluted in RPMI-1640 (10, 30, and 100 μM; Arava®, Sanofi, France) and/or uridine (30, 100, and 300 μM; Sigma-Aldrich, St. Louis, MO, USA) in the presence of anti-CD3 (3 μg/ml) and anti-CD28 (1.5 μg/ml). The proliferation of CD4 T cells was determined by dye dilution in flow cytometry analysis. The results were expressed as the percentage of suppression using the following formula: [proliferation of CD4 T cells only – (proliferation of T CD4 cells with LEF or LAP)/proliferation of CD4 T cells only] × 100.

Collagen-induced arthritis (CIA)

Male DBA/1 J mice were injected i.d. at the base of the tail with 200 μg bovine type II collagen (CII; a gift from Dr. David D. Brand, University of Tennessee Health Science Center) emulsified in Freund's complete adjuvant (CFA) on day 0. Mice were boosted i.d. with CII (200 μg emulsified in Freund's incomplete adjuvant (IFA)) on day 21. Mice were monitored daily for signs of arthritis. Scores were assigned based on erythema, swelling, or ankylosis present in each paw on a scale of 0 to 3, giving a maximum score of 12 per mouse. After arthritis induction, mice were treated orally with LAP (3 mg/kg and 10 mg/kg) or LEF (3 mg/kg) or saline daily. The clinical score was addressed every day after collagen boost. All mice were euthanized for histologic assessment of the hind limbs 4 weeks after the boost.

Histological analysis

Femur-tibial joints were collected 4 weeks after CII boost, fixed in 4% (vol/vol) buffered formalin and decalcified in 10% EDTA for 2–3 weeks. The tissues were then trimmed, dehydrated in ethanol, and embedded in paraffin for the preparation of the slides. Histological assessment was carried out following routine staining. Joint sections were stained with hematoxylin and eosin (H&E) to analyze synovitis (inflammatory cell influx and synovial hyperplasia) or Safranin-O to visualize proteoglycan depletion and cartilage destruction. The severity of the joint damage was scored according to the criteria described by Wang et al. [22]: 0 = no destruction; 1 = minimal erosion; 2 = slight to moderate erosion in a limited area; 3 = more extensive erosion; 4 = general destruction. The degree of synovial pathology (i.e., synovitis) was scored using a scoring system that measured the thickness of the synovial cell layer on a scale of 0–3 (0 = 1–2 cells, 1 = 2–4 cells, 2 = 4–9 cells, and 3 = 10 or more cells) and cellular density in the synovial stroma on a scale of 0–3 (0 = normal cellularity, 1 = slightly increased cellularity, 2 = moderately increased cellularity, and 3 = greatly increased cellularity) [23].

Cytokine quantification

Interleukin (IL)-17 and interferon (IFN)-γ cytokines were measured by enzyme-linked immunosorbent assay (ELISA) from hind paw homogenate of an individual mouse using antibodies according to the manufacturer's instructions (R&D Systems, Minneapolis, MN, USA). The results were expressed as pg of cytokine/mg of tissue.

Myeloperoxidase assay

Myeloperoxidase (MPO) activity in tissue homogenates was used as an index of neutrophil infiltration into paws from CIA mice as previously described [24].

Measurement of liver enzymes

Serum concentrations of aspartate aminotransferase (AST) or alanine aminotransferase (ALT) were measured using commercial kits according to the manufacturer's instructions (ID Labs Biotechnology Inc., London, Canada).

Antigen-induced arthritis (AIA)

Mice were immunized with methylated bovine serum albumin (mBSA; Sigma-Aldrich, St. Louis, MO, USA) as described previously [25]. Briefly, mice were immunized with subcutaneous injection of an emulsion with mBSA (500 μg; Sigma-Aldrich, St. Louis, MO, USA) and CFA (2 mg/ml of inactivated *Mycobacterium tuberculosis*; Sigma-Aldrich, St. Louis, MO, USA). Booster injections of mBSA in IFA were given at 7 and 14 days after the first immunization. On day 21 after the first immunization, arthritis was induced by an intra-articular injection of mBSA (30 μg). During the AIA protocol, LAP (10 mg/kg) or saline (vehicle) was given orally every day from 12 to 21 days after first immunization.

Determination of joint leucocyte infiltration

Leucocyte infiltration into the joints was assessed 6 h after intra-articular challenge with mBSA as previously described [26]. Briefly, articular infiltration of leukocytes was determined by washing the femur-tibial joint three times with 3.3 μl phosphate-buffered aline (PBS) + EDTA (0.2 M) and subsequent cell counting was performed in a Neubauer chamber. The results were expressed as the numbers of leucocyte × 10^4 (mean ± SEM)/joint.

Anti-mBSA antibody titer measurement

The titers of serum anti-mBSA antibody were measured by ELISA as previously described [26].

Recall experiments

Cell suspension (1 × 10^5 cells) of draining lymph nodes (inguinal) and spleen from naive and mBSA-immunized (treated or not with LAP) mice were stimulated in a 96-well round-bottom plate with mBSA (100 μg/ml) for 96 h. Next, the supernatant was collected to measure the levels of IL-17A, IFN-γ, and IL-4 by ELISA (R&D Systems, Minneapolis, MN, USA).

Statistical analysis

Statistical analyses were performed using one-way nonparametric analysis of variance (ANOVA) followed by Bonferroni's t test (for three or more groups) comparing all pairs of columns, or two-tailed Student's t test (for two groups). $P < 0.05$ was considered statistically significant. Statistical analysis was performed with GraphPad Prism (GraphPad Software, San Diego, CA, USA).

Results

Synthesis, molecular modeling, and ability of LAP to inhibit DHODH activity

LAP was synthetized using lawsone as the starting material in a one-pot methodology involving initial Knoevenagel condensation followed by formic acid catalyzed reduction in 78% yield. To increase the solubility of LAP, this naphthoquinone was treated with NaOH for 24 h to afford the LAP sodium salt in 95% yield (Fig. 1a). The structure of the salt was confirmed by ^1H and ^{13}C NMR and high-resolution mass spectrometry. Analysis of the LAP sodium salt stability on plasma and acid media (similar to the stomached conditions) was carried out using ultra-performance liquid-chromatography tandem mass spectrometry (UPLC-MS/MS) and it confirmed the instantaneous conversion of LAP sodium salt into a neutral molecule of LAP. The individual plasma profiles of LAP and LAP sodium salt after intravenous administration were identical and were best described by a two-compartmental open model, with a volume of distribution of 0.19 ± 0.03 l/kg, a total clearance of 0.04 ± 0.01 l/h/kg, and a half-life of 4.1 ± 1.1 h (Additional file 1: Figure S1; Additional file 2: Table S1). Linear pharmacokinetics were observed in the dose range investigated (2–25 mg/kg). Plasma profiles after oral administration of LAP and LAP sodium salt (at two different doses) were best described by the one-compartmental model, with bioavailabilities of 55–77% and 42%, respectively (Additional file 1: Figure S1; Additional file 3: Table S2).

Subsequently, we performed a computational analysis for the LAP molecule to propose a binding model in the active site of human DHODH (hDHODH), using a flexible docking approach implemented in the GOLD software [18]. As a control, we used the crystallographic binding mode of the active metabolite A771726 inside the hDHODH active site (PDB ID:1D3H). The binding model for LAP inside the hDHODH active site, proposed by docking, indicates that the hydrophobic pocket of hDHODH would be able to allow an accommodation of the prenyl (in hydrophobic contact with Phe98) and naphthoquinone moieties (in hydrophobic contact with Val134 and Val143) of LAP (Fig. 1b). Additional hydrogen bonds would be formed between the two carbonyl groups of such an inhibitor and Arg136 and Tyr356 of hDHODH, residues well conserved amongst the mammalian enzymes. The same polar contacts are also observed between these two hDHODH residues and the crystallographic inhibitor A771726 (PDB id: 1D3H) (Additional file 4: Figure S2) [5]. Next, to address whether LAP inhibits the DHODH activity, we carried out a cell-free DHODH activity assay by measuring the reduction of DCIP [12]. The hDHODH activity was significantly inhibited by LAP sodium salt with an IC_{50} value of 0.13 μM (Fig. 1c), indicating that LAP is a potent inhibitor of the hDHODH activity.

LAP inhibits lymphocyte proliferation through inhibition of pyrimidine biosynthesis

We next assessed the antiproliferative effect of LAP. To this end, freshly isolated mouse CD4 T cells were labelled with Dye Efluor 670 and stimulated with anti-CD3/CD28 in the presence of LAP or LEF (10, 30, and 100 μM) for 4 days. As shown in Fig. 2a, LAP or LEF inhibited the proliferation of murine CD4 T cells in a dose-dependent manner. We

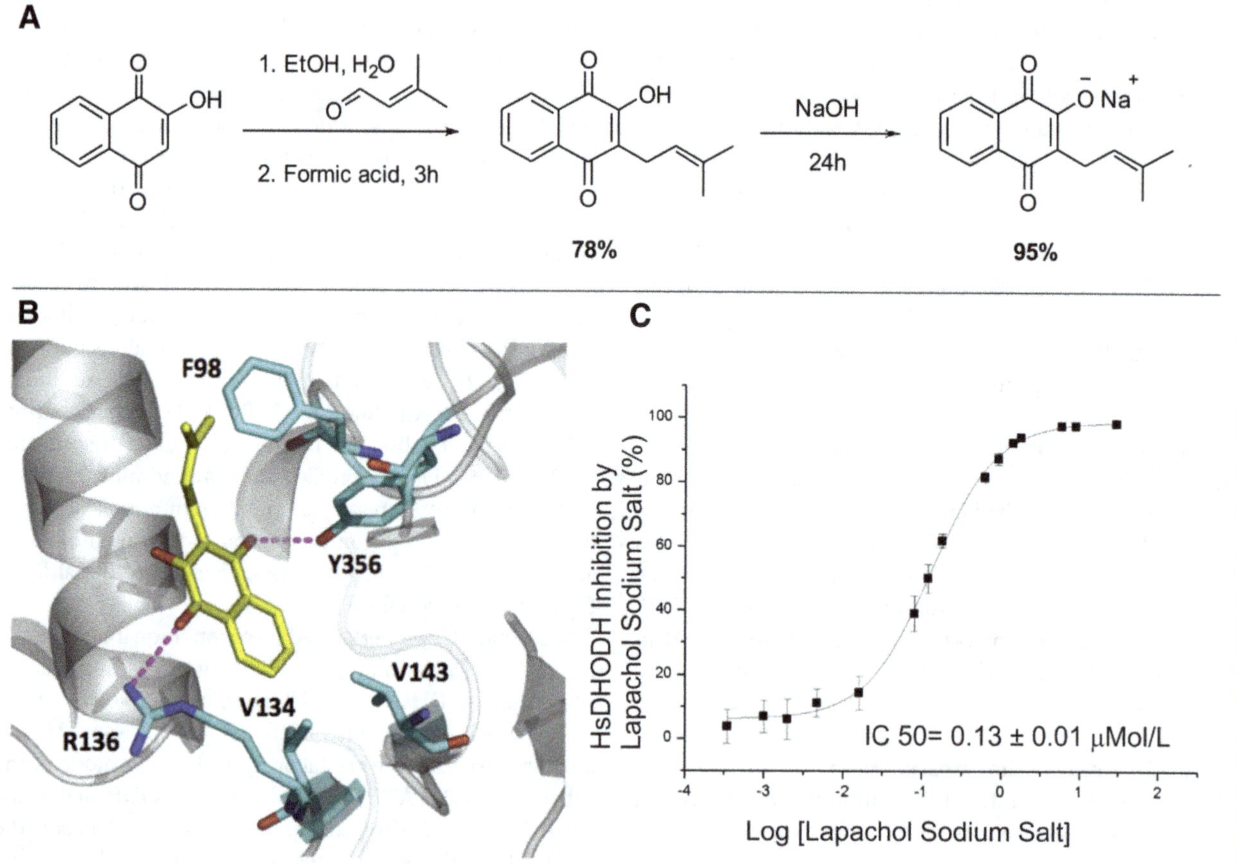

Fig. 1 LAP is a potent inhibitor of DHODH activity. **a** Synthetic strategy for developing LAP sodium salt from lawsone. **b** The top-ranked GOLD solution for LAP is shown inside the hDHODH active site, in hydrophobic and polar contacts with selected residues of the enzyme. Hydrogen bonds are here represented by *dashed magenta lines*. **c** Inhibitory effect of LAP on human dihydroorotate dehydrogenase (*hDHODH*). Half maximal inhibitory concentration (*IC_{50}*) determination of LAP based on DCIP colorimetric assay

also investigated the effect of LAP in human CD4 T cells isolated from the peripheral blood of healthy donors. Similar to that observed with murine cells, we also found a dose-dependent inhibition of human T-cell proliferation in the presence of LAP or LEF (Fig. 2b). However, we found that LAP exhibited a greater ability to suppress the proliferation of human and murine CD4 T cells than was observed with LEF at the same equivalent concentrations (Fig. 2a and b). Additionally, we performed annexin-V/propidium iodide (PI) staining of human CD4 T cells treated with LAP or LEF to assess apoptotic cell death. While LEF showed no toxic effects at all concentrations, flow cytometric analysis revealed that only the highest concentration of LAP (100 μM) was toxic (Additional file 5: Table S3). Thus, the reduction of T-cell proliferation by LAP below 100 μM was primarily due to inhibition of the proliferative response rather than a reduction of cellular viability by toxicity.

The antiproliferative effect of LEF is completely reversed by supplementation of uridine, supporting that DHODH is the target for LEF [4]. We then investigated whether the antiproliferative effect of LAP is also due to targeting DHODH. To this end, human CD4 T cells were pretreated with LAP in the presence of different concentrations of uridine. As shown in Fig. 2c, uridine was able to reverse the antiproliferative effect of LAP in a dose-dependent manner. Of note, uridine alone had a minimal effect on the proliferative response of anti-CD3-stimulated T cells.

LAP reduces the severity of experimental arthritis

We next examined the therapeutic potential of LAP in two experimental models of arthritis. The first model was collagen-induced arthritis (CIA), a well-established T cell-dependent preclinical model for RA [27]. Treatment with LAP was started just after booster injection with collagen on day 21 after the first immunization. Mice were orally treated with LAP (3 mg/kg and 10 mg/kg) once a day for 4 weeks. LAP was well tolerated without apparent side effects based on observations of the general symptoms of toxicity, including piloerection, diarrhea, weight loss, and prostration. We also found that treatment with LAP did not alter the serum levels of ALT or AST during the CIA protocol (Additional file 6: Figure S3), indicating that it

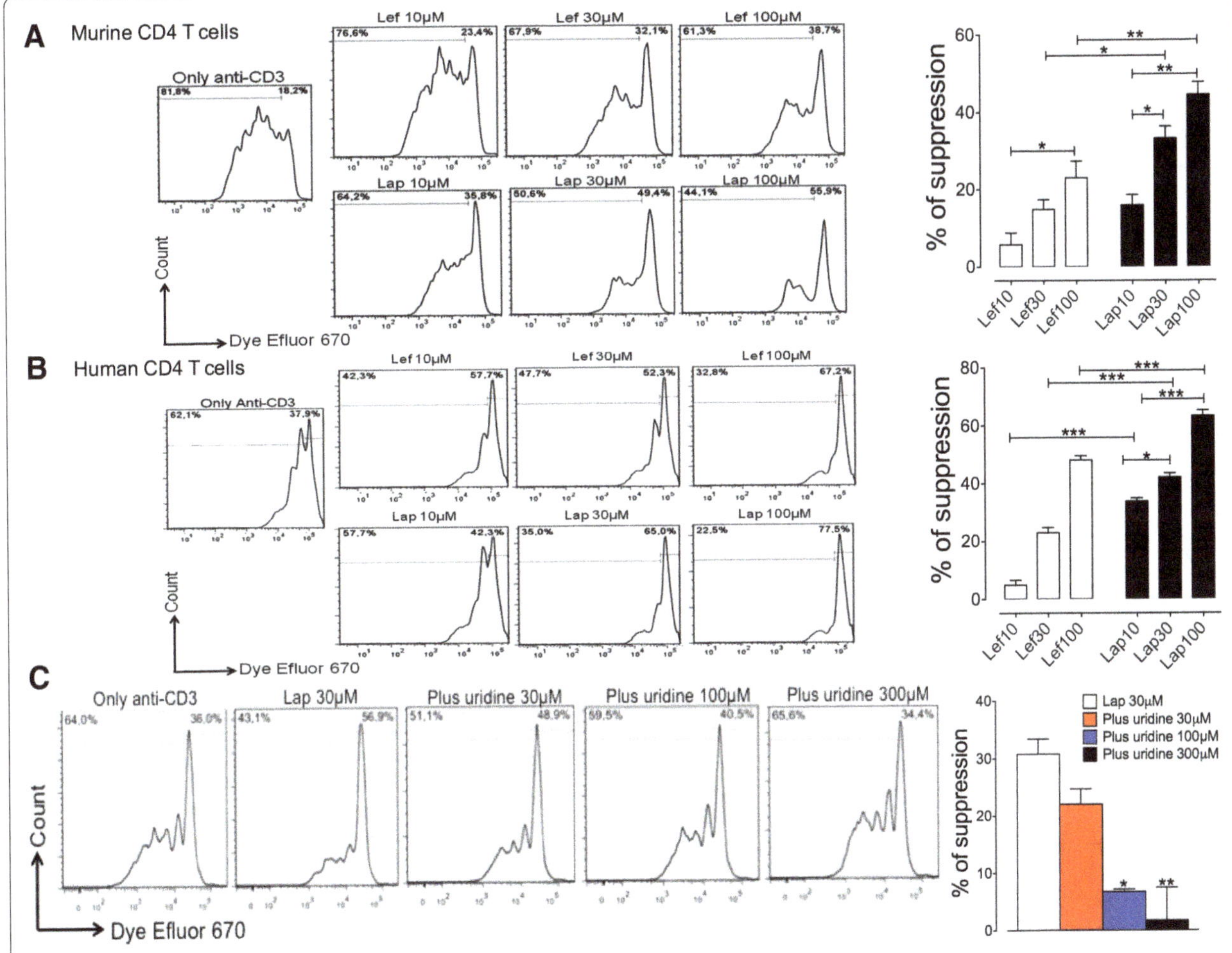

Fig. 2 LAP modulates lymphocyte proliferation in a dependent pyrimidine biosynthesis manner. Murine CD4 T cells were purified from lymph nodes of naive C57BL/6 male mice and labeled with 1 μM Dye Efluor® 670 for 15 min at 37 °C and stimulated for 4 days in the presence of anti-CD3 (3 μg/ml) and anti-CD28 (1.5 μg/ml). Cells were concomitantly incubated in the presence of lapachol (*Lap*) or leflunomide (*Lef*) (10, 30 and 100 μM). **a** The percentage of suppression was assessed by the proliferation of murine CD4 T cells assessing dye dilution in flow cytometry analysis. Human CD4 T cells were purified from blood of healthy volunteers and labeled with 1 μM Dye Efluor® 670 for 15 min at 37 °C and stimulated for 4 days in the presence of anti-CD3 (3 μg/ml) and anti-CD28 (1.5 μg/ml). Cells were concomitantly incubated in the presence of LAP or LEF (10, 30 and 100 μM). **b** The percentage of suppression was assessed by the proliferation of human CD4 T cells assessing dye dilution in flow cytometry analysis. Human CD4 T cells were purified from blood of healthy volunteers and labeled with 1 μM Dye Efluor® 670 for 15 min at 37 °C and stimulated for 4 days in the presence of anti-CD3 (3 μg/ml) and anti-CD28 (1.5 μg/ml). Cells were concomitantly incubated or not with LAP (10, 30, and 100 μM) and/or uridine (30, 100, and 300 μM). **c** The percentage of suppression was assessed by the proliferation of human CD4 T cells assessing dye dilution in flow cytometry analysis. The results were expressed using the following formula: [proliferation of CD4 T cells only – (proliferation of CD4 T cells with LEF or LAP)/proliferation of CD4 T cells only] × 100. Data are shown as mean ± SEM, $n = 5$ per group. $^{*}P < 0.05$, $^{**}P < 0.01$, $^{***}P < 0.001$

was not hepatotoxic at the doses used. As a positive therapeutic control, mice were treated with LEF (3 mg/kg) using the same treatment schedule. The doses of LEF and LAP used in this therapeutic protocol were based on previous reports [28]. Clinical arthritis scores were recorded from booster injection (day 0) and graded on a scale of the magnitude of paw swelling, erythema, and ankylosis (as described in the Methods section). We found that LAP, at both doses used, markedly attenuated the severity of arthritis in CIA mice, similar to those observed in mice treated with LEF, as evidenced by a reduction of clinical score and the number of affected paws (Fig. 3a). Histopathological analysis of knee joint sections from vehicle-treated mice stained with H&E and Safranin-O revealed inflammatory cell infiltration, pannus formation, and cartilage loss when compared to naive mice (Fig. 3b and c). Notably, LAP markedly reduced all histopathological features of arthritis severity when compared to the vehicle-treated group. No significant differences in histopathological features were observed between mice treated with LAP and LEF (Fig. 3b and c). Additionally, we measured the levels of inflammatory cytokines and MPO activity, which indirectly reflects neutrophil infiltration, in the hind paws from CIA mice treated or not with LAP or LEF.

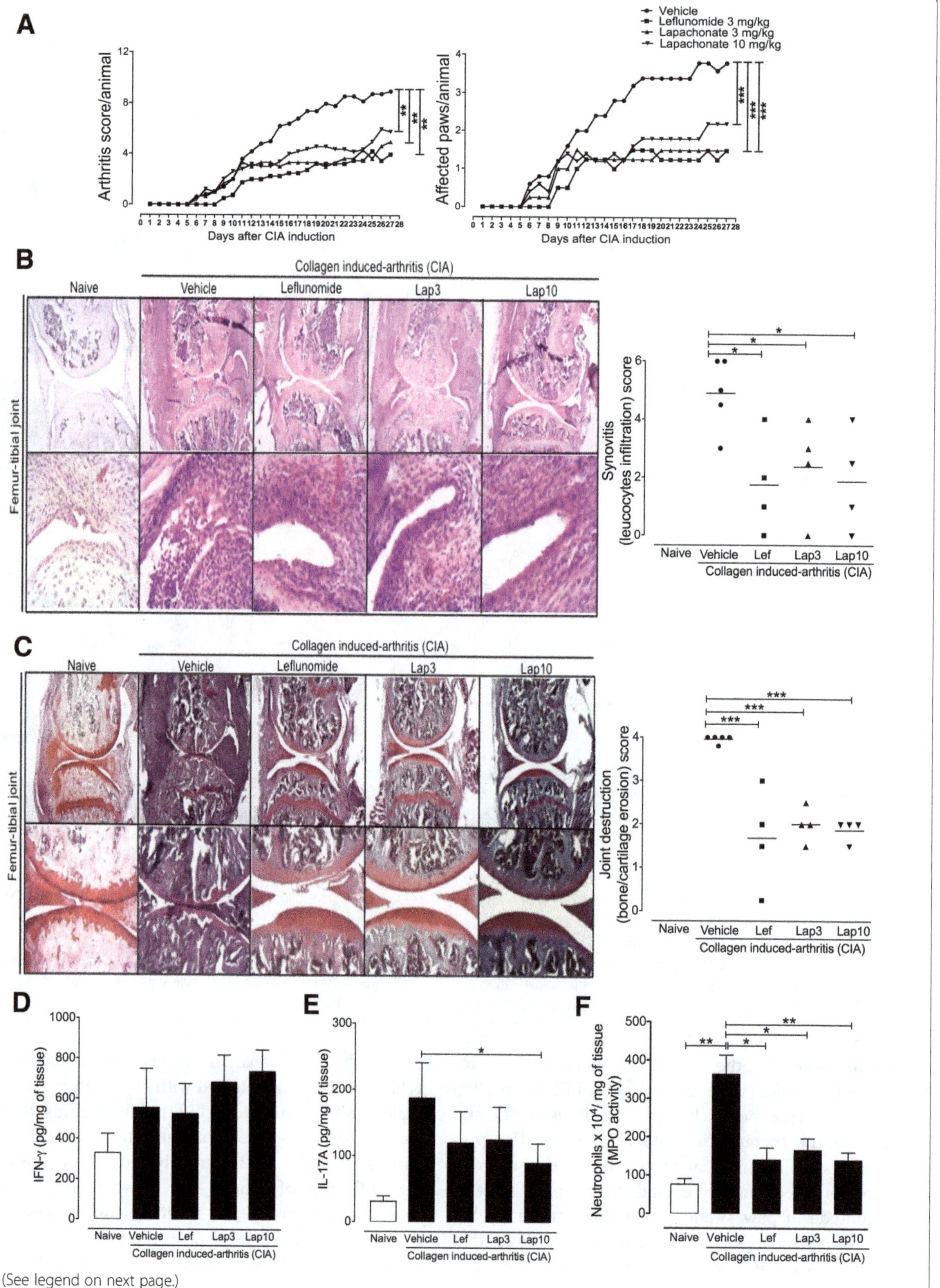

Fig. 3 (See legend on next page.)

(See figure on previous page.)
Fig. 3 Immunomodulatory effects of LAP on collagen-induced arthritis (CIA). DBA1/J male mice were injected i.d. at the base of the tail with 200 μg CII emulsified in CFA on day 0. Mice were boosted i.d. with CII (200 μg emulsified in IFA) on day 21. After arthritis induction, mice were treated orally with lapachol (*Lap*) (3 mg/kg and 10 mg/kg) or leflunomide (*Lef*) (3 mg/kg) or saline daily. **a** Clinical score/mouse (*left panel*) and affected paws/mouse (*right panel*) were addressed daily after arthritis induction. Data represent mean, $n = 5$ mice per group. *$P < 0.05$, **$P < 0.01$, ***$P < 0.001$. **b, c** Histological analysis of CIA mice treated with LAP (3 mg/kg and 10 mg/kg) or LEF (3 mg/kg). Representative images of knee joint sections stained with H&E (**b**) or Safranin-O (**c**) and respective histopathological scores. Magnification for H&E: *upper row* 100×; *lower row* 400×; Safranin-O: *upper row* in 100×; *lower row* in 250×. Data represent mean, $n = 5$ in the vehicle and naive groups, $n = 4$ in Lef, Lap3 and Lap10 groups. *$P < 0.05$, **$P < 0.01$. Production of interferon gamma (*IFN-γ*) (**d**) and interleukin-17A (*IL-17A*) (**e**) tissue levels from paws of CIA mice at 4 weeks after the boost with CII. **f** Myeloperoxidase (*MPO*) activity from paws of CIA mice at 4 weeks after the boost with CII. Data represent mean ± SEM, $n = 5$ mice per group. *$P < 0.05$, **$P < 0.01$

We did not found any significant differences in IFN-γ levels among all groups (Fig. 3d). However, CIA mice treated with LAP with the dose of 10 mg/kg showed a significant reduction in IL-17A levels (Fig. 3e). Moreover, we found that mice treated with LAP or LEF showed reduced MPO activity compared to vehicle-treated CIA mice (Fig. 3e).

Finally, we investigated the immunomodulatory effects of LAP in a second model of experimental arthritis. To this end, we employed the antigen-induced arthritis (AIA) model in C57BL/6 mice, which also requires a T-cell response for the generation of the acute articular inflammation [29]. Briefly, mice were treated orally with LAP (10 mg/kg) once a day over 9 days, beginning 12 days after the first immunization with the antigen mBSA. On day 21 after the first immunization, arthritis was induced by intra-articular injection of mBSA into the knees of immunized mice. We did not find differences in the serum levels of anti-mBSA total IgG between mBSA-immunized mice treated or not (vehicle) with LAP (Additional file 7: Figure S4). However, mice treated with LAP exhibited a remarkable reduction in leucocyte infiltration into the knee joint 6 h after mBSA challenge when compared to vehicle-treated mice (Fig. 4a). We then evaluated the recall responses by cells from mBSA-immunized mice treated or not with LAP. The mBSA-specific production of IL-17 and IFN-γ by draining lymph node cells and splenocytes was significantly reduced in mice treated with LAP (Fig. 4b and c). IL-4 was not detected in the supernatant of stimulated cells (data not shown). Collectively, these findings show the marked immunomodulatory effects of LAP in two models of experimental arthritis.

Discussion

In the present study, we conducted a series of in silico, in vitro and in vivo studies describing the biological activity and pharmacokinetic properties of LAP, which is a novel immunosuppressive drug that attenuates experimental autoimmune arthritis through inhibition of DHODH activity. Firstly, we synthetized LAP and performed chemical modifications to improve its solubility in water. In accordance with a previous report [9], we found that LAP can inhibit the enzymatic activity of hDHODH in vitro. Moreover, we also provided a convincing model for the interaction of LAP with hDHODH by computational docking studies, indicating similar interactions observed with A771726, the active metabolite of LEF. Specifically, the narrow and relatively good hydrophobic pocket of hDHODH allows a suitable accommodation of hydrophobic prenyl and aromatic moieties from LAP. In this case, the analyses predicted a consensual binding mode amongst all the poses calculated for LAP, which additionally interacts by hydrogen bonds with Arg136 and Tyr356 of hDHODH, residues well conserved amongst the mammalian enzymes [5].

LAP is a naturally occurring naphthoquinone that has been reported to exhibit antitumor, anti-inflammatory, and antimicrobial activities, but the molecular mechanism underlining these effects is poorly understood [9–15]. It was previously reported that some naphthoquinones derivatives, including LAP, can inhibit DHODH activity [9], but the biological relevance of this observation was not investigated. DHODH is a mitochondrial enzyme that catalyzes the rate-limiting step of the de novo pyrimidine synthesis [5]. Using lymphocyte proliferation assays, we demonstrated that LAP has a potent immunosuppressive activity on human and murine lymphocytes. Supplementation with uridine, which overcomes the inhibition of pyrimidine synthesis, reversed the antiproliferative activity of LAP on lymphocytes in vitro, demonstrating that the molecular mechanism underlying the antiproliferative effect is mainly due to DHODH inhibition. Importantly, we found that LAP exhibits a greater ability to suppress the proliferation of T cells than observed with LEF in vitro. These results suggest that LAP has immunosuppressive activity on lymphocytes through its direct ability to block DHODH activity and, consequently, inhibit pyrimidine synthesis.

In the pathogenesis of RA, it is well accepted that the influx and proliferation of T cells in the synovial space play a critical role in the articular inflammation and joint destruction [1, 27, 30]. In fact, autoreactive activated T cells in the joint stimulate plasma cells, mast cells, macrophages, and synovial fibroblasts to produce inflammatory mediators, which in turn stimulate matrix degradation [4]. Therefore, compounds that inhibit T-cell proliferation have been introduced into the therapeutic schedule of RA [2]. LEF is a widely used antiproliferative and immunosuppressive drug for treatment of RA that targets DHODH [4]. However, around 30–40% of RA patients do not have an appropriate response to LEF [7]. Thus, identification of new small

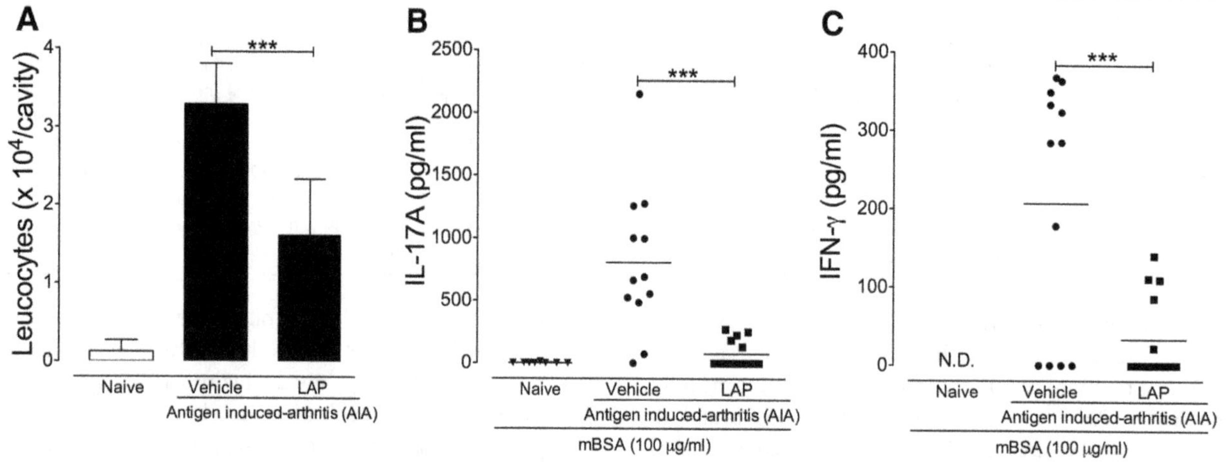

Fig. 4 Immunomodulatory effects of LAP on antigen-induced arthritis (AIA). Methylated bovine serum albumin (*mBSA*)-immunized C57BL/6 mice were treated orally with lapachol (*LAP*) (10 mg/kg) once a day over 9 days, beginning 12 days after the first immunization. On day 21 after the first immunization, mice were challenged with an intra-articular injection of 30 µg mBSA. **a** Leucocyte infiltration into the knee joint analyzed 6 h after mBSA challenge. **b**, **c** A pool of cell suspension of draining lymph nodes (inguinal) and spleen from naive or mBSA-immunized mice treated or not with LAP stimulated with mBSA (100 µg/ml) for 96 h. Production of interleuking-17A (*IL-17A*) (**b**) and interferon gamma (*IFN-γ*) (**c**) by splenic and draining lymph node cells in response to mBSA stimulation measured by ELISA in the culture supernatant. Data represent mean ± SEM, naive ($n = 8$), vehicle ($n = 12$), and LAP ($n = 14$). ***$P < 0.001$. *N.D.* not determined

molecule inhibitors targeting DHODH constitutes an attractive therapeutic approach for RA. Taking into account that LAP shows a great ability to inhibit DHODH in vitro, we hypothesized that LAP could have a therapeutic potential in the context of arthritis by interfering with T-cell proliferation. In accordance with its immunosuppressive activity in vitro, we found that LAP effectively attenuated arthritis development and progression in two well-established T cell-dependent models of autoimmune arthritis. Moreover, mice treated with LAP showed a reduction in joint inflammation and articular damage at similar effectiveness as LEF.

Synovial tissue infiltrating inflammatory cells from RA patients are more resistant to apoptotic events, contributing to their accumulation and, consequently, the persistence of inflammation [31]. The exact mechanism that drives the leucocyte resistance to apoptosis in RA remains unclear, but it is believed that proinflammatory cytokines released in the synovial fluid microenvironment are responsible for this phenomenon [32]. Since LAP is reducing the production of T cell-dependent proinflammatory cytokines in vivo, it could be indirectly interfering with the apoptosis of inflammatory cells. Thus, LAP and its derivate comprise a potential option for the development of novel lead candidates for treating RA based on DHODH inhibition. Indeed, β-lapachone, a closely related secondary metabolite of LAP, is a promising drug candidate currently in Phase II clinical trials for the treatment of cancer based on its ability to inhibit DHODH (ClinicalTrials.gov identifier: nCT01502800; ClinicalTrials.gov identifier: nCT02514031). However, further studies are needed to determine whether LAP will be effective in inhibiting proliferation of T cells from RA patients who show an inadequate response to LEF.

Conclusions

In summary, this study demonstrated that LAP is a novel immunosuppressive drug that attenuates experimental autoimmune arthritis through inhibition of DHODH activity. Therefore, LAP could be considered as a potential immunosuppressive lead candidate with potential therapeutic implications for RA.

Additional files

Additional file 1: Figure S1. Mean concentration–time profiles of lapachol after (A) 2 mg/kg i.v., (B) 10 mg/kg oral, and (C) 25 mg/kg oral administration to rats. Data points are mean ± standard deviation. (PDF 146 kb)

Additional file 2: TableS1. LAP and LAP sodium salt pharmacokinetic parameters determined by noncompartmental and compartmental approaches after i.v. administration of 2 mg/kg in Wistar rats. (PDF 93 kb)

Additional file 3: Table S2. Pharmacokinetic parameters after oral administration of lapachol (10 mg/kg and 25 mg/kg) and LAP sodium salt (30 mg/kg) in Wistar rats. (PDF 79 kb)

Additional file 4: Figure S2. Superimposition of the crystallographic hDHODH inhibitor A771726 (PDB id:1D3H, carbon atoms in cyan) and the top-ranked docking solution (carbon atoms in yellow), inside the active site. (PDF 458 kb)

Additional file 5: Table S3. Evaluation of the toxicity of lapachol in proliferating CD4 T cells. (PDF 224 kb)

Additional file 6: Figure S3. Serum levels of GPT and AST in LAP-treated mice during CIA protocol. (PDF 518 kb)

Additional file 7: Figure S4. Serum titers of anti-mBSA antibodies in LAP-treated mice on antigen-induced arthritis (AIA). (PDF 767 kb)

Abbreviations

AIA: Antigen-induced arthritis; ALT: Alanine aminotransferase; AST: Aspartate aminotransferase; AUC: Area under the curve; CFA: Complete Freund's adjuvant; CIA: Collagen-induced arthritis; CII: Type II collagen; Cmax: Peak plasma concentration; DCIP: 2,6-Dichloroindophenol; DHODH: Dihydroorotate dehydrogenase; DMARD: Disease-modifying antirheumatic drug; DMSO: Dimethyl sulfoxide; EDTA: Ethylenediaminetetraacetic acid; ELISA: Enzyme-linked immunosorbent assay; H&E: Hematoxylin and eosin; hDHODH: Human dihydroorotate dehydrogenase; i.v.: Intravenous; IC_{50}: Half maximal inhibitory concentration; IFA: Incomplete Freund's adjuvant; IFN: Interferon; IL: Interleukin; LAP: Lapachol; LEF: Leflunomide; mBSA: Methylated bovine serum albumin; MPO: Myeloperoxidase; MRT: Mean residence time; MSC: Model selection criterion; NCA: Noncompartmental approach; PBMC: Peripheral blood mononuclear cell; RA: Rheumatoid arthritis; t1/2: Half-life; ULPC-MS/MS: Ultra-performance liquid chromatography tandem mass spectrometry; Vdss: Volume of distribution

Acknowledgements

We thank Daniel Callejon for the help in the pharmacokinetic studies, and Sergio Rosa, Ieda Schivo, Ana Katia Santos, and Giuliana Bertozi for the technical support.

Funding

The research leading to these results received funding from the European Union Seventh Framework Programme (FP7-2007-2013) under grant agreement n° HEALTH-F4-2011-281608 (TIMER), from the São Paulo Research Foundation (FAPESP) under grant agreements n° 2009/54014-7, 2011/1967-0, 2012/25075-0, 2014/50265-3, 2012/20990-2 and 2013/08216-2 (Center for Research in Inflammatory Diseases), and from the University of São Paulo NAP-DIN and NPPNS under grant agreement n° 11.1.21625.01.0 and 2012.1.17587.1.1, respectively.

Authors' contributions

RSP conceived and designed the study, planned and performed in vitro and in vivo experiments, analyzed the data, and drafted the manuscript. GBS planned the experiments and performed the synthesis of LAP sodium salt and revised the manuscript. NTC contributed to the in vitro and in vivo experiments and analyzed the data. VAPJ performed the inhibition assays of DHODH and analyzed the data. MN performed the pharmacokinetic studies and analyzed the data. BGST analyzed the data from the pharmacokinetic experiments. GB performed the pharmacokinetic studies and analyzed the data. CHTPS performed the molecular docking analysis and revised the manuscript. TDC performed the pharmacokinetic studies and revised the manuscript. NPL contributed to the study's conception and performed the pharmacokinetic studies, and revised the manuscript. MCN planned the experiments, performed the inhibition assays of DHODH, and revised the manuscript. FSR performed the blind histopathological analysis, and revised the manuscript. PLJ contributed to the study's conception and revised the manuscript. TMC contributed to the study's conception and revised the manuscript. FQC conceived and designed the study, and drafted the manuscript. FSE conceived and designed the study, and drafted the manuscript. JCAF conceived and designed the study, supervised the study, and drafted the manuscript. All authors read and approved the final manuscript.

Competing interests

The authors declare that they have no competing interests.

Author details

[1]Department of Pharmacology, Ribeirão Preto Medical School, Center of Research in Inflammatory Diseases (CRID), University of São Paulo, Avenida Bandeirantes, 3900, Ribeirão Preto, São Paulo CEP: 14049-900, Brazil. [2]Department of Pharmaceutical Sciences, Faculty of Pharmaceutical Sciences of Ribeirão Preto, University of São Paulo, Avenida do Café s/n, Ribeirão Preto CEP: 14040-903, Brazil. [3]NPPNS, Department of Physics and Chemistry, Faculty of Pharmaceutical Sciences of Ribeirão Preto, University of São Paulo, Avenida do Café s/n, Ribeirão Preto, Brazil. [4]Pharmaceutical Sciences Graduate Program, Faculty of Pharmacy, Federal University of Rio Grande do Sul, Sarmento Leite 521, Porto Alegre, Brazil. [5]Department of Pathology, Ribeirão Preto Medical School, University of São Paulo, Avenida Bandeirantes 3900, Ribeirão Preto, Brazil. [6]Department of Internal Medicine, Ribeirão Preto Medical School, Center of Research in Inflammatory Diseases (CRID), University of São Paulo, Avenida Bandeirantes 3900, Ribeirão Preto, Brazil.

References

1. McInnes IB, Schett G. The pathogenesis of rheumatoid arthritis. N Engl J Med. 2011;365:2205–19.
2. Singh JA, Saag KG, Bridges SL, Akl EA, Bannuru RR, Sullivan MC, et al. 2015 American College of Rheumatology guideline for the treatment of rheumatoid arthritis. Arthritis Rheumatol (Hoboken, NJ). 2016;68:1–26.
3. Smolen JS, Kalden JR, Scott DL, Rozman B, Kvien TK, Larsen A, et al. Efficacy and safety of leflunomide compared with placebo and sulphasalazine in active rheumatoid arthritis: a double-blind, randomised, multicentre trial. European Leflunomide Study Group. Lancet. 1999;353:259–66.
4. Breedveld FC, Dayer JM. Leflunomide: mode of action in the treatment of rheumatoid arthritis. Ann Rheum Dis. 2000;59:841–9.
5. Liu S, Neidhardt EA, Grossman TH, Ocain T, Clardy J. Structures of human dihydroorotate dehydrogenase in complex with antiproliferative agents. Structure. 2000;8:25–33.
6. Singer O, Gibofsky A. Methotrexate versus leflunomide in rheumatoid arthritis: what is new in 2011? Curr Opin Rheumatol. 2011;23:288–92.
7. Emery P, Breedveld FC, Lemmel EM, Kaltwasser JP, Dawes PT, Gömör B, et al. A comparison of the efficacy and safety of leflunomide and methotrexate for the treatment of rheumatoid arthritis. Rheumatology (Oxford). 2000;39:655–65.
8. Hussain H, Krohn K, Ahmad VU, Miana GA, Green IR. Lapachol: an overview. Arkivoc. 2007;2007:145–71.
9. Knecht W, Henseling J, Löffler M. Kinetics of inhibition of human and rat dihydroorotate dehydrogenase by atovaquone, lawsone derivatives, brequinar sodium and polyporic acid. Chem Biol Interact. 2000;124:61–76.
10. Kathawate L, Joshi PV, Dash TK, Pal S, Nikalje M, Weyhermüller T, et al. Reaction between lawsone and aminophenol derivatives: synthesis, characterization, molecular structures and antiproliferative activity. J Mol Struct. 2014;1075:397–405.
11. Oramas-Royo S, Torrejón C, Cuadrado I, Hernández-Molina R, Hortelano S, Estévez-Braun A, et al. Synthesis and cytotoxic activity of metallic complexes of lawsone. Bioorganic Med Chem. 2013;21:2471–7.
12. Baggish AL, Hill DR. Antiparasitic agent atovaquone. Antimicrob. Agents Chemother. 2002;46:1163–73.
13. Duarte DS, Dolabela MF, Salas CE, Raslan DS, Oliveiras AB, Nenninger A, et al. Chemical characterization and biological activity of Macfadyena unguis-cati (Bignoniaceae). J Pharm Pharmacol. 2000;52:347–52.
14. Epifano F, Genovese S, Fiorito S, Mathieu V, Kiss R. Lapachol and its congeners as anticancer agents: a review. Phytochem Rev. 2014;13:37–49.
15. Souza MA, Johann S, dos Santos Lima LAR, Campos FF, Mendes IC, Beraldo H, et al. The antimicrobial activity of lapachol and its thiosemicarbazone and semicarbazone derivatives. Mem Inst Oswaldo Cruz. 2013;108:342–51.
16. Balassiano IT, De Paulo SA, Silva NH, Cabral MC, Carvalho MC. Demonstration of the lapachol as a potential drug for reducing cancer metastasis. Oncol Rep. 2005;13:329–33.
17. Müller K, Sellmer A, Wiegrebe W. Potential antipsoriatic agents: lapacho compounds as potent inhibitors of HaCaT cell growth. J Nat Prod. 1999;62: 1134–6.
18. Verdonk ML, Cole JC, Hartshorn MJ, Murray CW, Taylor RD. Improved protein-ligand docking using GOLD. Proteins Struct Funct Genet. 2003;52: 609–23.
19. Hartshorn MJ, Verdonk ML, Chessari G, Brewerton SC, Mooij WTM, Mortenson PN, et al. Diverse, high-quality test set for the validation of protein-ligand docking performance. J Med Chem. 2007;50:726–41.
20. Maeda M, Murakami M, Takegami T, Ota T. Promotion or suppression of experimental metastasis of B16 melanoma cells after oral administration of lapachol. Toxicol Appl Pharmacol. 2008;229:232–8.
21. FDA Guidance for industry, bioanalytical method validation US Department of Health and Human Services Food and Drug Administration, Center for Drug Evaluation and Research (CDER), 2001.

22. Wang YZ, Sun SQ, Zhou YB. Extract of the dried heartwood of Caesalpinia sappan L. attenuates collagen-induced arthritis. J Ethnopharmacol. 2011;136: 271–8.
23. Lewis JS, Hembree WC, Furman BD, Tippets L, Cattel D, Huebner JL, et al. Acute joint pathology and synovial inflammation is associated with increased intra-articular fracture severity in the mouse knee. Osteoarthr Cartil. 2011;19:864–73.
24. Moreno SE, Alves-Filho JC, Bertozi G, Alfaya TM, Theze J, Ferreira SH, et al. Systemic administration of interleukin-2 inhibits inflammatory neutrophil migration: role of nitric oxide. Br J Pharmacol. 2006;148:1060–6.
25. Veras FP, Peres RS, Saraiva ALL, Pinto LG, Louzada-Junior P, Cunha TM, et al. Fructose 1,6-bisphosphate, a high-energy intermediate of glycolysis, attenuates experimental arthritis by activating anti-inflammatory adenosinergic pathway. Sci Rep. 2015;5:15171.
26. Pinto LG, Talbot J, Peres RS, Franca RF, Ferreira SH, Ryffel B, et al. Joint production of IL-22 participates in the initial phase of antigen-induced arthritis through IL-1beta production. Arthritis Res Ther. 2015;17:235.
27. Brand DD, Latham KA, Rosloniec EF. Collagen-induced arthritis. Nat Protoc. 2007;2:1269–75.
28. Yamaguchi T, Kakefuda R, Tanimoto A, Watanabe Y, Tajima N. Suppressive effect of an orally active MEK1/2 inhibitor in two different animal models for rheumatoid arthritis: a comparison with leflunomide. Inflamm Res. 2012; 61:445–54.
29. Asquith MJ, Boulard O, Powrie F, Maloy KJ. Pathogenic and protective roles of MyD88 in leukocytes and epithelial cells in mouse models of inflammatory bowel disease. Gastroenterology. 2010;139:519–529.
30. McInnes IB, Schett G. Cytokines in the pathogenesis of rheumatoid arthritis. Nat Rev Immunol. 2007;7:429–42.
31. Raza K, Scheel-Toellner D, Lee C-Y, Pilling D, Curnow SJ, Falciani F, et al. Synovial fluid leukocyte apoptosis is inhibited in patients with very early rheumatoid arthritis. Arthritis Res Ther. 2006;8:1–7.
32. Ottonello L, Frumento G, Arduino N, Bertolotto M, Mancini M, Sottofattori E, et al. Delayed neutrophil apoptosis induced by synovial fluid in rheumatoid arthritis: role of cytokines, estrogens, and adenosine. Ann N Y Acad Sci. 2002;966:226–31.

19

Development of three-dimensional prints of arthritic joints for supporting patients' awareness to structural damage

Arnd Kleyer[1], Laura Beyer[1†], Christoph Simon[1†], Fabian Stemmler[1], Matthias Englbrecht[1], Christian Beyer[1], Jürgen Rech[1], Bernhard Manger[1], Gerhard Krönke[1], Georg Schett[1] and Axel J. Hueber[1,2*]

Abstract

Background: Rheumatoid arthritis (RA) and psoriatic arthritis (PsA) result in severe joint destruction and functional disability if left untreated. We aim to develop tools that help patients with RA and PsA to understand and experience the impact of inflammatory joint disease on the integrity of their (juxta-articular) bone and increase adherence to medical treatment. In this study, we used high-resolution peripheral quantitative computed tomography (HR-pQCT) to develop 3D prototypes of patients' finger joints.

Methods: HR-pQCT (XtremeCT, Scanco) measurements were performed in healthy individuals and patients with inflammatory joint disease, followed by a 3D print using the objet30 printer. Healthy participants (n = 10), and patients (n = 15 with RA and 15 with PsA) underwent a detailed, standardized interview with demonstration of printed joints.

Results: Utilizing HR-pQCT images of metacarpophalangeal (MCP) heads, high quality and exact 3D prints as prototypes were created. Erosions in different sizes and the trabecular network printed in detail were visualized, demonstrating structural reduction in arthritic vs. healthy bone. After demonstration of 3D prints (healthy vs. erosive joint, visual and haptic) 26/39 (66%) participants (including healthy volunteers) were deeply affected, often quoting "shock". Of the patients with RA and PsA, 13/15 (86%) and 11/15 (73%), respectively, stated that they would rethink their attitude to medication adherence. More importantly, 21/24 patients with RA or PsA (87.5%) expressed that they would have wished to see such 3D prints during their first disease-specific conversations.

Conclusion: Using arthro-haptic 3D printed prototypes of joints may help to better understand the impact of inflammatory arthritides on bone integrity and long-term damage.

Keywords: Arthritis, 3D Printing, Adherence, Bone

Background

Rheumatoid arthritis (RA) and psoriatic arthritis (PsA) are inflammatory diseases, which lead to joint destruction and functional disability if not adequately treated [1–3]. In RA, autoantibodies such as rheumatoid factor or anti-citrullinated peptide antibodies (ACPA) are typical serologic findings and are strongly associated with erosive disease [4]. Aside from bone erosion, pathognomonic features of RA comprise articular and periarticular bone loss and loss of trabeculation [5, 6]. In PsA no immune factor has been described yet, and clinically joint-associated bone changes include erosive disease and juxta-articular bone remodeling [2, 7–10].

A panel of highly effective and approved immunosuppressive drugs is available to treat inflammation and to avoid joint damage [3]. Despite these treatment opportunities, recent studies demonstrated poor adherence to these drugs [11, 12]. The reasons for this are multifactorial; however, it is mainly influenced by medical beliefs and lack of understanding of the disease [13]. Current tools for patients comprise leaflets and brochures, digital tools such as apps and website content and patient communities.

* Correspondence: axel.hueber@uk-erlangen.de
†Equal contributors
[1]Department of Internal Medicine 3 – Rheumatology and Immunology, Friedrich-Alexander-University Erlangen-Nürnberg (FAU) and Universitätsklinikum Erlangen, Ulmenweg 18, 91054 Erlangen, Germany
[2]Department of Internal Medicine 3 and Institute for Clinical Immunology, University of Erlangen-Nuremberg, Ulmenweg 18, 90154 Erlangen, Germany

Most of these tools have either not been evaluated scientifically or have not improved adherence when tested in clinical trials [14].

Focusing on the damage induced by inflammatory arthritis, radiographic techniques can be used to visualize bone changes. To date, conventional radiographs of the hands and feet are the gold standard in detecting and monitoring erosions; however, this method captures images only two dimensions and only larger sized erosions are depicted. High-resolution peripheral quantitative computed tomography (HR-pQCT) is approved to determine bone mineral density in human radial and tibial bone [15]. In recent years HR-pQCT has been shown to be a feasible instrument to evaluate bone microstructure such as erosions, osteophytes, articular trabecular network and the cortical border of arthritic finger joints. In contrast to conventional radiographs, HR-pQCT allows three-dimensional visualization of the scanned bone and exact separation of trabecular and cortical bone compartments, at a resolution of 82 μm [6, 16–19]. Generation of computed tomography (CT) images is complex, and not easily usable for day-to-day patient contacts, because 3D features are not available on every desktop computer.

Three-dimensional (3D) printing allows prototyping with almost any material. It is a rapid emerging technology, easy to use and quickly accessible. Different printing methods are available, with main principles in common: the generation of a 3D printed prototype model on the basis of a computer-aided design (CAD) model is transformed into a standard triangulation language (STL) file and after transfer to the 3D printer is printed by either polyjet, stereolithography or other procedures [20]. Different materials such as plastic or metal can be used. So far, medical approaches to 3D printing include planning for surgery, implant devices and bioprinting of tissue structures [21–24].

In this experimental study, we tested (1) the feasibility to generate exact 3D printed prototypes of arthritic and healthy joints from cross-sectional HR-pQCT data and in longitudinal HR-pQCT of a patient with RA, captured in a video to explain the development of erosion, and (2) whether patients accept such prototypes and if these lead to improvement in understanding disease.

Methods

Patient characteristics and image selection

HR-pQCT (XtremeCT, Scanco) measurements were performed as previously described in other studies [5, 6]. For 3D printing we selected images of healthy individuals and patients with RA at different stages of disease ranging from erosive, destructive disease to non-erosive bone alterations. To explain the course of different types of bone erosions we chose a female, ACPA-positive patient with RA, treated with a biologic disease-modifying antirheumatic drug (DMARD). To test the acceptance and understanding of printed joints in interviews, 40 people were selected comprising 10 healthy participants, 15 patients with RA and 15 patients with PsA. All datasets were pseudonymized.

Three-dimensional printing of joints from HR-pQCT data

For 3D printing we chose the objet30 Printer from Stratasys due to its extraordinary resolution at 24 μm. As the data source for our concept models we chose HR-pQCT (Xtreme CT, Scanco) images of the metacarpal heads. In contrast to magnetic resonance imaging (MRI), HR-pQCT acquires images at a much higher resolution and depicts bone microstructure [19]. Furthermore, compared to clinical CT the radiation dose is considerably lower. After motion grade assessment using sixfold zoom of the head of the metacarpophalangeal (MCP) joint the respective bone area was contoured and segmented. The segmented bone was used as the source for STL file creation with SCANCO software. Files were exported and repaired with Netfabb basic (Ver. 5.2.1) and Meshmixer (Ver. 10.8.126) and a final 3D printable file was generated and sent to the objet30 platform for 3D printing.

Movie production

For visualization of erosions and cystic structures that develop during the course of disease one ACPA-positive female patient (50 years of age) with RA was selected with a dataset covering 2 years of disease duration. The cystic erosive structure was artificially cut in a sagittal section using Netfabb basic (Ver. 5.2.1) and Meshmixer (Ver. 10.8.126) software. The video file was captured using the Canon EOS 5D Mark 3 and Canon EOS 650D and was modified using Adobe Premiere CC 2014.

Interview study design

To study the acceptance of 3D prints, 10 healthy participants (HP) (6 women and 4 men, average age 43.6 years), 15 patients with RA (11 women and 4 men, average age 56 years, average disease duration 14.3 years) and 15 patients with PsA (9 women and 6 men, average age 50 years, average disease duration 11.9 years, all of a Caucasian ethnic background) were interviewed. Healthy participants were informed about the diseases, using a national society brochure about arthritis.

The interviews were held in German, were audio-recorded, transcribed verbatim, translated into English and analyzed (for the complete interview guideline see Additional file 1). Interviews lasted about 10 to 20 minutes and were guided by an interview schedule developed in collaboration with a psychologist. Questions explored participants' opinions of therapy methods and their reactions to the demonstration of a 3D printed prototype of an erosive MCP joint (Figs. 1 and 2). The joints were also demonstrated as pictures, to allow a comparison. A detailed explanation of the joints

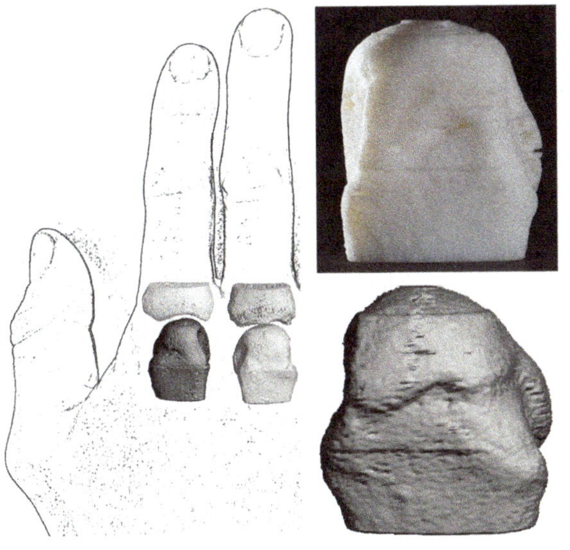

Fig. 1 Three-dimensional (3D) model prototype of the second metacarpophalangeal (MCP2) joint. Anatomical structure of MCP joints is depicted (*left panel*). *Lower right panel* demonstrates high-resolution peripheral quantitative computed tomography 3D reconstruction of a healthy MCP2 joint. *Upper right panel* 3D high-resolution model printed using a polyjet procedure (objet30, Stratasys)

was given to every participant afterwards. The coded interview data were analyzed using NVivo10 software.

Results

From CT images to production of 3D printed prototypes of finger joints

HR-pQCT images of a healthy intact second MCP (MCP2) head and arthritic joints in ACPA-positive patients with RA (n = 25) were used for prototype establishment. Following file repair, a high-quality and exact 3D model was created (Fig. 1, healthy joint).

For better visualization we chose an enlargement of 3:1 compared to the source data. Figure 2 displays representative printouts of MCP2 heads in three different angles (dorsal/radial/trabecular) in three different patients with pathognomonic bone alterations, for arthritic joints. Different-sized erosions and the trabecular network were visualized in detail, demonstrating a massive structural reduction in arthritic vs. healthy bone. A distinct pattern of localization was detected in erosions. The erosions were mainly found at a region close beneath the radial/ulnar or dorsal cartilage area (Fig. 2). No erosions were identified at the palmar location.

Motional visualization of erosive disease

Examining changes in the progression of disease is pivotal for understanding the pathogenesis of RA. Using longitudinal follow-up scans of the MCP joints, we observed the development of erosion in a representative patient. Artificial truncation through a cystic structure that defined erosion that was yet to develop separated the MCP head into two parts. This was 3D-printed for demonstration (Fig. 3) and filmed for motional visualization (Additional file 2). Interestingly, the print depicted two types of erosion. A dorsal porous structured cortical defect with irregularly shaped borders depicted erosion that usually could not be detected on conventional radiographs. In addition, a cystic structure that was also detected by MRI showed contrast enhancement (Fig. 3). At 2-year follow up the cystic structure contained new erosion; however, the borders showed signs of thickening. Thus, this video presented an illustration that was close to reality, of an arthro-haptic experience with a focus on joint architecture and bone changes over time.

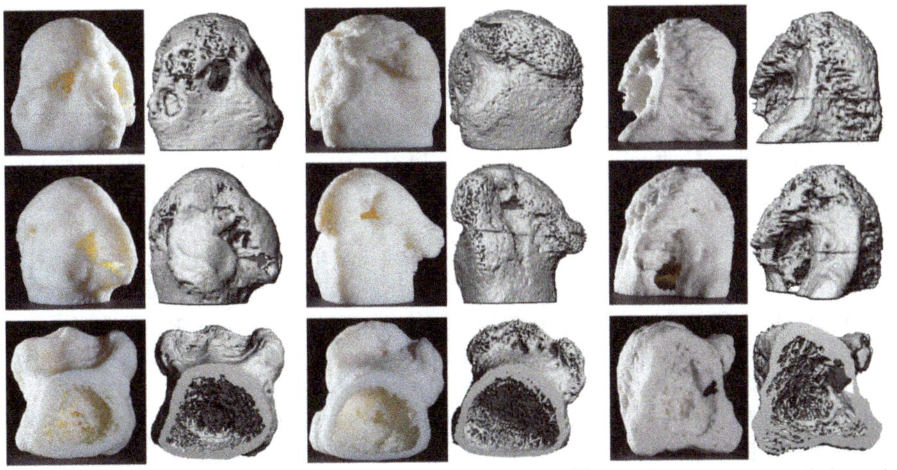

Fig. 2 Three-dimensional (3D) visualization of rheumatoid arthritis pathological change. Three individual metacarpophalangeal (MCP) heads in patients with rheumatoid arthritis are presented demonstrating erosive disease and osteophytes (*left, middle, right panel*). Further, loss of trabecular structure (*middle panel, bottom row*) and increased porosity are visible in all examples (in comparison to Fig. 1). 3D models exactly depict 3D high-resolution peripheral quantitative computed tomography reconstructions

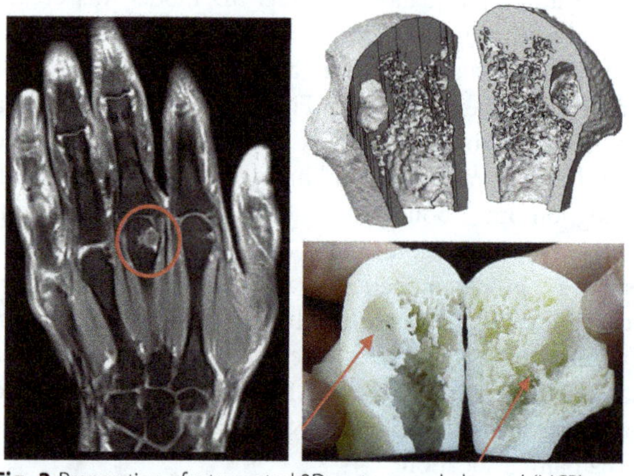

Fig. 3 Preparation of a truncated 3D metacarpophalangeal (MCP) head for video presentation. Magnetic resonance imaging (MRI) shows the cystic structure in the third MCP head in a patient with rheumatoid arthritis (*left panel, red circle*). In a 3D reconstruction this structure was artificially cut to demonstrate the internal bone formation (*right upper panel*). 3D prints of both halves resemble the cystic structure seen on MRI and computed tomography. Bottom *right panel*: *Left red arrow* shows the MRI corresponded cystic structure; right arrow connection tothe trabecular network. Video motion (Additional file 2) illustrates arthro-haptic experience for patient demonstration

Perception of 3D printed prototypes

Following the establishment of 3D prototypes we next sought to understand how implementation of 3D joints can be utilized for patient communication. Qualitative interviews were performed in healthy participants who had been informed about inflammatory joint disease. In this setting, this small sample simulates newly diagnosed patients.

After 3D demonstration (healthy joint vs. erosive joint, visual and haptic), healthy participants were asked for their emotional opinion. Nine out of ten healthy participants were deeply affected, often quoting "shock". Although they had been well-informed earlier, participants did not expect such an impressive impact of the demonstration (Table 1, quotes 1-5). Nevertheless, the demonstration was appreciated by 8 out of 10 participants (Table 1, quotes 6-8). One participant said that it might be too much of a shock and that a series of 3D printed prototypes with more intermediate versions could be superior (Table 1, quote 9).

Questioned about the difference between a 3D model and a computer animation, 9 out of 10 participants stated that they preferred the 3D model. Also the haptic demonstration was more concrete and seemed to emotionally affect participants on a larger scale. The less fictional 3D model could be advantageous, especially for older patients (Table 1, quotes 10-12). When questioned about their preference for either individual 3D joints or a representative model, 6 out of 10 participants expressed a preference for use of their own joints, while 2 participants were indifferent and 2 participants said that an example would be sufficient.

M-any patients with arthritis (19/30 (63%)) reported that they were shocked at the time of the first diagnosis and that the disease severely influenced their lives (Table 1, quotes 1-3). Being confronted with the 3D printed prototype, more than half of the patients were also deeply affected (17/29 (58.6%)), whereas another 7/29 (24%) valued the illustration demonstrated. Although most of them had seen schematic pictures of joint disease before, the direct comparison between the healthy and the erosive model, and the haptic experience, had an emotional impact on most of the patients (Table 1, quotes 4-8). Following the feedback from healthy participants on the advantages of a 3D model series (addition of an intermediate erosive disease model to the healthy and very erosive disease model), 11/11 patients with RA and 9/12 (75%) patients with PsA believed that a series of three models would have better effects (Table 1, quotes 9-10).

Comparing the difference between a 3D model and a computer animation, participants clearly preferred the 3D model (12/15 (80%) of the patients with RA and 10/15 (66%) of the patients with PsA) (Table 1, quotes 11-14). The possibility of touching the models, feeling the erosions and being able to turn it, was very important for internalization according to 22/30 (73%) patients (quotes 13, 14): 8/15 (53.3%) of the patients with RA and 8/12 (66.6%) of the patients with PsA indicated they would appreciate seeing their own joint as a 3D model. Some emphasized that it might increase adherence, as patients are personally confronted (Table 1, quote 15). Of the patients with RA, 13/15 (86%) and 11/15 (73%) of the patients with PsA stated that they would rethink their attitude to medication adherence after being confronted with the 3D printed prototypes (Table 1, quotes 16-18). More importantly, 21/24 (87.5%) of patients with RA or PsA said that they would have wished to see such 3D prints during their first disease-specific conversations. Thus, these interviews endorse the use of 3D prints for patient information and could have an impact on medication adherence.

Discussion

In this study, we introduced 3D printing in the context of rheumatology and inflammatory arthritis. First, we demonstrated the feasibility of bone prototyping using the combination of HR-pQCT and a desktop 3D printer. We created individual joint models with an extremely high resolution, which depict the trabecular network and erosive changes. Second, we demonstrated erosive change and development of erosions over time. Last, we tested patients' reactions and their views on future use of 3D prints in patient-doctor communication.

In the current study a poly-jet modeling procedure was used. Also stereolithographic 3D printers achieve high-resolution 3D prints in the range of microns (a set of 10 individual joints were printed as proof of concept, data not

Table 1 Selection of representative interview quotes

Healthy group			
Group and theme	Quote number	Participant	Quote
Theme 1: How does it make you feel to see this?			
	1	005	"Seeing the degeneration is frightening."
	2	006	"It shocks. I'd do anything to prevent it from worsening."
	3	005	"It would not scare me off, it would rather wake me up."
	4	009	"It's terrible. It clearly shows that the process is irreversible."
	5	005	"Wow, that's shocking- in some areas there is nothing left of the bone."
Theme 2: What do you think about the demonstration of the healthy and the erosive joint?			
	6	005	"To see it from the inside [...] to realize what it looks like under my skin- it's on the one hand macabre, but [...] it would affect me more and therefore I would not forget my medication. Because I have now seen what could happen to my joints if I don't do anything about it."
	7	006	"You know, sometimes it's difficult for us as ordinary people to understand what the doctor is trying to tell you. But with this model-it's the same thing with a car crash: when I see where the damage is, I can come up with something to fix it. I know what to do, how to repair it. Having seen this damage (because of RA and PsA) and the doctor telling me what to do about it- it's just obvious and not anonymous anymore."
	8	013	"The diagnosis scares anyway, so I guess it's better to know what you're dealing with and what might happen. Being left in the dark is even scarier. And since you can't change anything about it anymore, you have to cope with it, if you want to stop it from proceeding. So yes, I would prefer being informed with such a 3D model."
	9	012	"[...] 3 models is a reasonable option, because it shows, that one hasn't reached the final stage yet, and that one can still do something about it."
Theme 3: What would be the difference between a computer animation or a 3D model?			
	10	006	"It's (the 3D model) more real, not as abstract"
	11	012	"I think that some people don't take their medication, because they don't understand it, they don't have a relation to it and I am sure, that this 3D model could somehow reach patients easier than the more distanced computer animation."
	12	011	"I believe that especially older patients, who don't deal with computers that often, might prefer the 3D model."

Table 1 Selection of representative interview quotes *(Continued)*

Patient group			
Group and theme	Quotation number	Patient number	Quote
Theme 1: What did the diagnosis mean for you?			
	1	2.0	"It was a shock. Embarrassing, that everybody could see the dandruff. I didn't wear black any longer."
	2	1.1.4	"I try to put my better hand above the distorted fingers on pictures so that not everybody will see it immediately."
	3	2.5	"You're going to laugh, but I was relieved that I finally knew what was going on and a spade was a spade. I was moving like an old man and was simply glad to have found somebody who told me what was happening to me."
Theme 2: "What do you feel like, being confronted with the 3D print model?"			
	4	2.1	"There is always this fear. If I take a look at the degenerated one, I just think-great, if I don't watch out, mine will look exactly as degenerated."
	5	2.2	"I've got to be serious. I didn't think it was that bad."
	6	2.6	"I'm just glad that my joints haven't degenerated as far."
	7	3.3	"I think it might be especially helpful for patients who have just been diagnosed or who would not deal with it reasonably."
	8	2.0	"The 3D model is simply very close. I appreciate that. Seeing this affects, because I know that it could be me and that it might get worse one day."
Theme 3: "Would you prefer a series of 3 models, instead of 2, so that the process could be demonstrated in a more precise way?"			
	9	2.5	"I think this would be great, especially for rather sensitive people, who can be sloppy as well and who could benefit from the demonstration."
	10	1.1.1	"That would be great, because it could wake up, but wouldn't shock too much all the same."
Theme 4: "What would be the difference between a computer animation and the 3D print model?			
	11	2.4	"It is always better to hold something than to see it on pictures only. Especially for older people who don't deal with computers that often."
	12	2.5	"A 3D model is closer [...] and the impression lasts longer. We live in a society that deals a lot with computers and I think we have learnt how to turn out things we don't want to look at. The print is more impressive, more gripping."
	13	2.9	"Reality is always better."
	14	1.4	"It's just a different feeling, I can hold it and feel it."

Table 1 Selection of representative interview quotes *(Continued)*

Theme 5: "Would you prefer being confronted with an example joint or your own joint as a 3D print model?"		
15	2.3	"Seeing my own would motivate me even more. Because I have just seen my very own joint and that is worse than seeing someone else's."
Theme 6: "Could this demonstration increase patients' adherence?"		
16	1.1.6	"I definitely think that [it would be adherence supportive], yes. If I wouldn't already take my medicine, I would by now."
17	1.1.2	"Well, I think if you'd show this to someone, who doesn't know much about medicine, you could [...] make him understand and take the medication to avoid the degeneration."
18	2.6	"Especially if the patient thinks, that the pills are only against the pain and if he doesn't realize what else is going to happen [...], that there is a real, degenerative change in his body and the process is irreversible."

shown). The printing material allowed the creation of very durable samples. Printing took 4 to 8 hours depending on the size of the prototype, the resolution and the type of printer. Although 3D STL file creation of joints was simple due its implementation in the HR-pQCT software, moderate effort was necessary to repair and correct the file for error-free printing. Modern platforms already provide STL files for various objects (e.g. thingiverse.com). Also bones such as the tibia or full hands are available on such systems. However, lack of resolution and pathologic changes negate the utility of the files offered for demonstration.

Theoretically and in practice, other imaging 3D files could also be printed, such as in MRI or 3D ultrasound. Disadvantages are limited resolution (MRI) and lack of intra-osseous structure (ultrasound). Although the technical setup already exists, the realization demands a certain program user skill [25]. We predict that in due course future technical compound and software connections will be able to print different medical 3D imaging files by plug-and-play setups [20]. As a prototype example, we were able to visualize different types of erosions, which cannot be seen on conventional radiographs due to the anatomical distribution and small size. Demonstrating the formation of erosion from an MRI contrast-enhanced cystic structure depicts the power of this approach to exactly localize and quantify newly occurring structural damage in patients with arthritis.

In the patient interviews, the limitation of this study was the lack of comparison of 3D prints with 3D images or computer animations. Although we asked about participants preferences, we did not show the alternatives. Furthermore, we did not include a comparator in this study.

Focusing on feasibility, individualized 3D prints demand the image of the individual patient. HR-pQCT imaging is nearly as cost-intensive as common CT imaging. With the further file correction and print processing this process exceeds the simple presentation of conventional radiography and/or ultrasound.

Another drawback for individualized prints is the limited access to HR-pQCT. However, using showcase 3D prints can provide a cheap solution (approximately 1–10) demonstrating different stages of diseases on representative joint constructs. In this study a qualitative approach was chosen to gather crucial points from the patient's perspective. This limitation of lack of quantifiable data needs to be addressed in further studies. Despite the abstract visualization of enlarged MCP joints, patients recognized the prototypes as bone models and appreciated the added value for future patient-doctor communication. We experienced frequent requests for our 3D models to be used in daily practice after demonstration to rheumatologists.

Conclusions

This manuscript provides a new approach utilizing 3D printing techniques to demonstrate joint disease. Moreover, we were able to prototype reconstructions of early to late-stage destruction of the finger joints. In summary, using individual arthro-haptic joint constructs will address a gap in patient education and disease understanding. In the future, we will set up a platform for downloadable 3D joints for home/office-based printing.

Abbreviations

3D: 3-Dimensional; ACPA: Anti-citrullinated peptide antibodies; CAD: Computer aided design; CT: Computed tomography; HR-pQCT: High-resolution peripheral quantitative computed tomography; MCP: Metacarpophalangeal; MRI: Magnetic resonance imaging; PsA: Psoriatic arthritis; RA: Rheumatoid arthritis; STL: Standard triangulation language

Acknowledgements

Thanks to Patrick Lindner (Spirit Link Medical) and Michael Distler (Fotisto) for support in video and photographic production. We acknowledge support by Deutsche Forschungsgemeinschaft and Friedrich-Alexander-Universität Erlangen-Nürnberg (FAU) within the funding programme Open Access Publishing.

Funding

This study was supported by a conditional grant from Pfizer (WI197606) and the FP7 HEALTH program under the grant agreement FP7-HEALTH-F2-2012-305549 (EUROTEAM).

Authors' contributions

AK, LB, CS, ME, FS, CB and AJH collected the data. AK, LB, CS, JR, BM, GK, GS and AJH analyzed and interpreted the data. AK, CB, GS and AJH prepared and revised the manuscript. AK, ME und AJH designed the study. All authors read and approved the final manuscript.

Competing interests

The authors declare that they have no competing interests.

References

1. McInnes IB, Schett G. The pathogenesis of rheumatoid arthritis. N Engl J Med. 2011;365(23):2205–19.
2. Scarpa R, Ayala F, Caporaso N, Olivieri I. Psoriasis, psoriatic arthritis, or psoriatic disease? J Rheumatol. 2006;33(2):210–2.
3. Smolen JS, Aletaha D, McInnes IB. Rheumatoid arthritis. Lancet (London, England). Lancet. 2016;388(10055):2023-38. doi:10.1016/S0140-6736(16)30173-8. Epub 2016 May 3.
4. Schett G, Gravallese E. Bone erosion in rheumatoid arthritis: mechanisms, diagnosis and treatment. Nat Rev Rheumatol. 2012;8(11):656–64.
5. Kleyer A, Finzel S, Rech J, Manger B, Krieter M, Faustini F, Araujo E, Hueber AJ, Harre U, Engelke K, et al. Bone loss before the clinical onset of rheumatoid arthritis in subjects with anticitrullinated protein antibodies. Ann Rheum Dis. 2014;73(5):854–60.
6. Stach CM, Bauerle M, Englbrecht M, Kronke G, Engelke K, Manger B, Schett G. Periarticular bone structure in rheumatoid arthritis patients and healthy individuals assessed by high-resolution computed tomography. Arthritis Rheum. 2010;62(2):330–9.
7. Conigliaro P, Chimenti MS, Triggianese P, Sunzini F, Novelli L, Perricone C, Perricone R. Autoantibodies in inflammatory arthritis. Autoimmun Rev. 2016; 15(7):673–83.
8. Simon D, Faustini F, Kleyer A, Haschka J, Englbrecht M, Kraus S, Hueber AJ, Kocijan R, Sticherling M, Schett G, et al. Analysis of periarticular bone changes in patients with cutaneous psoriasis without associated psoriatic arthritis. Ann Rheum Dis. 2016;75(4):660–6.
9. Finzel S, Englbrecht M, Engelke K, Stach C, Schett G. A comparative study of periarticular bone lesions in rheumatoid arthritis and psoriatic arthritis. Ann Rheum Dis. 2011;70(1):122–7.
10. Finzel S, Sahinbegovic E, Kocijan R, Engelke K, Englbrecht M, Schett G. Inflammatory bone spur formation in psoriatic arthritis is different from bone spur formation in hand osteoarthritis. Arthritis Rheumatol. 2014;66(11):2968–75.
11. Rauscher V, Englbrecht M, van der Heijde D, Schett G, Hueber AJ. High degree of nonadherence to disease-modifying antirheumatic drugs in patients with rheumatoid arthritis. J Rheumatol. 2015;42(3):386–90.
12. Waimann CA, Marengo MF, de Achaval S, Cox VL, Garcia-Gonzalez A, Reveille JD, Richardson MN, Suarez-Almazor ME. Electronic monitoring of oral therapies in ethnically diverse and economically disadvantaged patients with rheumatoid arthritis: consequences of low adherence. Arthritis Rheum. 2013;65(6):1421–9.
13. Horne R, Chapman SC, Parham R, Freemantle N, Forbes A, Cooper V. Understanding patients' adherence-related beliefs about medicines prescribed for long-term conditions: a meta-analytic review of the Necessity-Concerns Framework. PLoS One. 2013;8(12):e80633.
14. Nieuwlaat R, Wilczynski N, Navarro T, Hobson N, Jeffery R, Keepanasseril A, Agoritsas T, Mistry N, Iorio A, Jack S, et al: Interventions for enhancing medication adherence (Review). Cochrane Db Syst Rev. 2014;(11):CD000011. doi:10.1002/14651858.CD000011.pub4.
15. Boutroy S, Bouxsein ML, Munoz F, Delmas PD. In vivo assessment of trabecular bone microarchitecture by high-resolution peripheral quantitative computed tomography. J Clin Endocrinol Metab. 2005;90(12):6508–15.
16. Fouque-Aubert A, Boutroy S, Marotte H, Vilayphiou N, Bacchetta J, Miossec P, Delmas PD, Chapurlat RD. Assessment of hand bone loss in rheumatoid arthritis by high-resolution peripheral quantitative CT. Ann Rheum Dis. 2010;69(9):1671–6.
17. Feehan L, Buie H, Li L, McKay H. A customized protocol to assess bone quality in the metacarpal head, metacarpal shaft and distal radius: a high resolution peripheral quantitative computed tomography precision study. BMC Musculoskelet Disord. 2013;14:367.
18. Barnabe C, Finzel S, Stok KS, Geusens P. High-resolution peripheral quantitative CT in rheumatology. Nat Rev Rheumatol. 2015;11(2):123.
19. Geusens P, Chapurlat R, Schett G, Ghasem-Zadeh A, Seeman E, de Jong J, van den Bergh J. High-resolution in vivo imaging of bone and joints: a window to microarchitecture. Nat Rev Rheumatol. 2014;10(5):304–13.
20. Chae MP, Rozen WM, McMenamin PG, Findlay MW, Spychal RT, Hunter-Smith DJ. Emerging applications of bedside 3D printing in plastic surgery. Front Surg. 2015;2:25.
21. Arealis G, Nikolaou VS. Bone printing: new frontiers in the treatment of bone defects. Injury. 2015;46 Suppl 8:S20–22.
22. Fedorovich NE, Alblas J, Hennink WE, Oner FC, Dhert WJ. Organ printing: the future of bone regeneration? Trends Biotechnol. 2011;29(12):601–6.
23. Mandrycky C, Wang Z, Kim K, Kim DH. 3D Bioprinting for engineering complex tissues. Biotechnol Adv. 2016;34(4):422–34.
24. Wyatt MC. Custom 3D-printed acetabular implants in hip surgery–innovative breakthrough or expensive bespoke upgrade? Hip Int. 2015;25(4):375–9.
25. Fastermann P. 3D-Druck/Rapid Prototyping. Berlin: Xmediapress Springer-Verlag; 2012.

Circulating and synovial antibody profiling of juvenile arthritis patients by nucleic acid programmable protein arrays

David S Gibson[1,2*†], Ji Qiu[3†], Eliseo A Mendoza[3], Kristi Barker[3], Madeleine E Rooney[1] and Joshua LaBaer[3]

Abstract

Introduction: Juvenile idiopathic arthritis (JIA) is a heterogeneous disease characterized by chronic joint inflammation of unknown cause in children. JIA is an autoimmune disease and small numbers of autoantibodies have been reported in JIA patients. The identification of antibody markers could improve the existing clinical management of patients.

Methods: A pilot study was performed on the application of a high-throughput platform, the nucleic acid programmable protein array (NAPPA), to assess the levels of antibodies present in the systemic circulation and synovial joint of a small cohort of juvenile arthritis patients. Plasma and synovial fluid from 10 JIA patients was screened for antibodies against 768 proteins on NAPPAs.

Results: Quantitative reproducibility of NAPPAs was demonstrated with > 0.95 intra-array and inter-array correlations. A strong correlation was also observed for the levels of antibodies between plasma and synovial fluid across the study cohort (r = 0.96). Differences in the levels of 18 antibodies were revealed between sample types across all patients. Patients were segregated into two clinical subtypes with distinct antibody signatures by unsupervised hierarchical cluster analysis.

Conclusion: The NAPPAs provide a high-throughput quantitatively reproducible platform to screen for disease-specific autoantibodies at the proteome level on a microscope slide. The strong correlation between the circulating antibody levels and those of the inflamed joint represents a novel finding and provides confidence to use plasma for discovery of autoantibodies in JIA, thus circumventing the challenges associated with joint aspiration. We expect that autoantibody profiling of JIA patients on NAPPAs could yield antibody markers that can act as criteria to stratify patients, predict outcomes and understand disease etiology at the molecular level.

Introduction

Juvenile idiopathic arthritis (JIA) is an autoimmune disease and the second most common disease of childhood after diabetes, affecting approximately one in every 1,000 children [1]. JIA consists of a clinically heterogeneous group of arthritic disorders that begin before age 16 years and persist for more than 6 weeks. The cause and pathogenesis of JIA are still poorly understood. Chronic inflammation of joints is the only common denominator for all JIA patients. Of the seven subsets of JIA identified according to the International League Against Rheumatism classification, oligoarticular, extended oligoarticular and polyarticular are the most common [2]. Adverse outcomes can present to varying degrees regardless of the disease subtype [3]. In approximately 25% of children with oligoarticular JIA the disease spreads over time to involve many joints, a condition known as extended oligoarticular disease [4]. A number of major challenges exist in the management of JIA, including a clear and timely diagnosis of JIA, identification of patients at risk of an aggressive disease course, and prediction of response to standard treatment. In overcoming these challenges the central aim is to prevent joint and periarticular damage.

Although clinical manifestations imply the involvement of adaptive immunity in JIA, research into the

* Correspondence: david.gibson@ucdenver.edu
† Contributed equally
[1]Arthritis Research Group, Centre for Infection and Immunity, Health Science Building, Queen's University of Belfast, 97 Lisburn Road, Belfast BT9 7BL, UK
Full list of author information is available at the end of the article

range of autoantigens that drive the humoral response has significantly lagged behind that of genetic analyses. Genetic associations between JIA subtypes and HLA or non-HLA molecules are known to be related to immune response and associated with other autoimmune diseases [5,6]. Autoimmune phenomena such as autoreactive T cells and autoantibodies can be detected readily in most JIA subgroups [7-9]. In contrast to the majority of circulating proteins, autoantibodies are easy to measure, less subject to variation in the blood, remarkably stable in serum samples, and readily detected with well-validated secondary reagents. Autoantibody tests for anti-cyclic citrullinated antibody, rheumatoid factor (RF) and anti-nuclear antigen (ANA) status have been adopted into clinical practice, and their role in diagnosis is well established in adult autoimmune diseases [10].

Autoantibody study in JIA has generally followed in the wake of research into adult rheumatoid arthritis (RA) by testing the performance of RA autoantigen targets in JIA patients. Even though the evidence provided by this approach has been limited, these studies have provided a glimpse of the heterogeneous molecular mechanisms that contribute to the pathogenesis of various subtypes of JIA. The heterogeneity of JIA is exemplified by the fact that findings from RA can only be applied to a few specific subgroups of JIA patients. RF, which has a sensitivity of ~80% in RA, is present only in a small subgroup of patients with polyarticular-onset JIA [11]. The discovery of RA-specific autoantibodies against citrullinated proteins prompted tremendous interest in their performance in JIA patients. Autoantibodies against citrullinated proteins (anti-cyclic citrullinated protein), which are highly specific for RA, can only be detected in RF-positive JIA patients [12,13], but are associated with a higher risk of joint erosion, more aggressive disease and therapeutic resistance [14,15]. Circulating immune complexes containing citrullinated fibrinogen have been identified in only a small subset of JIA patients [16]. Antinuclear antibodies, in contrast, are present in a significant proportion of children with oligoarticular, extended oligoarticular and polyarticular disease, and their presence, to some extent, predicts the development of uveitis.

Although reliable and sensitive, the ELISA is not practical as a high-throughput platform for screening large numbers of autoantibodies. Protein microarrays, on the other hand, provide a multiplexed, high-throughput platform to profile thousands of antibodies in parallel. Despite the potential of harnessing information on the humoral immune response in JIA, protein microarrays have only recently been used to investigate JIA [17]. The current study applies an innovative protein array platform, the nucleic acid programmable protein array (NAPPA), to provide initial evidence of the true variety of autoantibodies present in JIA patients. The NAPPA overcomes some challenges associated with conventional high-density protein arrays in terms of cost and programmability, and makes it possible to screen hundreds of samples for the discovery phase and to design customized arrays for the validation phase [18,19].

As an exploratory study into the autoantibody complement of early-stage juvenile arthritis, the goals were to determine whether NAPPAs are reproducible enough for autoantibody screening of JIA patients, whether plasma can be used in place of synovial fluid to reflect autoantibodies pertinent to joint pathology, and whether distinct autoantibody expression patterns can be observed for specific clinical subtypes. Both plasma and joint (synovial) fluid were therefore analyzed, and results were compared between duplicate spots within individual arrays, within the same sample type across different patients, and between sample types to highlight potential correlations and differences in autoantibody levels. This strategy highlights the performance characteristics and exhibits the inter-sample and intra-sample comparison abilities of the NAPPA platform. Associations with existing clinical decision-making criteria such as C-reactive protein (CRP) and functional ontology of autoantigens with differentially expressed autoantibodies were also explored.

Materials and methods

Patient samples

Ten patients with newly diagnosed untreated JIA according to International League Against Rheumatism criteria entered this study and were followed for 1 year. At the time of initial sampling there were six children with oligoarticular arthritis and four with polyarticular arthritis (three of whom were RF-negative). At 1 year, three oligoarticular cases had been reclassified as having extended oligoarticular JIA. All patients were examined by a consultant rheumatologist (MER), who confirmed their diagnosis. For the purposes of this study, only initial synovial fluids from children with disease duration < 6 months and untreated disease were studied. Arthrocentesis and joint steroid injection were performed according to clinical need.

Clinical details recorded included the subtype of JIA, age, sex, erythrocyte sedimentation rate (ESR) and CRP. Local inflammation was defined both as joint swelling and/or pain and tenderness with a reduced range of movement on physical examination. All synovial fluids were aspirated using an aseptic technique; plasma was obtained at the same visit. Samples were immediately centrifuged (5,000×g, 15 minutes, 4°C), aliquoted and stored (at -80°C) for at least 1 year to allow for clinical reclassification. Medical Ethics Committee approval was obtained for this study at Green Park Healthcare Trust, and patient assent and parent informed consent were given (Office for Research Ethics Committees Northern Ireland 408/03).

Nucleic acid programmable protein array production

A total of 768 sequence-verified full-length human genes in pANT7_cGST or pLDNT7_nFLAG were obtained from the Center for Personalized Diagnostics at the Arizona State University and are publicly available [20]. The 768 genes were selected to reflect a broad variety of physiological and pathological pathways (Tables S1 and S2 in Additional File 1). The high-throughput preparation of high-quality supercoiled DNA for cell-free protein expression was performed as described [19]. Briefly, *Escherichia-coli*-bearing expression plasmids were grown in 1.5 ml terrific broth for 24 hours with appropriate antibiotics. Plasmid DNA was purified with the NucleoPrep II anion exchange resin (Macherey-Nagel Inc., Bethlehem, PA, USA) using a Biomek FX (Beckman Coulter, Inc., Fullerton, CA, USA) automated laboratory workstation. Automated addition of all solutions was accomplished using a Matrix WellMate (Thermo Scientific, Hudson, NH, USA) rapid bulk liquid-dispensing instrument. Purified DNA was precipitated by addition of 0.6 volumes of isopropanol, followed by centrifugation at 5,000 ×*g* for 30 minutes. The DNA pellet was washed with 200 µl of 80% ethanol, centrifuged at 5,000 ×g for 15 minutes, dried and resuspended in deuterated water.

Plasmid DNA was supplemented with capture antibody (50 µg/ml anti-glutathione *S*-transferase (anti-GST) antibody (GE Healthcare Biosciences, Piscataway, NJ, USA) or anti-FLAG antibody (Sigma-Aldrich, St Louis, MO, USA)), protein cross-linker (2 mM BS3; Pierce, Rockford, IL, USA) and BSA (3 mg/ml; Sigma-Aldrich) prior to printing onto the array surface. All samples were printed using a Genetix QArray2 with 300 µm solid tungsten pins on aminosilane-coated glass slides. Arrays were stored in an airtight container at room temperature until use. The printed DNA was transcribed and translated *in situ* using previously published protocols [19]. The quality of DNA printing was assessed by PicoGreen staining (Invitrogen, Carlsbad, CA, USA) and protein expression using anti-GST mAb (Cell Signaling, Danvers, MA, USA) diluted at 1:200.

Detection of sample antibodies

For autoantibody profiling, printed arrays were after expression incubated with plasma or synovial fluid diluted 1:600 in the dilution buffer (5% milk with 0.2% Tween 20 in PBS) at 4°C overnight with gentle mixing. Human antibodies reacting with expressed proteins on array were detected by Cy5-labeled anti-human IgG (Jackson ImmunoResearch Laboratories, West Grove, PA, USA). Slides were scanned with a Tecan powerscanner and the images were quantified using ArrayPro Image analysis software. The highly immunogenic Epstein-Barr virus-derived antigen (Epstein-Barr virus nuclear antigen 1) was included as the positive control antigen. Negative controls included empty vectors and no DNA controls. Registration spots for array alignment were printed purified human IgG proteins.

Differential expression and unsupervised cluster analysis

Ten plasma samples and 10 matched synovial fluid samples from JIA patients were screened on 768 antigens displayed in NAPPA format. The normalized volume for each spot on each array was calculated by first removing the background signal estimated by the first quartile of the nonspots, and then log-transformation of the spot volumes was used to generate normally distributed data. The log-normalized volume was used to compare spot abundance. Differential spot analysis was performed across the two sample types with Prism 5.03 software (GraphPad Software Inc., La Jolla, CA, USA). Each comparison was filtered to find spots having > 1.45-fold change in average normalized volume expression between the sample types.

Expression data were analyzed using Epclust, a generic data clustering, visualization and analysis tool [21]. Unsupervised hierarchical analysis reordered protein expression patterns in an agglomerative fashion, using the unweighted pair-group average with arithmetic mean clustering procedure. Euclidean ranked correlation was the similarity measure used to group or separate the expression data. A heatmap was produced, accompanied by dual dendrograms depicting the extent of similarity between different patients and autoantibody levels in the samples. Information on the functional ontology of target antigens was mined from the UniProt archive version 2011.03.11 [22].

Serine/threonine kinase-10 antibody ELISA

As the NAPPA is a novel platform and is not routinely used for clinical measurements, independent verification of patient antibody levels to a protein randomly selected from Table 1 was performed by ELISA. GST protein fused to the full-length serine/threonine kinase-10 gene was expressed using the rabbit reticulocyte lysates, as above. Serine/threonine kinase-10-GST protein was applied to an anti-GST-coated ELISA plate (GE Biosciences, Pittsburgh, PA, USA) overnight at 4°C. Plates were washed in PBS-0.05% Tween and blocked with PBS-Tween with 2% milk, overnight at 4°C. After washing, the plate was incubated with 1:300 diluted plasma or synovial fluid samples and the presence of autoantibodies against serine/threonine kinase-10 was detected by incubation with horseradish peroxidase-labeled anti-human IgG secondary antibody (Zymax; Invitrogen). Tetramethyl benzidine substrate

Table 1 Autoantibodies differentially expressed between circulation and joint

Expression	Autoantigen	UniProt accession	Gene name	Functional ontology biological process
Higher in PL (> 45%)	C-terminal binding protein 1	Q13363	CTBP1	Differentiation, host-virus interaction, transcription regulation
	Guanine nucleotide binding protein (G protein), alpha 13	Q14344	GNA13	Cellular component movement, platelet activation
	Presenilin associated, rhomboid-like protein	Q9H300	PARL	-
	Trans-2,3-enoyl-CoA reductase	Q9NZ01	GPSN2	Fatty acid biosynthesis, lipid synthesis
	Cas-Br-M (murine) ecotropic retroviral transforming sequence b	Q13191	CBLB	Ubiquitin conjugation pathway
	Abhydrolase domain containing 16A	O95870	BAT5	-
	Tubulin, gamma complex associated protein 3	Q96CW5	TUBGCP3	Microtubule nucleation at the centrosome
	Modulator of apoptosis 1	Q96BY2	MOAP1	Apoptosis
	Family with sequence similarity 76, member B	Q5HYJ3	FAM76B	-
	Thyroid hormone receptor, alpha	P10827	THRA	Nuclear hormone receptor, transcriptional regulation
	Apolipoprotein A-II	P02652	APOA2	Host-virus interaction, lipid transport
	Eyes absent homolog 2 (Drosophila)	O00167	EYA2	DNA damage and repair, transcription regulation
	IL-6 receptor	P08887	IL6R	Regulation of the immune response, acute-phase reactions and hematopoiesis
	G protein-coupled receptor 153	Q6NV75	GPR153	-
	Histone deacetylase 3	O15379	HDAC3	Anti-apoptosis, histone deacetylation, transcriptional regulation
	Actin related protein M1	Q9BYD9	ARPM1	-
	Natural killer cell group 7 sequence	Q16617	NKG7	-
	Mitogen-activated protein kinase kinase 7	O14733	MAP2K7	Activation of JUN kinases
	Ubiquitin-conjugating enzyme E2A (RAD6 homolog)	P49459	UBE2A	DNA damage and repair, ubiquitin conjugation pathway
	v-kit Hardy-Zuckerman 4 feline sarcoma viral oncogene homolog	P10721	KIT	-
	Pleckstrin homology domain containing, family O member 1	Q53GL0	PLEKHO1	Regulation of the actin cytoskeleton
	Adaptor-related protein complex 1, sigma 1 subunit	P61966	AP1S1	Endocytosis, protein transport
	neuregulin 1	Q02297	NRG1	Induces growth and differentiation of epithelial, glial, neuronal and skeletal muscle cells
	Peroxisomal biogenesis factor 5	P50542	PEX5	Protein transport
	Nuclear receptor subfamily 6, group A, member 1	Q15406	NR6A1	Transcriptional regulation, cell proliferation
	Serine/threonine kinase 10	O94804	STK10	Serine and threonine phosphorylation
	Eukaryotic translation initiation factor 1	P41567	EIF1	Protein biosynthesis through ribosomal complexes
	Zinc finger protein 36, C3H type-like 2	P47974	ZFP36L2	Cell proliferation, regulates response to growth factors
	Cartilage oligomeric matrix protein	P49747	COMP	Controls apoptosis and cell adhesion within extracellular matrix
Higher in SF (> 45%)	Actinin, alpha 1	A1L0V1	ACTN1	-
Similar levels in PL and SF (< 10%)	Protein phosphatase 2, catalytic subunit, beta isozyme	P62714	PPP2CB	Protein dephosphorylation

Table 1 Autoantibodies differentially expressed between circulation and joint *(Continued)*

	Peroxisomal biogenesis factor 10	O60683	PEX10	Peroxisome biogenesis
	mitogen-activated protein kinase kinase kinase 7	O43318	MAP3K7	Component of a protein kinase signal transduction cascade; Stimulates NF-κB activation and the p38 mitogen-activated protein kinase pathway
	3-Hydroxy-3-methylglutaryl-CoA synthase 1	Q01581	HMGCS1	Cholesterol, steroin and sterol biosynthesis; lipid synthesis
	TNF receptor-associated protein 1	Q12931	TRAP1	Chaperone that expresses an ATPase activity
	Troponin C type 1 (slow)	P63316	TNNC1	Regulatory protein of striated muscle contraction

Target antigen list of a select group of autoantibodies that were detected either at similar levels or with at least a 45% difference between synovial fluid (SF) and plasma (PL). The majority of the differentially expressed antibodies are raised in plasma; for example, apolipoprotein AII and cartilage oligomeric matrix protein (COMP) [Uniprot:P02652, Uniprot:P49747]. Only actinin alpha I targeted antibodies were detected at higher levels in SF within the 45% difference threshold [Uniprot:A1L0V1]. Six proteins to which mean antibody levels remained static between fluids have also been listed for comparison. The levels of antibodies against these proteins across individual patient samples are shown in Figure 2A and Figure 3C. STK10, serine/threonine kinase-10.

(Dako, Carpinteria, CA, USA) was then added and the reaction stopped with 1 M H_2SO_4. The 450 nm optical density signals were read on a SpectralMax plate reader (Molecular Devices Inc., Sunnyvale, CA, USA). Protein ELISA analyses were performed in duplicate for each of the 10 paired patient fluids. Mean absorbance readings were subjected to paired *t* test analyses to determine the significance of any variation in antibody levels between fluids.

Results

Patients

As measures of the acute-phase reaction, the plasma ESR and CRP reflect the status of patients when samples were collected (Table 2). When patients are ranked from those displaying the lowest levels of inflammation to the highest, two main groups could be defined: low-medium inflammation (Patients O3, E2, P3, O1, E1 and P1); and medium-high inflammation (Patients O2, P4, E3 and P2). With particular relevance to the study aim, one-half of the study patients were positive for routinely measured autoantibodies. RF was detected in only one patient (Patient P2), whereas ANA antibodies were present in four patients (Patients O1, O2, E1 and P4).

Intra-slide precision and inter-sample correlation

In total, 768 antigen NAPPAs were probed with plasma, synovial fluid, and the dilution buffer (to control for detection antibody specificity) (Figure 1A and 1B). Scatter plots of data that illustrate the correlation between duplicate protein antigen spots within the same incubated slide from a single patient for plasma (Patient O1, r = 0.98) and synovial fluid (Patient O1, r = 0.98) are shown in Figure 1C. Correlation values of intra-slide duplicate values for each patient sample (plasma and synovial fluid, n = 20) were plotted to illustrate the precision of measurements across the experiment. An average correlation coefficient of r = 0.98 is observed across all samples (range of r = 0.97 to 0.99) (Figure 1D).

A strong correlation of antibody-antigen spot signals exists between synovial fluid and plasma samples on a patient-by-patient basis. A wider range exists in inter-slide correlations, with an overall trend toward antibody predominance in plasma. Outliers evident within correlations indicate a select group of antibodies that are detected at higher levels in one sample type within specific individuals (that is, Patients O1, O2, P1, P3 and E3; Figure 2A). The overall mean correlation between fluids

Table 2 Patient demographics

Patient	JIA subgroup (at 1 year)	Sex	Age at sample (years)	WBC ($\times 10^6$ cells/l)	ESR (mm/hour)	CRP (mg/l)	RF	ANA titer
O1	Oligoarticular	Male	6.6	8.2	10.0	15.0	Negative	1:80
O2	Oligoarticular	Female	2.5	12.8	37.0	26.0	Negative	1:80
O3	Oligoarticular	Male	8.5	6.6	2.0	6.4	Negative	Negative
E1	Extended Oligoarticular	Female	7.5	9.5	22.0	9.0	Negative	1:80
E2	Extended Oligoarticular	Female	4.7	10.9	10.0	8.4	Negative	Negative
E3	Extended Oligoarticular	Female	11.0	9.1	62.0	66.5	Negative	Negative
P1	Polyarticular	Female	3.2	11.0	31.0	4.0	Negative	Negative
P2	Polyarticular	Female	16.6	11.8	110.0	72.0	231.0	Negative
P3	Polyarticular	Female	2.2	7.5	10.0	8.6	Negative	Negative
P4	Polyarticular	Female	2.6	10.1	45.0	19.1	Negative	1:320

Demographic characteristics and routine laboratory measures of the study subjects. ANA, antinuclear antigen; CRP, C-reactive protein; ESR, erythrocyte sedimentation rate; JIA, juvenile idiopathic arthritis; RF, rheumatoid factor; WBC, white blood cells.

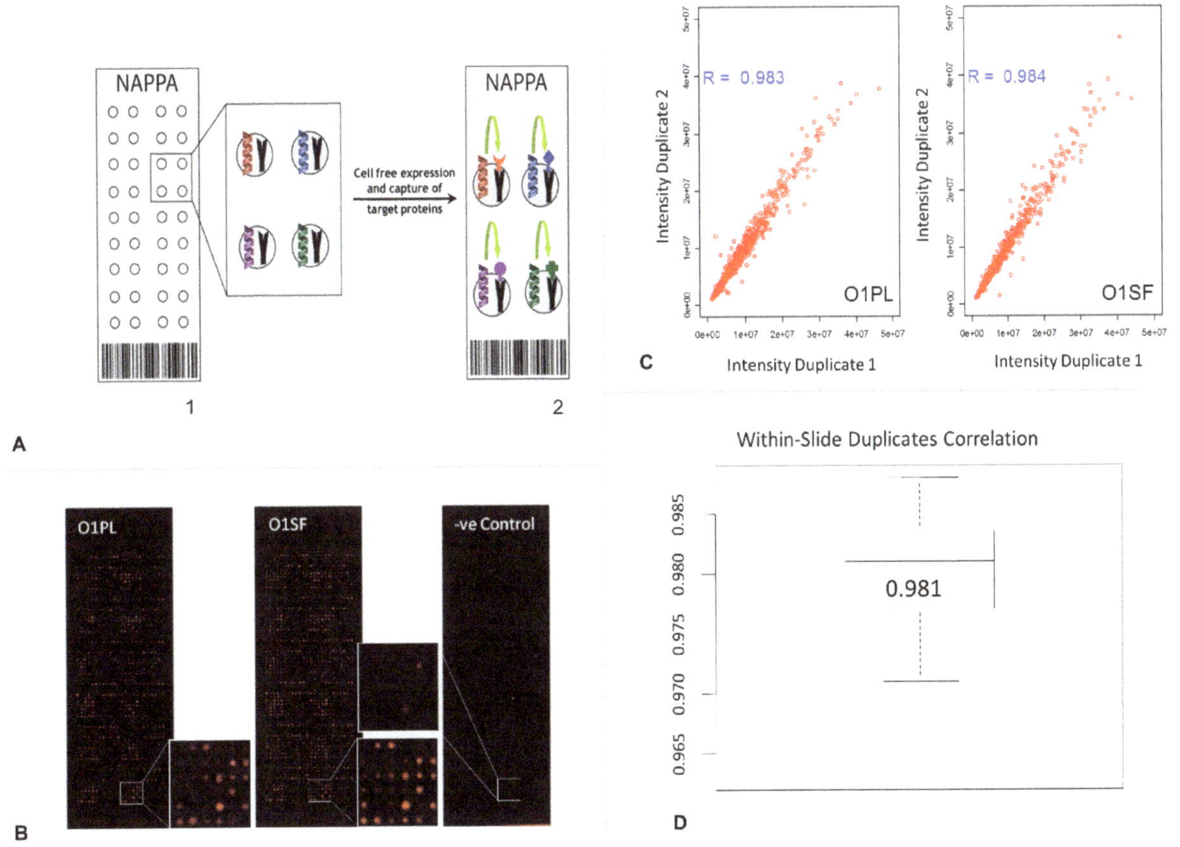

Figure 1 Intra-slide duplicate spot correlation. (A1) Nucleic acid programmable protein array (NAPPA) spotted with genes of interest. **(A2)** All proteins are tagged at the C-terminus to ensure only full-length translated proteins can be captured *in situ* by cospotted anti-tag antibodies. NAPPA has consistent protein amounts displayed at each spot; most are within twofold of the average [18,19]. Proteins are expressed just in time for assay, which eliminates concern of protein stability. **(B)** The 768 antigen NAPPAs incubated with plasma (O1PL), synovial fluid (O1SF) and PBS (to control for detection antibody specificity). Arrays were rinsed and incubated with a fluorophore conjugated anti-human IgG detection antibody, to probe for antigen-bound antibodies originating from the sample. **(C)** Scatter plots of data that illustrate the correlation between duplicate protein antigen spots within the same slide. Correlation of all 768 antigen duplicates from a single patient for plasma (O1PL; $r = 0.983$) and synovial fluid (O1SF; $r = 0.984$) incubated slides. **(D)** Correlation values of intra-slide duplicate values for each patient sample (plasma and synovial fluid, $n = 20$) plotted to illustrate the precision of measurements across the experiment. An average correlation coefficient of $r = 0.981$ is observed across all samples (range of $r = 0.971$ to 0.988). **{Figure 1D needed to be redrawn; please find new image for whole figure}**

across all antibodies detected within all samples is $r = 0.96$ (range of $r = 0.86$ to 0.98; Figure 2B).

Differential expression of antibodies between the circulation and joint

Unsupervised hierarchical cluster analysis of reactivity data against all 768 screened antigens based on the Euclidean distance measure (unweighted pair-group average with arithmetic mean) for both plasma and synovial fluid from all 10 patients revealed distinguishing expression patterns (Figure 3A). Constructed dendrograms for both antibody targets and individual patient samples indicate how the expression levels of proteins that are subject to similar regulatory pathways cluster and how these may relate to clinical subgroups within the study cohort. Tables S3 and S4 in Additional file 1 and Figure S1 in Additional file 2 list the proteins involved in regulating two clusters highlighted in Figure 3A. Cluster 1 proteins are more prevalent in Patients O2, P1, P3 and P4, whereas cluster 2 is elevated across the whole patient cohort. A given transcriptional regulator can impact upon multiple target genes - but it is interesting to note that even though each cluster contains the same number of proteins ($n = 49$), cluster 1 is subject to control by a smaller number ($n = 42$) of transcriptional regulators than those in cluster 2 ($n = 95$).

Patient samples were clustered into two key groupings: low antibody levels (Patients O1, O3, E1, E2, E3 and P3); and high antibody levels (Patients O2, P1, P2 and P4). It is intriguing that three of the four at-risk patients

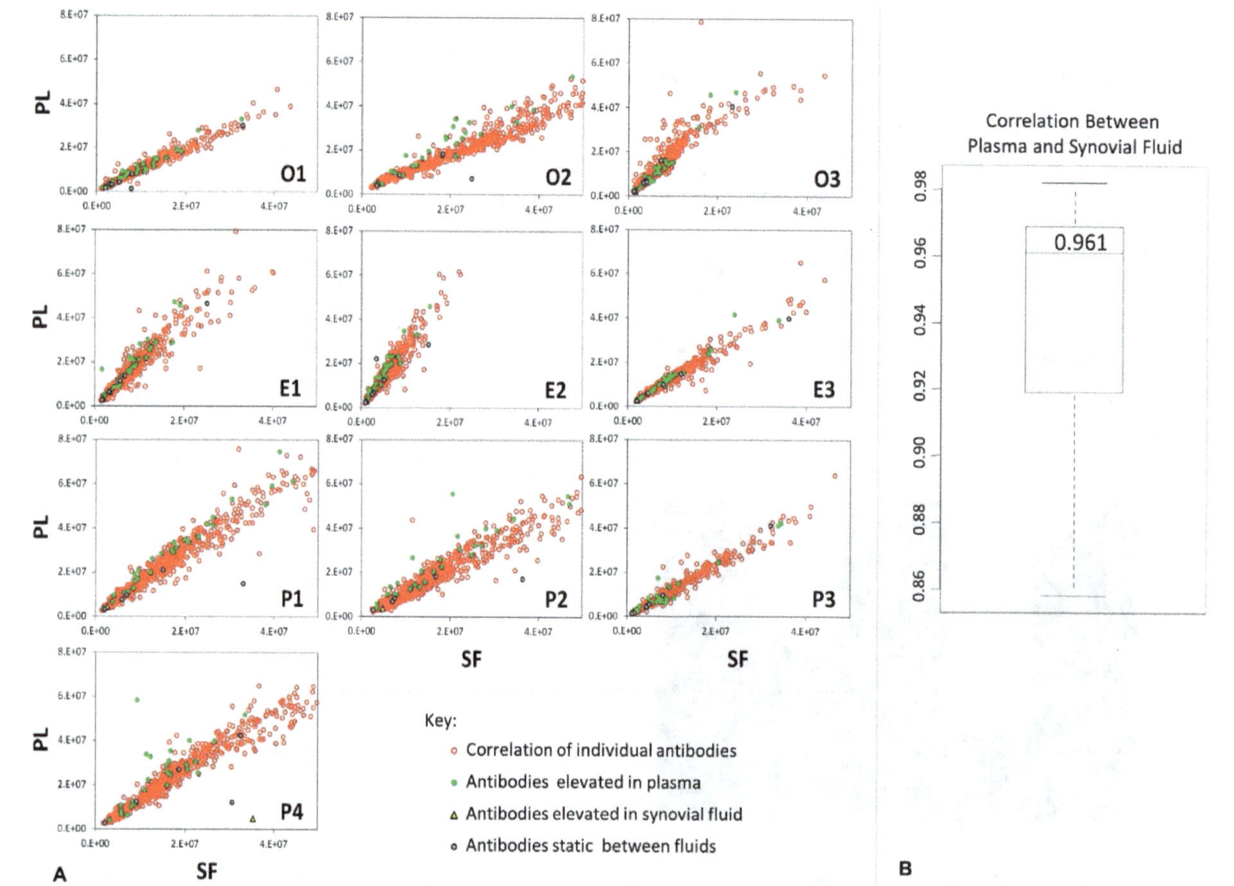

Figure 2 Inter-slide correlation between sample types. (A) Scatter plot correlation of antibody-antigen spot signal intensity between plasma (PL) and synovial fluid (SF) samples on a patient-by-patient basis. Across the study cohort, antibody prevalence in plasma is evident from the increased signal scale. Antibodies detected at ≤45% higher levels within plasma are indicated by green circular markers; those detected at ≤45% higher levels within synovial fluid are indicated by yellow triangular markers; a representative set detected at similar mean levels in both sample types are indicated by black circular markers. This subset of antibody targets is summarized in Table 1. **(B)** Overall mean correlation between fluids across all antibodies detected within all samples is $r = 0.961$ (range of $r = 0.859$ to 0.981).

previously identified with medium to high levels of CRP or ESR (Patients O2, P2 and P4) also cluster independently with high levels of antibodies relative to the remaining patients (Figure 3B). The trends observed do not reach statistical significance by Student's *t* test.

Unsupervised hierarchical cluster analysis of autoantibody levels detected with differences of at least 45% between synovial fluid and plasma is shown in Figure 3C. This difference threshold produced a workable list of 36 antibodies targeting specific antigens (Table 1). The majority of the differentially expressed antibody levels are elevated in plasma - that is, apolipoprotein AII, IL-6 receptor, thyroid hormone receptor alpha and G-protein coupled receptor 153 [Uniprot:P02652, Uniprot:P08887, Uniprot:P10827, Uniprot:Q6NV75]. Only actinin alpha I targeted antibodies were detected at higher levels in synovial fluid within the 45% difference threshold [Uniprot:A1L0V1]. The modest although significant increase in serine/threonine kinase-10 antibodies was independently confirmed by ELISA ($P = 0.038$; Figure 4) [Uniprot:O94804].

Discussion

The production of antibodies against self-antigens (autoantibodies) is a characteristic feature of many autoimmune diseases. At a clinical level, tests for specific autoantibodies - such as ANA positivity - are routinely employed to aid the diagnosis and to track the progress of these diseases. Traditionally, autoantibodies have been identified with a one-antigen-at-a-time, hypothesis-driven approach using methods such as immunofluorescence and ELISA.

In contrast, microarrays provide a particularly effective platform for the systematic study of thousands of proteins in parallel because they are sensitive and require low sample volumes [23,24]. Protein microarrays involve

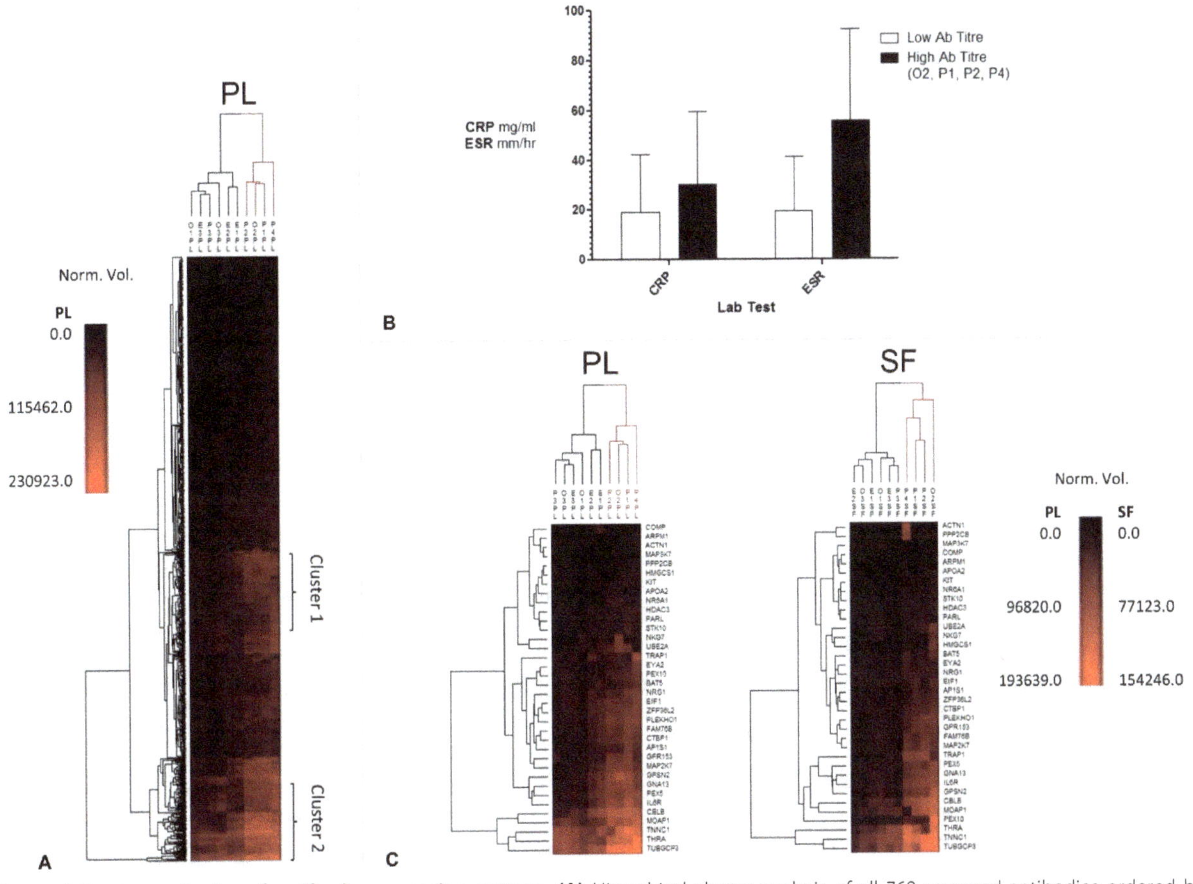

Figure 3 Heatmap display of antibody expression pattern. (A) Hiearchical cluster analysis of all 768 screened antibodies ordered by Euclidean distance measure (unweighted pair-group average with arithmetic mean) for plasma (PL) from all 10 patients, revealing distinguishing expression patterns. The degree of antibody binding is reflected in the color intensity of the heatmap, whereby the more intense the red, the more antibody is bound to a given antigen. Clustering and seriation of both antibody target ID's in rows and individual patient samples in columns segregates the study cohort by antibody expression levels. Two core patient clusters are revealed: lower antibody levels (Patients O1, O3, E1, E2, E3 and P3); and higher antibody levels (Patients O2, P1, P2 and P4) (red in patient sample dendrogram). **(B)** Levels of the conventional laboratory measures C-reactive protein (CRP) and erythrocyte sedimentation rate (ESR) are plotted for the study cohort with patients split into two groups defined above in (A) by low or high antibody levels. Error bars represent standard deviation; no significant difference exists between the two groups. **(C)** Hierarchical cluster analysis of autoantibody levels detected with differences of at least 45% between synovial fluid (SF) and PL. The majority of these antibodies are elevated in plasma relative to synovial fluid.

the display of thousands of different proteins with high spatial density on a microscopic surface. Protein microarrays have been applied to autoimmune biomarker studies focused on presymptomatic screening and diagnosis, clinical outcome prognosis and therapeutic response prediction [25-28]. In the field of autoimmune disorders, conventional printed arrays have been used to study RA, systemic lupus erythematosus, multiple sclerosis, hepatitis and encephalomyelitis [29-34].

The NAPPA is an innovative method to produce protein microarrays, where cDNAs encoding proteins of interest are spotted onto activated surfaces and proteins are produced *in situ* using mammalian *in vitro* expression systems [18,19]. The freshly made protein is captured by cospotted antibodies specific for a tag encoded at the end of the amino acid sequence. This approach circumvents the labor and cost considerations associated with conventional spotting of labile recombinant proteins into arrays. NAPPA technology recently revealed that ankylosing spondylitis patients' autoantibody responses were targeted towards connective, skeletal and muscular tissue, unlike those of RA patients [35].

The development of protein microarrays offers a compelling strategy to comprehensively screen antibodies. When properly executed, these microarrays allow thousands of full-length proteins to be tested simultaneously. NAPPA technology replaces printing proteins with a more reliable and less expensive process of printing DNA, circumventing the need to express, purify and store proteins. Additionally, this avoids concerns about

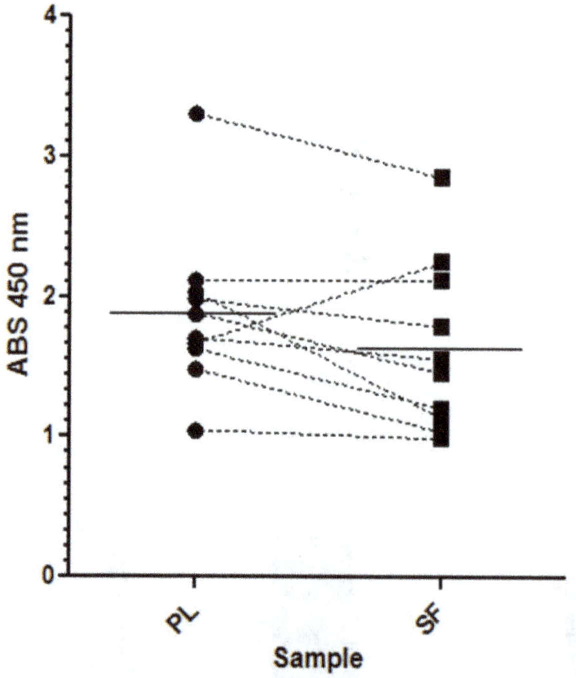

Figure 4 ELISA verification of serine/threonine kinase-10 antibody levels. The plasma concentrations of anti-serine/threonine kinase-10 antibodies were confirmed to be significantly higher in plasma (PL) than in synovial fluid (SL) by ELISA (paired *t* test $P = 0.038$). The paired PL (circular marker) and SF (square marker) samples from individual juvenile idiopathic arthritis patients are identified by a dashed line between points. The mean ELISA reading at 450 nm across the study cohort for each sample type is represented by a horizontal solid line.

protein stability because the proteins are expressed only at the time of assay. The responses are rapidly identified because the address of each protein is known in advance and there are no representation issues; all proteins, even rare ones, are represented equally (usually in duplicate). The proteins are arrayed on a single microscope slide requiring only a few microliters of plasma or serum per assay. An additional advantage of this approach is that the data can be evaluated to look for both informative individual antigens as well as for patterns of antigen responses with good predictive value [17,36,37]. Moreover, the coupling of clustering algorithms with the simultaneous comparison of many antigen responses lends itself well to the determination of antigens with concordant and independent responses.

In the current study, associations were found between at-risk patients with elevated CRP or ESR and elevated antibody levels. The trend is observed in both plasma and synovial fluid; and although no statistical significance can be tied to this association, future study with an expanded cohort could clarify any relationship. Given the relatively low prevalence of individual autoantibodies, large numbers of patient and control sera are needed to demonstrate statistical confidence in new markers. There is thus a strong need for quantitative reproducibility both within the array and from array to array so that data can be analyzed across arrays probed with samples on different days to draw statistical conclusions.

The current investigation clearly demonstrated quantitative reproducibility, differential reactivity against different proteins for individual samples, differential reactivity among different patients, and the potential to use plasma samples as a source for multiplex autoantibody discovery in JIA. The strong correlation between synovial fluid and plasma antibody levels represents a novel finding and provides confidence to use plasma for discovery of autoantibodies also found in the pathological joint, thus circumventing the challenges associated with joint aspiration. Certain antibodies were identified at elevated levels in plasma (relative to synovial fluid), suggesting that these may emanate either from immune cells within the circulation or from other tissues around which blood circulates. Additionally, these elevated antibodies were possibly produced just prior to sample collection, in response to stimulatory antigens, and have not yet reached homeostatic levels between the circulation and joint fluids. Intriguingly, in some cases there is a shift toward a higher signal in synovial fluid; however, this did not alter the relative abundances of individual species. One possible explanation of this variation in antibody concentration is the hydration status of the subjects in question. Overall, however, the relative abundance of specific antibody species correlates strongly in most cases.

A wealth of work exists based on conventional tests for solitary autoantibody species in plasma or serum across a number of arthritides, including JIA. ANAs are mainly associated with oligoarticular-onset JIA patients, but are also present in polyarticular and psoriatic subtypes [38,39]. Several reports have documented the association between the presence of ANAs and uveitis in JIA patients [40]. Distinct autoantigens that contribute to ANA positivity have not yet been identified. ANA testing is still performed by indirect immunofluorescence on HEp2 cells [41]. Antibodies against histones, HNRPA2 and nonhistone chromosomal proteins have been reported in JIA patients [42]. However, ANAs are present in patients with other autoimmune diseases as well as healthy individuals, and might be transiently increased during viral or bacterial infections. ANA testing to diagnose JIA is therefore limited due to its low disease specificity. Several other autoantigens, such as heat shock glomerular and endothelial proteins, have also been assessed in JIA, but the results are inconsistent and of limited value either for diagnosis or for understanding the disease pathological mechanism [43-45].

The unsupervised pair-wise clustering of antibody levels and clinical subtype, albeit in a small cohort, produced some interesting observations. The expression levels of antibodies directed at a select group of antigens appear to segregate patients into two clinically relevant clusters. The two defined patient groups are distinguished by the severity of disease, whereby a higher antibody titer is associated with an increase of the acute-phase indicators ESR and CRP. Additionally, a number of these high-antibody-titer patients tested ANA-positive or RF-positive, suggesting a trend - although this would require confirmation in a much larger patient cohort. Similarly, a recent protein array study demonstrated that juvenile arthritis patients can be stratified into distinct molecular subtypes based on the expression of antibody signatures [17]. Stoll and colleagues demonstrated that autoantibodies directed at the extracellular matrix and nuclear antigens are elevated in a subgroup of oligoarticular JIA patients that were less likely to attain clinical remission. Likewise, clinical subtyping of adult RA patients by arrays of 10 preselected antigens has been successfully demonstrated on an Immunological Multi-Parameter Chip Technology platform produced by Roche Diagnostics Corp., Indianapolis, IN, USA [46]. As a constituent of the observed elevated signature, antibodies against the IL-6 receptor, for example, may signal a distortion in the regulation of the immune and acute phase responses. In fact, synthetic humanized anti-IL-6 receptor embodies one of the highly selective biologic therapeutic tools now available to clinicians [47].

Conclusion

In the future we intend to move this work towards a statistically powered discovery study that will analyze a much larger cohort with healthy control subjects, to capture significant biological variance in antibody levels that correlate with clinically relevant outcomes. Pertinent clinical questions focused on the management of arthritis patients that remain unanswered include the prognosis of adverse outcome (for example, spread of inflammation to previously unaffected joints) and the timely prediction of which drugs could abrogate that outcome (for example, heterogeneity in response amongst JIA subgroups to expensive biologic drugs). Discovery findings should be considered a set of leads that then require meticulous validation, especially with respect to the utility of a multiplex antibody signature in a routine clinical setting.

In summary, autoantibody research in JIA has in general been hypothesis driven and often adapted from findings of adult RA and other autoimmune diseases. Unfortunately, even the most established findings in RA have not proven useful and relevant in all subtypes of JIA. A comprehensive profiling of the autoantigen repertoire in JIA patients will greatly improve our understanding of the molecular and cellular mechanisms that lead to the loss of immunological tolerance and production of autoantibodies.

Additional material

Additional file 1: Table S1, a complete list of NAPPA proteins, presenting the Entrez gene symbol, protein name, cellular location and molecule type for each protein produced on the NAPPA array within the current study; Table S2, functional networks of NAPPA proteins, listing the physiological and pathological functions of 25 networks constructed from the constituents of the NAPPA arrays used within the current study; Table S3, cluster 1 transcriptional regulation, listing the proteins responsible for transcriptional regulation of the target antigens within cluster 1 (Figure 3A**and** Additional File 2 **); and Table S4, cluster 2 transcriptional regulation, listing the proteins responsible for transcriptional regulation of the target antigens within cluster 2** (Figure 3A**and** Additional File 2).

Additional file 2: Figure S1, transcriptional regulation of antigen clusters, showing magnified sections of the hierarchical cluster analysis heatmap in Figure 3A**to illustrate two distinct clusters of 49 proteins targeted by antibodies within the plasma of study subjects**. The proteins responsible for transcriptional regulation of the target antigens within cluster 1 and cluster 2 are listed in Tables S3 and Table S4 in Additional File 1, respectively.

Abbreviations

ANA: antinuclear antigen; BSA: bovine serum albumin; CRP: C-reactive protein; ELISA: enzyme-linked immunosorbent assay; ESR: erythrocyte sedimentation rate; GST: glutathione-S transferase; IL: interleukin; JIA: juvenile idiopathic arthritis; mAb: monoclonal antibody; NAPPA: nucleic acid programmable protein array; PBS: phosphate-buffered saline; RA: rheumatoid arthritis; RF: rheumatoid factor.

Acknowledgements

DSG and MER would like to acknowledge the funding of this research by Arthritis Research UK in the form of a Project Grant (No. 18748). DSG would like to acknowledge support from Arthritis Research UK in the form of a Travelling Fellowship (No. 19250).

Author details

[1]Arthritis Research Group, Centre for Infection and Immunity, Health Science Building, Queen's University of Belfast, 97 Lisburn Road, Belfast BT9 7BL, UK. [2]Division of Endocrinology, Metabolism and Diabetes, School of Medicine, University of Colorado Denver, 12800 E. 19th Avenue, Aurora, CO 80045, USA. [3]Center for Personalized Diagnostics, Arizona State University, 1001 S. McAllister Avenue, Tempe, AZ 85287-6401, USA.

Authors' contributions

DSG designed the study, drafted the manuscript and performed statistical analysis. JQ helped conceive the study, participated in the image analysis of NAPPA slides and helped draft the manuscript. EAM participated in the printing and protein translation of NAPPA slides. KB carried out the immunoassays. MER collated the patient samples and demographic data. JL conceived the study and participated in its coordination and helped draft the manuscript. All authors read and approved the final manuscript.

Competing interests

The authors declare that they have no competing interests.

References

1. Symmons DP, Jones M, Osborne J, Sills J, Southwood TR, Woo P: **Pediatric rheumatology in the United Kingdom: data from the British Pediatric**

Rheumatology Group National Diagnostic Register. *J Rheumatol* 1996, **23**:1975-1980.

2. Petty RE, Southwood TR, Manners P, Baum J, Glass DN, Goldenberg J, He X, Maldonado-Cocco J, Orozco-Alcala J, Prieur AM, Suarez-Almazor ME, Woo P, International League of Associations for Rheumatology: **International League of Associations for Rheumatology classification of juvenile idiopathic arthritis: second revision, Edmonton, 2001.** *J Rheumatol* 2004, **31**:390-392.
3. Flato B, Lien G, Smerdel A, Vinje O, Dale K, Johnston V, Sorskaar D, Moum T, Ploski R, Forre O: **Prognostic factors in juvenile rheumatoid arthritis: a case-control study revealing early predictors and outcome after 14.9 years.** *J Rheumatol* 2003, **30**:386-393.
4. Huemer C, Malleson PN, Cabral DA, Huemer M, Falger J, Zidek T, Petty RE: **Patterns of joint involvement at onset differentiate oligoarticular juvenile psoriatic arthritis from pauciarticular juvenile rheumatoid arthritis.** *J Rheumatol* 2002, **29**:1531-1535.
5. Prahalad S, Glass DN: **A comprehensive review of the genetics of juvenile idiopathic arthritis.** *Pediatr Rheumatol Online J* 2008, **6**:11.
6. Rosen P, Thompson S, Glass D: **Non-HLA gene polymorphisms in juvenile rheumatoid arthritis.** *Clin Exp Rheumatol* 2003, **21**:650-656.
7. Macaubas C, Nguyen K, Milojevic D, Park JL, Mellins ED: **Oligoarticular and polyarticular JIA: epidemiology and pathogenesis.** *Nat Rev Rheumatol* 2009, **5**:616-626.
8. McGonagle D, Aziz A, Dickie LJ, McDermott MF: **An integrated classification of pediatric inflammatory diseases, based on the concepts of autoinflammation and the immunological disease continuum.** *Pediatr Res* 2009, **65**:38R-45R.
9. Wiegering V, Girschick HJ, Morbach H: **B-cell pathology in juvenile idiopathic arthritis.** *Arthritis* 2010, 759868.
10. Conrad K, Bachmann M: **Autoantibodies and systemic autoimmune diseases.** *Autoantibodies and Autoimmunity* Wiley-VCH Verlag GmbH & Co. KGaA, Weinheim, FRG; 2006, 225-245.
11. Ringold S, Seidel KD, Koepsell TD, Wallace CA: **Inactive disease in polyarticular juvenile idiopathic arthritis: current patterns and associations.** *Rheumatology (Oxford)* 2009, **48**:972-977.
12. Low JM, Chauhan AK, Kietz DA, Daud U, Pepmueller PH, Moore TL: **Determination of anti-cyclic citrullinated peptide antibodies in the sera of patients with juvenile idiopathic arthritis.** *J Rheumatol* 2004, **31**:1829-1833.
13. van Rossum M, van Soesbergen R, de Kort S, ten Cate R, Zwinderman AH, de Jong B, Dijkmans B, van Venrooij WJ: **Anti-cyclic citrullinated peptide (anti-CCP) antibodies in children with juvenile idiopathic arthritis.** *J Rheumatol* 2003, **30**:825-828.
14. Gilliam BE, Chauhan AK, Low JM, Moore TL: **Measurement of biomarkers in juvenile idiopathic arthritis patients and their significant association with disease severity: a comparative study.** *Clin Exp Rheumatol* 2008, **26**:492-497.
15. Syed RH, Gilliam BE, Moore TL: **Prevalence and significance of isotypes of anti-cyclic citrullinated peptide antibodies in juvenile idiopathic arthritis.** *Ann Rheum Dis* 2008, **67**:1049-1051.
16. Low JM, Chauhan AK, Gibson DS, Zhu M, Chen S, Rooney ME, Ombrello MJ, Moore TL: **Proteomic analysis of circulating immune complexes in juvenile idiopathic arthritis reveals disease-associated proteins.** *Proteomics Clin Appl* 2009, **3**:829-840.
17. Stoll ML, Li QZ, Zhou J, Punaro M, Olsen NJ: **Elevated IgG autoantibody production in oligoarticular juvenile idiopathic arthritis may predict a refractory course.** *Clin Exp Rheumatol* 2011, **29**:736-742.
18. Ramachandran N, Hainsworth E, Bhullar B, Eisenstein S, Rosen B, Lau AY, Walter JC, LaBaer J: **Self-assembling protein microarrays.** *Science* 2004, **305**:86-90.
19. Ramachandran N, Raphael JV, Hainsworth E, Demirkan G, Fuentes MG, Rolfs A, Hu Y, LaBaer J: **Next-generation high-density self-assembling functional protein arrays.** *Nat Methods* 2008, **5**:535-538.
20. **DNASU Plasmid Repository.** [http://dnasu.asu.edu/DNASU/].
21. **Expression Profile Data Clustering and Analysis Tool.** [http://www.bioinf.ebc.ee/EP/EP/EPCLUST/].
22. **UniProt manually annotated protein database.** [http://www.uniprot.org/].
23. MacBeath G, Schreiber SL: **Printing proteins as microarrays for high-throughput function determination.** *Science* 2000, **289**:1760-1763.
24. Zhu H, Bilgin M, Bangham R, Hall D, Casamayor A, Bertone P, Lan N, Jansen R, Bidlingmaier S, Houfek T, Mitchell T, Miller P, Dean RA, Gerstein M, Snyder M: **Global analysis of protein activities using proteome chips.** *Science* 2001, **293**:2101-2105.
25. Quintana FJ, Farez MF, Viglietta V, Iglesias AH, Merbl Y, Izquierdo G, Lucas M, Basso AS, Khoury SJ, Lucchinetti CF, Cohen IR, Weiner HL: **Antigen microarrays identify unique serum autoantibody signatures in clinical and pathologic subtypes of multiple sclerosis.** *Proc Natl Acad Sci USA* 2008, **105**:18889-18894.
26. Quintana FJ, Hagedorn PH, Elizur G, Merbl Y, Domany E, Cohen IR: **Functional immunomics: microarray analysis of IgG autoantibody repertoires predicts the future response of mice to induced diabetes.** *Proc Natl Acad Sci USA* 2004, **101(Suppl 2)**:14615-14621.
27. Hueber W, Kidd BA, Tomooka BH, Lee BJ, Bruce B, Fries JF, Sonderstrup G, Monach P, Drijfhout JW, van Venrooij WJ, Utz PJ, Genovese MC, Robinson WH: **Antigen microarray profiling of autoantibodies in rheumatoid arthritis.** *Arthritis Rheum* 2005, **52**:2645-2655.
28. Hueber W, Tomooka BH, Batliwalla F, Li W, Monach PA, Tibshirani RJ, Van Vollenhoven RF, Lampa J, Saito K, Tanaka Y, Genovese MC, Klareskog L, Gregersen PK, Robinson WH: **Blood autoantibody and cytokine profiles predict response to anti-tumor necrosis factor therapy in rheumatoid arthritis.** *Arthritis Res Ther* 2009, **11**:R76.
29. Hueber W, Kidd BA, Tomooka BH, Lee BJ, Bruce B, Fries JF, Sonderstrup G, Monach P, Drijfhout JW, van Venrooij WJ, Utz PJ, Genovese MC, Robinson WH: **Antigen microarray profiling of autoantibodies in rheumatoid arthritis.** *Arthritis Rheum* 2005, **52**:2645-2655.
30. Fattal I, Shental N, Mevorach D, Anaya JM, Livneh A, Langevitz P, Zandman-Goddard G, Pauzner R, Lerner M, Blank M, Hincapie ME, Gafter U, Naparstek Y, Shoenfeld Y, Domany E, Cohen IR: **An antibody profile of systemic lupus erythematosus detected by antigen microarray.** *Immunology* 2010, **130**:337-343.
31. Li QZ, Xie C, Wu T, Mackay M, Aranow C, Putterman C, Mohan C: **Identification of autoantibody clusters that best predict lupus disease activity using glomerular proteome arrays.** *J Clin Invest* 2005, **115**:3428-3439.
32. Somers K, Govarts C, Stinissen P, Somers V: **Multiplexing approaches for autoantibody profiling in multiple sclerosis.** *Autoimmun Rev* 2009, **8**:573-579.
33. Song X, Bandow J, Sherman J, Baker JD, Brown PW, McDowell MT, Molloy MP: **iTRAQ experimental design for plasma biomarker discovery.** *J Proteome Res* 2008, **7**:2952-2958.
34. Song Q, Liu G, Hu S, Zhang Y, Tao Y, Han Y, Zeng H, Huang W, Li F, Chen P, Zhu J, Hu C, Zhang S, Li Y, Zhu H, Wu L: **Novel autoimmune hepatitis-specific autoantigens identified using protein microarray technology.** *J Proteome Res* 2010, **9**:30-39.
35. Wright C, Sibani S, Trudgian D, Fischer R, Kessler B, Labaer J, Bowness P: **Detection of multiple autoantibodies in patients with ankylosing spondylitis using nucleic acid programmable protein arrays.** *Mol Cell Proteomics* 2012.
36. Anderson KS, Sibani S, Wallstrom G, Qiu J, Mendoza EA, Raphael J, Hainsworth E, Montor WR, Wong J, Park JG, Lokko N, Logvinenko T, Ramachandran N, Godwin AK, Marks J, Engstrom P, Labaer J: **Protein microarray signature of autoantibody biomarkers for the early detection of breast cancer.** *J Proteome Res* 2011, **10**:85-96.
37. Gibson DS, Finnegan S, Jordan G, Scaife C, Brockbank S, Curry J, McAllister C, Pennington S, Dunn M, Rooney ME: **Stratification and monitoring of juvenile idiopathic arthritis patients by synovial proteome analysis.** *J Proteome Res* 2009, **8**:5601-5609.
38. Felici E, Novarini C, Magni-Manzoni S, Pistorio A, Magnani A, Bozzola E, Buoncompagni A, Martini A, Ravelli A: **Course of joint disease in patients with antinuclear antibody-positive juvenile idiopathic arthritis.** *J Rheumatol* 2005, **32**:1805-1810.
39. Grassi A, Corona F, Casellato A, Carnelli V, Bardare M: **Prevalence and outcome of juvenile idiopathic arthritis-associated uveitis and relation to articular disease.** *J Rheumatol* 2007, **34**:1139-1145.
40. Heinz C, Mingels A, Goebel C, Fuchsluger T, Heiligenhaus A: **Chronic uveitis in children with and without juvenile idiopathic arthritis: differences in patient characteristics and clinical course.** *J Rheumatol* 2008, **35**:1403-1407.
41. Shin JI, Kim KH, Chun JK, Lee TJ, Kim KJ, Kim HS, Kim DS: **Prevalence and patterns of anti-nuclear antibodies in Korean children with juvenile idiopathic arthritis according to ILAR criteria.** *Scand J Rheumatol* 2008, **37**:348-351.

42. Nordal EB, Songstad NT, Berntson L, Moen T, Straume B, Rygg M: **Biomarkers of chronic uveitis in juvenile idiopathic arthritis: predictive value of antihistone antibodies and antinuclear antibodies.** *J Rheumatol* 2009, **36**:1737-1743.
43. Zlacka D, Vavrincova P, Hien Nguyen TT, Hromadnikova I: **Frequency of anti-hsp60, -65 and -70 antibodies in sera of patients with juvenile idiopathic arthritis.** *J Autoimmun* 2006, **27**:81-88.
44. Zhao J, Liu X, Wang Z, Li Z: **Significance of anti-CCP antibodies in modification of 1987 ACR classification criteria in diagnosis of rheumatoid arthritis.** *Clin Rheumatol* 2010, **29**:33-38.
45. Bloom BJ, Toyoda M, Petrosian A, Jordan S: **Anti-endothelial cell antibodies are prevalent in juvenile idiopathic arthritis: implications for clinical disease course and pathogenesis.** *Rheumatol Int* 2007, **27**:655-660.
46. Chandra PE, Sokolove J, Hipp BG, Lindstrom TM, Elder JT, Reveille JD, Eberl H, Klause U, Robinson WH: **Novel multiplex technology for diagnostic characterization of rheumatoid arthritis.** *Arthritis Res Ther* 2011, **13**:R102.
47. Nishimoto N, Yoshizaki K, Miyasaka N, Yamamoto K, Kawai S, Takeuchi T, Hashimoto J, Azuma J, Kishimoto T: **Treatment of rheumatoid arthritis with humanized anti-interleukin-6 receptor antibody: a multicenter, double-blind, placebo-controlled trial.** *Arthritis Rheum* 2004, **50**:1761-1769.

Permissions

All chapters in this book were first published in AR&T, by BioMed Central; hereby published with permission under the Creative Commons Attribution License or equivalent. Every chapter published in this book has been scrutinized by our experts. Their significance has been extensively debated. The topics covered herein carry significant findings which will fuel the growth of the discipline. They may even be implemented as practical applications or may be referred to as a beginning point for another development.

The contributors of this book come from diverse backgrounds, making this book a truly international effort. This book will bring forth new frontiers with its revolutionizing research information and detailed analysis of the nascent developments around the world.

We would like to thank all the contributing authors for lending their expertise to make the book truly unique. They have played a crucial role in the development of this book. Without their invaluable contributions this book wouldn't have been possible. They have made vital efforts to compile up to date information on the varied aspects of this subject to make this book a valuable addition to the collection of many professionals and students.

This book was conceptualized with the vision of imparting up-to-date information and advanced data in this field. To ensure the same, a matchless editorial board was set up. Every individual on the board went through rigorous rounds of assessment to prove their worth. After which they invested a large part of their time researching and compiling the most relevant data for our readers.

The editorial board has been involved in producing this book since its inception. They have spent rigorous hours researching and exploring the diverse topics which have resulted in the successful publishing of this book. They have passed on their knowledge of decades through this book. To expedite this challenging task, the publisher supported the team at every step. A small team of assistant editors was also appointed to further simplify the editing procedure and attain best results for the readers.

Apart from the editorial board, the designing team has also invested a significant amount of their time in understanding the subject and creating the most relevant covers. They scrutinized every image to scout for the most suitable representation of the subject and create an appropriate cover for the book.

The publishing team has been an ardent support to the editorial, designing and production team. Their endless efforts to recruit the best for this project, has resulted in the accomplishment of this book. They are a veteran in the field of academics and their pool of knowledge is as vast as their experience in printing. Their expertise and guidance has proved useful at every step. Their uncompromising quality standards have made this book an exceptional effort. Their encouragement from time to time has been an inspiration for everyone.

The publisher and the editorial board hope that this book will prove to be a valuable piece of knowledge for researchers, students, practitioners and scholars across the globe.

List of Contributors

Maja Bulatović Ćalasan, Oscar FC van den Bosch and Nico M Wulffraat
Department of Pediatric Immunology, Room KC 03.063.0, University Medical Center, Wilhelmina Children's Hospital, Utrecht 3508 AB, The Netherlands

Marjonne CW Creemers
Department of Rheumatology, Jeroen Bosch Hospital, 's-Hertogenbosch, The Netherlands

Martijn Custers
Department of Rheumatology, Woerden, Maartenskliniek, The Netherlands

Antonius HM Heurkens
Department of Rheumatology, Meander Medical Center, Amersfoort, The Netherlands

Jan Maarten van Woerkom
Department of Rheumatology, Gelre Hospitals, Apeldoorn and Zutphen, The Netherlands

Arnd Kleyer, Laura Beyer, Christoph Simon, Fabian Stemmler, Matthias Englbrecht, Christian Beyer, Jürgen Rech, Bernhard Manger, Gerhard Krönke and Georg Schett
Department of Internal Medicine 3 - Rheumatology and Immunology, Friedrich-Alexander-University Erlangen-Nürnberg (FAU) and Universitätsklinikum Erlangen, Ulmenweg 18, 91054 Erlangen, Germany

Axel J. Hueber
Department of Internal Medicine 3 - Rheumatology and Immunology, Friedrich-Alexander-University Erlangen-Nürnberg (FAU) and Universitätsklinikum Erlangen, Ulmenweg 18, 91054 Erlangen, Germany
Department of Internal Medicine 3 and Institute for Clinical Immunology, University of Erlangen-Nuremberg, Ulmenweg 18, 90154 Erlangen, Germany

Raphael S. Peres, Nerry T. Cecilio, Thiago M. Cunha, Fernando Q. Cunha and Jose C. Alves-Filho
Department of Pharmacology, Ribeirão Preto Medical School, Center of Research in Inflammatory Diseases (CRID), University of São Paulo, Avenida Bandeirantes, 3900, Ribeirão Preto, São Paulo CEP: 14049-900, Brazil

Gabriela B. Santos, Carlos H. T. P. Silva and Flavio S. Emery
Department of Pharmaceutical Sciences, Faculty of Pharmaceutical Sciences of Ribeirão Preto, University of São Paulo, Avenida do Café s/n, Ribeirão Preto CEP: 14040-903, Brazil

Valquíria A. P. Jabor, Michael Niehues, Gabriela Buqui, Norberto P. Lopes and Maria C. Nonato
NPPNS, Department of Physics and Chemistry, Faculty of Pharmaceutical Sciences of Ribeirão Preto, University of São Paulo, Avenida do Café s/n, Ribeirão Preto, Brazil

Bruna G. S. Torres and Teresa Dalla Costa
Pharmaceutical Sciences Graduate Program, Faculty of Pharmacy, Federal University of Rio Grande do Sul, Sarmento Leite 521, Porto Alegre, Brazil

Fernando S. Ramalho
Department of Pathology, Ribeirão Preto Medical School, University of São Paulo, Avenida Bandeirantes 3900, Ribeirão Preto, Brazil

Paulo Louzada-Júnior
Department of Internal Medicine, Ribeirão Preto Medical School, Center of Research in Inflammatory Diseases (CRID), University of São Paulo, Avenida Bandeirantes 3900, Ribeirão Preto, Brazil

Maria G. Ledesma-Colunga, Norma Adán, Georgina Ortiz, Mariana Solís-Gutiérrez, Fernando López-Barrera, Gonzalo Martínez de la Escalera and Carmen Clapp
Instituto de Neurobiología, Universidad Nacional Autónoma de México (UNAM), Campus UNAM-Juriquilla, 76230 Querétaro, México

Sabrina Gmuca and Timothy G. Brandon
Division of Rheumatology, Department of Pediatrics, The Children's Hospital of Philadelphia, Philadelphia, PA, USA

Rui Xiao
Department of Biostatistics and Epidemiology, Perelman School of Medicine, University of Pennsylvania, Philadelphia, PA, USA

Ilaria Pagnini
University of Florence and Anna Meyer Children's Hospital, Florence, Italy

Tracey B. Wright
University of Texas Southwestern Medical Center and Texas Scottish Rite Hospital of Children, Dallas, TX, USA

Timothy Beukelman
University of Alabama at Birmingham, Birmingham, AL, USA

Esi M. Morgan
Cincinnati Children's Hospital, Cincinnati, OH, USA

Pamela F. Weiss
University of Pennsylvania Perelman School of Medicine and Children's Hospital of Philadelphia, Philadelphia, PA, USA
Department of Pediatric Rheumatology, The Children's Hospital of Philadelphia, 34th Street and Civic Center Boulevard, Wood Building, Fourth Floor, Philadelphia, PA 19104, USA

Sergio Abrignani
DISCCO-Department of Clinical Science and Community Health Università degli Studi di Milano, 20122 Milan, Italy
INGM-National Institute of Molecular Genetics "Romeo ed Enrica Invernizzi", 20122 Milan, Italy

Alessandra Penatti
DISCCO-Department of Clinical Science and Community Health Università degli Studi di Milano, 20122 Milan, Italy
ASST-Gaetano Pini/CTO Orthopedic and Traumatology Specialist Center, Rheumatology and Orthopedic Department, 20122 Milan, Italy

Pier Luigi Meroni
DISCCO-Department of Clinical Science and Community Health Università degli Studi di Milano, 20122 Milan, Italy
ASST-Gaetano Pini/CTO Orthopedic and Traumatology Specialist Center, Rheumatology and Orthopedic Department, 20122 Milan, Italy
Laboratory of immuno-rheumatological researches, IRCCS Istituto Auxologico Italiano, 20149 Milan, Italy

Jong-Ho Lee
Brain Tumor Center and Department of Neuro-Oncology, The University of Texas MD Anderson Cancer Center, Houston, TX 77030, USA

Federica Facciotti, Moira Paroni, Massimiliano Pagani and Jens Geginat
INGM-National Institute of Molecular Genetics "Romeo ed Enrica Invernizzi", 20122 Milan, Italy

Paola Larghi
INGM-National Institute of Molecular Genetics "Romeo ed Enrica Invernizzi", 20122 Milan, Italy
Department of Pathophysiology and Transplantation, Università degli Studi di Milano, 20122 Milan, Italy

Antonella Murgo, Orazio De Lucia, Luca Pierannunzii and Marcello Truzzi
ASST-Gaetano Pini/CTO Orthopedic and Traumatology Specialist Center, Rheumatology and Orthopedic Department, 20122 Milan, Italy

Andreea Ioan-Facsinay
Department of Rheumatology, Leiden University Medical Center, 2300 Leiden, The Netherlands.

Roberta De Matteis
Laboratory of immuno-rheumatological researches, IRCCS Istituto Auxologico Italiano, 20149 Milan, Italy

Melissa B. Aldrich, Fred C. Velasquez, Sunkuk Kwon, Ali Azhdarinia, Kenneth Pinkston, Barrett R. Harvey, John C. Rasmussen and E. M. Sevick-Muraca
The Center for Molecular Imaging, The Brown Foundation Institute of Molecular Medicine, The University of Texas Health Science Center, Houston, TX 77030, USA

Wenyaw Chan
Department of Biostatistics, The School of Public Health, The University of Texas Health Science Center, Houston, TX 77030, USA

Russell F. Ross
Kimberly Clark Corporation, Atlanta, GA, USA

Caroline E. Fife
The Wound Care Clinic, CHI St. Luke's Health, The Woodlands Hospital, The Woodlands, TX 77382, USA

Edith M. Williams
Department of Public Health Sciences, Medical University of South Carolina, 135 Cannon Street, Suite CS303, Charleston, SC 29425, USA
Center for Health Disparities Research, Medical University of South Carolina, 135 Rutledge Avenue, Room 280H, Charleston, SC 29425, USA

Bongjun Kim, Won Jong Jin, Hong-Hee Kim and Zang Hee Lee
Department of Cell and Developmental Biology, Dental Research Institute, School of Dentistry, Seoul National University, 28 Yeongon-dong, Jongno-gu, Seoul 110-749, Republic of Korea

Hyunil Ha
Clinical Research Division, Korean Medicine-Based Herbal Drug Development Group, Korea Institute of Oriental Medicine, 483 Expo-Ro, Yuseong-Gu, Daejeon 305-811, Republic of Korea

Angela Mc Ardle, Brian Flatley and Stephen R. Pennington
Conway Institute of Biomedical Research, University College Dublin, Belfield, Dublin 4, Ireland

Oliver FitzGerald
Conway Institute of Biomedical Research, University College Dublin, Belfield, Dublin 4, Ireland
Department of Rheumatology, St Vincent's University Hospital, Elm Park, Dublin 4, Ireland

Lykke Midtbøll Ørnbjerg and Mikkel Østergaard
DANBIO registry and Copenhagen Center for Arthritis Research, Center for Rheumatology and Spine Diseases, Centre of Head and Orthopedics, Ndr. Ringvej 57, DK-2600 Glostrup, Denmark
Rigshospitalet, Department of Clinical Medicine, Faculty of Health and Medical Sciences, University

Trine Jensen
Department of Endocrinology, Hvidovre Hospital, Hvidovre, Denmark

Wolfgang Peter Bøhme
Department of Medicine, Hospital of South West Jutland, Esbjerg, Denmark

Ole Rintek Madsen
Department of Medicine and Rheumatology, Copenhagen University Hospital Gentofte, Gentofte, Denmark

Dongzhou Liu
Department of Rheumatology and Immunology, Shenzhen People's Hospital, the Second Clinical Medical College of Jinan University, Shenzhen, China

Åsa Andersson
Department of Drug Design and Pharmacology, Faculty of Health and Medical Sciences, University of Copenhagen, Universitetsparken 2, Copenhagen Ø DK-2100, Denmark

Yasumori Izumi, Shigeto Tohma, Fuminori Hirano, Haruko Ideguchi, Ryutaro Matsumura, Tomoya Miyamura, Shunsuke Mori, Takahiro Fukui, Nozomi Iwanaga, Yuka Jiuchi, Hideko Kozuru, Hiroshi Tsutani, Kouichirou Saisyo, Takao Sugiyama, Yasuo Suenaga, Yasumasa Okada, Masao Katayama, Kenji Ichikawa, Hiroshi Furukawa and Kenji Kawakami
Japanese National Hospital Organization (NHO) (Evidence-based Medicine Study Group), Higashigaoka 2-5-23, Meguro, Tokyo 152-8621, Japan

Kiyoshi Migita
Japanese National Hospital Organization (NHO) (Evidence-based Medicine Study Group), Higashigaoka 2-5-23, Meguro, Tokyo 152-8621, Japan
Department of Rheumatology, Fukushima Medical University, Hikarigaoka 1, Fukushima 960-1295, Japan

Manabu Akazawa
Department of Public Health and Epidemiology, Meiji Pharmaceutical University, Noshio 2-522-1, Kiyose, Tokyo 204-8588, Japan

Yukihiro Akeda
Research Institute for Microbial Diseases, Osaka University, Yamadaoka 3-1, Suita, Osaka 565-8563, Japan

Kazunori Oishi
Infectious Diseases Surveillance Center, National Institute of Infectious Diseases, Toyama 1-23-1, Shinjuku, Tokyo 162-8640, Japan

Trevor Faith
Department of Public Health Sciences, Medical University of South Carolina, 135 Cannon Street, Suite CS303, Charleston, SC 29425, USA

Daniëlle M Gerlag and Paul P Tak
Division of Clinical Immunology and Rheumatology, Academic Medical Centre, University of Amsterdam, Meibergdreef 9, 1105, AZ, Amsterdam, The Netherlands
University of Cambridge, U.K. Trinity Lane, Cambridge CB2 1TN, UK, and GlaxoSmithKline, Stevenage UK Gunnels Wood Road, Stevenage Herts SG1 2NY, UK

Thomas Vogl and Johannes Roth
Institute of Immunology, University of Münster, Münster, Germany

Leonard E. Egede
Center for Health Disparities Research, Medical University of South Carolina, 135 Rutledge Avenue, Room 280H, Charleston, SC 29425, USA
Division of General Internal Medicine and Geriatrics, Department of Medicine, Medical University of South Carolina, 96 Jonathan Lucas Street, Suite 803, Charleston, SC 29425, USA

Rebekah J. Walker
Center for Health Disparities Research, Medical University of South Carolina, 135 Rutledge Avenue, Room 280H, Charleston, SC 29425, USA
Division of General Internal Medicine and Geriatrics, Department of Medicine, Medical University of South Carolina, 96 Jonathan Lucas Street, Suite 803, Charleston, SC 29425, USA
Health Equity and Rural Outreach Innovation Center (HEROIC), Ralph H. Johnson Veterans Affairs Medical Center, 109 Bee Street, Charleston, SC 29401, USA

Theodoros Dimitroulas
4th Department of Internal Medicine, Hippokration Hospital, School of Medicine, Aristotle University of Thessaloniki, Thessaloniki, Greece
Department of Rheumatology, Russells Hall Hospital, Dudley Group NHS FT, Pensnett Road, DY1 2HQ Dudley, UK

Jacqueline Smith
Department of Rheumatology, Russells Hall Hospital, Dudley Group NHS FT, Pensnett Road, DY1 2HQ Dudley, UK

James Hodson
Institute of Translational Medicine, University Hospital Birmingham NHS Foundation Trust, Queen Elizabeth Hospital Birmingham, Mindelsohn Way, Birmingham B15 2WB, UK

Aamer Sandoo
School of Sport, Health and Exercise Sciences, Bangor University, George Building, Bangor, Gwynedd, Wales LL57 2PZ, UK

George D. Kitas
Arthritis Research UK Epidemiology Unit, University of Manchester, Oxford Road, Manchester M13 9PT, UK

J Sjef Verbeek
Human Genetics, Leiden University Medical Center, Leiden, The Netherlands

Irene Di Ceglie, Giuliana Ascone, Niels A. J. Cremers, Annet W. Sloetjes, Birgitte Walgreen, Fons A. J. van de Loo, Marije I. Koenders, Peter M. van der Kraan, Arjen B. Blom, Martijn H. J. van den Bosch and Peter L. E. M. van Lent
Experimental Rheumatology, Radboud university medical center, Geert Grooteplein Zuid 28, 6525 GA Nijmegen, The Netherlands

Man W Tang
Division of Clinical Immunology and Rheumatology, Academic Medical Centre, University of Amsterdam, Meibergdreef 9, 1105, AZ, Amsterdam, The Netherlands

Lei Zhao, Yasuto Yamaguchi, Xiaomei Ge, John Morser and Lawrence L. K. Leung
Department of Medicine, Division of Hematology, Stanford University School of Medicine, Stanford, CA 94305, USA
Veterans Affairs Palo Alto Health Care System, Room A4-131, Building 101, 3801 Miranda Avenue, Palo Alto, CA 94304, USA

William H. Robinson
Department of Medicine, Division of Endocrinology, Stanford University School of Medicine, Stanford, CA 94305, USA
Veterans Affairs Palo Alto Health Care System, Room A4-131, Building 101, 3801 Miranda Avenue, Palo Alto, CA 94304, USA
Department of Medicine, Division of Immunology and Rheumatology, Stanford University School of Medicine, Stanford, CA 94305, USA

Richard Partington, Toby Helliwell, Sara Muller, Alyshah Abdul Sultan and Christian Mallen
Arthritis Research UK Primary Care Centre, Primary Care Sciences, Keele University, Keele ST5 5BG, UK

Huihui Chi, Yue Sun, Qiongyi Hu, Honglei Liu, Xiaobing Cheng, Junna Ye, Hui Shi, Yufeng Yin, Mengru Liu, Xinyao Wu, Zhuochao Zhou, Jialin Teng, Chengde Yang and Yutong Su
Department of Rheumatology and Immunology, Ruijin Hospital, Shanghai Jiao Tong University School of Medicine, No. 197 Ruijin Second Road, Shanghai 200025, China

Thomas Litman, Troels Marstrand, Kristian Moller, Lars Svensson and Tord Labuda
Disease Pharmacology/Molecular Biomedicine, LEO Pharma A/S, Industriparken 55, Ballerup DK-2750, Denmark

Lisa GM van Baarsen, Maria C Lebre, Dennis van der Coelen, Saïda Aarrass and Tamara H Ramwadhdoebe
Division of Clinical Immunology and Rheumatology, Academic Medical Centre, University of Amsterdam, Meibergdreef 9, 1105, AZ, Amsterdam, The Netherlands
Department of Experimental Immunology, Academic Medical Centre, University of Amsterdam, Meibergdreef 9, 1105 AZ, Amsterdam, The Netherlands

Katja CM Denninger
Department of Drug Design and Pharmacology, Faculty of Health and Medical Sciences, University of Copenhagen, Universitetsparken 2, Copenhagen Ø DK-2100, Denmark
Disease Pharmacology/Molecular Biomedicine, LEO Pharma A/S, Industriparken 55, Ballerup DK-2750, Denmark

David S Gibson
Arthritis Research Group, Centre for Infection and Immunity, Health Science Building, Queen's University of Belfast, 97 Lisburn Road, Belfast BT9 7BL, UK
Division of Endocrinology, Metabolism and Diabetes, School of Medicine, University of Colorado Denver, 12800 E. 19th Avenue, Aurora, CO 80045, USA

Ji Qiu, Eliseo A Mendoza, Kristi Barker and Joshua LaBaer
Center for Personalized Diagnostics, Arizona State University, 1001 S. McAllister Avenue, Tempe, AZ 85287-6401, USA

Madeleine E Rooney
Arthritis Research Group, Centre for Infection and Immunity, Health Science Building, Queen's University of Belfast, 97 Lisburn Road, Belfast BT9 7BL, UK

Index

www.ingramcontent.com/pod-product-compliance
Lightning Source LLC
LaVergne TN
LVHW080707210926
848485LV00003B/431